ANNUAL PROGRESS IN CHILD PSYCHIATRY AND CHILD DEVELOPMENT 1989

ANNUAL PROGRESS IN CHILD PSYCHIATRY AND CHILD DEVELOPMENT 1989

Edited by

STELLA CHESS, M.D.

Professor of Child Psychiatry
New York University Medical Center

and

MARGARET E. HERTZIG, M.D.

Associate Professor of Psychiatry
Cornell University Medical College

BRUNNER/MAZEL, Publishers • New York

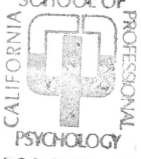

Library of Congress Card No. 68–23452
ISBN 0–87630–569–9
ISSN 0066–4030

Published by

BRUNNER/MAZEL, INC.
19 Union Square
New York, New York 10003

Manufactured in the United States of America

10 9 8 7 6 5 4 3 2 1

CONTENTS

A NOTE FROM ONE
OF THE EDITORS

Editing these annual volumes has been a labor of love for myself and Dr. Chess. This work has been arduous and exciting over the years, as we have reviewed an ever-increasing number of journals and witnessed the dramatic advances in the fields of child psychiatry and child development.

It is clear that this series should continue. However, each year we ourselves grow a year older. Therefore, several years ago we pursuaded a younger but mature colleague, Dr. Margaret Hertzig, to share in the increasing editorial responsibilities of *Annual Progress in Child Psychiatry and Child Development*. Her theoretical and clinical sophistication has been an asset for *Annual Progress* for several years. We are confident that her contribution will expand with succeeding years. Dr. Hertzig has now assumed a senior role as an editor and this issue is the fruit of collaboration of Dr. Chess and Dr. Hertzig. I have resigned as I am no longer needed as a co-editor.

I shall now, instead, together with my colleagues in the New York Longitudinal Study, make my primary commitment to the pursuit of new clinical and theoretical insights to be learned from the analyses of the massive data of this study.

Alexander Thomas, M.D.

ANNUAL PROGRESS IN CHILD PSYCHIATRY AND CHILD DEVELOPMENT 1989

Part I
INFANCY STUDIES

The world of the infant, once viewed as inaccessible to direct investigation, has become increasingly understandable and comprehensible as a consequence of innovative studies designed to enable even pre-verbal children to "tell us what they know." In the first paper in this section, Meltzoff illustrates this approach, in a carefully designed and controlled study of imitation in nine-month-old infants. The finding that some 50% of nine-month-olds are capable of imitating simple actions with novel objects even after a 24 hour delay, is a downward extension of this investigator's previous demonstration of the imitative capacities of 14-month-olds (see *Annual Progress, 1986*). The findings are of theoretical interest in suggesting a role for delayed as well as immediate imitation in the social development of children during the first year of life. Moreover, the powerful methodology has the potential of application to the study of recall and recognition memory in the pre-verbal child.

The second paper in this section, by Persson-Blennow, Binett, and McNeil, derives from an ongoing longitudinal study comparing the development of the offspring of psychotic women with that of low-risk control infants. In this report, the investigators examine aspects of mother-infant interaction at six ages during the first year of life in relation to the development of the infant's fear of strangers by 12 months of age in order to test the hypothesis that a failure to develop fear of strangers during the first year of life is related to negative mother-infant interaction characteristics. While the results provide some support for the hypothesis (within both high-risk and low-risk groups, mother-infant interaction was significantly more deviant and negative in cases where the infant subsequently failed to develop fear of strangers), the background characteristics associated with such failure were different in the index and control groups. In addition, the authors report little overlap between insecure attachment and fear of strangers. The findings underscore the complexity of factors influencing social development of infants and young children and the importance of longitudinal studies as clarifying research strategies.

1

Infant Imitation and Memory: Nine-Month-Olds in Immediate and Deferred Tests

Andrew N. Meltzoff

University of Washington

The ability of nine-month-old infants to imitate simple actions with novel objects was investigated. Both immediate and deferred imitation were tested, the latter by interposing a 24-hour delay between the stimulus-presentation and response periods. The results provide evidence for both immediate and deferred imitation; moreover, imitative responding was not significantly dampened by the 24-hour delay. The findings demonstrate that there exists some underlying capacity for deferring imitation of certain acts well under 1 year of age, and thus that this ability does not develop in a stagelike step function at about 18–24 months as commonly predicted. These findings also show that imitation in early infancy can span wide enough delays to be of potential service in social development; actions on novel objects that are observed one day can be stored by the child and repeated the next day. The study of deferred imitation provides a largely untapped method for investigating the nature and development of recall memory in the preverbal child.

The study of infant imitation has attracted theorists from a variety of orientations. Perceptual and cognitive developmentalists are interested in imitation because the reproduction of a target act can be used to measure percep-

Reprinted with permission from *Child Development*, 1988, Vol. 59, 217–225. Copyright 1988 by the Society for Research in Child Development, Inc.

This work was supported by grants from NICHD (HD-22514) and the John D. and Catherine T. MacArthur Foundation. The author thanks Craig Harris for assistance on all phases of this project and Pat Kuhl, Mike Kahn, and the reviewers for making valuable suggestions on an earlier version of this paper.

tion, motor control, the coordination of perception and action, and, under certain conditions, memory and representational abilities (Flavell, 1985; Meltzoff, 1985a, 1985b). Imitation has also attracted the interest of social-developmentalists, for it provides an efficient channel for early social learning. At least some of the skills of early childhood are learned via the observation of adult behavior, rather than through conditioning, trial and error, or individual maturational growth, and the origins and early development of such social learning warrant investigation (Bandura & Walters, 1963; Hartup & Coates, 1970). Finally, Piagetian psychology has focused on imitative development as playing a vital role in the transition from a purely sensorimotor level to a more representational form of intellectual organization (Flavell, 1985; Piaget, 1962).

For each of these approaches, deferred imitation takes on special importance. Cognitive theorists highlight deferred imitation as a way of investigating long-term memory in preverbal infants. Deferred imitation is relevant to social theorists because the infant or child will not always be able to reproduce each adult action as soon as it is demonstrated; thus, for imitation to fulfill its social utility, the infant or child must be capable of initiating imitation long after the target display has terminated. Finally, Piagetians focus on deferred imitation as a developmental milestone that first emerges at about 18–24 months (during sensorimotor stage 6) contemporaneously with pretend play and productive language as part of a general emergence of the "symbolic function" (Inhelder, 1971; Lézine, 1973; Piattelli-Palmerini, 1980; Sinclair, 1969, 1970).

Only recently have the origins and development of deferred imitation begun to be empirically investigated. McCall, Parke, and Kavanaugh (1977) tested for deferred imitation in 1–3-year-old children, and as predicted by Piagetian theory they found that infants first began to reproduce target actions after a delay at approximately 24 months. However, two other reports suggest that, at least under certain circumstances, such behavior can be elicited at younger ages. Meltzoff (1985b) found evidence for deferred imitation after a 24-hour delay in 14-month-old infants, and Abravanel and Gingold (1985) reported imitation after a 10-min delay in 12-month-olds. Nevertheless there are still questions about the nature of this ability before 18–24 months. It remains possible that deferred imitation before about 18–24 months is a sharply constrained phenomenon—severely limited in the number of acts that can be retained for later reproduction, and/or in the length of delay that can be tolerated.

The work reported here was designed to assess deferred imitation at a younger age than has been tested heretofore (9-month-old infants), using a long delay period (24 hours) and a variety of tasks (three items). In addition, immediate imitation was also assessed using the same age group and the same three tasks.

The immediate test was included both as a comparison with the deferred test and as a contribution in its own right because studies of immediate imitation at this particular age have not always incorporated the control conditions necessary to distinguish imitative versus nonimitative production of the target behaviors (e.g., Uzgiris & Hunt, 1975). To isolate imitative responding, control groups that do not see the target action are needed to assess the spontaneous rate of the behavior at issue, and imitation should be inferred only if these controls produce the target behavior less than do infants who are exposed to modeling. Without such controls, the production of the matching behavior after seeing the display is not unambiguous evidence for imitation because it could be produced by chance, be facilitated by the mere presence of the adult, and/or other possibilities that are best determined by the appropriate controls (see Meltzoff, 1985b; Meltzoff & Moore, 1983, for reviews).

STUDY 1

Method

Subjects. The sample consisted of 60 9-month-old infants who were identified through the local newspapers and recruited by a telephone call. Criteria for admission into the study were no known physical, sensory, or mental handicaps, normal length of gestation (over 37 weeks), and normal birthweight (2,500–4,500 grams). The mean age at the time of test was 38.78 weeks (SD = 0.73), and the mean birthweight was 3,645 grams (SD = 423). Equal numbers of males and females were used. One additional subject was tested but then eliminated from the study due to excessive crying.

Testing environment and apparatus. The test took place in a small room (3.2 × 2.2 m) that was unfurnished except for the experimental apparatus. During the test the infant was seated on his or her parent's lap across a small rectangular table (1.2 × .76 m) from the experimenter. Behind and to the left (1.0 m) of the experimenter was a video camera that was focused on the subject so as to include a record of the infant's torso, head, and most of the tabletop. A similar camera behind and to the right (1.0 m) of the infant recorded the adult. The videotape decks recording the experiment were housed in an adjacent viewing room to reduce auditory distractions. The experiment was electronically timed by a character generator that mixed elapsed time in 0.10-sec increments directly onto the videotaped records.

Stimuli. Three novel objects designed to be highly manipulable by infants of this age were constructed from materials around the laboratory. Each object involved a different action, as described below.

The first object was an L-shaped unpainted wooden construction composed of a wooden rectangle (9.2 × 10 cm) connected by a hinge to a larger rectangular base (15.3 × 23.5 cm). The action demonstrated was to reach out and push the vertical extension over so that it lay flat on top of the base. This required a push of moderate force (.7 kg · m/s^2), which was determined by pilot studies to be within the capacity of 9-month-olds. The second object was a small black box (5.4 × 15 × 16.5 cm) with a black button (2.2 × 3 cm) mounted in a recess so that it lay .6 cm below the top surface of the box. The action demonstrated by the adult was pushing the button, which then activated a switch inside the box and produced a beeping sound. The beep was a rapidly pulsating tone of about 2,000 Hz, and its intensity, measured at the approximate location of the infant's head, was 61 dB Sound Pressure Level. The third object was a small orange plastic egg (6.4 cm high and 4.5 cm in diameter at its widest point) cut laterally in half and filled with a few metal nuts so that it rattled when shaken. The action demonstrated was to pick up the egg and shake it.

The hinged toy was oriented with the edge of the vertical piece facing the infant and could be pushed flat by moving it from right to left. The black box was tilted up at a slight angle (30°) by wooden supports with the top directly facing the subject. During the response period these objects were set in velcro strips to prevent them from accidentally being pushed off the table by the infant while manipulating them. For all groups, the egg presented to the infants in the response period was identical to the one used by the model except that it did not contain any noisy fillings. This prevented any accidental rattling sounds from the infant just touching the toy.[1]

Procedure. Upon arriving at the university, infants and parents were escorted to a waiting room where they remained for about 10–15 min while the parents completed the necessary forms. They were then brought to the test room, and the infant and male experimenter interacted by handing rubber toys back and forth across the test table until the infant seemed comfortable with the experimenter and the room. This "warm-up" period usually required 1 to 3 min, and at that point the test began.

In the imitation group ($N = 24$), each infant was sequentially shown the three target actions (hinge folding, button pushing, egg rattling). The three test objects were shown one at a time in all possible test orders, balanced across the group. Each target action was demonstrated three times in a 20-sec modeling period. At the end of the three modeling periods, the infants were given

---

[1]It is possible that the infants in the imitation group might have expected the egg to make a sound when they shook it in the response period, but this should not have influenced the results because the first shaking motion was the only action scored.

a sequence of three response periods to assess whether they would reproduce the actions they saw. The objects were brought back one at a time in their original sequence and placed on a spot directly in front of the infant for a 20-sec response period starting from the infant's first touch of the toy. If the infant became distracted during the modeling or response period, the experimenter would say "look over here" or "oh, see what I have," but never used words relating to the tasks at hand, such as "push," "shake," "fold," "copy," or "imitate."

The control groups (totaling 36 subjects) proceeded identically to the imitation group except that they did not see the target actions modeled. To approximate different aspects of the display, three different control groups were used: a "baseline control," an "adult-touching control," and an "adult-manipulation control."

For the baseline condition ($N = 12$), the modeling periods were simply omitted and the infants were timed for the three sequential 20-sec response periods with the test objects; all else was identical to the imitation condition. This control assesses the spontaneous probability of infants producing the target actions in the absence of previous contact with the stimuli or the modeled action. In the adult-touching condition ($N = 12$), infants saw the adult reach out and hold each object three times in the modeling periods, but they were not shown the particular target actions. These control modeling periods were followed by a series of three 20-sec response periods, exactly as in the imitation and baseline conditions. This condition controls for the possibility that infants might somehow be induced into producing the target actions if they see the adult approach and touch the object, even if the exact target action was not modeled. The adult-manipulation control ($N = 12$) was conducted to mimic further aspects of the target display but still without demonstrating the critical action. Infants who see that objects have consequences, that they beep or rattle, may be more motivated to manipulate them. The adult-manipulation condition demonstrated such consequences without demonstrating the target actions. For example, infants were exposed to the beeping sound made by the black box during the modeling period (as were infants in the imitation group); however, this sound was produced by having the experimenter place both his hands on the sides of the box and surreptitiously use his thumb to activate a small switch in the back of the box that was invisible to the child. Similarly, infants were exposed to the rattling sound made by the egg during the modeling period; however, this was accomplished by having the adult use one finger to spin the egg in place so that it made the sound. Finally, regarding the third object, infants were shown that the small flap could move relative to the wooden base. This was accomplished by using a toy identical to that used in the imitation condition but without the metal hinge screwed on. Infants saw the object with the flap already placed in a horizontal position (the "end state" for the flap in the imitation group), and it was then moved toward the infant and back while being held between the experimenter's thumb and forefinger. The forward and back movement approximated the distance traversed by the arc of the flap in the imitation condition. At the end of the control modeling periods the objects were presented to the infants for the 20-sec response periods, following the same procedure as the other test conditions.

Although no differences in the production of the target behavior under the three control conditions (baseline, adult touching, adult manipulation) were anticipated (Meltzoff, 1985b, used a similar design and found no significant differences), taken together they provide an especially rigorous assessment of the probability of nonimitative production of the target behaviors and thus permit the inference of imitation if differentially more target behaviors are seen in the imitation versus control groups.

Response scoring. The videotape records of the response periods for the experimental and control infants were identical in the sense that all infants had a series of three 20-sec response periods. Thus there were no artifactual clues on the videotape as to whether or not the infant had been exposed to the target action. A scorer who was naive to group assignment viewed these response periods and provided a dichotomous yes/no code as to whether the infant produced the target action with each object. A "yes" for the button was recorded if the button was pushed in far enough to trigger the beeping sound automatically; a "yes" for the egg was recorded if the infant shook the object, where shake was defined as a quick bidirectional movement in which the trajectory retraced itself. A "yes" code for the hinge object was recorded if the vertical flap was folded down through an arc greater than 45° toward the baseplate. A randomly selected 25% of the subjects were rescored to assess both intra- and interobserver agreement on the number of target behaviors infants produced. Both a Pearson r and the kappa statistic, which is an index of agreement, ranging from 0 to 1.00, that incorporates a correction for chance (Applebaum & McCall, 1983; Cohen, 1960), were calculated and respectively yielded the following values: intraobserver agreement, .93, .91; interobserver agreement, .87, .91.

Results and Discussion

Each infant was presented with three test objects and therefore could duplicate 0–3 of the target behaviors. For the purposes of the main nonparametric analysis, each infant's response was classified as either "low" (0–1 target behaviors produced) or "high" (2–3 target behaviors produced), as shown in Table 1. A 4 × 2 chi-square test assessing the effects of the four experimental

TABLE 1

IMMEDIATE IMITATION (N = 60): NUMBER OF
INFANTS WITH HIGH VERSUS LOW TEST SCORES AS
A FUNCTION OF EXPERIMENTAL CONDITION

	TEST SCORES	
CONDITION	Low	High
Baseline control	9	3
Adult-touching control	12	0
Adult-manipulation control	12	0
Imitation.	12	12

Table 1. Immediate Imitation (N = 60): Number of Infants with High versus Low Test Scores as a Function of Experimental Condition

conditions on the infants' behavior reached significance, $\chi^2(3)$ = 16.00, $p <$ .01, with infants in the imitation condition producing more target behaviors than the controls. Because several of the expected frequencies in this Table are less than 5, these same data were also reanalyzed as a 2 × 2 table contrasting the imitation condition (N = 24) with the combined controls (N = 36). These results were also highly significant, $\chi^2(1)$ = 11.20, $p <$ .001. Although the underlying data are more amenable to nonparametric analysis, it is worth noting that the same pattern of results is also obtained using a one-way ANOVA, which shows that the number of target behaviors (possible range = 0–3) varies significantly as a function of experimental condition, $F(3,56)$ = 6.30, $p <$ .001. In accordance with the imitation hypothesis, a planned comparison between the imitation condition and the mean of the controls shows that infants produce significantly more target behaviors in the imitation than in the control conditions, $t(56)$ = 4.02, $p <$ .0001.

These data indicate that infants' behavior is influenced by the adult model. Infants in the control conditions are less likely to produce the target actions than those infants who see them performed. The inclusion of the controls allows us to infer that infants in the imitation group were not simply producing the target behaviors because they were aroused by seeing the adult approach and touch the toy or because they heard the consequences (beep, rattle) of the adult's manipulation. These possibilities were addressed by the types of controls used.

The results show that 9-month-olds can imitate certain simple actions with novel toys under conditions in which little delay is involved. Will imitative responding be dampened if a lengthy delay is interposed? Or, is deferred imitation wholly absent after a lengthy delay, perhaps tapping a significant constraint in the cognitive organization of young infants? These questions were addressed in Study 2.

STUDY 2

Method

Subjects. The subjects were 60 normal 9-month-old infants, including equal numbers of males and females. The criteria for admission into the study were 4the same as those used in Study 1. The mean age was 39.14 weeks (SD = 0.69) and mean birthweight was 3,499 grams (SD = 417). An additional seven infants were tested but eliminated from the study: five for not returning for the second test after the delay, one for crying, and one for a procedural error. These eliminated subjects were distributed approximately evenly across the test conditions.

Test environment, procedure, and scoring. The infants were tested in the same laboratory, using the same objects, under the same general procedure and design as Study 1. The studies differed only by the introduction of a 24-hour delay (actual range = 23.5–24 hours). The delay interval was interposed in the following manner. For the imitation condition, the three actions were sequentially modeled as before. The infants were then sent home and scheduled for a visit the next day. When they returned to the test laboratory, the experimenter engaged in a short warm-up with rubber toys (1–3 min) until the infants seemed comfortable. Next the sequence of three 20-sec response periods was presented exactly as had been done in the immediate imitation experiment. For the baseline control, infants came to the laboratory on day 1, entered the test room, and engaged in the rubber toy warm-up just as had the infants in the imitation group. They then were sent home. On day 2, they were treated identically to those infants in the imitation condition, that is, they were presented the sequence of three response periods. For the adult-touching and adult-manipulation controls, the procedure was the same except that infants saw the three control events (these were described in Study 1) on the first day before being sent home. On the second visit they were treated identically to those in the imitation condition.

The videotapes of the response periods were shown to an observer who remained blind to the infant's test condition and scored the data exactly as in Study 1. A randomly selected 25% of the subjects were rescored to assess both intra- and interobserver agreement on the number of target responses infants produced. A Pearson *r* and kappa statistic were both calculated and respectively yielded the following values: intraobserver agreement, .91, .86; interobserver agreement, .95, .82.

Results and Discussion

The results support the hypothesis that infants are capable of imitating after the 24-hour delay (Table 2). The 4 × 2 table assessing the effects of the four experimental conditions on infants' behavior reached significance, with infants in the imitation condition producing more target behaviors than the controls, $\chi^2(3) = 8.01$, $p < .05$. Due to small expected frequencies, the data were also reanalyzed as a 2 × 2 table contrasting the imitation condition ($N = 24$) with the combined controls ($N = 36$), $\chi^2(1) = 4.88$, $p < .05$. The outcome of the alternative parametric analysis is in line with these chi-square tests. A one-way ANOVA shows that the infants' test scores vary significantly as a function of experimental condition, $F(3,56) = 4.69$, $p < .01$, and a planned comparison shows that infants produce more target behaviors in the imitation condition than in the controls, $t(56) = 3.32$, $p < .005$.

It is of interest that the pattern of results is nearly identical either with the 24-hour delay (Study 1) or without it (Study 2). Inspection of Table 1 and Table 2 reveals that the imitation effect not only replicates, but that the profile of the results is essentially unaffected by the delay. A comparison of the results across the two studies can most easily be assessed statistically by comparing the two 2 × 2 contingency tables reported above. In the immediate test, 50% of the subjects in the imitation group received a high imitation score, as opposed to only 8.33% in the controls; in the deferred tests, the comparable comparison was 50% versus 19.44%. A chi-square test for the homogeneity of these two tables (Fleiss, 1981) reveals no significant difference

TABLE 2

DEFERRED IMITATION ($N = 60$): NUMBER OF
INFANTS WITH HIGH VERSUS LOW TEST SCORES AS
A FUNCTION OF EXPERIMENTAL CONDITION

CONDITION	TEST SCORES	
	Low	High
Baseline control	8	4
Adult-touching control	11	1
Adult-manipulation control	10	2
Imitation	12	12

Table 2. Deferred Imitation ($N = 60$): Number of Infants with High versus Low Test Scores as a Function of Experimental Condition

($p > .20$), and it is noteworthy that the data in the imitation conditions themselves were in fact identical (50%) whether infants responded immediately or after a delay.

The fact that the results are so similar across the two studies allows us to combine the studies meaningfully, and this larger sample size of 120 subjects in turn affords a further look at the effectiveness of imitation. It is striking that across the studies nearly 20% of the subjects in the imitation condition reproduced three of the target displays. These subjects retained and duplicated all three of the events they were shown. The control infants document that the production of the three target behaviors is highly improbable in the absence of seeing the relevant displays. Across both studies, 0 of the 72 control infants produced all three targets. The difference is highly significant ($p < .0005$, Fisher exact test). Once again, there is no effect of delay on this performance, inasmuch as five of the 24 infants in the deferred test reproduced all three behaviors and four of the 24 infants in the immediate test did so.

An alternative parametric analysis combining the results of the two studies involves a condition (4) × delay (2) ANOVA. The relevant means are displayed in Table 3. The main effect of condition is significant, $F(3,112) = 10.39$, $p < .001$, and a planned comparison shows that infants produced significantly more of the target behaviors in the imitation condition than in the controls, $t(116) = 5.22$, $p < .0001$. There was no main effect of delay, $F(1,112) = .34$. There was also no condition × delay interaction, $F(3,112) = .44$, indicating that the imitation effect was not dampened due to the 24-hour delay.

GENERAL DISCUSSION

These studies show that 9-month-old infants will imitate simple actions using novel toys both immediately and after a delay. Infants will close a wooden

MEANS AND STANDARD DEVIATIONS OF INFANTS' SCORES AS A FUNCTION OF DELAY AND
EXPERIMENTAL CONDITION

	DELAY					
	Immediate		Deferred		Combined	
CONDITION	Mean	SD	Mean	SD	Mean	SD
Baseline control	1.00	.74	1.17	.72	1.08	.72
Adult-touching control	.75	.45	.58	.67	.67	.57
Adult-manipulation control	.50	.52	.83	.72	.67	.64
Imitation	1.54	.93	1.58	.97	1.56	.94

NOTE.—Maximum score = 3.

Table 3. Means and Standard Deviations of Infants' Scores as a Function of Delay and Experimental Condition

flap after witnessing an adult do so, they will push a button after seeing this act, and they will duplicate the shaking of a small plastic egg. This work does not assess the degree to which more novel motor patterns, actions involving complex temporal or spatial sequencing, or activities with more symbolic or cognitive loadings will be imitated at this early age. On the basis of other research (Abravanel & Gingold, 1985; Killen & Uzgiris, 1981; McCabe & Uzgiris, 1983; McCall et al., 1977), it seems likely that there will be interesting constraints on the types of tasks such young infants will copy. For example, in the current study, as with virtually all experiments conducted to date with infants, the actions tested in the imitation condition occur with some nonzero probability in the controls. It would now be informative to test whether a behavior with truly a zero probability in the absence of modeling would be duplicated either immediately or after a delay. Similarly, it would be informative to probe the limits of imitation by testing the degree to which modeling can influence infants' behavior on more symbolic or problem-solving tasks such as object permanence (Wishart, 1986) or the categorization of objects (Gopnik & Meltzoff, 1987). However, even without these probes into the limiting conditions of imitation, the current research establishes several interesting things about what infants *can* do at this age and thus extends our current knowledge about early imitation. The findings have implications for social, Piagetian, and cognitive developmental theories, as discussed in turn below.

From a social viewpoint it is noteworthy that the design involved showing infants first one, and then a second, and finally a third act, and only then allowing them to respond. Generalizing from the laboratory to home interaction is difficult; however, it is possible to suggest how successful imitation under these circumstances might be of service in everyday life. Consider that parents and siblings do not always allow infants access to one toy before showing other potentially competing acts with different toys. The current findings show that at least by 9 months old these social realities are not in themselves enough to block the imitation of the now absent events. Evidently even these young infants can hold in mind more than one event for subsequent reproduction once they get access to the toy. These findings are thus compatible with the notion that imitation could be functional even between young infants and their siblings or other ''real-world'' models who do not always allow an immediate response before proceeding to display other behaviors.

The results are also relevant to Piagetian theory, for the experiments were carefully designed to be sensitive to three critical distinctions made in this theory. (1) The control groups eliminated the possibility that infants in the imitation condition produced the target behavior on day 2 solely because they were more comfortable with the toys, laboratory, or experimenter on the second day. The subjects in both the adult-touching and adult-manipulation controls were exposed to the same toys for the same length of time, and they too were brought back on a second day. Had such controls not been included, few theoretical implications could be drawn from the delay experiment. (2) It is noteworthy that nearly 20% of the subjects in the imitation condition, as opposed to 0% in the controls, reproduced all three of the target actions modeled. This indicates that at least some 9-month-olds could simultaneously keep in mind three different inputs over the 24-hour delay and provides a rather strong demonstration of deferred imitation in this age group. (3) The design ensured that the infant's reproduction on day 2 was based on a memory of the displays and not on a memory of the infant's *own action* from day 1.

This last issue has relevance for a general cognitive-developmental and especially a Piagetian viewpoint. Had infants been allowed to engage in immediate imitation, and then return for a subsequent deferred test, they could simply have been retaining and retrieving their own previously performed actions. It has been argued that the retention and duplication of one's previous acts is a lower-order cognitive task than is initiating a target behavior for the first time on the basis of a stored representation of the display (Piaget, 1952, 1954, 1962). An extreme case of the former is the reinitiation of a conditioned response after a delay, which has been demonstrated by Rovee-Collier, Sullivan, Enright, Lucas, and Fagen (1980) in 3-month-old infants and is generally not seen as addressing the narrower Piagetian concern.

Thus many theorists acknowledge that some form of memory is involved in the following sequence of events: immediate imitation followed by a delay and then a reinitiation of this imitation after the delay. However, this is not classically regarded as a pure case of deferred imitation, and its first appearance would not be predicted to occur only at sensorimotor "stage 6." The current study was designed to respect this theoretical distinction, and infants were not given the opportunity for immediate duplication before being tested in the deferred situation. As such, the findings suggest a downward revision in the age at which some form of legitimate deferred imitation can be performed.

The current work does not directly address the larger idea associated with Piaget's theory and others (Piaget, 1952, 1962; Piattelli-Palmarini, 1980) of a synchronous "stage 6" shift involving symbolic play, deferred imitation, manual search for invisibly displaced objects, and productive language, because these additional measures were not also taken on these same subjects. The results show, however, that at least some capacity for deferred imitation is present under 1 year of age, which is well before these other developments have been typically observed. This suggests that the initial ability to defer imitation for a lengthy delay may not emerge as a contemporaneous achievement with other aspects of the symbolic function and underscores the need for reexamining which cognitive achievements hang together with which during infancy and the transition to early childhood (Corrigan, 1979; Fischer, 1980; Gopnik & Meltzoff, 1984, 1986, 1987; Uzgiris, 1973).

The results also are informative for theories of infant memory, for the deferred imitation effects after 24 hours are virtually identical to those of immediate imitation. This finding, while at first somewhat surprising, is reminiscent of Fagan's (1973) report that infants' performances on a recognition-novelty task did not strikingly decline after 24-hour delays or even longer. Young infants may take longer to encode certain stimuli than older infants (Fagan, 1982; McCall & McGhee, 1977), but once the stimuli are encoded, they seem able to retain them over lengthy delay intervals. On the basis of this work and other ongoing studies in our laboratory (e.g., Meltzoff, 1985a, 1985b), it can be hypothesized that once an event is encoded, the retention interval per se is not a narrowly delimiting factor in early infancy, which in the context of studies of imitation translates into the suggestion that imitative development may not be characterized by a sudden stagelike shift in the raw ability to defer duplicative actions. The strong version of this hypothesis is that nearly any motor pattern that infants are capable of imitating immediately can also be imitated under carefully designed delay conditions. Having found that delay time under the present procedure did not reduce performance in the imitation tasks, it now becomes interesting to introduce systematic interference during the retention interval. By varying the type and content of the interfering stimuli, especially by introducing specific visual versus motor tasks during the delay, it should be possible to investigate the nature of the stored representation used as the basis of deferred imitation by young infants. Is the absent event stored in "visual," "motor," or in some other terms?

Finally, the relation between the present work on deferred imitation and previous work on infant visual memory (Cohen & Gelber, 1975; Fagan, 1982) bears mention, for they are different yet complementary in nature. The previous work has largely focused on "recognition" memory in which the infant's ability to make a perceptual distinction between a novel versus familiar perceptual pattern is tested over various delay intervals. The deferred imitation paradigm taps abilities more akin to "recall" than recognition memory. Infants must do more than perceptually discriminate between a familiar versus novel experience. In the deferred imitation case, they must guide their gross motor behavior to reproduce the act they saw 24 hours earlier, which illustrates a kind of nonverbal recall or cued recall memory (Flavell, 1985; Meltzoff, 1985b; Sophian, 1980; Watson, in press; Werner & Perlmutter, 1979). The deferred imitation test paradigm promises to be a useful new tool in investigating long-term recall memory in young infants.

REFERENCES

Abravanel, E., & Gingold, H. (1985). Learning via observation during the second year of life. *Developmental Psychology,* **21,** 614–623.

Applebaum, M. I., & McCall, R. B. (1983). Design and analysis in developmental psychology. In W. Kessen (Ed.), P. H. Mussen (Series Ed.), *Handbook of child psychology: Vol.* **1.** *History, theory and methods* (pp. 415–476). New York: Wiley.

Bandura, A., & Walters, R. H. (1963). *Social learning and personality development.* New York: Holt, Rinehart & Winston.

Cohen, J. A. (1960). A coefficient of agreement for nominal scales. *Educational and Psychological Measurement,* **20,** 37–46.

Cohen, L. B., & Gelber, E. R. (1975). Infant visual memory. In L. B. Cohen & P. Salapatek (Eds.), *Infant perception: From sensation to cognition* (Vol. **1,** pp. 347–403). New York: Academic Press.

Corrigan, R. (1979). Cognitive correlates of language: Differential criteria yield differential results. *Child Development,* **50,** 617–631.

Fagan, J. F. (1973). Infants' delayed recognition memory and forgetting. *Journal of Experimental Child Psychology,* **16,** 424–450.

Fagan, J. F. (1982). Infant memory. In T. Field et al. (Eds.), *Review of human development* (pp. 79–92). New York: Wiley.

Fischer, K. W. (1980). A theory of cognitive development: The control and construction of hierarchies of skills. *Psychological Review,* **87,** 477–531.

Flavell, J. H. (1985). *Cognitive development* (2d ed.). Englewood Cliffs, NJ: Prentice-Hall.

Fleiss, J. L. (1981). *Statistical methods for rates and proportions.* New York: Wiley.

Gopnik, A., & Meltzoff, A. N. (1984). Semantic and cognitive development in 15- to 21-month-old children. *Journal of Child Language,* **11,** 495–513.

Gopnik, A., & Meltzoff, A. N. (1986). Relations between semantic and cognitive development in the one-word stage: The specificity hypothesis. *Child Development,* **57,** 1040–1053.

Gopnik, A., & Meltzoff, A. N. (1987). The development of categorization in the second year and its relation to other cognitive and linguistic developments. *Child Development,* **58,** 1523–1531.

Hartup, W. W., & Coates, B. (1970). The role of imitation in childhood socialization. In R. A. Hoppe, G. A. Milton, & E. C. Simmel (Eds.), *Early experiences and the processes of socialization* (pp. 109–142), New York: Academic Press.

Inhelder, B. (1971). The sensory-motor origins of knowledge. In D. N. Walcher & D. L. Peters (Eds.), *Early childhood: The development of self-regulatory mechanisms* (pp. 141–155). New York: Academic Press.

Killen, M., & Uzgiris, I. C. (1981). Imitation of actions with objects: The role of social meaning. *Journal of Genetic Psychology,* **138,** 219–229.

Lézine, I. (1973). In J. I. Nurnberger (Ed.), *Biological and environmental determinants of early development* (pp. 221–232). Baltimore: Williams & Wilkins.

McCabe, M. A., & Uzgiris, I. C. (1983). Effects of model and action on imitation in infancy. *Merrill-Palmer Quarterly,* **29,** 69–82.

McCall, R. B., & McGhee, P. E. (1977). The discrepancy hypothesis of attention and affect in infants. In I. C. Uzgiris & F. Weizmann (Eds.), *The structuring of experience* (pp. 179–210). New York: Plenum.

McCall, R. B., Parke, R. D., & Kavanaugh, R. D. (1977). Imitation of live and televised models by children one to three years of age. *Monographs of the Society for Research in Child Development,* **42**(5, Serial No. 173).

Meltzoff, A. N. (1985a). The roots of social and cognitive development: Models of man's original nature. In T. M. Field & N. Fox (Eds.), *Social perception in infants* (pp. 1–30). Norwood, NJ: Ablex.

Meltzoff, A. N. (1985b). Immediate and deferred imitation in fourteen- and twenty-four-month-old infants. *Child Development,* **56,** 62–72.

Meltzoff, A. N., & Moore, M. K. (1983). The origins of imitation in infancy: Paradigm, phenomena, and theories. In L. P. Lipsitt (Ed.), *Advances in infancy research* (Vol. **2,** pp. 265–301). Norwood, NJ: Ablex.

Piaget, J. (1952). *The origins of intelligence in children.* New York: Norton.

Piaget, J. (1954). *The construction of reality in the child.* New York: Basic.

Piaget, J. (1962). *Play, dreams and imitation in childhood.* New York: Norton.

Piattelli-Palmarini, M. (1980). *Language and learning: The debate between Jean Piaget and Noam Chomsky.* Cambridge, MA: Harvard University Press.

Rovee-Collier, C. K., Sullivan, M. W., Enright, M., Lucas, D., & Fagen, J. W. (1980). Reactivation of infant memory. *Science,* **208,** 1159–1161.

Sinclair, H. (1969). Developmental psycholinguistics. In D. Elkind & J. H. Flavell (Eds.), *Studies in cognitive development: Essays in honor of Jean Piaget* (pp. 315–336). New York: Oxford University Press.

Sinclair, H. (1970). The transition from sensory-motor behaviour to symbolic activity. *Interchange,* **1,** 119–126.

Sophian, C. (1980). Habituation is not enough: Novelty preferences, search, and memory in infancy. *Merrill-Palmer Quarterly,* **26,** 239–257.

Uzgiris, I. C. (1973). Patterns of cognitive development in infancy. *Merrill-Palmer Quarterly,* **19,** 181–204.

Uzgiris, I. C., & Hunt, J. McV. (1975). *Assessment in infancy: Ordinal scales of psychological development.* Urbana: University of Illinois Press.

Watson, J. S. (in press). Memory in infancy. In J. Piaget, J. P. Bronkart, & P. Mounoud (Eds.), *Encyclopédie de la pléidade: La psychologie.* Paris: Gallimard.

Werner, J. S., & Perlmutter, M. (1979). Development of visual memory in infants. In H. W. Reese & L. P. Lipsitt (Eds.), *Advances in child development and behavior* (Vol. **14,** pp. 1–56). New York: Academic Press.

Wishart, J. G. (1986). Siblings as models in early infant learning. *Child Development,* **57,** 1232–1240.

2

Offspring of Women with Nonorganic Psychosis: Mother-Infant Interaction and Fear of Strangers During the First Year of Life

I. Persson-Blennow, B. Binett, and T. F. McNeil

University of Lund, Malmö, Sweden

Mother-infant interaction characteristics at six ages during the first year of life were studied in relationship to the developmen of the infant's fear of strangers (FOS) during the first year. Among 46 offspring of women with psychosis history, a failure to develop the expected FOS was associated with antecedent negative qualitative aspects of interaction such as increased maternal tension, reduced harmony in feeding and increased infant crying. Among 80 low-risk control infants, a failure to develop FOS was associated with an antecedent quantitative reduction in social contact within the mother-infant pair. At a case level, an absence of FOS overlapped little with anxious attachment to the mother, and these two developmental phenomena bear partially different relationships to the mother-infant interaction characteristics.

While infants show unselectively positive responses to both familiar and unfamiliar persons during the first half year of life, selective preference for familiar persons (usually the mother), coupled with negative response and withdrawal from strangers, appears during the second 6 months of life. This

---

Reprinted with permission from *Acta Psychiatr Scand*, 1988, Volume 78, 379–383. Copyright 1988.

This research has been supported by Grants No. 3793 and 6214 from the Swedish Medical Research Council, by Grant No. MH18857 from PHS, DHEW, USA, and by the W. T. Grant Foundation, U.S.A.

"fear of strangers" (FOS) or "eight-month anxiety", which appears on the average at 8 months of age,[1-4] is found in almost all infants by 12 months,[2,3,5] generally lasts for at least two consecutive months[6] and declines some time during the first half of the second year of life.[7] Smith & Sloboda[8] recently reported finding individual consistency in both positive and negative affective responses to different strangers.

Although disagreement exists about the underlying nature of FOS,[7,9,10] FOS is considered to be important by authors that represent very different theoretical schools, and a failure to develop FOS has been considered as clearly pathological.[4,11] An absence of FOS may possibly be related to risk for later psychopathology, as children with a high risk for serious psychopathology have been found to have had more frequent failure to develop FOS.[12]

In previous studies, the appearance of FOS has been found to relate to a wide range of biological, personal and environmental conditions[12] including infant-mother attachment.[2,4,13,14] It has been suggested that FOS signals the development of the infant's positive attachment to (typically) the mother. Deviations in infant attachment are known to be related to maternal behavior,[15] and many authors have assumed that the mother's behavior also influences the development of FOS. However, little empirical evidence exists to support this assumption.[7] In addition, Schaffer[16] found no relationship between the age of onset of FOS and social interaction variables such as maternal responsiveness to the child's needs or interaction with the child.

Given uncertainty about whether and how maternal behavior influences the development of FOS, further study was indicated. The current longitudinal study of the development of high-risk offspring of index women with a history of nonorganic psychosis, and low-risk offspring of control women[17] presented the opportunity to investigate the relationship between maternal and infant behavior in interaction during the first year of life and infant FOS during that period. In this study, mother-infant interaction was studied systematically at six ages during the first year[18], and infant FOS was investigated both through a standardized test at 1 year and through repeated maternal interviews during the first year.[12]

The hypothesis that was tested in this substudy was that a failure to develop FOS during the first year of life is related to negative mother-infant interaction characteristics. The current high-risk and low-risk groups have been found to differ from one another on both FOS and mother-infant interaction characteristics.[12,18] As the background factors related to the development of FOS may thus possibly be different between these two groups, the hypothesis was tested separately for the high-risk cases and for the low-risk cases.

MATERIAL AND METHODS

The basic samples and methods have been described previously.[12, 17–21] The subjects included in this sub-study were those 126 mother-infant pairs who participated in the longitudinal study and for whom data were obtained for both mother-infant interaction at any of the six observation occasions during the infant's first year, and infant FOS at 1 year. The maximum sample sizes were 46 index pairs and 80 control pairs; the sample sizes varied somewhat across the different interaction ages.

Interaction was observed in feeding on the maternity ward at 3 days after delivery and in both feeding and an unstructured play situation in the home at 3 and 6 weeks and 3.5, 6 and 12 months.[18–21] The maternal, infant and reciprocal variables employed in the current analyses were the same as those used in investigating the antecedents of anxious attachment, as described in [15].

FOS was investigated by a standardized method according to Schaffer & Emerson, as described in [12]. On the basis of the infant's behavior in the test situation, the infant was classified as evidencing strong, medium or no FOS. At the home visits at 3.5, 6 and 12 months, the mother was asked whether and when the infant had shown fear towards strangers encountered together with the mother in the course of everyday life. On the basis of data from both the observation and the interviews, the infants were divided into those who had never evidenced FOS (FOS-negative cases) and those who had evidenced FOS (FOS-positive cases).

The FOS-negative infants were compared with FOS-positive infants on the selected interaction variables investigated at each of the interaction study ages. Analyses were done separately within the index and control groups, in a manner described in[15]. The hypothesis indicated one-tailed analyses.

RESULTS

The results for selected variables are shown in Table 1 (the results for all variables analyzed here are available from the authors).

In both index and control groups, statistically significant differences on interaction characteristics were found between FOS-negative and FOS-positive cases from 6 weeks through 6 months (and also at 12 months in index cases). The greatest number of significant differences on interaction characteristics was found at 6 weeks, i.e., well in advance of the time of expected development of FOS. The interaction characteristics relating to FOS were entirely different in the index vs. control groups.

The interaction of FOS-negative (vs. FOS-positive) index cases was characterized by significantly less harmony in feeding (at 6 months, with a similar

Situation/age/group		Interaction variable					
		Harmony in feeding	Mother social contact	Mother tense/ uncertain	Child social contact	Amount of child crying	Reciprocal behaviors
3 days							
Feeding	Index	n.s.	0.10	n.s.	n.s.	n.s.	
	Control	n.s.	n.s.	n.s.	n.s.	n.s.	
3 weeks							
Feeding	Index	n.s.	n.s.	n.s.	n.s.	n.s.	n.s.
	Control	n.s.	n.s.	n.s.	n.s.	n.s.	n.s.
Play	Index		n.s.	n.s.	n.s.	n.s.	n.s.
	Control		n.s.	n.s.	0.10	n.s.	0.10
6 weeks							
Feeding	Index	n.s.	n.s.	0.05	n.s.	0.10	n.s.
	Control	n.s.	0.025	n.s.	0.10	n.s.	0.10
Play	Index		n.s.	0.01	n.s.	n.s.	n.s.
	Control		0.025	n.s.	0.01	n.s.	0.025
3.5 months							
Feeding	Index	0.10	n.s.	0.05	n.s.	n.s.	n.s.
	Control	n.s.	0.025	n.s.	n.s.	n.s.	• n.s.
Play	Index		n.s.	n.s.	n.s.	n.s.	n.s.
	Control		0.10	n.s.	n.s.	n.s.	0.10
6 months							
Feeding	Index	0.01	n.s.	0.10	n.s.	0.05	n.s.
	Control	n.s.	n.s.	n.s.	n.s.	n.s.	0.10
Play	Index		n.s.	0.10	n.s.	0.05	n.s.
	Control		n.s.	n.s.	n.s.	n.s.	0.005
12 months							
Feeding	Index	n.s.	n.s.	n.s.	n.s.	n.s.	n.s.
	Control	n.s.	n.s.	n.s.	n.s.	n.s.	n.s.
Play	Index		n.s.	0.05	n.s.	0.025	n.s.
	Control		n.s.	n.s.	n.s.	n.s.	n.s.

Table 1. Significance (*P*) of Comparisons of FOS-Negative Vs. FOS-Positive Infants on Mother-Infant Interaction Characteristics (Selected Variables).

tendency at 3.5 months), greater maternal tension/uncertainty (at 6 weeks, 3.5 months and 12 months, with a similar tendency at 6 months) and more child crying (at 6 and 12 months, with a similar tendency at 6 weeks); none of these variables were significantly different for FOS-negative vs. FOS-positive control cases.

In contrast, the interaction of FOS-negative (vs. FOS-positive) control cases was characterized by reduced maternal social contact (at 6 weeks and 3.5 months, with a similar trend at 3 days), reduced child social contact (at 6 weeks, with a similar trend at 3 weeks) and reduced mother-infant reciprocal behaviors (at 6 weeks and 6 months, with similar trends at 3 weeks and 3.5 months).

In neither index nor control cases was the appearance of FOS significantly related at any age to maternal body contact, mother's response to child's verbal contact, mother's consideration for child's needs in play, child's motor activity, child's nonnutritive sucking or child's response to mother's verbal contact.

The results thus provide some support for the hypothesis, but differently in index and control groups.

DISCUSSION

Within both high-risk and low-risk groups, mother-infant interaction was significantly more deviant and negative in cases where the infant subsequently failed to develop fear of strangers during the first year of life. However, the background characteristics were different in high- and low-risk groups: Among the low-risk control cases, an absence of FOS was associated with a quantitative reduction in social contact within the pair (i.e., in maternal, infant and reciprocal social behaviors); this reduction was strongest at 6 weeks, but tendencies were found as early as 3 weeks, and significant differences continued at 3.5 and 6 months. Among the high-risk index cases, an absence of FOS was associated with more qualitative aspects of interaction, i.e., with increased maternal tension/uncertainty, reduced harmony in feeding and increased infant crying; these characteristics were strongest at 6 months, but they were found from 6 weeks to 1 year of age.

The reason why the development of FOS in high-risk cases was not sensitive to reduced social contact is unknown. The total high-risk group (vs. control) had an increased rate of low social contact[18-21], but in spite of this, reduced social contact was related to the absence of FOS only among control cases.

As FOS has been considered to signal the development of attachment to the mother, a comparison of background factors associated with anxious attachment vs. with an absence of FOS seems warranted. Our earlier study of the background for anxious attachment in these same samples[15] showed only some overlap with the current results. Anxious attachment in index offspring was preceded by reduced harmony in feeding and increased offspring crying (as was also found here for absence of FOS); however, greater maternal tension/ uncertainty did not precede anxious attachment, increased tension being associated with attachment first at 1 year. Furthermore, anxious attachment in index offspring was also anteceded by less maternal consideration for child's needs, less infant social contact and less reciprocal behavior, none of which was found as a significant antecedent of the absence of FOS in index cases. Among controls, reduced maternal social contact preceded both anxious attachment and absence of FOS, while reduced harmony in feeding and less consideration for the child's needs preceded anxious attachment but not absence of FOS.

Some of the differences in background for attachment vs. FOS may reflect the fact that anxious attachment and absence of FOS overlap very little with each other at the individual subject level. Among the 46 index subjects, 13 had anxious attachment and 14 had absence of FOS but only five had both anxious attachment and absence of FOS; among the 80 controls, only one had both anxious attachment and absence of FOS (among a total of 14 with anxious attachment and 12 with absence of FOS). At this operational level of study, anxious attachment to the mother and failure to develop FOS appear to represent different aberrations in emotional development, with partially different precedents in mother-infant interaction characteristics.

REFERENCES

1. Spitz R A. Anxiety in infancy: a study of its manifestations in the first year of life. Int J Psychoanal 1950:*31*:138–143.
2. Schaffer H R, Emerson P E. The development of social attachments in infancy. Monogr Soc Res Child Dev 1964:*29*:No. 94, pp. 5–77.
3. Morgan G A, Ricciuti H N. Infants' responses to strangers during the first year. In: Foss B M, ed. Determinants of infant behaviour. IV. London: Methuen, 1969:253–272.
4. Stevens A G. Attachment behaviour, separation anxiety, and stranger anxiety in polymatrically reared infants. In: Schaffer H R, ed. The origins of human social relations. London: Academic Press, 1971:137–146.
5. Tennes K H, Lampl E E. Stranger and separation anxiety in infancy. J Nerv Ment Dis 1964:*139*:247–254.
6. Emde R N, Gaensbauer T J, Harmon R J. Emotional expression in infancy. A biobehavioral study. Psychol Issues 1976:*10*:No. 37.
7. Décarie T G. Manifestations, hypotheses, data. In: Décarie T G, ed. The infant's reaction to strangers. New York: International Universities Press, 1974:7–55.
8. Smith P K, Sloboda J. Individual consistency in infant-stranger encounters. Br J Dev Psychol 1986:*4*:83–91.
9. Solomon R, Décarie T. Fear of strangers: a developmental milestone or an overstudied phenomenon? Can J Behav Sci 1976:*8*:351–362.
10. Sroufe L A. Really a matter of data: a reply to Solomon. Child Dev 1980:*51*:260–261.
11. Benjamin J D. Some developmental observations relating to the theory of anxiety. J Am Psychoanal Assoc 1961:*9*:652–668.
12. Näslund Binett B, Persson-Blennow I, McNeil T F, Kaij L, Malmquist-Larsson A. Offspring of women with nonorganic psychosis: fear of strangers during the first year of life. Acta Psychiatr Scand 1984:*69*:435–444.
13. Ainsworth M D S. The development of infant-mother attachment. In: Caldwell B M, Ricciuti H N, eds. *Review of child development research.* Vol. 3. Chicago: University of Chicago Press, 1973:1–94.
14. Bowlby J. *Attachment and loss.* Vol. II. *Separation. Anxiety and anger.* New York: Basic Books, 1973.

15. Persson-Blennow I, Binett B, McNeil T F. Offspring of women with nonorganic psychosis: antecedents of anxious attachment to the mother at one year of age. Acta Psychiatr Scand 1988:78:66–71.
16. Schaffer H R. The onset of fear of strangers and the incongruity hypothesis. J Child Psychol Psychiatry 1966:7:95–106.
17. McNeil T F, Kaij L, Malmquist-Larsson A, et al. Offspring of women with nonorganic psychoses: development of longitudinal study of children at high risk. Acta Psychiatr Scand 1983:68:234–250.
18. Persson-Blennow I, Näslund B, McNeil T F, Kaij L. Offspring of women with nonorganic psychosis: mother-infant interaction at one year of age. Acta Psychiatr Scand 1986:73:207–213.
19. Persson-Blennow I, Näslund B, McNeil T F, Kaij L, Malmquist-Larsson A. Offspring of women with nonorganic psychosis: mother-infant interaction at three days of age. Acta Psychiatr Scand 1984:70:149–159.
20. Näslund B, Persson-Blennow I, McNeil T F, Kaij L. Offspring of women with nonorganic psychosis: mother-infant interaction at three and six weeks of age. Acta Psychiatr Scand 1985:71:441–450.
21. McNeil T F, Näslund B, Persson-Blennow I, Kaij L. Offspring of women with nonorganic psychosis: mother-infant interaction at three-and-a-half and six months of age. Acta Psychiatr Scand 1985:71:551–558.

Part II
DEVELOPMENTAL STUDIES

The papers in this section span a wide range of issues relevant to the development of children and to their status as adults. In the first paper, Angoff considers an old issue, the nature-nurture debate over intelligence and aptitude, from a new perspective. He argues that the relevant issue, in the context of a consideration of group differences, is not whether intelligence is largely genetic or environmentally determined, but rather whether or not intelligence can be changed. A thoughtful review of the relevant recent literature leads him to reject the commonly held position that high heritability necessarily connotes immutability and that low heritability necessarily connotes changeability. Rather, under appropriate conditions, changes in the aptitude and intelligence of groups can and do occur. While this observation has been made in the past—Gordon's studies of Canal Boat children in Britain (Gordon, H., *Mental and Scholastic Tests Among Retarded Children.* London: Board of Education, Education Pamphlet No. 44, 1923) and Klineberg's investigations of intelligence among Blacks living in the South and in the Northern United States (Klineberg, O., *Race Differences.* New York: Harper, 1935), its restatement at this time serves to re-legitimize the study of factors influencing intelligence and aptitude in disadvantaged populations. Sandra Scarr's paper in this volume, "Race and Gender as Psychological Variables," provides another perspective on this issue.

Judy Dunn is a leading researcher in the area of sibling relationships. Her succinct and authoritative review considers sibling influences on child development from a variety of perspectives, including aggression and conflict; cooperation, friendliness, and empathy; socio-cognitive capacities; factors influencing the quality of the sibling relationship; and the influence of disabled and chronically ill siblings. Dunn concludes that although the influence of siblings on one another constitutes an important source of environmental influence on the development of individual differences, evidence of sibling influence that is clearly independent of other family factors is rare. Rather, differences in sibling relationships are closely linked to differences in other family relationships, and to the emotional quality of the family. Nevertheless, it appears as if siblings play a causal role in the development of aggressive behavior, in children's style of conflict behavior, and in cooperative fantasy play.

In the next paper, Thomas Horner extends his revision of the traditional psychoanalytic view of the psychic life of the young infant (*Annual Progress,*

1986) to the toddler years, focusing on what Mahler has characterized as the rapprochement sub-phase of the process of separation-individuation. As reframed by Horner, rapprochement reflects not the culmination of steps taken by the infant from symbiotic union with the mother to an established sense of separateness as Mahler originally proposed, but rather, a process of reattaining basic love and security when frustrations and resistance, with their correlated affects, have been effectively handled. The revision is consistent with the growing body of evidence indicating that the infant is born with innate capacities that permit him or her to function as an active partner in social interactions that occur within the context of the regulation of physiological functions, and never to experience a period of total self/other undifferentiation. While acknowledging the utility of the rapprochement concept as a metaphor for describing the specific conflicts, defensive maneuvers, and characterological dynamics of older children and adults, Horner notes that clinical reconstructions, despite their thematic persuasiveness, are methodologically inferior means of studying the specific dynamics of earlier periods of development. Moreover, all positive attachment relationships possess the means to avoid many conflicts and to restore basic states of love and security when unavoidable conflicts arise. Rapprochement, or reconciliation following a disruption of relations, applies equally to all developmental stages.

Bullock and Lütkenhaus address development during the toddler years from a somewhat different vantage point. This elegantly designed study examines the developmental course of volitional behavior between 15 and 35 months of age. In these authors' view, active volitional competence is the hallmark of a goal-directed self. While a rudimentary capacity for intentional behavior is most probably present during infancy, successful attainment of outcomes becomes increasingly likely as the child develops skills necessary to regulate behavior. The methodology permits the analysis of several components of volitional behavior: the ability to engage in task-directed behavior; to monitor, correct, and control activities; and to express positive affect in association with the outcome of actions were observed. Clear developmental gradients are identified. Children under a year and a half of age are primarily activity, rather than outcome, oriented. Attention to producing a specific outcome, defined by an external standard, first becomes evident at 26 months, and is not consistent across different tasks until 32 months of age. By the beginning of the third year of life, most children consistently regulate their activities by attending to task demands, monitoring and correcting errors, inhibiting ongoing actions when a task is completed, and expressing pleasure in association with successful mastery. That, in older children, the expression of positive affect comes increasingly to be associated with producing outcomes that match a standard, is of particular importance to our understanding of the role of affect in the development of an explicit sense of agency and competence.

The findings of Oppenheim, Sagi and Lamb's study, "Infant-Adult Attachments on the Kibbutz and Their Relation to Socioemotional Development 4 Years Later," illustrates the complexities involved in interpreting responses to the "Strange Situation." Their study was initiated in an attempt to clarify the meaning of C-type (resistant) attachment among kibbutz-raised infants who, as a group, are significantly more likely to exhibit this pattern than are those raised in the United States. Aspects of the socioemotional development of children whose attachments to mothers, fathers, and metaplot (caregivers) were assessed in the Strange Situation when they were 11 to 14 months old, were examined at age five years. The measures of socioemotional development reflected the children's behavior in the children's house at the kibbutz, but not at home or with their parents. Although the authors anticipated that classifications of infant-mother, infant-father, and infant-metapelet relationships would have equivalent effects on the children's later social and emotional behavior, neither infant-mother nor infant-father classifications were significantly associated with the chosen outcome measures. However, infants who had B-type (secure) attachments to their metapelet were later found to be less ego controlled and more empathic, dominant, purposive, achievement-oriented and independent than C-group (resistant) subjects. Although the similarity of the correlates of infant-metapelet attachment characteristics to those found for infant-mother attachment in the United States may be a reflection of the central importance of the metapelet in the early social life of kibbutz infants, this interpretation is constrained by the situation specificity of the outcome measures. The data strongly suggest that Strange Situation classifications assess the relationships between infants and specific adults rather than individual "traits." The exploration of the developmental significance of attachment relationships with different significant adults is an important area for future research.

The final paper in this section broadens the sweep of prediction to adult life. Clarke and Clarke note that development is characterized by both constancy and change. The interactions between biological and social factors are complex, and their complexity is further increased by the fact that an individual is not a passive recipient of environmental influences, but a participant in transactional interactions, the nature of which shape behavioral responses. A selective review of adult outcomes of severe mental retardation, autism, conduct disorders, mild mental retardation, and adjustment disorders of childhood illustrates the proposition that the presence of an organic component narrows the range of reaction between constitution and environment. Thus, a highly dependent life path is inevitable in cases of severe mental retardation, and the "escape rate" in cases of autism is very small. About half of conduct disordered children have a very poor outcome as adults, and only one-third of those administratively classified as mildy retarded in childhood continue to require special services after school-leaving age. However, adjustment disorders of childhood only rarely show continuities into adult life. This model of interacting trajectories—the biological and the social—during the whole life span leads to the prediction that as social and familial disruptions become more common, conduct disorders, mild mental retardation and adjustment problems during childhood will become more prevalent, while the incidence of severe mental retardation will decrease in association with advances in biomedical technology.

3

The Nature-Nurture Debate: Aptitudes and Group Differences

William H. Angoff

Educational Testing Service, Princeton, New Jersey

The thesis of this article is that the debate over whether intelligence is largely genetically or largely environmentally determined is actually irrelevant in the context of group differences. The real issue is whether intelligence can be changed, an issue that does not at all go hand in hand with the issue of heritability. Many inherited characteristics are changeable, and conversely, many environmentally acquired characteristics are extremely resistant to change.

The political nature of this dispute has had serious consequences in the attitudes of psychologists toward important and useful constructs like academic aptitude, which seems in some quarters to have been rejected because of its partially hereditary character and its presumed imperviousness to change. However, several studies have shown that under appropriate conditions aptitude and intelligence can and do change. These studies have important implications for the future performance of minorities in this society.

Like few other scientific and social issues, the matter of the heritability of intelligence has been the subject of intense debate since the beginning of this century. In recent years, the debate has become especially heated, following the appearance of the 1969 article by Jensen in the *Harvard Educational Review* and the 1971 article by Herrnstein in the *Atlantic* magazine. What I am suggesting here is that the debate over whether intelligence is largely genetically or largely environmentally determined is actually misplaced, even irrelevant, in the context of group differences and that the question of heritability is not really an issue here at all. The real issue, the one that should instead be

Reprinted with permission from *American Psychologist,* 1988, Vol. 43, No. 9, 713–720. Copyright 1988 by the American Psychological Association, Inc.

the focus of debate in this context, is whether intelligence can be *changed,* and if so, how, and under what circumstances.

It is not hard to see why the debate has become so keen in recent years and why the connection between heritability and changeability is so crucial to it. Very likely the most important aspect of the issue is that aptitude (i.e., *academic* aptitude) and intelligence are in fact thought by many to be largely innate (i.e., inherent in the individual at the time of birth) and to a considerable extent inherited, and *therefore* unchangeable both within a given lifetime and across generations. If one holds to the view that the two concepts—heritability and changeability—are indeed closely connected and if one also recalls that minorities in this society, especially Blacks, score much lower on aptitude and intelligence tests than Whites and have, over the years, been generally lower achieving than Whites, it is an easy leap to conclude that Blacks are innately, even genetically, inferior. Moreover, the conclusion that is thought to follow from the heritable and presumed immutable nature of aptitude, or intelligence, is that the low scores (and by inference, the low aptitude and intelligence) of Black parents will be followed by the low scores of their children and that the disparity of the present will be a continuing fact of the future. That these inferences rest on faulty premises and are therefore unwarranted is not always to the point. The inferences nevertheless are drawn, and curiously enough, the same faulty premise—that high heritability necessarily connotes immutability and that low heritability necessarily connotes changeability—is often held by people at opposite ends of the social-political spectrum. Indeed, it is their shared belief in the validity of these connotations that is at the root of the heredity-environment controversy.

The foregoing picture of the future of Black people in our society is not an unreasonable extension of the views of some of the extreme hereditarians today. It resembles the kind of thinking advanced by some of the well-known and highly respected psychologists in the early decades of this century, who were supporters of, or at least fellow travelers in, the American eugenics movement. Those who challenged the view (and many who challenge it today) did so by disputing the work of the hereditarians instead of challenging the connection between heritability and immutability. Their claim is that intelligence is not inherited but is largely or entirely environmental in origin. Some of them also argue that the so-called intelligence tests are invalid measures of intelligence and that the race differences they reveal are artificial and spurious.

Strangely enough, both parties to the controversy seem generally willing to accept the assumption that inherited traits are not subject to change, at least not readily. This is the assumption that deserves attention.

Several years ago, an article in the *New York Times* by Henry Scott Stokes (Stokes, 1982, p. 16E) caught my eye. The article gave the results of a study of intergenerational change in stature conducted by the Ministry of Health and Welfare in Japan and reported that between 1946 or so and 1982 the average height of young adult males increased by about four inches. Clearly, this is a dramatic increase, one that does not, or should not, go unnoticed. I tried to track the study down, writing first to Stokes himself, then, eventually to the Japanese Ministry. After some months, I received a photocopy of a page from the report, indicating that indeed there was a gain in those 36 years, but it was closer to 3⅓ inches, still not inconsiderable by anyone's standards. We have seen evidence of and heard of secular changes in height many times, but we have not often heard of changes of this magnitude. Casual, admittedly uncontrolled observations of our own almost without exception lead us to the conclusion that the heights of adults also have increased over the generations in this country, especially over the last generation or so.

These observations are, in fact, supported by voluminous sources of data that demonstrate that inherited characteristics, even those with heritability coefficients approaching unity, have changed, sometimes dramatically, from one generation to the next and certainly over the course of several generations. The data may violate some preconceived notions of heritability, but in one respect, at least, they should not: The statistics from which one calculates indexes of heritability and from which one infers heritability are only coefficients of correlation between the measured characteristics of family members (e.g., Falconer, 1981; Taylor, 1980); and correlations have nothing to say about mean (or variability) differences between the variables. Thus, the correlations between the heights of fathers and the heights of their sons would be unaffected whether the sons were two, three, or five inches taller, or shorter, than their fathers. Indeed, changes in height over generations and across comparable cohorts in different geographical locations have been documented in many places, for example, Carter and Marshall (1978), Damon (1974), Greulich (1957, 1977), Roche (1979), and Tanner (1962, 1970). All of these writers have reported secular changes in physical characteristics, including, especially, height. Tanner (1962), for example, reported that British and American adolescents are half a foot taller today on the average than their predecessors of a century ago. Particularly interesting are the studies that compare American-born children of Japanese parents with their native-born Japanese contemporaries in Japan. Greulich (1957), for example, reported on a study of 898 American-born Japanese children in California and found that the California children were "taller, heavier, more advanced skeletally, and, during the prepubertal period, distinctly longer-legged than the children in Japan."

What makes the reference to secular changes in height particularly interesting in this context is that height has been consistently regarded as an example of a trait with an extremely high heritability index, close to 1.0. The fact that it displays intergenerational change appears, however, to be entirely irrelevant to the heritability coefficient itself. What is perhaps more to the point is that if a trait with this degree of heritability is so changeable, then certainly other traits, like intelligence, which are acknowledged to have lower heritability coefficients, may also be changeable.

This is certainly not the first time that the connection—rather, the lack of connection—between heritability and immutability has ever received attention. Several writers, including the geneticists Erlenmeyer-Kimling and Jarvik (1963) and also James Crow (1969), one of the respondents to Jensen's 1969 article in the *Harvard Educational Review,* have had their say about this issue. Crow wrote that the heritability index

> does not directly tell us how much improvement in IQ to expect from a given change in environment. In particular, it offers no guidance as to the consequences of a new kind of environmental influence. For example, conventional heritability measures for height show a value of nearly 1.0. Yet because of identified environmental influences, the mean heights in the United States and Japan have risen by a spectacular amount. (p. 306)

Sandra Scarr and Robert Plomin, two of the most prominent and productive developmental behavioral geneticists in America today, have had the same things to say. Scarr (1981a) has written, "A . . . faulty . . . conclusion is that, if genetic differences contribute more than environmental differences due to the variance of IQ scores, then IQ is considered to be not very malleable. The myth of heritability limiting malleability seems to die hard" (p. 53). In another place (1981a), she has said, "Even if the heritability for IQ in a population were 1.0, meaning that present environmental differences contributed nothing to individual phenotypic differences, a change in environment could dramatically shift the mean of the entire phenotypic distribution" (p. 53). In yet another place (1981b) she has said,

> The most common misunderstanding of the concept "heritability" relates to the myth of fixed intelligence. If h^2 [heritability coefficient] is high, this reasoning goes, then intelligence is genetically fixed and unchangeable at the phenotypic level. This misconception ignores the fact that h^2 is a population statistic, bound to a given set of environmental conditions at a given point in time. Neither intelligence nor h^2 estimates are fixed. (p. 73)

Robert Plomin (1983) has offered the same kinds of observations. He noted that there is some difficulty in "shaking the mistaken notion that genetic differences begin prior to birth and remain immutable ever after" (p. 253). He said that "we need to pry apart the close association that the adjectives 'genetic' and 'stable' have come to share: Longitudinally stable characters are not necessarily hereditary, nor are genetically influenced characters necessarily stable over time. . . . genetic does not mean immutable" (p. 254).

I should add that Scarr and Plomin have not been alone in making these assertions. Anastasi (1982, p. 350) and Crawford (1979) have made precisely the same points, as, incidentally, has Stephen Jay Gould (1981, p. 156) on the one hand, and Arthur Jensen (1969, p. 45) and Richard Herrnstein (1973, p. 58) on the other, writers who are generally known to occupy quite different positions in the hereditary-environment debate. Crawford (1979) has made the interesting observation that many of us implicitly associate genetics with determinism and environmentalism with free will—clearly, a gross extrapolation of a common view.

The controversy over differential change becomes closely identified with the nature-nurture controversy as a consequence of the further assumption that there is a fixed and permanent blueprint for the development of inherited traits in the gene pattern, causing these traits to be resistant to change at *any* age. Why this view is held is hard to say. Several writers—for example, Bereiter (1970, p. 289), Cronbach (1969), Erlenmeyer-Kimling and Jarvik (1963), Jensen (1969), and Rose (1976, p. 124)—have all mentioned that the effects of phenylketonuria, an inherited metabolic defect, are now quite tractable as a consequence of dietary control. This is similarly true of inherited diseases such as hemophilia, diabetes, and galactosemia, as well as many others, including heart disease and even the tendency to develop dental caries. In a news article on the subject of environmental interventions in the control of inherited diseases, Harold Schmeck (1984) wrote,

> Rapid advances are occurring in research aimed at making gene therapy possible. Natural viruses are being modified to act as efficient carriers of the genes, and more and more genes that might usefully be transplanted are being identified and grown in laboratories. (p. C1)

Conversely, it is well known that some environmentally acquired habits and attitudes are extremely resistant to change. These include not only the physically addictive habits like smoking, drinking, and drug addiction, but also racial, national, and religious prejudices; attitudes toward crime, money, and marriage; attitudes of authoritarianism, and even voting behavior.

But what of the index of heritability itself? The variations in the estimates of this construct are nothing less than astonishing, extending from estimates of near zero reported by Schwartz and Schwartz (1974) and denials by Kamin (1974) of the validity of any source of evidence that intelligence is inherited, to estimates of .80 and higher offered by Burt (1958) and Jensen (1969). Jensen seems to have lowered his estimates since his 1969 article. In his 1980 volume, *Bias in Mental Testing* (p. 244), he reported .75 as the central tendency of empirical studies of the heritability index; and in *Straight Talk About Mental Tests* (1981, p. 103), he reported that estimates of variance due to genetic factors range from .60 to .80, averaging .70, and suggested that recent estimates may be even lower. Plomin (1986) and Scarr and Weinberg (1978) have reported their estimates in similarly conservative ways. Plomin has estimated that IQ heritability in adulthood appears to be in the range .40 to .60 (p. 262). Scarr and Weinberg have also offered a range, .40 to .70. In all these sets of estimates, the numbers are clearly rounded and approximate, confirming the views of all three sets of authors that the question of the size of the heritability coefficient defies a specific, precise answer. Indeed, Scarr (1974) has wisely pointed out that the question itself is a "pseudo-question," offering answers that depend on a variety of considerations, including the ethnic composition of the population, the nature of the abilities and skills measured and how they are tested, the ages of the individuals studied, and the genetic and environmental composition of the population under consideration. Clearly, in an environmentally homogeneous group, heritability coefficients are likely to be inflated; in an environmentally heterogeneous group, the opposite is likely to be true.

Finally, as further evidence that this question has not been neglected, Bouchard and McGue (1981), in an updated comprehensive summary of 111 studies assembled in a survey of world literature on familial resemblances in measured intelligence, have been willing to say that there is clear evidence for partial genetic determination of IQ, but unlike others, they have hesitated to evaluate the strength of the effect.

In another connection, Scarr (Scarr-Salapatek, 1971) has made the observation that

> even if the heritabilities of IQ were extremely high in all races, there is still no warrant for equating within-group and between-group heritabilities. There are examples in agricultural experiments of within-group differences that are highly heritable but between-group differences that are entirely environmental. Draw two random samples of seeds from the same genetically heterogeneous population. Plant one sample in uniformly good conditions, the

other in uniformly poor conditions. The average height difference
between the populations of plants will be entirely environmental,
although the individual differences in height within each sample
will be entirely genetic. (p. 1226)

This illustration makes an excellent point and is particularly apt in the
present circumstance because it describes a set of conditions closely analogous
to the historic differences in the lives of Black and White people in this country. Virtually all of the Blacks who were brought here from Africa arrived
under the most abject conditions. They spent their first 200 years or more
enslaved and the next 120 years segregated and directly or indirectly deprived
of the educational opportunities commonly afforded Whites. For example, in
virtually every slave state it was a criminal offense for a slave to learn to read
and write, and it was a criminal offense for a White to provide that opportunity (Webber, 1978). There were, to be sure, many violations of the law, some
flagrant and some minor and quietly ignored, but the law was official, and it
was often harshly enforced, especially when the violations were thought to be
too conspicuous and flagrant. In any case, it was seldom to the advantage of
the slave owners to educate their field hands, and for the very large part,
slaves were kept ignorant, illiterate, and deprived of access even to the most
rudimentary cognitive skills and knowledges. It is also well known that these
conditions did not change rapidly after the Emancipation, and even today full
equality of educational opportunity is certainly not the norm.

What is so puzzling is that despite these many years of denial of normal
access to educational opportunity and what these years of denial have undoubtedly done to curb the motivations and ambitions of Blacks to enter into the
educational mainstream, many of our colleagues were, and some still are,
willing to believe that the disparities in measured intelligence are simply the
result of a different, if not an inferior, gene pool. This is all the more striking
when one considers how few heritability studies have been done on Black populations and how few studies have been done with equally mixed Black and
White populations.

The point that is worth repeating here, however, is that the notion of heritability in connection with group differences in this society has not advanced
our thinking in this area, but in fact has distracted and confused it, even retarded it. Whatever the "true" heritability coefficient for intelligence is (if,
indeed, there is such a thing), whether it is high or low, and what factors affect
its calculation, the essential point is that in the context of group differences
and what these differences connote, its numerical value is irrelevant. What is
relevant is whether these group differences can be changed, with what means,
and with what effect. It has been amply demonstrated that changeability, or as

Scarr would have it, "malleability," is not a function of the genetic or nongenetic origin of intelligence. This being the case, it is certainly time to separate these two notions and deal with them individually.

Apparently, this has not been an easy thing to do. Moreover, the notion of the heritability of intelligence and aptitude has produced other outcomes, including an unfortunate and important spin-off of the nature-nurture dispute, causing some to cast doubt and suspicion on the usefulness of the constructs of intelligence and aptitude themselves. Indeed, the acrimony of the debate regarding these constructs and their heritability has sometimes reached levels of stridency that go far beyond those observed in conventional scientific debate. It entails little discernment to conclude that the heat has been generated as a consequence of the political, rather than the scientific, implications of the views expressed about heritability—specifically, what the presumed immutability of intelligence and aptitude signifies for the future of minorities in this society.

But the constructs of intelligence and aptitude are, in fact, useful and valid, and it is important to consider them here. They have been invented quite legitimately to account for the fact that individuals who have been exposed to the same educational stimuli nevertheless consistently display stable and predictable differences in achievement. Despite the fact that such differences are commonly observed, however, these concepts and their amenability to valid measurement have been the subject of considerable debate for some time. The debate has been given new form in recent years by the appearance of additional (or to use Anastasi's, 1975, word "surplus," i.e., unwarranted and probably invalid) meanings and implications that have attached themselves to the notion of aptitude and by the invalid uses to which aptitude tests have sometimes been put. The implications of these surplus meanings are often articulated in popular discussions, where they have caught the attention and interest of the general public.

Let us leave the social and political issues aside for the time being (however crucial they are in other contexts) and examine here some of the facets of the concept of aptitude that eventually need to be clarified before considering its usefulness in its own right. One of these has to do with its distinctiveness as a construct separate from the construct of achievement. Quite apart from this, but related to it, is the question of whether the measurement of aptitude can be satisfactorily distinguished from the measurement of achievement. A second has to do with the changeability of aptitude and the nature of that changeability, either within the individual or across cohorts of individuals. Finally, a third question concerns the role of the genetic origins of aptitude in the matter of changeability, an issue already alluded to in some detail. Each of these are large subjects, and they deserve much more detailed discussion than can be given to them here. At the same time, it may be useful to examine at least the first two, however briefly.

Before doing so, we should observe again that given the same amount of exposure to education, both inside and outside the classroom, some individuals seem to be able to solve problems; understand the significance of events, facts, and connections; and draw inferences, generalizations, and deductions that others seem unable to do at all, or at least not as readily. It seems to be true that although some individuals can learn the same material as others can, they do so more slowly and with more effort.

There is little question that these observations lend considerable validity to the concept of academic aptitude as a legitimate construct. Yet, there is a great unwillingness to accept it as such. Anastasi (1984), for example, has spoken of some of the distinctions that are made between aptitude and achievement as an "indestructible strawperson," and has said that she would, if she could, excise the word *aptitude* from our vocabulary (1980). This is curious, in a sense. We seem to have no difficulty accepting other aptitudes—such as athletic aptitude, musical aptitude, mechanical aptitude, and artistic and dramatic aptitude—as valid and useful constructs. And just as with academic aptitude, there are vast differences among individuals with respect to rates of learning in these various areas. Yet, although these other aptitudes are generally accepted as valid constructs, somehow the construct of academic aptitude appears to be harder to accept, at least in some quarters.

In an effort to clarify the concept, some attempts have been made to develop what are thought to be clear distinctions between academic aptitude and academic achievement. For example, the College Entrance Examination Board, whose tests since its founding in 1900 had been specifically developed and used only to evaluate the student's acquired knowledge of particular secondary school subjects, introduced the Scholastic Aptitude Test (SAT) in 1926. This test was conceived as a supplement to the existing achievement test battery and was intended to provide a broad measure of the student's general ability to pursue *any* academic program successfully. Similarly, in 1952 the Graduate Record Examinations (GRE) developed a system of aptitude and achievement tests—the former, to measure general academic promise, and the latter, to assess what the students had learned in particular college courses. In recent years, however, in an effort to disclaim what are thought to be some of the "surplus," or unintended and false meanings associated with aptitude, the College Board (e.g., 1981) has included a statement in its bulletin, *Taking the SAT,* to the effect that the SAT is not a test of some "inborn and unchanging" capacity—incidentally, marrying the two unrelated notions, as other writers have done, as though they bore a synonymous, even synergistic, relationship to each other. With similar purpose, the GRE Board took action not long ago to rename its Aptitude Test the GRE General Test.

It is certainly true that the distinctions between aptitude and achievement are often unclear and difficult to make. I would submit, however, that the proposed solution of playing with semantics (as for example, in substituting the term *developed abilities* for *aptitude*) is not at all helpful, for it only serves to blur the distinctions further. The fact is, *both* aptitude and achievement are developed abilities; and so is any other cognitive trait that changes progressively with age. It is often the case that constructs are easily confused with the instruments that are designed to measure them, with the result that we often presume to judge the validity of a construct when in fact we are actually judging the adequacy of the instruments we use to measure it. This, I believe, is the case here. It is certainly true that some tests (e.g., verbal and mathematical tests) can often be classified as either aptitude or achievement. But it is at least equally true that there are a host of other tests—tests of physics, Slavic literature, chemistry, French, and automobile repair, for example—that cannot by any stretch of the imagination be considered aptitude tests. The problem, one suspects, lies in the insufficiency of our conception of aptitude as a general construct and in our construction of measures to fit that conception.

Nevertheless, in spite of these inadequacies in the measures of aptitude, many investigators (e.g., Bereiter, 1974; Carroll, 1974) would argue that the construct of academic aptitude "deserves a conceptual status distinct from achievement," as Bereiter (p. 53) put it, and should not be abandoned simply because of the confusions and tensions that we have experienced in defining it. The same confusions, one might argue, are present in the definitions of other types of aptitudes. It does suggest, however, that we must continue to search for measures that are distinctly different from achievement, items that focus more on process that on content, and items that vary in difficulty and discriminate over a wide range of talent but depend on material learned only at the very elementary levels.

But we do make several distinctions between the concepts and the instruments:

1. Growth in achievement results from more-or-less formal exposure to a particular subject or area of content and is typically quite rapid. Aptitude, on the other hand, grows slowly as a consequence of ordinary living, both outside the formal learning environment as well as inside it, often developing through "undefined and uncontrolled learning" (A. Anastasi, personal communication, September 29, 1987).

2. Aptitude tends to resist short-term efforts to hasten its growth, whereas achievement is much more susceptible to such efforts.

3. It has often been said that scores on achievement tests are to be taken as a measure of the amount learned; aptitude tests are thought to provide a measure (or prediction) of the rate of future learning.

4. Humphreys (1974) has held, as have others, that aptitude and achievement tests differ only in degree and that specific tests of these two concepts fall on a continuum. He has gone on to make essentially the following observations: Aptitude tests draw their items from a wide range of human experience. (Intelligence tests, which are a close relative of aptitude tests, draw their items from an even wider, and often different, range of experiences and include a much wider variety of items than do achievement tests.) When aptitude tests do make use of subject matter learned in formal course work, they typically draw on content learned several years earlier by most individuals, content presumably equally familiar to almost everyone. Achievement test items, on the other hand, are more circumscribed. They are necessarily drawn from the restricted subject matter of a particular course of training, usually a recent one. Correspondingly, aptitudes are generalizable to a wide range of endeavor, whereas the knowledges and skills represented in an achievement test normally apply to a narrower sphere of activity.

5. Inasmuch as achievement tests are based on a relatively narrow domain, known and understood best by those who have been exposed to that domain, they (obviously) cannot be used for evaluating the educational outcomes for individuals who have not been exposed to it. Aptitude tests, however, draw from much wider domains, not confined to the material learned in the classroom, and are presumably within the actual, or accessible, experiences of all individuals. Therefore, unlike achievement tests, aptitude tests can be used to make general intellectual evaluations for all who share a common culture regardless of their particular classroom experiences. On the other hand, because their coverage is not classroom specific, aptitude tests cannot be used, as achievement tests can, to evaluate the quality of particular educational programs.

6. Aptitude is by its nature prospective—indeed, the word aptitude itself has implications for the success of future learning. Thus, scores on an aptitude test are typically used for predicting future success in the general domain of that aptitude. Not only is the sense of aptitude prospective, it sometimes implies that the learner whose aptitude is being evaluated has not yet been exposed to the subject matter to be learned and therefore cannot yet be tested on it. Achievement is by its nature retrospective, which is also implied by the word, and achievement tests are typically used to evaluate the level of accomplishment in prior learning experiences. This is not to say that achievement tests cannot or have not been used to predict future success. They have, and they are very useful for that purpose. Past achievement is always a good predictor of future achievement, often a better predictor than aptitude.

The idea seems to be held that inasmuch as aptitudes as we conceive of them today are (appropriately) thought to be developed abilities, frequently in continuous change, therefore they cannot be innate. That they are developed, and developing, abilities in continuous change, especially during the very early years, cannot be denied; raw scores and some types of scaled scores on aptitude and intelligence tests increase rapidly during that time. Even the claim of IQ constancy is an implicit admission that mental ability changes but that the change is indexed to the change in chronological age. One does not follow from the other, however; change in the level of aptitude is not by itself evidence that it is not genetically determined. There is, we are compelled to admit, and as already discussed, considerable evidence that aptitude, or intelligence, does have a substantial genetic component. There are many characteristics, known to be innate, that are also acknowledged to change within a lifetime, some even with external intervention—for example, stature, hirsuteness, reproductive ability, and most other physical characteristics. The genetic pattern is laid down at the time of conception, but the characteristics themselves change continuously, sometimes not even appearing until later in life, often not until adulthood.

Thus, it appears that the issue for useful consideration is not whether aptitude is innate; indeed, it bears repeating that the issue of innateness is irrelevant in the context of group differences. Nor is the fact of ordinary change (i.e., predictable change associated with change in age) a useful issue in this context. What is at issue is whether there can be differential change across cohorts of individuals and/or differential change in the individual; that is, whether and to what extent differential environmental experiences, including special intervention strategies, can exert a differential impact on scores. Currently, the predominant view is that within the normal range of intelligence, aptitudes are indeed susceptible to differential cognitive training, but that the training must begin very early in life and continue for an extended period through the formative years and beyond, and further, that the cognitive training must be carried out in a continuously supportive and motivating atmosphere.

It has already been pointed out that what makes the concept of aptitude particularly difficult to deal with objectively are some of its implications, as some see them, for the present and future status of minority groups in our society. The thesis here is that there is no justification at all for such implications. In order to understand better the mechanisms that are characteristic of aptitude and what they do imply, other urgent questions have developed— whether, for example, scores on aptitude tests do in fact rise or fall differentially as a function of ordinary intervening experience or of special educational or environmental interventions.

Several different kinds of efforts have been undertaken to study changes in IQ. Of special note are the studies designed to raise the IQs of retarded children. A recently published, highly useful book, authored by Spitz (1986), summarizes the best known of these efforts and comes to the dismal conclusion that they have been uniformly failures—some of them even reporting fraudulently positive results.

But what of changes within the normal range of intelligence? These appear to be more encouraging, especially in those instances in which changes can be effected in the kinds of environmental conditions that, at least in theory, tend to impede the development of intellectual processes. These studies are of two types: those that observe changes in the cohorts and those that observe changes in individuals for whom special educational programs have been developed. Those of the first sort appear to be more numerous.

Tuddenham (1948) reported having administered the Wells Revision (Form 5) of the Army Alpha to a representative sample of 768 White enlisted men of the World War II draft and found that their median performance on the Army Alpha fell at about the 83rd percentile of the corresponding World War I population. He concluded that a large part of the difference between the two populations was attributable to more and better education for the more recent group. In any case, it is noted that this cohort change, which took place over a *single* generation, amounted to very nearly a full standard deviation, a substantial increase by any standard.

A similar investigation was carried out on a more restricted population in Eastern Tennessee by Wheeler (1942). Group IQ tests were administered in 1940 to over 3,200 children in 40 schools. Comparison of these results was made with results obtained with children coming from the same areas and largely from the same families, who had similarly been tested in 1930. During the intervening 10-year period, the social, economic, cultural, and educational conditions in these communities had improved substantially. The mean IQs rose from 82 in 1930 to 93 in 1940, over 88% of a standard deviation, also a major effect.

Lyle Jones (1983) examined Black-White group differences on the verbal sections of the National Assessment of Educational Progress (NAEP) and found that the difference between the groups in percentage correct on the NAEP items generally declined in the 1960s and 1970s. He noted a similar "reduction of the gap" between Black and White groups on the verbal sections of the SAT and the GRE.

Similar findings are observable on the mathematical sections: There is a comparable and consistent decline in the average differences between the two groups at every age. There are also considerably higher levels of performance for Black children born since the middle 1960s than for those born earlier. It is interesting, moreover, that the findings from the SAT, which is administered to a self-selected population, are consistent with those from the National Assessment population, which is a nationally representative sample of the nation's children. It is also interesting that studies of writing, science, and social studies support the studies of reading and mathematics.

Jones and his associates (Burton and Davenport) also found a correlation between the difference in the amount of math taken by Black and White students and the discrepancy in their means, suggesting that school factors associated with the amount of study of math may have a real effect on the math performance of Black students. Jones speculated that these changes are part of a larger change, especially in the Southeastern United States, where Black people previously had little if any opportunity for social, educational, political, or economic contact with the mainstream population. Since then, there have been profound changes in all these areas, which, he suggested, "might be expected to elevate the aspirations of Black youngsters and to provide evidence that school achievement will enhance prospects for career success."

Then what can be said for special studies that were designed to raise IQ? Honzik, Macfarlane, and Allen (1948) studied 222 children over a period of 12 years, from age 6 to age 18. Over this span of years, a large number of the children, about 58%, showed increases of 15 or more IQ points, and 35% showed increases of 20 or more points. In this study (the California Guidance Study), detailed investigations of the home, when the participants had reached the age of 30, revealed that home conditions that were characterized by parental care, affection, and concern with achievement were likely to promote higher levels of ability and achievement in their children. These findings were supported in a follow-up study several years later by Honzik (1967).

These are some of the better known studies of intergenerational and intra-individual change in IQ. True, they are not numerous, in part because intergenerational data are hard to come by and in part because intra-individual studies are so difficult to design and control without losing masses of data.

Although it is quite well understood, it will bear repeating that changes in the individual are much more easily effected if efforts to make them are instituted in early childhood. They are not, however, easily effected if the efforts to make them are delayed until adolescence or later. By way of confirmation of this generalization, I would like to mention a recent study by Angoff and Johnson (in press), in which they collected a sample of almost 23,000 cases of GRE General Test examinees who had also taken the SAT four or five years earlier. Although the principal purpose of the study was to examine the differential impact of curriculum on GRE scores, they also calculated the intercorrelations of all the variables under study. What was interesting was that even though the total sample was a highly self-selected one, consisting only of students applying for graduate study, the correlation of the SAT-verbal with GRE-verbal was as high as .86; the correlation of the SAT-mathematical and GRE-quantitative was equally high—also .86. This is not to say that there are no differences between verbal and quantitative aptitudes, in particular with respect to their susceptibility to curricular effects, but it is also clear that at this stage of life changes in aptitude are not always made very easily.

Nevertheless, aptitude *is* subject to change if the conditions are right—if, as suggested earlier, the cognitive training begins early in life and continues for an extended period through the formative years and beyond, and if it is carried out in a continuously supportive and motivating atmosphere. If there is any hope of closing the Black-White gap, such an effort will have to be buttressed by a broad program of educational, psychological, cultural, and economic types of interventions targeted not only at the child but also at the child's parents, his or her extended family, and indeed, the entire community. The difference we see today between Black and White populations developed after centuries of neglect; it is not likely to be eliminated without an effort of substantial proportions.

REFERENCES

Anastasi, A. (1975). Harassing a dead horse. [Review of *The aptitude-achievement distinction*]. *The Review of Education, I.* 356–362.

Anastasi, A. (1980). Abilities and the measurement of achievement. In W. B. Schrader (Ed.), *New directions for testing and measurement* (pp. 1–10). San Francisco: Jossey-Bass.

Anastasi, A. (1982). *Psychological testing* (5th ed.). New York: Macmillan.

Anastasi, A. (1984). Aptitude and achievement tests: The curious case of the indestructible strawperson. In B. S. Plake (Ed.), *Social and technical issues in testing: Implications for construction and usage* (pp. 129–140). Hillsdale, NJ: Erlbaum.

Angoff, W. H., & Johnson, E. G. (in press). *A study of the differential impact of curriculum on aptitude test scores.* Princeton, NJ: Educational Testing Service.

Bereiter, C. (1970). Genetics and educability: Educational implications of the Jensen debate. In J. Hellmuth (Ed.), *Disadvantaged child: Vol. 3. Compensatory education* (pp. 279–299). New York: Brunner-Mazel.

Bereiter, C. (1974). Comments on Burket's paper: Eliminating an inconsistency in Burket's time-distance model. In D. R. Green (Ed.), *The aptitude-achievement distinction* (pp. 49–53). Monterey, CA: CTB/McGraw-Hill.

Bouchard, T. J., & McGue, M. (1981). Familial studies of intelligence: A review. *Science, 212.* 1055–1059.

Burt, C. (1958). The inheritance of mental ability. *American Psychologist, 13.* 1–15.

Carroll, J. B. (1974). The aptitude-achievement distinction: The case of foreign language aptitude and proficiency. In D. R. Green (Ed.), *The aptitude-achievement distinction* (pp. 286–303). Monterey, CA: CTB/McGraw-Hill.

Carter, C. D., & Marshall, W. A. (1978). The genetics of adult stature. In F. Faulkner & J. M. Tanner (Eds.), *Human growth: Vol. I: Principles of prenatal growth* (pp. 299–305). New York: Plenum Press.

College Board. (1981). *Taking the SAT: A guide to the Scholastic Aptitude Test and Test of Standard Written English.* New York: Author.

Crawford, C. (1979). George Washington, Abraham Lincoln, and Arthur Jensen: Are they comparable? *American Psychologist, 34,* 664–672.

Cronbach, L. J. (1969). Heredity, environment, and educational policy. *Harvard Educational Review, 39,* 338–347.

Crow, J. F. (1969). Genetic theories and influences: Comments on the value of diversity. *Harvard Educational Review, 39,* 301–309.

Damon, A. (1974). Larger body size and earlier menarche: The end may be in sight. *Social Biology, 21.* 8–11.

Erlenmeyer-Kimling, L., & Jarvik, L. F. (1963). Genetics and intelligence: A review. *Science, 142,* 1477–1478.

Falconer, D. S. (1981). *An introduction to quantitative genetics* (2nd ed.). New York: Longman.

Gould, S. J. (1981). *The mismeasure of man.* New York: W. W. Norton.

Greulich, W. W. (1957). A comparison of the physical growth and development of American-born and Japanese children. *American Journal of Physical Anthropology, 15,* 489–515.

Greulich, W. W. (1977). Some secular changes in the growth of American-born and native Japanese children. *American Journal of Physical Anthropology, 45,* 553–568.

Herrnstein, R. J. (1971). IQ. *The Atlantic, 228,* 43–64.

Herrnstein, R. J. (1973). *IQ in the meritocracy.* Boston: Little, Brown.

Honzik, M. P. (1967). Environmental correlates of mental growth: Prediction from the family setting at 21 months. *Child Development, 38,* 337–364.

Honzik, M. P., Macfarlane, J. W., & Allen, L. (1948). The stability of mental test performance between two and eighteen years. *Journal of Experimental Education, 17,* 309–324.

Humphreys, L. G. (1974). The misleading distinction between aptitude and achievement tests. In D. R. Green (Ed.), *The aptitude-achievement distinction* (pp. 262–274). Monterey, CA: CTB/McGraw-Hill.

Jensen, A. R. (1969). How much can we boost IQ and scholastic achievement? *Harvard Educational Review, 39,* 1–123.

Jensen, A. R. (1980). *Bias in mental testing.* New York: Free Press.

Jensen, A. R. (1981). *Straight talk about mental tests.* New York: Free Press.

Jones, L. V. (1983, November). *White-black achievement differences: The narrowing gap.* Invited address presented at the meeting of the Federation of Behavioral, Psychological, and Cognitive Sciences, Washington, DC.

Kamin, L. J. (1974). *The science and politics of IQ.* Potomac, MD: Erlbaum.

Plomin, R. (1983). Developmental behavioral genetics. *Child Development, 54,* 253–259.

Plomin, R. (1986). *Development, genetics, and psychology.* Hillsdale, NJ: Erlbaum.

Roche, A. P. (1979). Secular trends in stature, weight, and maturation. *Monographs of the Society for Research in Child Development, 44,* 3–27.

Rose, S. (1976). Scientific racism and ideology: The IQ racket from Galton to Jensen. In H. Rose & S. Rose (Eds.), *The political economy of science* (pp. 112–141). London: Macmillan Press.

Scarr, S. (1974). Some myths about heritability and IQ. *Nature, 251.* 463–465.

Scarr, S. (1981a). Genetics and the development of intelligence. In S. Scarr (Ed.), *Race, social class, and individual differences in IQ* (pp. 3–59). Hillsdale, NJ: Erlbaum.

Scarr, S. (1981b). Unknowns in the IQ equation. In S. Scarr (Ed.), *Race, social class, and individual differences in IQ* (pp. 61–74). Hillsdale, NJ: Erlbaum.

Scarr, S., & Weinberg, R. A. (1978). The influence of "family background" on intellectual attainment. *American Sociological Review, 43,* 674–692.

Scarr-Salapatek, S. (1971). Unknowns in the IQ Equation. [Review of *Environment, heredity, and intelligence; The IQ Argument;* and *IQ*]. *Science, 174,* 1223–1228.

Schmeck, H. M. (1984, April 10). Treatment is nearing for genetic defects. *New York Times,* p. C1.

Schwartz, M., & Schwartz, J. (1974). Evidence against a genetic component to performance on IQ tests. *Nature, 248,* 84–85.

Spitz, H. (1986). *The raising of intelligence: A selected history of attempts to raise retarded intelligence.* Hillsdale, NJ: Erlbaum.

Stokes, H. S. (1982, October 17). Life and limbs are growing longer in Japan. *New York Times,* p. 16E.

Tanner, J. M. (1962). *Growth at adolescence* (2nd ed.). Oxford: Blackwell Press.

Tanner, J. M. (1970). Physical growth. In P. H. Mussen (Ed.), *Manual of child psychology* (3rd ed., pp. 77–155). New York: Wiley.

Taylor, H. F. (1980). *The IQ Game.* New Brunswick, NJ: Rutgers University Press.

Tuddenham, R. (1948). Soldier intelligence in World Wars I and II. *American Psychologist, 3,* 54–56.

Webber, T. L. (1978). *Deep like the rivers: Education in the slave quarter community, 1831–1865.* New York: W. W. Norton.

Wheeler, L. R. (1942). A comparative study of the intelligence of East Tennessee mountain children. *Journal of Educational Psychology, 33,* 321–344.

4

Annotation:
Sibling Influences on
Childhood Development

Judy Dunn

Pennsylvania State University, University Park

The relationship between young siblings is distinctive in its emotional power and intimacy, its qualities of competitiveness, ambivalence, and of emotional understanding that can be used to provoke or to support. On common sense grounds these qualities, and the high frequency of interaction and imitation between siblings, suggest that the relationship will be of developmental importance—both through the direct impact of siblings upon one another, and through the indirect effects of the siblings' relationships with the parents. On theoretical grounds, the sibling relationship has been stressed as potentially important by psychologists who regard the interaction between children as important (following Piaget, 1965 and Sullivan, 1953), by clinicians (e.g. Adler, 1959; Levy, 1937; Winnicott, 1977), family systems theorists (Minuchin, 1985), and most recently by developmental behavior geneticists (Plomin & Daniels, 1987; Rowe & Plomin, 1981; Scarr & Grajek, 1982). How far and in what ways does systematic research support these hypotheses about sibling influence, and what, in particular are the implications of recent research on siblings for clinicians and those concerned with the care of children?

In the last few years there has been an upsurge of interest in the study of siblings. This interest has been focussed on a number of different but related issues implicating sibling influence: Two of these have clear relevance for cli-

Reprinted with permission from the *Journal of Child Psychology and Psychiatry*, Vol. 29, No. 2, 119–127. Copyright 1988 by the Association for Child Psychology and Psychiatry, Pergamon Journals Ltd.

nicians. The first concerns the individual differences between sibling pairs in the quality of their relationship and the factors that influence these, especially the connections between parent-child and sibling-child relationships. The second concerns the special problems experienced by children with handicapped or disabled siblings. Of the other themes in recent work on siblings, one in particular has made striking contributions to our understanding of normal developmental principles, and will be briefly referred to in this annotation; this is research focussed on the question of why siblings are so different from one another.

Before considering the findings of this research on siblings, one general point should be noted. Rarely can we conclude from the research that there is evidence of sibling influence that is clearly independent of other family factors, since differences in sibling relationships are closely linked to differences in other family relationships, and to the emotional climate of the family (Brody & Stoneman, 1988). The same point is of course equally applicable to discussions of the influence of parental relationships, or of marital relationships upon children; in each case there are close connections between the relationships (Dunn, 1987).

INDIVIDUAL DIFFERENCES IN SIBLING RELATIONSHIPS

Aggression and Conflict

Studies of siblings—whether focussed on infancy, the preschool period, middle childhood or adolescence—report both a marked range of individual differences between sibling pairs in measures of friendliness, conflict, rivalry, and dominance, and that such dimensions are relatively independent of one another (Abramovitch, Pepler & Corter, 1982; Dunn, 1983; Furman & Buhrmeister, 1985). Of most concern to parents and clinicians is the frequent aggression and conflict shown by some siblings (Baskett & Johnson, 1982; Clifford, 1959; Newson & Newson, 1970). Two questions are at issue here. First, does aggression from a sibling influence the behavior and adjustment of the recipient—is the experience of a hostile sibling relationship associated with the development of aggressive or problem behavior? Second, what factors influence the development of such hostile sibling relationships?

Studies of siblings from the second year through middle childhood report correlations between frequent aggressive or hostile behavior of one sibling and that of the other (Beardsall, 1987; Brody, Stoneman & Burke, 1987; Dunn & Munn, 1986a). Moreover, detailed behavioral observations within the family by Patterson and his group (Patterson, 1984, 1986) indicate that siblings do indeed play a shaping role in the development of aggressive behavior in both clinic and normal populations. Patterson's results indicate that coercive behavior by siblings makes a substantial contribution to the development of coercive behavior that is independent of the contribution of parental behavior. Other studies show that siblings not only exert an influence on the frequency of coercive behavior, but also influence the style of conflict behavior. The incidence of teasing, bossing, conciliation, physical aggression, and reasoned argument in conflict by secondborn children was found to be correlated with the behavior of their older siblings at an earlier time point in preschool children (Dunn & Munn, 1986a) and in 6–7-year-olds (Beardsall, 1987).

How far the development of a hostile relationship between siblings is related to other aspects of problem behavior, or disturbed behavior outside the family is an issue on which evidence is at present suggestive rather than definitive. First, there is evidence from Patterson's group that coercive behavior by a sibling towards a target child is systematically linked to the target child having problems with peers outside the family [peer rejection as assessed by parents, peers and teachers (Dishion, 1986)]. Second, epidemiological studies have reported poor relations with siblings to be more common in children with other behavior problems; thus Richman, Stevenson and Graham (1982) reported that poor relationships with siblings at 4 years old were related not only to other problems at the time but also to a clinical rating of disturbance four years later. However, the question of whether the poor sibling relationship plays a formative role in disturbed behavior in other contexts, or whether it is one manifestation of more general disturbance needs more research attention. Similarly, there is evidence for similarities between siblings in truant behavior (Neilson & Gruber, 1979), delinquent behavior (Patterson, 1986; Wadsworth, 1979; West & Farrington, 1973), but not clear evidence that the sibling relationship has causal influence independent of other family factors.

The factors contributing to the development of conflict between siblings are considered below.

Cooperation, friendliness and empathy. The extent to which friendliness, cooperation and affection are shown by siblings appears to be an independent dimension from the dimensions of conflict and rivalry—whether the siblings studied are preschoolers (Abramovitch *et al.*, 1982; Dunn & Munn, 1986b), in early childhood (Dunn, Stocker & Plomin, 1987) or middle childhood (Furman & Buhrmeister, 1985). In early childhood, correlational data shows that friendly, sympathetic and cooperative behavior by older siblings is associated with similar behavior by younger siblings at the time, and 6–12 months later (Dunn & Munn, 1986b). Such correlational data do not establish cause, and it is likely that the behavior of the mother is also implicated in the development of empathic behavior (Radke-Yarrow, Zahn-Waxler & Chapman, 1983). However, it is possible that siblings influence some aspects of prosocial behavior quite independently of their parents: cooperative play and especially cooperative social fantasy play is more commonly shown by children whose older siblings have been very friendly towards them. Mothers very rarely take part in such social pretend play (Dunn & Dale, 1984) and there is no evidence that they influence the development of capabilities of cooperation in play with other children.

Socio-cognitive capabilities. The interaction between children and their peers is thought to be of special significance in the development of social understanding (see for e.g. Damon, 1977; Hartup, 1983; Piaget, 1965; Sullivan, 1953). If this argument has plausibility, then it is likely that siblings are of special significance in these aspects of development, given the intimacy and intensity of the relationship. There is now some evidence that differences in the behavior of older siblings are indeed associated with differences in the socio-cognitive abilities of later-born siblings. In the preschool period the development of teasing, references to social rules, conciliation and early participation in social role play (Dunn & Munn, 1986a,b) and socio-cognitive abilities more formally assessed (Light, 1979) is related to earlier behavior of the older sibling; in middle childhood, associations have been reported between older siblings' behavioral style and 6-year-olds' affective perspective taking and social reasoning abilities (Beardsall, 1987). Again, the direction of causal influence cannot be inferred. Gender role identification has been linked—for later-born siblings—to the presence (and presumably behavior) of older siblings (Sutton-Smith & Rosenberg, 1970).

FACTORS INFLUENCING THE QUALITY OF THE SIBLING RELATIONSHIP

Given the evidence for associations between the quality of sibling relationships and aggressive behavior, rejection by peers, early development of cooperative capabilities in play and aspects of socio-cognitive development, the question of what factors influence individual differences in siblings' behavior to one another assumes some importance. On the development of conflict and aggression between siblings, research within normal families has shown first, that such conflict is very common (Newson & Newson, 1970); second, that family structure variables such as age gap and gender show no consistent relations to sibling conflict (Abramovitch *et al.,* 1982; Dunn & Munn, 1986a; Furman & Buhrmeister, 1985; Stoneman, Brody & McKinnon, 1984); third, that the temperament of the siblings is systematically linked to differences in conflict (Brody *et al.,* 1987; Munn & Dunn, 1988); fourth, that the emotional climate of the family is related to frequency and intensity of conflict between siblings (Brody & Stoneman, 1988).

Fifth, the behavior of parents towards siblings in conflict is related to the frequency of such conflict (Brody & Stoneman, 1987; Brody *et al.*, 1987; Dunn & Munn, 1986a). Two issues need to be considered here. The first concerns parental intervention in conflict. It is frequently maintained that parental intervention increases sibling conflict—on the grounds either that children chiefly quarrel to gain parental attention (Dreikurs, 1964), and/or that parental intervention deprives children of the opportunity to learn how to resolve conflicts. Indeed Schachter and Stone (1987) have argued that if children are deprived of the experience of resolving sibling conflict, this can in certain families lead to serious pathological consequences, with the development of bullying, self-seeking, impulsive and anti-social individuals. However, the direction of effects in the parent intervention/sibling conflict connection is by no means clear. Small-scale intervention studies (Kelly & Main, 1979; Leitenberg, Burchard & Stoneman, 1983) have been interpreted as supporting the argument against parental intervention (Brody & Stoneman, 1988). Of course it is likely that if parents "stay out" of sibling disputes they are less likely to distribute blame and comfort—and thus are less likely to behave differentially towards the children.

This brings us to the second issue—one of real significance: differential behavior shown by parents towards siblings is clearly implicated in conflict frequency. Consistent evidence that differential maternal behavior is related to the quality of the siblings' relationship is reported in every study that has included assessment of maternal behavior to both siblings. Thus an association between differential maternal behavior and negative behavior between the siblings, reported by Bryant and Crockenberg (1980) for sisters between 6 and 9 years, has also been found by Brody and colleagues (Brody *et al.*, 1987), by Stocker, Dunn and Plomin in a study of 160 siblings in early childhood (1987), by Hetherington and her colleagues in siblings studied after divorce (1987), and by McHale and Gamble (1988) for children with disabled siblings (see below), and in studies of siblings of cancer patients (Cairns, Clark, Smith & Lansky, 1979). It appears that for families under stress the link is particularly strong. The significance of parental differential behavior towards siblings is underlined by the finding that emotional adjustment differences in adolescent siblings are associated with perceived differences in parental behavior towards siblings (Daniels, Dunn, Furstenberg & Plomin, 1985).

Less is known about what factors influence the positive aspects of sibling relationships. Correlations have been found between maternal discussion of feelings and needs of one sibling with the other, and later friendly behavior by both siblings (Dunn & Kendrick, 1982); such findings echo the results of

Yarrow and Zahn-Waxler's study showing that altruistic behavior is fostered by maternal child-rearing characterized by discussion of others' feelings (Radke-Yarrow *et al.*, 1983). The evidence for associations between family structure variables (age gap, gender) and friendly cooperative behavior between siblings is not consistent. However it appears that during the first two years of life, second-born children's behavior towards their older siblings is significantly influenced by the first-borns' interest and affection towards them (Dunn & Kendrick, 1982).

The Influence of Disabled and Chronically Sick Siblings

The question of whether the experience of having a disabled or sick sibling influences children's adjustment and development is one of obvious practical and social importance. There is an extensive literature on the development and adjustment of the siblings of handicapped or sick children; for recent reviews of research on siblings of handicapped children see Brody and Stoneman (1983), Lobato (1983), McHale, Simeonsson & Sloan (1984), Rodger (1985); for reviews on siblings of chronically sick children see Drotar and Crawford (1985) and McKeever (1983), Van Dongen-Melman and Sanders-Woudstra (1986); see also a special issue of the *Journal of Children in Contemporary Society,* 1987. The literature on families with handicapped children documents the extent of emotional adjustment in the normal siblings and its relation to socioeconomic factors (Farber, 1959; Gath, 1974; Grossman, 1972), family structure variables such as gender, ordinal position and age gap (Breslau, Wietzman & Messenger, 1981; Cleveland & Miller, 1977; Farber, 1959; Farber & Ryckman, 1965; Gath, 1974; Grossman, 1972), parental attitudes (Caldwell & Guze, 1960; Grossman, 1972), quality of marital and parent-child relationships (Ferrari, 1984; McHale & Gamble, 1988) and extent of handicap (Breslau, Weitzman & Messenger, 1981; Grossman, 1972).

However the issue of how far normal siblings directly influence their disabled or sick siblings, or vice versa, remains unclear from the bulk of this research, for two reasons. First, it is evident that the presence of a disabled or sick child can have a number of complex and different effects on family relationships, and it is likely that any or all of these may contribute to the outcome of normal children within the family. Few of the studies reviewed were designed to assess separately the different contributing effects; research that does—for instance Ferrari (1984)—has shown that the quality of a mother's support system and the marital relationship are importantly related to child outcome. Thus while indirect effects of the presence of a disabled sibling are clear, direct effects are rarely described.

Second, very few of the studies include direct observation or documentation of sibling interaction and its relation to child outcome. The value of those that do is notable: Thus McHale and Gamble's (1988) study of the siblings of disabled children which included detailed telephone interview information about daily interactions provides a test of many of the hypotheses concerning sibling influence in such families. First, it gives support for the view established with interviews (Ferrari, 1984) and retrospective data (Cleveland & Miller, 1977; Farber & Jenne, 1963) that children with disabled siblings are more considerate and kind to their siblings, suggesting a connection with the reported high incidence of altruism, tolerance and humanistic concerns in adults who had grown up with a handicapped sibling (Grossman, 1972). Second, the study showed that while problems in interaction between the siblings was not more frequent than in a normal control group, such interaction was perceived to be more difficult by the siblings of the disabled. Third, the study showed that children's attributions concerning the behavior and problems of the disabled sibling were linked to the children's adjustment, thus paralleling the evidence from children with chronically sick siblings that even with very young children such attributional processes are important (Sourkes, 1987). Fourth, it tests the hypothesis that adjustment problems in the normal siblings are due in part to the increased caring and household responsibilities placed on them [an account offered as interpretation of the origins of the greater vulnerability of girls with disabled siblings to adjustment problems (Cleveland & Miller, 1977; Farber, 1959; Grossman, 1972)]. Documentation of the activities of the children showed that extent of household and child care activities was not associated with psychological adjustment; rather, the behavior of the disabled sibling towards the normal child, and (especially for girls) the relationship with the mother were the important factors. Most importantly, the differential behavior of the mother towards both children was shown to be linked to the adjustment of the normal child.

As several of the reviewers note, there is a clear need for further research that includes direct description of the interaction and relationship of the siblings, that takes account of the connections between family relationships, and that includes consideration of possible beneficial influence—bidirectional—of the siblings upon one another. Rarely have researchers considered the question of whether the interaction between normal and disabled child has positive effects on the latter, yet a parallel could be drawn with the few small-scale studies of siblings trained to be "therapists" of children with behavior problems or disablement; these have shown that normal siblings can indeed have a positive influence on their disabled siblings (Laviguer, 1977; Miller & Cantwell, 1976; Weinrott, 1974).

SUMMARY

To summarize the main points concerning sibling influence:

1. That siblings play a causal role in the development of aggressive behavior, in children's style of conflict behavior and in cooperative fantasy play is strongly suggested by recent research.
2. Marked problems in the sibling relationship are indicative of other problems, but a causal role for siblings is not established, other than for aggressive behavior.
3. Family factors are closely involved in the quality of sibling relationships—and thus in sibling influence, namely differential parental behavior, and the emotional climate of the family. That is, it is important not to consider the sibling relationship in isolation from other family relationships.
4. Studies of families under stress indicate heightened importance of these family factors.
5. It is likely, but not yet established, that later-born siblings are influenced by first-born in socio-cognitive development and gender identity.
6. Finally it should be noted that an important theme in current research on siblings is a concern with the question of why siblings develop to be so different from one another. It has been shown that the major source of environmental influence on the development of individual differences is within-family rather than between-family differences in experience (Plomin & Daniels, 1987). The different experiences each sibling may have within their relationship is one potential source of such differential environmental influence. Thus documenting the influence of siblings upon each other takes on added significance: By clarifying the extent and nature of this influence we will gain not only useful clinical information but illumination on a developmental principle of very general significance.

REFERENCES

Abramovitch, R., Pepler, D. & Corter, C. (1982). Patterns of sibling interaction among preschool-age children. In M. E. Lamb & B. Sutton-Smith (Eds), *Sibling relationships across the life span: Their nature and significance* (pp. 61–86). Hillsdale, NJ: Erlbaum.

Adler, A. (1959). *Understanding human nature.* New York: Premier.

Baskett, L. M. & Johnson, S. M. (1982). The young child's interactions with parents versus siblings: A behavioral analysis. *Child Development, 53*, 643–650.

Beardsall, L. (1987). *Conflict between siblings in middle childhood.* Unpublished Ph.D. dissertation, University of Cambridge.

Breslau, N., Wietzman, M. & Messenger, K. (1981). Psychologic functioning of siblings of disabled children. *Pediatrics, 67,* 344–353.

Brody, G. H. & Stoneman, Z. (1983). Children with atypical siblings. In B. Lahey & A. Kazden, (Eds), *Advances in clinical child psychology* (Vol. 6) (pp. 285–326). New York: Plenum.

Brody, G. H. & Stoneman, Z. (1988). Sibling conflict, individual child characteristics, and family transactions. *Journal of Children in Contemporary Society.*

Brody, G. H., Stoneman, Z. & Burke, M. (1987). Child temperaments, maternal differential behavior, and sibling relationships. *Developmental Psychology, 23,* 354–362.

Bryant, V. B. & Crockenberg, S. (1980). Correlates and dimensions of prosocial behavior: A study of female siblings with their mothers. *Child Development, 51,* 529–544.

Cairns, N., Clark, G., Smith, S. & Lansky, S. (1979). Adaptation of siblings to childhood malignancy. *The Journal of Pediatrics, 95,* 484–487.

Caldwell, B. M. & Guze, G. B. (1960). A study of the adjustment of parents and siblings of institutionalized and noninstitutionalized retarded children. *American Journal of Mental Deficiency, 64,* 849–861.

Cleveland, D. & Miller, N. (1977). Attitudes and life commitment of older siblings of mentally retarded adults: An exploratory study. *Mental Retardation, 3,* 38–41.

Clifford, E. (1959). Discipline in the home: A controlled study of parental practices. *Journal of Genetic Psychology, 95,* 45–82.

Damon, W. (1977). *The social world of the child.* San Francisco: Jossey-Bass.

Daniels, D., Dunn, J., Furstenberg, F. & Plomin, R. (1985). Environmental differences within the family and adjustment differences within pairs of adolescent siblings. *Child Development, 56,* 764–774.

Dishion, T. (1986, November). *Peer rejection.* Seminar to Oregon Learning Centre.

Dreikers, R. (1964). *Children: the challenge.* New York: Hawthorne Books.

Drotar, D. & Crawford, P. (1985). Psychological adaptation of siblings of chronically ill children: Research and practice implications. *Developmental and Behavioral Pediatrics, 6,* 335–362.

Dunn, J. (1983). Sibling relationships in early childhood. *Child Development, 54,* 787–811.

Dunn, J. (1988). Relation among relationships. In S. Duck (Ed.), *Handbook of personal relationships.* New York: Wiley (in press).

Dunn, J. & Dale, N. (1984). I a daddy: 2-year-olds' collaboration in joint pretend with sibling and with mother. In I. Bretherton (Ed.), *Symbolic play: The developing of social understanding* (pp. 131–158). New York: Academic Press.

Dunn, J. & Kendrick, C. (1982). *Siblings: Love, envy, and understanding.* Oxford: Blackwells/Cambridge, MA: Harvard University Press.

Dunn, J. & Munn, P. (1986a). Sibling quarrels and maternal intervention: Individual differences in understanding and aggression. *Journal of Child Psychology and Psychiatry, 27,* 583–595.

Dunn, J. & Munn, P. (1986b). Siblings and the development of prosocial behavior. *International Journal of Behavioral Development, 9,* 265–284.

Dunn, J., Stocker, C. & Plomin, R. (1987). *Assessing sibling relationships in childhood*. Submitted for publication.

Farber, B. (1959). Effects of a severely mentally retarded child on family integration. *Monographs of the Society for Research in Child Development, 21*, (2 Serial No. 75).

Farber, B. & Jenne, W. C. (1963). Family organization and parent-child communication: Parents and siblings of a retarded child. *Monographs of the Society for Research in Child Development, 28*, (7, Serial No. 91).

Farber, B. & Ryckman, D. B. (1965). Effects of severely mentally retarded children on family relationships. *Mental Retardation Abstracts, 2*, 1–17.

Ferrari, M. (1984). Chronic illness: Psychosocial effects on siblings—I. Chronically ill boys. *Journal of Child Psychology and Psychiatry, 25*, 459–476.

Furman, W. & Buhrmeister, D. (1985). Children's perception of the qualities of sibling relationships. *Child Development, 56*, 448–461.

Gath, A. (1974). Sibling reactions to mental handicap: A comparison of the brothers and sisters of mongol children. *Journal of Child Psychology and Psychiatry, 15*, 187–198.

Grossman, F. K. (1972). *Brothers and sisters of retarded children.* Syracuse: Syracuse University Press.

Hartup, W. (1983). Peer relations. In P. Mussen (Ed.) & E. M. Hetherington (Vol. Ed.), *Handbook of child psychology—Vol. IV. Socialization, personality, and social development* (pp. 103–196). New York: Wiley.

Hetherington, E. M. (1987). Parents, children, and siblings six years after divorce. In R. A. Hinde & J. Stevenson-Hinde (Eds), *Relations among relationships*. Oxford: Oxford University Press (in press).

Kelly, F. D. & Main F. O. (1979). Sibling conflict in a single-parent family: An empirical case-study. *American Journal of Family Therapy, 7*, 39–47.

Lavinguer, H. (1977). The use of siblings as an adjunct to the behavioral treatment of children in the home with parents as therapists. *Behavior Therapy, 7*, 602–613.

Leitenberg, H., Burchard, J. D., Burchard, S. N., Fuller, E. J. & Lysaght, V. V. (1977). Using positive reinforcement to suppress behavior: Some experimental comparisons with sibling conflict. *Behavior Therapy, 8*, 168–182.

Levi, A. M., Buskia, M. & Gerzi, S. (1977). Benign neglect: Reducing fights between siblings. *Journal of Individual Psychology, 33*, 240–245.

Levy, D. M. (1937). Studies in sibling rivalry. *American Orthopsychiatric Association Research Monographs, 2*.

Light, P. (1979). *The development of social sensitivity*. Cambridge: Cambridge University Press.

Lobato, D. (1983). Siblings of handicapped children: A review. *Journal of Autism and Developmental Disorders, 13*, 347–364.

Mash, E. J. & Johnson, C. (1983). Sibling interactions of hyperactive and normal children and their relationship to reports of maternal stress and self-esteem. *Journal of Clinical Child Psychology, 12*, 91–99.

McHale, S. & Gamble, W. C. (1988). Sibling relationship and adjustment of children with disabled brothers and sisters. *Journal of Children in Contemporary Society* (in press).

McHale, S., Simeonsson, R. J. & Sloan, J. L. (1984). Children with handicapped brothers and sisters. In E. Schopler & G. B. Mesibov (Eds), *The effects of autism on the family* (pp. 327–342). New York: Plenum.

McKeever, P. (1983). Siblings of chronically ill children: A literature review with implications for research and practice. *American Journal of Orthopsychiatry*, **53**, 209–218.

Miller, N. B. & Cantwell, D. (1976). Siblings as therapists: A behavioral approach. *American Journal of Psychiatry*, **133**, 447–450.

Minuchin, P. (1985). Families and individual development: Provocations from the field of family therapy. *Child Development*, **56**, 289–302.

Munn, P. & Dunn, J. (1988). *Temperament and the developing relationship between siblings*. Submitted for publication.

Neilson, A. & Gruber, D. (1979). Psychosocial aspects of truancy in early adolescence. *Adolescence*, **14**, 312–326.

Newson, J. & Newson, E. (1970). *Four years old in an urban community*. Harmondsworth, U.K.: Penguin Books.

Patterson, G. R. (1984). Siblings: Fellow travellers in coercive family processes. *Advances in the Study of Aggression*, **1**, 173–214.

Patterson, G. R. (1986). The contribution of siblings to training for fighting: A microsocial analysis. In D. Olweus, J. Block & M. Radke-Yarrow (Eds), *Development of antisocial and prosocial behavior: Research, theories and issues* (pp. 235–261). New York: Academic Press.

Piaget, J. (1965). *The moral judgement of the child*. New York: Free Press.

Plomin, R. & Daniels, D. (1987). Why are children within the same family so different from one another? *Brain and Behavioral Sciences*, **10**, 1–16.

Radke-Yarrow, M., Zahn-Waxler & Chapman, M. (1983). Children's prosocial dispositions and behavior. In P. Mussen (Ed.) & E. Hetherington (Vol. Ed.), *Handbook of child psychology. Vol. IV. Socialization, personality and social development* (pp. 469–545). New York: Wiley.

Richman, N., Stevenson, J. & Graham, P. (1982). *Pre-school to school: A behavioral study*. London: Academic Press.

Rodger, S. (1985). Siblings of handicapped children: A population at risk? *The Exceptional Child*, **32**, 47–56.

Rowe, D. C. & Plomin, R. (1981). The importance of non-shared (E_1) environmental influences in behavioral development. *Developmental Psychology*, **17**, 517–531.

Scarr, S. & Grajek, S. (1982). Similarities and differences among siblings. In M. E. Lamb & B. Sutton-Smith (Eds), *Sibling relationships: Their nature and significance across the life span* (pp. 357–381). Hillsdale, NJ: Erlbaum.

Schachter, F. F. & Stone, R. K. (1987). Comparing and contrasting siblings: Defining the self. *Journal of Children in Contemporary Society* (in press).

Sourkes, B. M. (1987). Siblings of the child with a life-threatening illness. *Journal of Children in Contemporary Society* (in press).

Stocker, C., Dunn, J. & Plomin, R. (1987). Maternal differential behavior and the relationship between young siblings (submitted for publication).

Stoneman, Z., Brody, G. H. & McKinnon, C. (1984). Naturalistic observations of children's activities and roles while playing with their siblings and friends. *Child Development*, 55, 617–627.

Sullivan, H. S. (1953). *The interpersonal theory of psychiatry*. New York: Norton.

Sutton-Smith, B. & Rosenberg, B. G. (1970). *The sibling*. New York: Holt, Rinehart, & Winston.

Van Dongen-Melman, J. E. W. M. & Sanders-Woudstra, J. A. R. (1986). Psychosocial aspects of childhood cancer: A review of the literature. *Journal of Child Psychology and Psychiatry,* **27,** 145–180.

Wadsworth, M. E. J. (1979). *Roots of delinquency: Infancy, adolescence, and crime.* Oxford: Robertson.

Weinrott, M. R. A. (1974). A training program in behavior modification for siblings of the retarded. *American Journal of Orthopsychiatry,* **44,** 362–375.

West, D. J. & Farrington, D. P. (1973). *Who becomes delinquent?* London: Heinemann.

Winnicott, D. W. (1977). *The Piggle.* London: Hogarth/Institute of Psychoanalysis.

PART II: DEVELOPMENTAL STUDIES

5

Rapprochement in the Psychic Development of the Toddler: A Transactional Perspective

Thomas M. Horner

University of Michigan, Ann Arbor

The concept of rapprochement, central to separation-individuation theory, is examined and reinterpreted from a transactional perspective. A range of naturally occurring confrontations and conflicts between toddlers and their caregivers is addressed to advance the idea that rapprochement is a continuing rather than phase-specific process of early development.

With the acquisition of upright, free locomotion and with the closely following attainment of that stage of cognitive development that Piaget regards as the beginning of representational intelligence. . . . the human infant has emerged as a separate and autonomous person. These two powerful "organizers" . . . constitute the midwives of psychological birth. In this final stage of the "hatching" process, the toddler reaches the first level of identity—that of being a separate individual entity. (*Mahler, Pine, & Bergman, 1975, p. 77*)

Thus did Mahler introduce the codified form of the rapprochement subphase covering the period of 15 or 16 months to 24 months (*see also Mahler, 1972; Mahler & McDevitt, 1980*). Rapprochement is the culmination of steps taken by the infant from symbiotic union with the mother to an established sense of separateness and personal identity, the apotheosis of which

---

Reprinted with permission from the *American Journal of Orthopsychiatry*, 1988, Vol. 58, No. 1, 4–15. Copyright 1988 by the American Orthopsychiatric Association, Inc.

This paper is a revised version of a paper presented to the American Academy of Child and Adolescent Psychiatry, Los Angeles, 1986.

is the phase of consolidated individuality and emotional object constancy directly following the subphase of rapprochement. It is a period of waning imperviousness to frustration and increased displays of separation anxiety. The key element is the child's acute awareness of separateness, an awareness that is stimulated on the one hand by maturationally-acquired abilities to move away from the mother, and on the other hand by cognitive growth.

Rapprochement connotes a process of detente and reconciliation following a rupture in relations (*Mahler, 1961, p. 413*). The toddler acts according to the aroused senses of separateness and ambivalence that form around the looming poles of autonomy-independence and loss. Because in the previous subphase (Practicing) the infant's need for closeness has been of its own accord "held in abeyance" (*Mahler, Pine, & Bergman, p. 78*), the child's putative increased frequency of approaches to the mother during the Rapprochement subphase, along with greater degrees of clamor in this respect, warrant the term that is assigned to this subphase.

The major affect constellation during rapprochement is depression coupled with anxiety concerning re-engulfment. To be sure, there are pleasures connected to experiences of new things, and elations at independent discoveries and pursuits. But central to the period is the child's acute experience of separateness and what Mahler et al. convey as the correlated loss of omnipotence, and these account for significant portions of the child's vulnerability to depression and anxiety.

> At the very height of mastery, toward the end of the practicing period, it has already begun to dawn on the junior toddler that the world is *not* his oyster, that he must cope with it more or less "on his own," very often as a relatively helpless, small, and separate individual, unable to command relief or assistance merely by feeling the need for it, or even by giving voice to that need.
>
> [While] individuation proceeds very rapidly and the child exercises it to the limit, he also becomes more and more aware of his separateness and employs all kinds of mechanisms in order to resist and undo his actual separateness from the mother. . . . [No] matter how insistently the toddler tries to coerce the mother, she and he can no longer function effectively as a dual unit—that is to say, the child can no longer maintain his delusion of [shared] parental omnipotence, which he still at times expects will restore the symbiotic status quo [ante]. . . . He must gradually and painfully give up the delusion of his own grandeur, often by way of dramatic fights with the mother . . . (*Mahler, Pine, & Bergman, pp. 78–79*).

The painful nature of this process has been repeatedly emphasized. Bergman (*1978*) stated that the toddler in the rapprochement subphase "is repeatedly faced with feelings of helplessness" (*p. 158*). According to Blanck and Blanck (*1979*), the "writers of the Bible put it more poetically—Paradise is Lost" (*p. 8*). According to Mahler and McDevitt (*1980*),

> the three basic fears in early development—the fear of loss of the object, loss of the object's love, and castration anxiety—all come together during this subphase. (*p. 405*).

The child, they assert, is specifically threatened with a collapse of self-esteem (*p. 404*). Accordingly, the child:

> employs all kinds of mechanisms to resist and undo this painful sense of separateness from his mother, while, at the same time, he experiences a great desire to expand his newly developing auton-omy. He is torn between the wish to stay near mother and a com-pulsion to move away from her, between the desire to please her and the anger directed against her, the latter being brought on by the jealousies and possessiveness characteristic of the anal phase, as well as by reactions to the anatomical sexual differences, partic-ularly in the little girl at this age. (*Mahler & McDevitt, 1980, pp. 404–405*).

Mahler (*1961, 1966*) fashioned a whole fabric of loss and grief around this psychological situation.

Two behavior patterns, then, epitomize the rapprochement subphase: shad-owing and darting away. They "indicate both [the child's] wish for reunion with the love object and his fear of re-engulfment by it." (*Mahler, Pine, & Bergman, p. 79*).

At the foundation of the rapprochement concept is the belief that the child's original condition of object-related psychic life is one of symbiotic unity and omnipotence. Following the allegorical prose of Ferenczi (*1913*) and others in the psychoanalytic movement who wrote similarly, Mahler and her followers emphasized the terrible losses bestowed by the rapprochement period. The ma-jor developmental task is "to renounce [sic] symbiotic omnipotence" (*Mahler, Pine, & Bergman, p. 107*).

> This realization [of separateness] greatly challenge[s] the feeling of grandeur and omnipotence of the practicing period, when the little fellow had felt "on top of the world". . . . What a blow to the

hitherto fully-believed omnipotence, what a disturbance to the bliss of dual unity! (*Mahler, Pine, & Bergman, p. 90*).

The acuteness and magnitude of the polarity of separateness and union account for what Mahler termed the *rapprochement crisis.* Much of the theoretical connection between rapprochement and later clinical phenomena rests with reconstructions of early childhood events and conditions that have been made from adult forms of psychopathology, particularly their intrapsychic concomitants (*Hartcollis, 1977; Lax, Bach, & Burland, 1980; Masterson, 1982*). Disagreement exists within the psychoanalytic community over the degree to which direct translations between early experiences, or experiential paradigms, and present personality organization can be made (*Etchagoyen, 1982; Schafer, 1982; Segal, 1982; Solnit, 1982*).[1] Following Spence (*1982, 1986*), I believe that while reconstructions may serve the therapeutic aim of developing thematic continuities between hypothetical early object relations paradigms and experiences on the one hand, and current adjustment patterns and problems on the other, from the standpoint of the scientific standards needed for establishing *actual* continuities, reconstruction is simply unsound.

From a number of vantage points, including those of observable infant social interactive behavior, epistemology, and logic, the attributions of symbiosis and omnipotence as cardinal features of infant psychic life have been effectively dismissed (*Hamilton, 1982; Klein, 1981; Peterfreund, 1978; Stern, 1985*). Against prevalent positions anchored in both the child and adult psychoanalytic literature, and citing relevant empirical studies, I recently emphasized what I believe the psychic life of the infant to be (*Horner, 1985*), summarized as follows:

1. The original psychic condition of life is one of sensory, perceptual, and cognitive distinctions, thereby making a theory of naturally-occurring symbiotic fusion (which is, epistemologically considered, not the same as nondifferentiation) unserviceable if not untenable.

2. The objective position of the infant is one of competence to engage the world both socially and instrumentally with regard to the inanimate object world. Its subjective position is one of experiencing the pleasures of mastery and the frustrations of impediments imposed by the physical and social worlds

---

[1]While few doubt that global and perhaps even some specific continuities exist between early and later development periods (*Emde & Harmon, 1984; Rutter, 1984; Hinde, 1982*), except for various thematic and formal resemblances which risk false or moot inferences about continuities (*Spence, 1982*) they are extremely elusive. Certainly, as Kagan (*1984a, 1984b*) has pointed out, there are strong culturally-anchored philosophical biases toward seeking and finding continuities. Perhaps, as Kagan suggests, the emergence of self awareness (which is not the same as the loss of a symbiotic condition) in the second year allows for continuities to become more apparent. (*Brim & Kagan, 1980*).

of experience. Although feelings of consummation, triumph, elation, and exaltation are within the range of pleasures that can be objectifiably discerned in infants, it is theoretically unserviceable and untenable to ascribe to the infant a basic subjective position of omnipotence.

3. Clinical reconstructions, no matter how thematically persuasive, are methodologically inferior means of ascertaining either the action or validity of specific dynamics in earlier periods of development. It was once appropriate to comment that, because of its lack of language, the psychic life of the infant was inaccessible except by the indirect method of reconstruction. But with the powerful observational and measurement paradigms that have been developed in the past two decades this assertion must be greatly altered, if not rejected.

TRANSACTIONAL FACTORS

Naturally Occurring Conflicts

From its extrauterine outset, human life is characterized by a dialectic of tensions and congruencies within relationships. This dialectic is based on instinctual and acquired needs, as well as on collective patterns of interpersonal exchange. Freud saw this dialectic in terms of the individual *vs* culture/civilization. He centered neurosis, as well as development in general, on the internalized version of this basic condition of conflict. Trivers (*1974*) has discussed the dialectic from a sociobiological perspective, citing natural processes of competition and conflict in parent-offspring relations. He wrote that offspring are "psychological manipulators," that is, they possess capacities actively to affect parental behavioral states that are in direct and biologically determined conflict with them. Although Trivers's discussion is constructed along the lines of dynamically operating predispositions in primates, particularly at the point of weaning, it applies to the human condition quite as well. The conflicting nature of parent and infant interests inevitably permeates the lifespan of each, rendering no unique status in this respect to the period of so-called rapprochement.

The affectional and competence moorings of successful and self-fulfilled development are rooted (but not guaranteed) in positive attachment relationships established with caregivers early in life (*Bowlby, 1969*). Although many positive affects occur within such a context, love and the basic sense of security that devolves from emotionally available caregivers play key organizing roles in the formation and deepening of positive relationships. They are the basis of the individual's being able to withstand the naturally occurring doses of frustration that arise in the course of everyday life, and they are the basis of a condition of solidified attachment that psychoanalysis has long defined as object constancy—that is, loyalty to the love object despite that person's frustrating properties (*Fraiberg, 1969*).

The parent also establishes a condition of constancy toward the infant, who is an object of love, and, as such, is also a natural source of periodic frustration that is withstood by the parent through the operation of that very same condition of love-anchored loyalty.

Love, the center of the early caregiving relationship, is thus a two-way process and has regulating and security-engendering functions with respect to each partner's capacity to frustrate the other. For the parent, love is the wellspring of authentic soothing, the mainstay of authentic forbearance, and the foundation-piece of authentic, confident expectation that life's impasses can be overcome. For the infant it is the crucible of self-engendered positive impacts on the caregiving environment.

Equipped with cognitive-memory acquisitions (*Kagan, 1984a, 1984b*), the toddler gives ground much less readily than heretofore to parent-induced distractions and is thus an increasingly formidable adversary in situations of conflict. As a result, conflicts are likely to be more intense, protracted, and requiring of parent compromise than during the first year of the child's life. The social context in which a conflict arises plays a significant role in its course and outcome. Who, for example, has not observed a toddler achieve victory over a forbidding parent in the market check-out line only because of the latter's wish not to create a public scene? Who, also, has not observed a toddler vanquished in the same context by a mother who was not inhibited by the idea of public display of her control. Finally, who has not observed the tactics of older toddlers who have discerned that some settings (*e.g.,* grandparents' homes) are naturals for pushing some issues beyond the limits that have been otherwise established?

Whereas infant care entails a series of parental compromises from the outset, toddlerhood ushers in new levels of compromise. In the first year of the child's life, parents compromise for the infant's well-being in view of the child's dependent status and lack of significant comprehension of interpersonal situations. With the onset of toddlerhood there occurs a shift in the parents' perception of the child's capacities and dispositions for intentional behavior. Parents now experience (with justification, it seems, when developmental research is brought to bear) the child as more calculating in its self-assertions than before. Among other things, the most important of which is continuation of mutual love and attachment, the toddler and parents assert their respective and sometimes conflicting aims. On the parents' side this typically entails socialization agendae and establishment of authority; on the child's side the agenda is likely to be more concrete and immediate to the conflict at hand. The process of achieving developmental compromise, then, requires an understanding, accommodating adult and a temperamentally compliant child whose capacities for control and resilience (*Block & Block, 1980; Waters & Sroufe, 1983*) are developing in pace with parental expectations and tolerance levels.

Given the putative dynamics of its symbiotic pre-stages, rapprochement is a logical term to characterize the period in which the child makes its first significant departures from symbiotic ties with the mother. Rapprochement connotes reconciliation after a rupture. It therefore takes into account the tensions that naturally exist between caregiver and child. But its assignment to a specific developmental period (in which the tensions are connected specifically to the simultaneous needs to dissolve and recapture the symbiotic union, and to avoid the loss of the individuated self) must be justified by appropriate subjective factors within the child. Moreover, rapprochement connotes a more critical period for this process than is warranted, for it implies that there have never been such conflicts before and that, barring arrest or fixation, they will never occur in quite the same way again. To be sure, in Mahlerian terms the critical aspect of the rapprochement period is vitally connected to the child's specific self-representational status, but with that status now revised (*Horner, 1985; Stern, 1985*) the concept of it as critical—that is, phase-specific—is dismissed.

Certainly there are losses in the toddler's life—the toddler reported by one parent, for example, to be sad because she could no longer put on panties she had outgrown; or the young toddler from whom the breast or bottle is now withheld. Certainly, also, there are individuating landmarks. But the central organizing feature of this developmental period is not the loss of symbiotic union and the correlated fear of self- and autonomy-destroying reattainment *per se,* but the dynamic of individually distributed and separately felt interests and needs for the child and caregiver that are in varying states of conflict and resolution. Each member of the caregiving dyad is both subject and object of the aforesaid dialectic virtually from the full-term newborn period. (The achievement of infant-maternal rapport following the early period of homeostatic regulation, which both Sander [*1975*] and Greenspan [*1981*] have recognized as part of an original transactional condition of infancy, could with equal logic be termed a period of rapprochement—and often is when the period has been stormy, *e.g.,* characterized by colic.) This is why Stern's (*1984, 1985*) concept of early affect attunement is so important. It allows two subjectivities to remain a part of our thinking, not only about disturbances and their etiological and transactional course, but also about normal patterns of development and adjustment.

The Infant's Perspective

From a point in time that is much closer to full-term birth than traditionally estimated by psychoanalytic theorists, infants make sensory, perceptual, and cognitive distinctions. These warrant the assumption of an abiding condition of subjectivity around which maturationally or experientially derived expansions in mental capacity are unified, and in regard to which experiences of nonsubjective events are processed as such (*Stern, 1985*). Two corollaries to this are that *1*) from the outset of full-term extrauterine life there is an active, engaging nature in humans which operates according to a unifying capacity; and *2*) there are tensions elemental to being human (one of the most significant of which is being someone else's experience) which can impair or grossly affect the course and eventual security of the unifying capacity. In this respect, the basic principle governing the positive social behavior of individuals in each other's company is the maintenance of a sense of well-being derived from the experiences, security, and control of conditions and events in which one is ensconced.

The infant's principal subjective experience of the other, particularly the parent, is as mediator or, as Spitz conceived it, auxiliary ego. Unfortunately, too much has been made of this role as an actual part (hence symbiotically organized) of the infant's ego-self. Not enough emphasis has been placed on its auxiliary nature: from the very young infant's standpoint others are externally located and perceived sources of help. The still-face studies of Tronick, Als and Adamson (*1979*) as well as our own maternal distraction studies (*Horner & Carlson, 1985*) demonstrate how much, even at very young ages (3–4 months), infants try to overcome barriers to interaction imposed by the mother. Field's (*1977*) studies of same-aged infants' responses to patterns of maternal intrusion bear similar testament to behavioral controls (gaze aversion) exerted by infants to withstand that intrusion.

The subjective experience of the infant, then, is one built of direct and self-induced contacts and resistances around interpersonal events. As such, the experience entails distinctions, not mergings (*Horner, 1985; Stern, 1985*).

The Caregiver's Perspective

With regard to the alleged omnipotence felt by the infant in the Symbiotic and Practicing subphases of separation-individuation development, four sources of ascription are stimulated in adults by infants that are in their day-to-day care (*Horner, 1985, pp. 338–339*): *1*) Infants' failures, indisposition, or inabilities to follow the organized routines expected or demanded by the adult. *2*) Infants' nondeliberate capacities to thwart the intents and efforts of the adult through their egocentrically-governed persistences and insistencies. *3*) Adults' (particularly single caregivers') vulnerabilities to feeling enslaved by the involvement demands of the infant. *4*) Adults' inclinations to exalt or idealize the condition of infancy, which may be compensatory or part of an existential or spiritual contemplation of mortality. These forces continue to operate throughout toddlerhood. The second and third enumerated sources are salient in this regard because frustration of parental aims can now be deliberate as well as incidental, and because the toddlers' new horizons, which expand their range of demands, heighten the vulnerable parent's potential for feeling enslaved. These new horizons are opened on the one hand by basic maturational changes that adduce widening competence, and on the other hand by socialization pressures exerted by adults. The first have a great deal to do with inducing (through signals of readiness) the latter, and include abilities to walk and climb, to use words to communicate, and to use affects instrumentally toward desired ends. The latter cluster around parental emphases on cooperative, obedient, and increasingly extended interactions with others, including agemates.

COMPETENCE AND SOCIALIZATION

With the toddler's acquisitions of self-locomotion, verbal and intentional affect communication, and organized sustained social interactions with agemates, the adult's view of the child's status vis-a-vis others undergoes a powerful transition. This transition sees the gradual rise of parental expectations or demands, resting on two assumptions: that the toddler has a rudimentary capacity to comply; and that the child possesses a unified self-construct that is increasingly accessible verbally and in quasi-logical terms. These in turn foster new levels of expectation by the parent, especially with respect to behavioral self-regulation.

Walking and Climbing

In elaborating separation-individuation theory, Mahler made special mention of the impact of maturation on the separation-individuation process. The impact of walking, for example, she held to be the extension of the range of infant activity, bringing with it new domains to conquer. "The world is the toddler's oyster" became a catch-phrase used to describe that expansion. The onset of rapprochement behavior was viewed largely as a response to the increased sense of separateness induced by the toddler's extended geographical forays. But the parental side of this separation experience has frequently been overlooked, even though it is a ubiquitous part of the developmental landscape.

The onset of walking delights parents, too; they spend a lot of time inducing this milestone, and the excitement of first steps, as many a home movie proves, is keen and mutual. But self-locomotion has other important results besides the impact of the specific sense of separateness it engenders. Walking and climbing increase the risk of injury to the child, thus heightening the parent's vigilance and precautionary (sometimes prohibitive) stance toward exploration. Walking and climbing also increase the chances of the child's getting into things that are forbidden but which have little to do with personal safety—valuables that might be broken or other people's possessions.

The toddlers' ability to walk, coupled with increasing weight and size, stimulates adults to carry them less; this, in turn, stimulates many toddlers to cling. The regulation of physical contact between parents and young children has no precise course. Yet clinging is one form of contact maintenance that parents may actively resist for a variety of reasons, including the fostering of independence and the onset of sheer fatigue.

Toddlers sometimes cling in this period because of increasing external demands, sometimes against their inclinations, on their powers of locomotion. Some may come to resent their otherwise joyfully consummated walking skill if these demands exceed their capacity or their tolerance. There is little change in the child from previous phases in use of clinging to maintain contact. But maturation induces and expands opportunities and motives to use it as a way of altering the adult's behavior. In other words, to employ the ethological framework cited above (*Trivers, 1974*), the child's possibly coercive clinging is stimulated, not by an intrinsic sense of separateness (coming out of symbiosis), but by the extrinsic push toward self-reliant behavior. It has little or nothing to do with who is who (the individuation model) but very much to do with who does, or insists on, what. Persistent clinging by the toddler can therefore be experienced as tyrannical by the parent.

Walking and climbing can thus result in greater parental frustration and prohibition. If heavily taxed, parents may become hostile, introducing the problem of parental aggression in both direct and indirect forms.[2]

---

[2]Mahler drew attention to the darting behavior enabled by the toddler's walking and running, and found it significant of ambivalent wishes to flee the mother's engulfing potential and to be swept up by her. The descriptions she and her followers have made of this common "game" in toddlerhood imply that it arises as the toddler's *own* solution to the felt ambivalence. Setting aside the natural pleasure the game frequently affords toddlers and their parents, one wonders, in those cases where it has become compulsive, how much has been determined by the putative fusion-separateness dilemma and how much by a pre-established pattern of infant-parent interchange where parental aggression—direct or indirect—is a key factor in its genesis. Moreover, how much does the game derive from the familiar mother-led one of "Gonna getchu [get you]!" frequently instigated in the first year of the child's life?

Self-locomotion spawns widened geographical reaches which may in turn precipitate separation anxiety. They also elicit parental forms of behavior which, protective as they may be from the parent's perspective, are either prohibitive or fearsome from the child's perspective. As climbing is added to the behavioral repertoire, parental remonstration may increase in order to protect either the child or property, purposes which are beyond the child's understanding. The child's increasing capacity to remember locations of desired hidden objects compounds this situation, particularly since it may increase the toddler's demands. Hidden or out-of-reach objects include not only "things put away for now" (food, items that can only be used at special times, etc.) and dangerous or valuable items, but also those private things that the parent simply does not want the child to know about or use. Until consistent parameters are defined and enforced (whether benignly or aggressively) the toddler may continue to be insistent and therefore thwarted. Toddlers whine and coerce, then, largely as a function of parents' refusals and prohibitions.

Verbal Communication

Like walking, the period in which talking arises is special to both child and parent. The child's abilities to express and comprehend verbally portend a simpler future for matters of communication, particularly in the area of behavioral control. The self-control merits attention here, not so much from the standpoint of the child's actual capacity to exert it, but from the standpoint of the adult's expectation that the child is now (or is fast becoming) able to comply with verbal commands. How much simpler for the parent to be able to say "Stop that!" or "Don't do that!" than to have to use physical coercion. The onset of the infant's verbal capacities, then, can cause premature expectations of compliance based on verbal commands alone. Thus, the toddler is again in a precarious position vis-a-vis parental aggression.

Affect as Communication

When can the individual feign an affect state (or at least exaggerate an authentic affect state) for ulterior purposes? Are all attributions made by parents about their toddlers' manipulative abilities false? If not, how does one tell the difference? There is evidence that intentional communications by infants toward parents arise during the last quarter of the first year (*Dore, 1983; Golnikoff, 1983a,b; Greenfield, 1980*) and that intentional (*i.e.*, goal-directed) behavior of a social nature occurs as early as three months (*Horner, 1985; Horner & Carlson, 1985*). By toddlerhood there is a demonstrated capacity to manipulate communications to overcome passive or active resistance to a social intent (*Golnikoff, 1983a, 1983b; Greenfield, 1980*).

Klinnert, Sorce, Emde, Sternberg, and Gaensbauer (*1984*) adduced significant convergent data from two surveys (one cross-sectional, one longitudinal) of mothers' perceptions of their infants' affect expression patterns over the first 18 months of life. At about nine months of age, a quarter of the mothers began to see their infants' expressions of anger as containing elements of willful aggression. Between 12 and 18 months, most mothers described what Klinnert et al. termed a *surge of aggressiveness* in their children. Coordinately, the mothers reported behavior in themselves that paralleled that of the infant:

> when the infant's expressions of anger changed so did the mother's behavior. Across all the ages, the primary cause which mothers reported for anger was frustration of wants or needs. Therefore, when infants cried angrily at three months of age, mothers' most frequently reported response was a sense of urgency to alleviate the cause or, if it could not be alleviated, to comfort the infants. But by the time infants had reached 12 months of age, the mothers' responses had shifted. Instead of hurrying to remove the frustration or meet the need, mothers reported that they most frequently distracted, ignored, or disciplined the infants. (*Klinnert et al., 1984, pp. 348–349*).

The authors then speculated:

> Presumably, the infants began to see their mothers as the source of frustration, while the mothers began to experience the infants as obstructive. Also of great import was the infants' increased capacity for goal-directed behavior, which allowed them to show their anger in a manner that was previously not possible. . . . [In] the anger system the babies' new instrumental skills put them into conflict with an environment that was heretofore primarily nurturant. By nature, the instrumental or intentional behaviors that characterize anger are aggressive acts, and as the aggression began to show itself, mothers initiated a deliberate socialization process by attempting to decrease or eliminate such emerging intentional behaviors. . . . *The nurtured partner suddenly turns the previously unfocused anger on the heretofore primarily nurturing partner, eliciting either patient restraint or outright anger! (Klinnert et al., 1984, p. 349, emphasis added).*

The authors supposed that the described process was connected to the infant's increased feelings of separateness (*p. 352*). As much to the point, however, is the child's increasing sense of not prevailing in conflicts with the parent (perhaps conflicts previously settled in the child's favor), a sense that is likely to augment any level of preexisting ambivalence.

Observations and reports such as those by Klinnert et al. validate many parents' assertions that their toddlers attempt to manipulate them with affect states; and, indeed, the parent is likely to feel less able to manipulate the infant's affect states without resistance. Persistent children will make the adult feel pressed hard to yield and, thus, thwarted.

Consider whining, the vocal counterpart, and sometimes accompaniment, of clinging. It is a vocal signal of discomfort, often over an unfulfilled want; it is an insistent, often angry, demand. It is inevitable in the course of normal toddlerhood and, even without an operational definition, every parent and experienced child watcher recognizes it when it occurs. Whining is obviously used instrumentally by the older child to achieve desired ends, which include fulfillment of the original want or a palliative. Located on the continuum of fussiness, whining has its developmental onset at just about the time that parents alter their responses to the angry or otherwise insistent demands made by the toddler at points of conflict. Those temper tantrums that do not belong to any predisposing condition of temperament probably originate then as well.

Social Interest and Skills

Finally, the infant's expanding repertoire of social interests and skills, enhanced on the one hand by opportunities introduced by parents for contacts with agemates in various preschool and play-group settings, and on the other hand by the toddler's rapidly increasing competence to carry out cooperative interchanges with peers (*Eckerman & Stein, 1982; Ross, Lollis, & Elliott, 1982*), opens up additional forces which gently but decisively dilute the toddler's direct involvements with the parent. Parents begin to present to the child (and gradually to enforce) paradigms of cooperation and altruism. These may coincide with or contradict the desired dynamics of other parents in the vicinity.

The self-directed activities and socially motivated pursuits of the toddler offer the parent tempting and enlarged respites from the ebb and flow of demands made by the toddler throughout the day, and from day to day. Satisfied with the personal opportunities afforded by such respites, the mother teeters at times on a fulcrum of divided interests and motives whose affective dynamics cannot be entirely missed by the increasingly affect-sensitive and social-referencing toddler (*Clyman, Emde, Kempe, & Harmon, 1986; Klinnert, Campos, Sorce, Emde, & Svejda, 1983*).

REFOCUSING THE ISSUE

Rapprochement as a specific sequela of symbiosis conveys a misleading sense of toddlers' actual experiences of their caregiving worlds. Lacking a specifically transactional focus, the concept omits important factors operating within the adult that affect infants and toddlers.

The utility of the rapprochement concept as a metaphor for describing and framing the specific conflicts, defensive maneuvers, and characterological dynamics of older children and adults is widely acknowledged. Rapprochement can be regarded as a useful fiction for establishing clinical-empathic links with personalities that have made alternating states of object closeness (usually hostile dependence) and distance (usually hostile rejection) their principal method of adjustment to the world of other people, or whose capacities for maintaining continuity of relationship are impaired.

In rejecting the theory of infantile symbiosis and omnipotence as a general framework for considering developmental phenomena, one need not abandon the possibility that transient subjective states that entail feeling merged with the other (quasi-symbiosis), feeling alone (loss of partner's investment), or feeling elated over mastery (quasi-omnipotence) are indeed within the range of affective capacities of infants and toddlers (*Pine, 1985, 1986*). Thus, the search for significant factors, perhaps even some that are etiologically central in severe personality disturbance, need not be shunted entirely away from the developmental period to which rapprochement refers. Nor is there any need to dismiss attempts to discover meanings in the ubiquitous behavior of toddlers: they *do* cling, they *do* coerce, they *do* oscillate between independence and dependence in ways often tyrannical to adults, their actions *do* frequently so exceed their comprehension as to seem motivated by a sense of omnipotence or magic, they *do* exalt themselves at moments of personal triumph and mastery, and they *do* protest and grieve their losses.

Transactional (or organizational) models have been used increasingly to conceptualize both the complexities of organism-milieu dynamics (*Sameroff & Chandler, 1975*) and the intricacies of interpersonal dynamics (*Cicchetti & Aber, 1986; Emde, Harmon, & Good, 1986; Sander, 1975; Sroufe & Walters, 1977*). It does not take sophisticated experimental paradigms to demonstrate the dynamics described in this presentation. Visits to public settings containing infants and toddlers, and unobtrusive observations of infants and parents in more intimate circumstances, generally provide ample opportunities to observe them.

Positive attachment relationships possess unique, intrinsically organized means to avoid many conflicts and to restore basic states of love and security when unavoidable conflicts arise. Withal, resistance and occasional hostility toward each other are natural features in the relationship of toddler and parent. Viewed from this standpoint, rapprochement is not a process of dealing with lost symbiotic bliss but a process of restoring positive equilibrium following perturbations in the relationship—a process of re-attaining basic love and security when frustrations and resistance, with their correlated affects, have been effectively dealt with. It is a process, then, that applies to infancy, toddlerhood, and all the stages of development thereafter.

REFERENCES

Bergman, A. (1978) From mother to the world outside: The use of space during the separation-individuation phase. In S. A. Grolnick, L. Barkin, & W. Muensterberger (Eds.), *Between fantasy and reality: Transitional objects and phenomena.* New York: Aronson.

Blanck, G., & Blanck, R. (1979). *Ego psychology II: Psychoanalytic developmental psychology.* New York: Columbia University Press.

Block, J., & Block, J. (1980). The role of ego-control and ego-resiliency in the organization of behavior. In W. A. Collins (Ed.), Development of cognition, affect, and social relations. *Minnesota Symposia on Child Development* (Vol 13, pp. 39–101). Hillsdale, NJ: Erlbaum.

Bowlby, J. (1969). *Attachment and loss: Vol 1. Attachment.* New York: Basic Books.

Brim, O. G., & Kagan, J. (1980). Constancy and change: A view of the issues. In O. G. Brim, & J. Kagan (Eds.), *Constancy and change in human development* (pp. 1–26). Cambridge, MA: Harvard University Press.

Cicchetti, D., & Aber, J. L. (1986). Early precursors of later depression: An organizational perspective. In I. P. Lipsitt, & C. Rovee-Colher (Eds.), *Advances in infancy research* (Vol 4, pp. 88–137). Norwood, NJ: Ablex.

Clyman, R. B., Emde, R. N., Kempe, J., & Harmon, R. J. (1986). Social referencing and social looking among twelve-month-old infants. In T. B. Brazelton, & M. W. Yogman (Eds.), *Affective development in infancy* (pp. 75–94). Norwood, NJ: Ablex.

Dore, J. (1983). Feeling, form, and intention in the baby's transition to language. In R. M. Golnikoff (Ed.), *The transition from pre-linguistic to linguistic communication* (pp. 167–190). Hillsdale, NJ: Erlbaum.

Eckerman, C. O., & Stein, M. R. (1982). The toddler's emerging interactive skills. In K. H. Rubin, & H. S. Ross (Eds.), *Peer relationships and social skills in childhood* (pp. 41–72). New York: Springer-Verlag.

Emde, R. N., & Harmon, R. J. (1984). Entering a new era in the search for developmental continuities. In R. N. Emde, & R. J. Harmon (Eds.), *Continuities and discontinuities in development* (pp. 1–11). New York: Plenum.

Emde, R. N., Harmon, R. J., & Good, W. (1986). Depressive feelings in children. In M. Rutter, C. E. Izard, & P. B. Read (Eds.), *Depression in young people: Developmental and clinical perspectives* (pp. 135–162). New York: Guilford.

Etchagoyen, R. H. (1982). The relevance of the "here and now" transference interpretation to the reconstruction of early psychic development. *International Journal of Psychoanalysis, 63,* 65–76.

Ferenczi, S. (1913). Stages in the development of the sense of reality. In *Selected papers of Sandor Ferenczi* (Vol 1). New York: Basic Books.

Field, T. M. (1977). Effects of early separation, interactive deficits and experimental manipulations on infant-mother face-to-face interaction. *Child Development, 48,* 763–771.

Fraiberg, S. (1969). Libidinal object constancy and mental representation. *Psychoanalytic Study of the Child, 24,* 9–47.

Golnikoff, R. M. (1983a). Infant social cognition: Self, people, and objects. In L. Liben (Ed.), *Piaget and the foundations of knowledge.* Hillsdale, NJ: Erlbaum.

Golnikoff, R. M. (1983b). Preverbal negotiation of failed messages: Insights into the transition period. In R. M. Golnikoff (Ed.), *The transition from prelinguistic to linguistic communication* (pp. 57–78). Hillsdale, NJ: Erlbaum.

Greenfield, P. M. (1980). Towards an operational analysis of intentionality: The use of discourse in early child language. In D. Olson (Ed.), *The social foundations of language and thought* (pp. 254–279). New York: Norton.

Greenspan, S. I. (1981). *Psychopathology and adaptation in infancy and early childhood.* New York: International Universities Press.

Hamilton, V. (1982). *Narcissus and Oedipus: The children of psychoanalysis.* Boston: Routledge and Kegan.

Hartcollis, P. (Ed.) (1977). *Borderline personality disorders.* New York: International Universities Press.

Hinde, R. A. (1982). *Ethology.* London: Fontana.

Horner, T. M. (1985). The psychic life of the infant: Review and critique of the psychoanalytic concepts of symbiosis and infantile omnipotence. *American Journal of Orthopsychiatry, 55,* 324–344.

Horner, T. M., & Carlson, G. (1985, October). *Social interactive initiatives in 12- and 18-week-old infants: Intrinsically motivated systems for maintaining affective involvement with caregivers.* Paper presented at the meeting of the American Academy of Child and Adolescent Psychiatry, San Antonio, TX.

Kagan, J. (1984a). Continuity and change in the opening years of life. In R. N. Emde, & R. J. Harmon (Eds.), *Continuities and discontinuities in development* (pp. 15–39). New York: Plenum.

Kagan, J. (1984b). *The nature of the child.* New York: Basic Books.

Klein, M. (1981). On Mahler's autistic and symbiotic phases: An exposition and evaluation. *Psychoanalysis and Contemporary Thought, 4,* 64–105.

Klinnen, M. D., Campos, J. J., Sorce, J. F., Emde, R. N., & Svejda, M. (1983). Emotions as behavior regulators: Social referencing in infancy. In R. Plutchik & H. Kellerman (Eds.), *Emotion: Theory, research, and development, Vol 2: Emotions in early development.* New York: Academic Press.

Klinnert, M. D., Sorce, J. F., Emde, R. N., Sternberg, C., & Gaensbauer, T. (1984). Continuities and change in early emotional life: Maternal perceptions of surprise, fear, and anger. In R. N. Emde, & R. J. Harmon (Eds.), *Continuities and discontinuities in development* (pp. 339–354). New York: Plenum.

Lax, R. F., Bach, S., & Burland, J. A. (1980). *Rapprochement: The critical subphase of separation-individuation.* New York: Aronson.

Mahler, M. S. (1961). On sadness and grief in infancy and childhood: Loss and restoration of the symbiotic love object. *Psychoanalytic Study of the Child, 16,* 332–351.

Mahler, M. S. (1972). Rapprochement subphase of the separation-individuation process. *Psychoanalytic Quarterly, 41,* 487–506.

Mahler, M. S., & McDevitt, J. B. (1980). The separation-individuation process and identity formation. In S. I. Greenspan, & G. H. Pollock (Eds.), *The course of life: Psychoanalytic contributions toward understanding personality development, Vol. I: Infancy and early childhood* (pp. 395–406). Washington, DC: U.S. Dept. of Health and Human Services.

Mahler, M. S., Pine, F., & Bergman, A. (1975). *The psychological birth of the human infant.* New York: Basic Books.

Masterson, M. F. (1981). *The narcissistic and borderline disorders.* New York: Brunner/Mazel.

Peterfreund, E. (1978). Some critical comments on psychoanalytic conceptualization of infancy. *International Journal of Psychoanalysis, 59,* 427–441.

Pine, F. (1985). *Developmental theory and clinical process.* New Haven: Yale University Press.

Pine, F. (1986). On symbiosis and infantile omnipotence [Letter to the Editor]. *American Journal of Orthopsychiatry, 56,* 166–167.

Ross, H. S., Lollis, S. P., & Elliott, C. (1982). Toddler-peer communication. In K. H. Rubin, & H. S. Ross (Eds.), *Peer relationships and social skills in childhood* (pp. 73–98). New York: Springer-Verlag.

Rutter, M. (1984). Continuities and discontinuities in socioemotional development: Empirical and conceptual perspectives. In R. N. Emde, & R. J. Harmon (Eds.), *Continuities and discontinuities in development* (pp. 41–68). New York: Plenum.

Sameroff, A. J., & Chandler, M. (1975). Reproductive risk and the continuum of caretaking casualty. In F. Horowitz (Ed.), *Review of child development research* (Vol 4, pp. 187–244). Chicago: University of Chicago Press.

Sander, L. (1975). Infant and caregiving environment. In E. J. Anthony (Ed.), *Explorations in child psychiatry.* New York: Plenum.

Schafer, R. (1982). The relevance of the "here and now" transference interpretation to the reconstruction of early psychic development. *International Journal of Psychoanalysis, 63,* 77–82.

Segal, H. (1982). Early psychic development as reflected in the psychoanalytic process: Steps in integration. *International Journal of Psychoanalysis, 63,* 15–22.

Solnit, A. (1982). Early psychic development as reflected in the psychoanalytic process. *International Journal of Psychoanalysis, 63,* 23–38.

Spence, D. P. (1982). *Narrative truth and historical truth.* New York: Norton.

Spence, D. P. (1986). When interpretation masquerades as explanation. *Journal of the American Psychoanalytic Association, 34,* 3–22.

Sroufe, L. A., & Walters, E. (1977). Attachment as an organizational construct. *Child Development, 55,* 17–29.

Stern, D. N. (1984). Affect attunement. In J. D. Call, E. Galenson, & R. L. Tyson (Eds.), *Frontiers of infant psychiatry* (Vol 2, pp. 3–14). New York: Basic Books.

Stern, D. N. (1985). *The interpersonal world of the infant.* New York: Basic Books.

Trivers, R. L. (1974). Parent-offspring conflict. *American Zoologist, 14,* 249–264.

Tronick, E., Als, H., & Adamson, L. (1979). Structure of early face-to-face communicative interactions. In M. Bullows (Ed.), *Before speech* (pp. 349–374). New York: Cambridge University Press.

Waters, E., & Sroufe, L. A. (1983). A developmental perspective on competence. *Developmental Review, 3,* 79–97.

6

The Development of Volitional Behavior in the Toddler Years

Merry Bullock and Paul Lütkenhaus
Max Planck Institut für psychologische Forschung,
München, West Germany

In order to generate a description of early volitional skills, tod-dlers' abilities to match their activities to externally defined task standards and to monitor and control activities with respect to out-comes were studied. Children between 15 and 35 months were ob-served as they engaged in a series of play and clean-up tasks. The results showed that there is a consistent developmental pattern in the extent to which children focus on producing outcomes (rather than on acting for its own sake), the extent to which they monitor, correct, and control activities, and the frequency with which they react to their outcomes with positive affect. These patterns are in-terpreted in terms of changes in the representation of actions, self-regulation abilities, and the active involvement of the self in actions.

Much of human activity is volitional: one acts in order to achieve a partic-ular outcome or goal. Although intentional behaviors most likely begin in early infancy, successful attainment of outcomes becomes more likely as the child develops the skills to regulate behavior with respect to intended goals. This article is concerned with toddlers' intentional actions in a laboratory set-ting where they were requested to produce outcomes across several tasks. We were interested in the extent to which children directed and monitored their own goal-directed behavior.

Reprinted with permission from *Child Development*, 1988, Vol. 59, 664–674. Copyright 1988 by the Society for Research in Child Development, Inc.

The authors gratefully thank Heinz Heckhausen, who commented on earlier phases of this work, Irmgard Hagen, who served as experimenter, Angelika Fritz, who helped with the data scoring, and the parents and children who participated. Some of these data were presented at the biennial meetings of the Society for Research in Child Development, Baltimore, 1987.

Conceptually, one may distinguish different abilities necessary for attaining intended outcomes or goals. First, the actor must be able to anticipate a not yet attained goal state and must understand that this goal can be reached through some specific activity. Second, the actor must represent the means-end relation between activities and their outcomes. For many actions, the representation of the goal state will also include a criterion (or standard) defining an appropriate end state that can be used to compare the momentary and anticipated outcomes. We consider the ability to represent actions in terms of standards and means-and-ends as a necessary but general prerequisite to attaining intended goals.

Beyond such representational abilities, however, additional skills, that we will label volitional skills, are necessary for translating knowledge into successful action. Generally, volitional skills involve remaining task oriented, that is, keeping the anticipated goal in mind, and monitoring progress toward an anticipated goal state. This includes waiting or searching for appropriate opportunities to act, resisting distractions, overcoming obstacles, correcting actions, and stopping acting when a goal is reached. Although general representational and memory abilities are necessary prerequisites for these activities, it is their active use within the context of goal-directed actions that is our focus.

The toddler years appear to be an important transition period in the development of the components of volitional competence. Although one can infer the beginnings of volitional behavior, including a rudimentary focus on producing effects in infants from such everyday activities as sucking (e.g., Bruner & Bruner, 1968), secondary circular reactions (Piaget, 1954), or contingency learning (e.g., Rovee-Collier & Gekoski, 1979; Watson, 1972), these activities are relatively limited in their complexity and sequence. In contrast, during the second year of life, children's understanding of events and actions becomes more differentiated: they are able to recall past experiences (Ashmead & Perlmutter, 1980; Daehler & Greco, 1985), to represent and recall the sequences of common events (Mandler, 1983; O'Connell & Gerard, 1985), to imitate novel events at a later time (Piaget, 1954), and to react to some activities in terms of standards of performance (Gopnik & Meltzoff, 1984; Kagan, 1981). The presence of such capacities suggests that the general representational and memory abilities necessary for successfully attaining less proximal intended goals are available. Further, children in the second year begin to act more systematically in problem-solving tasks (e.g., DeLoache, Sugarman, & Brown, 1985; Spungen & Goodman, 1983) and begin to meet the compliance requests of others (e.g., Golden, Montare, & Bridger, 1977; Kopp, 1982; Vaughn, Kopp, & Krakow, 1984), suggesting that some degree of control and monitoring is available.

In addition to the above skills, the nature of a child's intentional actions may be affected by the child's changing concept of the self, and by motivational changes in the importance of self-produced outcomes. Part of the definition of volitional action is that attainment of a goal is perceived to be the result of one's own activity. This implies that the actor at least implicitly represents the self as an active agent. In terms of developmental changes in volitional competence, the extent to which the child actively regulates his or her own behavior may require an active concept of agency.

It is not known when active awareness of agency emerges, although research on self-recognition and on the conditions that activate self-assertion and self-related emotions suggests that this awareness is available by the third year. Certainly, by the end of the second year, most children show evidence of explicit self-recognition (see Bertenthal & Fischer, 1978; Brooks-Gunn & Lewis, 1984; Levine, 1983), and in the third year they begin to refer to themselves as agents of action in everyday speech (Geppert & Küster, 1983; Huttenlocher, Smiley, & Charney, 1983; Lütkenhaus, 1984). More indirect evidence for the emergence of an active "self-as-originator" (Heckhausen, 1981) comes from observations that during the second year children begin to demand to perform activities independently (Geppert & Küster, 1983; Heckhausen, 1984) and increasingly derive pleasure from producing outcomes rather than from simply engaging in attractive activities (Hetzer, 1931). In addition, the emergence of resistance to compliance (e.g., Wenar, 1982) and emotional reactions to success and failure (e.g., Geppert & Gartmann, 1983; Heckhausen & Roelofsen, 1962; Lütkenhaus, Grossmann, & Grossmann, 1985) suggest that outcomes are increasingly perceived as relevant to one's sense of agency.

Although the relation between different aspects of volitional competence in toddlers has received some theoretical attention (e.g., Kagan, 1981; Kopp, 1982; Wenar, 1976), for the most part they have been investigated separately, either in the context of cognitive development (e.g., DeLoache et al., 1985) or of self-control (e.g., Golden et al., 1977; Vaughn et al., 1984), or of self-recognition (e.g., Brooks-Gunn & Lewis, 1984). The purpose of this study was to gather information about the interrelations among different aspects of volitional competence. We were particularly interested in asking whether and when toddlers are focused on the outcomes of their activities, rather than on the activities themselves; in when they begin to monitor their ongoing activities with respect to an anticipated outcome; in when they begin to focus on meeting specific, external task standards; and in whether an orientation toward outcomes is reflected in affective, self-related responses. Studying the interrelations among knowledge, control, and self-related components of intentional actions may allow a better description of how volitional competence changes over development: increased representational and regulatory skills may allow the child to monitor and control activities in order to achieve intended outcomes and to compare achieved outcomes to "standards" of performance, as defined by social others or as inherent in the task itself. A growing awareness that one is the originator of one's actions and a growing sense of pleasure derived from mastering outcomes (see White, 1959) may alter the motivational basis of volitional activities and provide the child with the impetus and opportunities to develop and practice volitional skills.

To elicit intentional actions in a laboratory situation, we presented two block-building tasks and one clean-up task to 15- to 35-month-old children. We chose activities that would be well within the manual capacity of this age range according to norms from infant tests (e.g., stacking blocks, filling a container, wiping with a sponge) and that would be engaging enough to capture the children's interest. For each task, a specific outcome was requested. To make some amount of control necessary, we constructed the tasks so that it would be easy for children to become involved in the activity itself and hence distracted from producing the outcome. Performance across the three tasks was used to make a general assessment of children's attention to producing outcomes, of their attention to matching specific task standards, and of one aspect of action control, stopping when an outcome was reached. One of the block-building tasks was analyzed in detail to assess other aspects of volitional competence, including monitoring and affective responses to producing an outcome.

METHOD

Subjects

A total of 82 children, 40 boys and 42 girls between the ages of 15 and 35 months, participated. The children were divided into four age groups: 15–18 months ($N = 22$, $M = 17$ months), 19–22 months ($N = 21$, $M = 20$ months), 23–28 months ($N = 20$, $M = 26$ months), and 29–35 months ($N = 19$, $M = 32$ months), with approximately equal numbers of boys and girls in each group. An additional eight children, equally distributed across age groups, were excluded from the sample because of technical errors, or because of missing data on one or more of the tasks. The sample, recruited by contacting parents through birth announcements listed in the local newspaper and through toddler play groups, represented a mixed but predominantly middle-class group. All children were tested with a parent or caretaker present.

Tasks

Tower building. The task consisted of constructing a figure (e.g., a house) from three blocks. The figure was separated into three clear components (e.g., a door, a window, a roof) each painted on separate blocks, and each block had the same part painted on four of its sides. There were five trials, each with a different three-block figure (tree, giraffe, stick figure, house, and girl) presented in the same order. To begin each trial, the experimenter showed the child a colored cardboard box that had a picture on it illustrating the figure the blocks inside would make when stacked into a tower. The experimenter labeled the picture, then opened the box and took out the blocks one at a time. As she did so, she named each block (e.g., "door," "window," "roof"), slowly stacked them, and pointed out that the tower made a figure ("Now it is finished. There is a house."). She then said to the child, "You build that, too," and laid the figure blocks on the table next to three unpainted extra blocks. The extra blocks served as distractors, and enabled us to assess whether the child would restrict the tower to the relevant figure blocks, or would incorporate the unpainted blocks into the tower, either haphazardly (ignoring the standard of building a figure) or after the figure blocks were stacked together (not stopping when the outcome was reached). Prior to the figure-building trials, children were given one warm-up trial with three unpainted blocks to be sure they understood and could produce the expected activity (e.g., stacking blocks into a tower).[1]

Blackboard cleaning. The experimenter showed the child a blackboard with chalk scribbling on the right third of its surface, provided a small bowl containing a sponge and water, and, pointing to the board generally, said "the blackboard is dirty—you make it clean." Earlier in the procedure the experimenter had demonstrated cleaning the blackboard with the same sponge and water. In this task, the activities of wetting and wringing out the sponge and wiping the board were sufficiently attractive in themselves to serve as distractors.

Figure dressing. Children were shown a wooden figure (e.g., a clown) whose body comprised a box, filled with four square blocks, painted red, yellow, green, and blue. The experimenter explained that the figure was dressed with the blocks to keep him warm. She then turned the figure over, dumping the blocks on the table, and said to the child, "Dress him so that he is not cold." The inside of the box was painted with four color patches that matched the colors of the blocks and could serve as implicit guides for where the blocks should go. There were two trials, each with a different figure. On the first trial, only four blocks were available to fill the figure. On the second trial, the experimenter put four extra blocks, painted the same colors as the first four, on

[1]A thoughtful reviewer noted that the warm-up trial might have biased children to think that they needed to use the unpainted blocks in some way. To ask whether this was so, in a subsequent study the experimenter explicitly said that the unpainted blocks were not necessary for building as she built a demonstration tower for each trial. We found that this extra cue made no difference in the quality of children's control.

the table with the set of blocks available for filling the figure. These extra blocks served as distractor material and allowed us to assess whether the child stopped the activity when the figure was filled.

Measures and Scoring

Standards and stopping. Each child's performance on each task was coded into one of five categories, reflecting differences in attention to standards and control over stopping. For the Tower task, this was the highest category shown on at least two of the five trials, and for the Blackboard and Figure tasks it was derived from the overall performance. The categories were as follows:

Category 1: No attention to standards. This included unsystematic manipulation of the materials (e.g., blocks banged together, playing with the sponge in the water) or haphazard products (towers in which the painted and unpainted blocks were mixed together; failing to fill the clown figure without a prompt; random swiping at the blackboard).

Category 2: Attention to a rudimentary (but not correct) standard and no evidence for stopping. The activities were task oriented, but the outcome was not correct, and extra materials were used. On the Tower task, the rudimentary standard was building with three painted blocks together; for the Figure task, it was filling the clown with at least four blocks on the first trial; for the Blackboard task, it was directing more attention to the dirty than the clean part of the blackboard, measured in terms of the frequency and order of swipes.

Category 3: Attention to a rudimentary (but not correct) standard and stopping. The rudimentary standards were as described for Category 2. In the Tower task, stopping was coded when the child built with just three painted blocks (or made separate towers of painted and unpainted blocks); in the Figure task, stopping was coded when the child used just four blocks to fill the clown figure on the second trial; and in the Blackboard task, stopping was coded when the child spontaneously stopped wiping the board (otherwise the experimenter later intervened to stop the trial).

Category 4: Correct outcome and no evidence for stopping. The outcome produced was correct, but the child continued the activity after it was attained. The correct outcome for the Tower task was to stack the painted blocks in the correct order; for the Figure task, to place the blocks in the same color sequence as that painted inside the figure; and for the Blackboard task, to clean all the chalk marks off the board.

Category 5: Correct outcome and stopping. The child produced the outcome precisely as demonstrated/requested by the experimenter.

Estimates of scoring reliability for these and subsequent measures were computed by comparing the ratings from a second coder who was blind to any hypotheses. Reliability was computed for at least 25% of the sample (range, 25%–100%). There was 99% agreement for the Tower task (kappa = .98), 89% for the Blackboard task (kappa = .83), and 91% for the Figure task (kappa = .88). Disagreements for these and subsequent measures were resolved by discussion and review of the videotaped records.

Monitoring. Performance on the Tower task was used to assess three measures of task monitoring, each of which pertained to the child's active, ongoing regulation of activity during building. Two of the measures concerned how the towers were built: (*a*) Single Block Care was scored when the child attended to or corrected the alignment between at least two blocks in a tower on at least one trial (91% agreement, kappa = .82); (*b*) Tower Care was scored when the child carefully stacked all the blocks in a tower on at least one trial (91% agreement, kappa = .82); the third measure, (*c*) Corrections concerned what was built, and were scored when the child made any of the following corrections: took an unpainted block out of the tower, began to add an unpainted block and then refrained from doing so, corrected the orientation of a painted block, or corrected the order of the painted blocks (97% agreement, kappa = .95).

Affect measure. Facial and postural gestures during the Tower task were used to provide an assessment of whether children showed a specific emotional reaction at the end of their building activity (an ''outcome reaction''). To do this, we first coded any ''clear affective response specific to building'' on the basis of a global judgment for each trial. We chose to use a global judgment as the basis for the ratings because preliminary work, in which we coded facial expressions (e.g., smile, frown) and postural gestures (e.g., hands in the air, quick straightening of the body, slumping, etc.) independently, did not seem to adequately specify the children's emotional reactions. We then noted when such reactions occurred: to the experimenter's building, during, or at the end of the child's activity. We scored those reactions that occurred at the end of building activity as ''outcome reactions.'' The prototypical outcome reaction consisted of a smile and an abrupt movement of the arms and hands, made just as a tower was completed. However, a smile was not always necessary, and postural gestures might be quite minimal. We should note that although we intended to include both positive and negative outcome reactions (analogous to ''success'' and ''failure'' reactions) as variables, we did not observe any clear negative reactions to building in this age group. Agreement for the outcome reaction scores was 85% (kappa = .71).

Procedure

Overall, we attempted to create a ''natural'' order of events that would maximize the child's interest and understanding of the tasks. After a warm-up period, during which the child and experimenter looked through a picture-book or played with a stacking game, the Tower, Blackboard, and Figure tasks were presented in the same order to all children. These tasks were part of a longer procedure that included other measures pertaining to self-recognition reported elsewhere (see Bullock & Lütkenhaus, in preparation). The entire procedure took about half an hour (it ranged from 20 to 60 min) and was videotaped for later transcription and analysis.

RESULTS

The performance on each of the three tasks for each age group is presented in Table 1. The top half shows the percentage of children who fell into each of the five performance categories. From these data, we looked at three summary variables: outcome-oriented behavior (at least Level 2 performance), correct outcomes according to the externally defined task standard (Levels 4 and 5), and stopping (Levels 3 and 5). For each measure, we performed a repeated-measures analysis of variance with age and sex as between- and task as within-subjects factors. These were followed up with Tukey post hoc tests (alpha levels were set at $p < .05$) to assess particular group differences. Because there were neither main effects nor interactions due to sex, this variable will not be discussed further.

Outcome-oriented behavior. The frequency of outcome-oriented behavior increased with age, $F(3,78) = 23.7$, $p < .01$, and varied across tasks, $F(2,156) = 10.2$, $p < .01$. The 26- and 32-month groups did not differ and

TABLE 1

PERCENTAGE OF CHILDREN IN EACH PERFORMANCE CATEGORY ON THE TOWER BUILDING (T), FIGURE DRESSING (F), AND BLACKBOARD (B) TASKS

	AGE GROUP											
	17 Months (N = 22)			20 Months (N = 21)			26 Months (N = 20)			32 Months (N = 19)		
	T	F	B	T	F	B	T	F	B	T	F	B
Performance category:												
1. No standard	41	50	86	33	29	62	...	15	25	...	5	...
2. Simple standard, no stop	14	41	14	29	62	14	30	35	...	11	11	5
3. Simple standard, stop	41	9	...	38	10	10	60	30	10	42	32	...
4. Correct, no stop	...	...	...	...	...	10	...	5	20	...	16	26
5. Correct, stop	5	...	...	...	...	5	10	15	45	47	37	68
Summary variables:												
Outcome orientation	59	50	14	67	71	38	100	85	75	100	95	100
Correct outcome	5	...	...	...	...	14	10	20	65	47	53	95
Stopping	45	9	...	38	10	14	70	45	55	90	68	68

Table 1. Percentage of Children in Each Performance Category on the Tower Building (T), Figure Dressing (F), and Blackboard (B) Tasks

were outcome-directed in nearly all of the tasks (M = 2.6, SD = .6 and M = 2.9, SD = .2 across the three tasks for the two groups, respectively). The 20-month group showed less frequent outcome-oriented behavior (M = 1.8, SD = .8), as did the 17-month group (M = 1.2, SD = .97). Overall, children were more likely to be outcome oriented on the Tower (80%) and Figure (74%) tasks than on the Blackboard task (55%).

Correct outcomes. The frequency of correct outcomes, that is, success in matching a particular, externally defined task standard, also showed age, $F(3,78)$ = 47.7, $p < .01$, and task, $F(2,156)$ = 20.3, $p < .01$, differences. The 32-month group was correct on the majority of the tasks (M = 1.9, SD = .7) significantly more than the 26-month group (M = .95, SD = .8) or the younger groups, who produced virtually no correct outcomes. Attention to the precise task standard was more likely on the Blackboard task (41% of the children produced correct outcomes) than on the Tower (15%) or Figure (17%) tasks.

Stopping. Stopping the activity when an outcome was reached showed similar main effects as the other measures. Stopping was age, $F(3,78)$ = 24.1, $p < .01$, and task, $F(2,156)$ = 12.3, $p < .01$, related. The oldest group stopped on more tasks (M = 2.3, SD = .7) than all other groups, and the 26-month group stopped more frequently (M = 1.7, SD = .9) than the two younger groups (M = .6, SD = .8 and M = .5, SD = .6, respectively). The pattern of task differences showed that the Tower task was the easiest, with 60% of the children stopping, compared with 32% and 33% on the Figure and Blackboard tasks. In addition, stopping was more frequent when children produced correct outcomes (75%) than when they attended to a more simple standard (50%), $\chi^2(2,N$ = 172) = 9.1, $p < .01$.

Monitoring measures. In Table 2 we list the percentage of children who showed Single Block Care, Tower Care, and Corrections at least once during the Tower task trials. There were age differences for all three measures,

TABLE 2

PERCENTAGE OF CHILDREN IN EACH AGE GROUP WHO SHOWED EACH OF THREE
MONITORING BEHAVIORS DURING THE TOWER TASK

	AGE GROUP			
	17 Months (N = 22)	20 Months (N = 21)	26 Months (N = 20)	32 Months (N = 19)
Single Block Care	45	71	95	100
Tower Care	9	29	85	95
Corrections	5	14	40	58

Table 2. Percentage of Children in Each Age Group Who Showed Each of Three Monitoring Behaviors During the Tower Task

$F(3,78) = 16.1, p < .01$, for Single Block Care, $F(3,78) = 29.4, p < .001$, for Tower Care, and $F(3,78) = 7.2, p < .001$, for Corrections. Although some of the children in the two younger age groups did monitor their activities, this tended to be restricted to the manipulation of single blocks, not to the tower as a unit. In contrast, virtually all the children in the two older age groups monitored their towers as a whole (e.g., their towers were carefully stacked). Corrections, which we considered to reflect monitoring the outcome rather than the activity, were infrequent overall and restricted primarily to the two older age groups.

Not surprisingly, monitoring was related to the outcome produced. A trial × trial comparison of towers at Level 2 (rudimentary standard, no stopping), Level 3 (rudimentary standard and stopping), and Levels 4 and 5 (correct towers) showed that Tower Care increased with tower level, $F(2,273) = 5.32, p < .01$ (43%, 56%, and 75% careful building, respectively) as did Corrections, $F(2,273) = 11.02, p < .01$ (2%, 12%, and 32% corrections, respectively).

Affective reactions to an outcome. Fifty-six children (68% of the sample) showed an affective reaction at least once during the Tower task. Of these, 49 reacted only to their own building, four to both their own and the experimenter's building, and three to the experimenter's tower only, a reliable difference, $\chi^2(1,N = 56) = 24.64, p < .01$. The specificity of the reaction was somewhat related to age: of the seven children who showed a reaction to at least one of the experimenter's demonstration towers, four were in the 17-month group (and three of the four showed no reaction to their own building). Affective reactions specific to outcomes were also age related. The percentage of children in the four age groups whose affective reactions were produced at the end of their own building activity on at least one trial was 36, 62, 75, and 90, a reliable age difference, $F(3,78) = 6.7, p < .01$. The increase in outcome reactions over age and the restriction of this reaction to the child's own building suggest that it is reasonable to take outcome reactions as a measure of involvement of the self in activities, the expression of which becomes more coherent and more specific with age.

In addition to age differences, we were interested in the extent to which an affectively positive reaction reflects some sort of evaluation of one's own outcome or effort (e.g., a "success" reaction). We accordingly asked whether the outcome reactions of individual children were associated with building trials where they were relatively more successful or where they expended relatively more effort. In order to tap goal-directed effort as broadly as possible, we derived a composite "product orientation" score for each trial. This measure was computed by giving the child 1 point each for outcome-oriented behavior, stopping, tower care, and corrections, producing a score that could vary from 0 to 4 for each trial. We then performed a repeated-measures analysis of variance on the mean product orientation scores for trials with an outcome reaction (reaction trials) and trials where there was no outcome reaction (no-reaction trials). For this analysis, we retained all children who showed an outcome reaction to their own towers at least once, with two exceptions: one child who showed an outcome reaction on every trial, and one who showed an outcome reaction on one trial but then simply manipulated the blocks on the other trials. The analysis showed that performance on reaction trials (M = 2.2, SD = .99) was reliably higher than on no-reaction trials (M = 1.9, SD = 1.2), $F(1,50)$ = 6.16, $p < .02$. This difference was repeated at each age level, although significant only for the youngest group. The means for reaction and no-reaction trials were 1.9 and .96 for the 17-month group, 1.44 and 1.03 for the 20-month group, 2.35 and 2.05 for the 26-month group, and 2.78 and 2.72 for the 32-month group. These data show that, independent of overall building level (which increased predictably across the age groups), an outcome reaction was more likely when a child built a better tower.

DISCUSSION

Overall, the data concerning toddler's actions showed a consistent pattern. We will first discuss each of our several measures and then turn to the implications of these data for characterizing the growth of volitional skills.

Task standards were generally not incorporated into the younger children's actions. Although children in the 17-month group did perform the activity appropriate to the requested outcome (e.g., washing, building), this activity was outcome-directed for fewer than half the children. The 20-month group was more outcome-directed, although the outcomes they produced tended to be those afforded by the materials, not the task instructions. Attention to producing a specific outcome, one defined by an external standard, was first evident in the 26-month group, but consistent across tasks only in the 32-month group. These data on children's performance may be compared with reports from others who have, directly or indirectly, looked at children's understanding of standards. Kagan (1981), for example, reported that children as young as 19 months noted when toys seemed to violate normative standards (the toys were flawed or dirty), and also that 19–20-month-olds evaluated their own abilities to meet a standard of performance set in an experimental task. Similarly, Gopnik and Meltzoff (1984) reported that 14-month-olds noted a failure to achieve a particular task outcome. Our results suggest a more differentiated account of what it means to "understand" standards. Although children focused on producing outcomes by 20 months, consistent with Kagan's findings, this represents only the most rudimentary appreciation of task standards. A more stringent criterion for understanding, defined in our study as producing correct outcomes, was evident only in the two older age groups. Although it is possible that our sample would have demonstrated earlier understanding of standards with different or easier tasks, we believe that the age differences across the studies reflect an important distinction between passively recognizing a standard and actively incorporating that knowledge into one's ongoing behavior. In our tasks, demonstrating an understanding of standards required that the child not only recognize the standard (all that was required in Kagan's or Gopnik & Meltzoff's studies), but also use this knowledge within an activity. In this sense, the measure of understanding we have used is not "pure" but is interwoven somewhat with the ability to regulate actions with respect to task knowledge. It is most likely that children can recognize whether standards are obtained or not well before they can act to achieve them. And, indeed, several younger children seemed to recognize a standard (e.g., on the Tower task, they labeled the parts of the figure; on the clown task they named the colors) even when their product did not achieve it.[2] The effects of recognizing a standard that one cannot successfully produce are not known. Kagan (1981) suggests that this discrepancy leads to distress in 20-month-olds, because children in his studies refused to imitate a series of symbolic acts, or became distressed when asked to do so. We did not observe any such distress.

The data on stopping indicate that control over beginning and ending an action is not guaranteed by task understanding. For example, the Tower and Figure tasks both consisted of building with blocks and were equivalent with respect to attending to task standards. Stopping on the Figure task, though, was more difficult than on the Tower task. In this task, it was as though the demands offered by a container, even an already filled one, were such that the children found it very difficult to leave the extra blocks out. Indeed, many children filled the figure, but then found themselves with one of the extra blocks in their hands, took out a block already in the figure, and replaced it with the one in their hand. This, of course, did not solve the problem, because there was still a block in the hand. The typical solution was to continue taking

---

[2]In an attempt to separate the ability to recognize a standard and the ability to incorporate a standard into one's activity, we looked at two additional sources of information. In a subsequent study, also using a tower-building task, we included a task to see whether children could discriminate correctly and incorrectly built towers. We found that most of the 24-month-olds and a majority of 18-month-olds who built incorrect towers could nevertheless discriminate correctly and incorrectly built figures. Our second source of information came from an informal test of four 17-month-olds in which we asked whether they had the understanding necessary for producing correct outcomes in the Figure and Tower tasks. Specifically, we asked whether they could match the colored blocks used in the Figure task with their respective colors, and whether they could match the painted blocks used in the Tower task with their respective figures. All of the children passed our criterion for matching figures, and half passed the criterion for color matching, suggesting that a younger child who is outcome-oriented could, in principle, produce a correct outcome.

out and putting in blocks until the experimenter intervened to end the trial. Similar perseverance was noted for the Blackboard task, but for different reasons. Here it was the activity itself that was appealing, and many of the children seemed to lose sight of the goal of cleaning the chalk marks in the press of wiping the board. We would argue that toddlers' control problems are not simply a reflection of lack of knowledge about the task goals, although of course knowledge of what to do is a necessary ingredient. Rather, the problem lies in avoiding distractions from materials or activities that press for their own expression. When children failed to stop, it tended to be because they fell prey to the press of the activity or materials. These observations and the corresponding age trends are consistent with other reports of children's spontaneous completion of everyday clean-up activities (e.g., Rheingold, 1982), as well as control in laboratory situations, such as control over delay (e.g., Golden et al., 1977; Vaughn et al., 1984).

Action control requires an ability to monitor activities with respect to an anticipated outcome as well as stopping. Our observations on the frequency and type of monitoring in the Tower task suggest that at first such control begins to be exercised with respect to *how* an activity is performed (Single Block and Tower Care), and then, as standards become more explicitly defined, with respect to *what* is produced (Corrections). It is as though the unit of action changes from one of separate, isolated activities to one in which the activities are subjugated to an anticipated outcome. Informal observations of differences in how children performed the Blackboard task support this idea: the younger children were much more focused on the particular acts of wiping than the older, even when they were applying the sponge to the clean part of the board (or to the wall behind).

Our findings that children produce affective responses selectively to their own outcomes is consistent with other reports suggesting an increase in the active involvement of the self during the toddler years. Geppert and Küster (1983), for example, report analogous increases in the frequency with which children protest when their activities are interrupted or when they are offered unbidden help, and Hetzer (1931) reported that when children completed an activity they "regarded their work" with positive affect, a pattern she and others (e.g., Heckhausen, 1981) interpret as a "success" reaction. Because outcome reactions were more likely when children, in fact, showed more monitoring and experienced greater relative success (in comparison with their other trials), we interpret them also as an indication of the active involvement of the self in actions. We had expected that the degree to which outcome reactions were differentially made to better or more effortful products would increase with age; however, it did not. There are two possible clarifications for this surprising result. One is that the more narrow range in the older children's product-orientation scores allowed less room for divergence. A more interesting possibility is that differences in the psychological difficulty of the task may have masked developmental changes in outcome-reaction specificity. Although all children could perform the task (whether correctly or not), our impression was that it was less challenging for the older children, perhaps making their self involvement less intense than it would be with a more challenging task. To fully test the specificity hypothesis, it is necessary to devise tasks that are equivalently challenging across the age range.

The overall pattern of results is consistent with the following developmental sequence: children younger than a year and a half are primarily activity, rather than outcome, oriented. This means that they focus their attention more on the flow of activities than on the ends or consequences their activities lead to (see Spangler, Bräutigam, & Stadler, 1984). Although even younger infants also work to produce effects (e.g., contingency learning, secondary circular reactions), these must be in close temporal proximity to the child's actions to evoke their pleasure and interest (e.g., Millar & Watson, 1979). The younger infant's focus on effects may be due more to a motivating sense of a contingency between actions and their effects than to a focus on the specific outcome produced. One indication of this difference in activity versus outcome orientation is that children below 18 months rarely show an affective reaction that is specific to their own outcomes, although they do show pleasure on controlling the effects of their activities (e.g., Lewis, Sullivan, & Brooks-Gunn, 1985; Watson, 1972). Consistent with this pattern, when children younger than 18 months monitor their actions, this monitoring serves only the immediate goal of continuing the action. By 20 months, children begin to pay attention to producing outcomes per se, and react to these with pleasure, perhaps reflecting a change in their sense of mastery. However, at this point outcomes are still unspecific and produced without much control (e.g., stopping) or monitoring of the products. It is as though a beginning orientation toward outcomes conflicts with a focus on the attractive activity, reflected in the difficulties children have in stopping or in remaining task oriented.

With the beginning of the third year, there is a change: most children have begun to consistently regulate their activities with respect to producing outcomes (e.g., they pay attention to simple standards, monitor their activities with respect to such standards, and stop), suggesting that actions are more clearly represented as a unit, defined in terms of some anticipated outcome. However, the skills to manipulate the separate pieces of this unit, that is, to direct and correct activities in midstream, are infrequent until after 30 months. We suspect that the improved performance of the 32-month group arose from at least two independent sources. First, their understanding of the precise standard was more articulated, providing a different criterion for an "outcome" than for the younger children, and allowing them to plan their actions with respect to this criterion. Second, when they did err, the older children were more able to manipulate and correct the separate components of their actions. For example, in the Tower task, some of the younger children built incorrect towers, noted that they were incorrect by pointing or verbalizing, but then did nothing to make a correction. In contrast, the older children were more likely to spontaneously manipulate and rearrange the blocks during and after the course of building. The increased ability to correct errors, not just to avoid them, has been noted by other investigators (e.g., DeLoache et al., 1985) as well. The abilities to insert new or different actions into an ongoing sequence, or to correct an outcome after it has been completed, are examples of volitional skills that require both an integration of separate activities under the guidance of specific task standards, and a flexible representation, allowing manipulation of the components of these constructed units.

The age and trial effects concerning outcome reactions suggest that there may be a change in the underlying motivational basis of actions as well: outcome responses increase in frequency before children are consistently outcome-oriented, suggesting that one impetus for practicing action skills is the pleasure found in producing outcomes. However, at all ages, pleasure was most likely when the child produced an outcome that required attention or effort or that posed an action "problem." These results provide an explanation for the infrequency of mastery "pleasure" in the first year (see Morgan & Harmon, 1984) and for the subsequent increase of affective responses to "challenging tasks." Changes in the conditions that elicit pleasure are consistent with the claim that, although affective expressions per se do not alter much with development, what does change are the conditions under which they are emitted and their meaning for the actor (e.g., Sroufe, 1979). We would argue that over the toddler years, affect comes to be differentially associated with producing outcomes that match a standard. An affective reaction specific to autonomous achievement of a goal may be an indication of the first active relation between the experience of mastery and the self. This experience may be one of the ingredients necessary for the development of an explicit sense of agency and competence (e.g., a psychological self).

Although the present data allow only speculation, it seems that the 20-month group shows the greatest discrepancy between appreciation of task standards, control over meeting them, and active involvement of the self, a result consistent with characterizations of the "terrible twos" as stemming from frustration at the difference between what one wants to do and what one is able to do. Kagan (1981) has suggested that the hallmark of the end of the second year is the emergence of an active, goal-directed self. It is necessary to know a great deal more before we can precisely describe what this self is, and how it emerges. We suspect that changes in the child's ability to monitor increasingly coherent units of action and to correct activities in midstream are some of the important changes that contribute to active volitional competence, the essence of a goal-directed self.

REFERENCES

Ashmead, D., & Perlmutter, M. (1980). Infant memory in everyday life. In M. Perlmutter (Ed.), *Children's memory: New directions for child development* (Vol. **10**, pp. 1–17). San Francisco: Jossey-Bass.

Bertenthal, B. I., & Fischer, K. W. (1978). Development of self-recognition in the infant. *Developmental Psychology,* **14**, 44–50.

Brooks-Gunn, J., & Lewis, M. (1984). Early self-recognition. *Developmental Review,* **4**, 215–239.

Bruner, J., & Bruner, B. (1968). On voluntary action and its hierarchical structure. *International Journal of Psychology,* **3**, 239–255.

Daehler, M., & Greco, C. (1985). Memory in very young children. In M. Pressley & C. Brainerd (Eds.), *Cognitive learning and memory in children* (pp. 49–79). New York: Springer-Verlag.

DeLoache, J., Sugarman, S., & Brown, A. (1985). The development of error correction strategies in young children's manipulative play. *Child Development,* **56**, 928–939.

Geppert, U., & Gartmann, D. (1983). *The emergence of self-evaluative emotions as consequences of achievement actions.* Poster presented at the seventh biennial meetings of the International Society for the Study of Behavioral Development, Munich.

Geppert, U., & Küster, U. (1983). The emergence of "wanting to do it oneself": A precursor of achievement motivation. *International Journal of Behavior Development,* **6**, 355–369.

Golden, M., Montare, A., & Bridger, W. (1977). Verbal control of delay behavior in two-year-old boys as a function of social class. *Child Development,* **48**, 1107–1111.

Gopnik, A., & Meltzoff, A. N. (1984). Semantic and cognitive development in 15- to 21-month-old children. *Journal of Child Language,* **2**, 495–513.

Heckhausen, H. (1981). Developmental precursors of success and failure experience. In G. d'Ydewalle & W. Lens (Eds.), *Cognition in human motivation and learning* (pp. 15–32). Hillsdale, NJ: Erlbaum.

Heckhausen, H. (1984). Emergent achievement behavior: Some early developments. In J. Nicholls (Ed.), *Advances in achievement motivation* (pp. 1–32). Greenwich, CT: JAI.

Heckhausen, H., & Roelofsen, I. (1962). Anfänge und Entwicklung der Leistungsmotivation: I. Im Wetteifer des Kleinkindes [Beginnings and development of achievement motivation: I. Competition in toddlers]. *Psychologische Forschung,* **26**, 313–397.

Hetzer, H. (1931). *Kind und Schaffen* [Child and creation]. Jena: Gustav Fischer.

Huttenlocher, J., Smiley, P., & Charney, R. (1983). Action categories in the child. *Psychological Review,* **90**, 72–93.

Kagan, J. (1981). *The second year: The emergence of self-awareness*. Cambridge, MA: Harvard University Press.

Kopp, C. B. (1982). Antecedents of self-regulation: A developmental perspective. *Developmental Psychology*, **18**, 199–214.

Levine, L. E. (1983). Mine: Self-definition in 2-year-old boys. *Developmental Psychology*, **19**, 544–549.

Lewis, M., Sullivan, M., & Brooks-Gunn, J. (1985). Emotional behavior during the learning of a contingency in infancy. *British Journal of Developmental Psychology*, **3**, 307–316.

Lütkenhaus, P. (1984). Pleasure derived from mastery in three-year-olds: Its function for persistence and the influence of maternal behavior. *International Journal of Behavioral Development*, **7**, 343–358.

Lütkenhaus, P., Grossman, K. E., & Grossmann, K. (1985). Transactional influences of infant's orienting ability and maternal cooperation on competition in three-year-old children. *International Journal of Behavioral Development*, **8**, 257–272.

Mandler, J. M. (1983). Representation. In J. H. Flavell & E. M. Markman (Eds.), P. H. Mussen (Series Ed.), *Handbook of child psychology: Vol. 3. Cognitive development* (pp. 420–494). New York: Wiley.

Millar, W. S., & Watson, J. S. (1979). The effect of delayed feedback on infant learning reexamined. *Child Development*, **50**, 747–751.

Morgan, G., & Harmon, R. (1984). Developmental transformations in mastery motivation. In R. N. Emde & R. M. Harmon (Eds.), *Continuities and discontinuities in development* (pp. 263–291). New York: Plenum.

O'Connell, B., & Gerard, A. B. (1985). Scripts and scraps: The development of sequential understanding. *Child Development*, **56**, 671–681.

Piaget, J. (1954). *The construction of reality in the child*. New York: Basic.

Rheingold, H. L. (1982). Little children's participation in the work of adults, a nascent prosocial behavior. *Child Development*, **53**, 114–125.

Rovee-Collier, C., & Gekoski, M. (1979). The economics of infancy: A review of conjugate reinforcement. *Advances in Child Development and Behavior*, **13**, 195–246.

Spangler, G., Bräutigam, I., & Stadler, R. (1984). Handlungsentwicklung in der frühen Kindheit und ihre Abhängigkeit von der kognitiven Entwicklung und der emotionalen Erregbarkeit des Kindes [Action development in early childhood and its relation to children's cognitive development and emotional excitability]. *Zeitschrift für Entwicklungspsychologie und Pädagogische Psychologie*, **16**, 181–193.

Spungen, L., & Goodman, J. (1983). Sequencing strategies in children 18–24 months: Limitations imposed by task complexity. *Journal of Applied Developmental Psychology*, **4**, 109–124.

Sroufe, A. (1979). Emotional development. In J. Osofsky (Ed.), *Handbook of infant development* (pp. 462–518). New York: Wiley.

Vaughn, B. E., Kopp, C. B., & Krakow, J. B. (1984). The emergence and consolidation of self-control from eighteen to thirty months of age: Normative trends and individual differences. *Child Development*, **55**, 990–1004.

Watson, J. (1972). Smiling, cooing and the game. *Merrill-Palmer Quarterly*, **18**, 323–329.

Wenar, C. (1976). Executive competence in toddlers: A prospective, observational study. *Genetic Psychology Monographs*, **93**, 189–285.

Wenar, C. (1982). On negativism. *Human Development*, **25**, 1–23.

White, R. (1959). Motivation reconsidered: The role of competence. *Psychological Review*, **66**, 297–334.

PART II: DEVELOPMENTAL STUDIES

7

Infant-Adult Attachments on the Kibbutz and Their Relation to Socioemotional Development Four Years Later

David Oppenheim
University of Utah and University of Haifa, Israel
Abraham Sagi
University of Haifa, Israel
Michael E. Lamb
*National Institute of Child Health and Human Development,
Bethesda, Maryland*

The predictive validity of Strange Situation classifications was studied in a sample of infants raised on kibbutzim in Israel. C-type (resistant) attachments are frequently found on Israeli kibbutzim, but the long-term correlates of this "insecure" pattern have not been identified. Fifty-nine kibbutz children, whose attachments to mothers, fathers, and metaplot were assessed in the Strange Situation when they were 11 to 14 months old, were seen again when they were 5 years old to assess their socioemotional development. There were no significant associations between infant-mother and infant-father attachment classifications and indices of later child

Reprinted with permission from *Developmental Psychology*, 1988, Vol. 24, No. 3, 427–433. Copyright 1988 by the American Psychological Association.

This research was supported by the School of Social Work at the University of Haifa and by the Levin Center for Research on Normal and Pathological Development at the Hebrew University, Jerusalem. This article is based on a thesis submitted to the University of Haifa in partial fulfillment of the requirements for a master's degree.

The authors are grateful to Ronit Bogler, Rachel Dvir, David Estes, Kathleen Sternberg, Tineke Pollak, and Ronit Shoham for assistance with data collection, and to the parents, children, metaplot, and preschool teachers for their cooperation and assistance.

Much of the research reported here was completed while Michael Lamb was at the University of Utah.

> *development, but infants who had B-type attachments to their meta-*
> *plot were later less ego controlled and more empathic, dominant,*
> *purposive, achievement-oriented, and independent than C-group*
> *subjects. All these group differences were in the direction predicted*
> *on the basis of prior research on the correlates of infant-mother*
> *attachment. All the measures of socioemotional development re-*
> *flected the children's behavior in the children's house at the kib-*
> *butz but not at home or with their parents. This may explain, in*
> *part, the relatively strong predictive power of attachment status*
> *with metapelet as opposed to attachment status with mother and*
> *father. Moreover, the results may underscore the central impor-*
> *tance of the metapelet (careprovider) as a key figure in the early*
> *social life of kibbutz infants. The findings thus raise questions re-*
> *garding the developmental significance of attachment relationships*
> *with various significant adults.*

Continuity between early attachment and aspects of later socioemotional development has been assessed in several American studies (see Lamb, 1987,
and Lamb, Thompson, Gardner, & Charnov, 1985, for a review), although few
researchers have attempted predictions beyond the age of 3 years. Using a
modified Strange Situation procedure, Waters, Wippman, and Sroufe (1979)
found B-group (secure) subjects to be more competent with their peers at 42
months of age. Arend, Gove, and Sroufe (1979) reported that B-group children
were more ego-resilient and curious than non-B children. Pastor (1981) found
that at the age of 21 months, A- (avoidant) and B-group children from economically disadvantaged backgrounds were significantly more persistent, en-
thusiastic, and compliant; and relied less on mothers for support than did C-
group (resistant) subjects. Using an overlapping sample, Sroufe (1983; Sroufe,
Fox, & Pancake, 1983) found that, at 4 to 5 years of age, B-group subjects
scored higher than non-B subjects on ego resiliency, self-esteem, agency, positive affect, and positive behavior, and scored lower on negative affect and
dependency. In addition, B-group subjects ranked higher in social competence,
number of friends, popularity, social skills, compliance, and empathy. Data on
the 40 children described by Sroufe (1983) were later combined with data on
56 other children by Erickson, Sroufe, and Egeland (1985). Measures of
agency, dependency, social skills, compliance hostility, frustration tolerance,
impulsiveness, and withdrawal revealed differences between B and non-B infants in the expected direction. In Holland, van IJzendoorn and his colleagues
(van IJzendoorn & Tavecchio, 1987; van IJzendoorn, van der Veer, & van
Vliet-Vissor, 1987) reported that C-group children were later more ego-
controlled than B-group children. Overall, attachment classifications do, in

certain circumstances, predict later differences between B and non-B subjects. By preschool age, children who had been B-group infants are often better adjusted than non-B-group children on a variety of measures, provided there has been continuity in family circumstances (Lamb et al., 1985). A- and C-group infants do not appear to differ in any consistent way.

On many of the occasions on which Ainsworth's Strange Situation procedure has been used outside the United States, the distribution of infants among the three major categories of attachment has differed significantly from the distribution typically found in the United States. Especially salient in several foreign studies is the high proportion of infants belonging to Group A (avoidant attachment) or Group C (resistant attachment). In the United States, 60%-70% of the infants observed are typically assigned to Group B (secure attachment), with 20%-25% in Group A and 10%-15% in Group C (Ainsworth, Blehar, Waters, & Wall, 1978). In Germany, by contrast, Grossmann, Grossmann, Spangler, Suess, and Unzner (1985) placed only 33% of their subjects in the B group, whereas 49% were classified in the A group. Miyake, Chen, and Campos (1985) classified 72% of their Japanese infants in the B group, with 28% in the C group and none in the A group, whereas Sagi et al. (1985) classified 56% of the infants from Israeli kibbutzim in the B group, with 33% in the C group. The high frequencies of A- or C-group infants may reflect a higher prevalence of insecure relationships in these societies, but they may also be due to cultural differences in child-rearing goals and practices. The purpose of this study was to clarify the meaning of C classifications in kibbutzim by determining whether there was an association between early attachment and later assessments of the children's socioemotional development. Of course, this focus on predictive validity does not vitiate the need for research on the associations between prior rearing conditions and Strange Situation behavior—both types of studies play an important role in investigating the validity of the Strange Situation procedure (Lamb et al., 1985). In our study, the validity of the C classifications would be supported if associations between early classifications and indices of later development corresponded to the relations found in the United States. A lack of convergence would raise questions about the appropriateness of using the Strange Situation to make inferences about the future behavior of kibbutz-reared children.

On the basis of attachment theory and the research reviewed above, we predicted that B-group infants would be more socially competent with peers and more empathic as kindergartners than C-group children. We expected that the B-group children would be characterized by greater ego resilience, less ego control (given that C-group children appear overcontrolled), and a more internal locus of control than would C-group children. B-group children were expected to perceive their parents as less punitive and more nurturant than C-group children on the basis of extensive research on the antecedents of individual differences in Strange Situation behavior (see Ainsworth et al., 1978, and Lamb et al., 1983, for reviews). Consistent with previous studies, we expected no differences between attachment groups in their cognitive level, and if such differences were found we planned to statistically control for them so that any differences between B- and C-group subjects on measures of socioemotional development could be attributed to factors other than cognitive level.

No predictions were made regarding the differential contributions of attachment relationships with the three attachment figures: mothers, fathers, and metaplot (careproviders; *metapelet* is the singular form). There is no necessary similarity between infant attachments to fathers and mothers (Lamb et al., 1985), implying that Strange Situation classifications assess the relationships between infants and specific adults rather than individual "traits," but attachment theorists have not specified how the effects of the different attachments are integrated (Bretherton, 1985). Main and her colleagues (Main, Kaplan, & Cassidy, 1985; Main & Weston, 1981) have reported that infant-mother relationships predict behavior better than infant-father relationships, but such findings were not obtained in Sweden by Lamb, Hwang, Frodi, and Frodi (1982), and it is in any event not clear that this finding should be generalized from studies of traditional U.S. families to the very different kibbutz society. Our working hypothesis was that classifications of infant-mother, infant-father, and infant-metapelet relationships would have equivalent effects on the children's later social and emotional behavior.

METHOD

Subjects

Fifty-nine subjects (34 boys and 25 girls) from the Sagi et al. (1985) study were relocated when they were between 56 and 58 months of age. The subjects belonged to 15 kibbutzim in the northern part of Israel, 7 kibbutzim from the United Kibbutz Movement (Takam) and 8 kibbutzim from the Arzi movement. Table 1 presents the distribution of subjects across attachment groups.[1] Although only 59 of the original 86 subjects were retested at follow-up, the distribution across attachment categories of the subjects in this subsample was

---

[1]Several researchers, including some of the present authors, have questioned the designation of B_4 infants as members of the "secure" B group (Sagi et al., 1985; van IJzendoorn, Goosens, Kroonenberg, & Tavecchio, 1984), but the issue remains unresolved. Consistent with widely accepted practices, therefore, the B_4 infants were placed in the B group for the analyses reported here.

Table 1

Distribution of 5-Year-Old Subjects (Groups A; B, and C)
According to Their Attachment Classifications
at 11 to 14 Months of Age

	Avoidant (A)		Secure (B)		Resistant (C)	
Attachment figure	N	%	N	%	N	%
Mother (N = 56)	4	7 (8)	30	53 (56)	22	39 (33)
Father (N = 55)	6	11 (11)	36	64 (65)	13	23 (22)
Metapelet (N = 58)	7	12 (15)	29	49 (52)	22	38 (32)

Note. Figures in parentheses refer to the distribution at 11 to 14 months
for the complete sample.

Table 1. Distribution of 5-Year-Old Subjects (Groups A, B, and C) According to Their
Attachment Classifications at 11 to 14 Months of Age

quite similar to the distribution in the full sample. Insufficient numbers of
children who had been classified in the A group (4, 6, and 7 with mother,
father, and metapelet, respectively) were retested, and it was not advisable to
combine the A and C groups because this might mask effects if the groups had
contrasting scores. As a result, the analyses that we report involved fewer than
59 subjects, because A-group children were not included. Thirty metaplot and
30 kindergarten teachers provided descriptions of the 59 children included in
the follow-up.

Procedure

Details about the Strange Situation sessions, which took place when the
infants were between 11 and 14 months of age, were provided by Sagi et al.
(1985). The follow-up observational and test data describing the 5-year-old
subjects was collected during the morning hours in the children's living quarters, which is the place where they spend most of their days and (in kibbutzim
with communal sleeping arrangements) their nights too. First, the children
were observed unobtrusively during free play. Thereafter, the kindergarten
teacher introduced the researcher to the target child. Testing took place in a
separate room of the children's house, with tests administered in the following
order: Kagan Parent Role Test (KPRT; Kagan & Lemkin, 1960), WPSSI IQ test
(Lieblich, 1974), Interpersonal Awareness Test (IAT; Borke, 1971), and Stanford Preschool Internal-External Scale (SPIES; Mischel, Zeiss, & Zeiss, 1974).
During their free time, the kindergarten teachers and metaplot were instructed
in the use of the California Child Q-Set (CCQ; Block & Block, 1979, 1980),
and the Preschool Behavior Q-sort (PBQ; Baumrind, 1968, 1971), respec-

tively. They subsequently completed these Q-sort descriptions of each child. Restrictions on the amount of time during which we had access to the teachers and metaplot prevented us from having both adults complete both the CCQ and PBQ, as might have been ideal. Instead, each completed only one Q-sort. In no case was either inventory completed by the same individual with whom attachment was earlier assessed: In the kibbutz system, children are routinely assigned to new metaplot as they grow older. By design, kindergartners on kibbutzim are cared for (i.e., are awoken, dressed, fed breakfast and lunch, and supervised outside class) by metaplot, whereas kindergarten teachers assume responsibility for classroom education. All metaplot and kindergarten teachers had had responsibility for the children they rated for at least 6 months.

The following are descriptions of the various measures and instruments used:

Peer Play Scale. The Peer Play Scale (Howes, 1980; personal communication, 1984) was used to code the interaction between the subjects and their peers during the approximately 25 min-long free-play session. The scale distinguishes seven levels of play: (a) parallel play, (b) parallel play with mutual regard, (c) simple social play, (d) complementary and reciprocal play with mutual awareness, (e) complementary and reciprocal play (as in Level d) with social bids (as in Level c), (f) role assignment play, and (g) games with external rules. Prior to the data collection, it was found necessary to add intermediate levels between the play levels originally defined. For example, a 1.5 score was given when the subject looked at her partner but the latter did not look back. The observation session was divided into eighty 15-s time units, in each of which the highest level of social play was coded. The child's mean level of play during the observation was used to index level of play for analytic purposes. Interrater reliability was computed during observations prior to the beginning of data collection. In addition, every seventh observation during the data collection process was conducted by two observers to ensure maintenance of adequate reliability: Scores based on the two observers' ratings were highly correlated, $r = .99$. When corrected for chance agreement using Cohen's kappa, the mean coefficient was .85.

Kagan Parent Role Test. Kagan's Parent Role Test (KPRT; Kagan & Lemkin, 1960) was used to assess the subject's perceptions of their parents. The test consists of 23 statements (e.g., "Someone is giving the little boy/girl an ice cream cone") about each of which the child was asked to indicate whether the statement applied more to father or mother by responding verbally or pointing to a mother or father silhouette. The statements pertain to three constructs: punitiveness, nurturance, and salience. The scores for each parent on each dimension were computed by counting the number of relevant items (i.e., pertaining to punitiveness, nurturance, or salience) that the subject assigned to mother or father. The KPRT has been successfully used in both the

United States (e.g., Kagan & Lemkin, 1960; Radin, 1982; Radin & Sagi, 1982) and Israel (Sagi, 1982) to measure children's perceptions of their parents. In the United States, Kagan and Lemkin reported that, as predicted, 3- to 8-year-olds perceived their mothers to be more nurturant and less punitive than their fathers. (The salience score was added later.) Radin found that scores on the Kagan and Lemkin index of paternal nurturance were positively associated with scores on an independent measure of paternal nurturance. Radin also found that paternal punitiveness, as assessed using the KPRT, was positively associated with an index of paternal decision making. In Israel, Sagi (1982) predicted, and found, that children with more highly involved fathers would perceive their fathers to be more nurturant, more salient, and less punitive than did children with less involved fathers. Prior research thus established the construct validity of the KPRT scores.

WPPSI IQ Test. In order to prevent the testing battery from lasting more than an hour, only 4 of the 10 subtests (Information, Comprehension, Block Design, and Picture Completion) of the Israeli version of the WPPSI (Lieblich, 1974) were chosen, on the basis of the high correlations of these verbal and performance subtests with the verbal and performance total scores, respectively (Lieblich, 1974). An IQ index was generated by summing each subject's standard scores (adjusted for age) on the 4 subtests. This index was used to detect differences in the cognitive level of B- and C-group subjects and to control statistically for the differences when they occurred.

Interpersonal Awareness Test (IAT). The IAT (Borke, 1971) was used to assess the child's empathy, operationally defined as the ability to perceive the feelings of another child. The first part of the test includes seven short vignettes in which another child is subjected to emotion-provoking situations. The subject can either respond verbally, naming the emotion the other child might feel, or point toward one of four pictures showing a happy, sad, angry, or frightened child of the same sex. In the second part of the test, eight short statements describe the subject interacting with another child in a way that may provoke happiness, sadness, or anger. Again, the subject can describe the other child's feelings verbally or nonverbally. The subject's score is the sum of all the correct responses. Using the IAT, Borke (1971) demonstrated that children as young as 3 to 4 years of age were capable of interpersonal awareness, contrary to Piaget's claims. Although developed in the United States, a Hebrew translation of the IAT has previously been used in Israel; Sagi (1982) reported, consistent with his prediction, that greater father involvement was associated with greater empathy in children.

Stanford Preschool Internal External Scale (SPIES). The SPIES (Mischel et al., 1974) is a 14-item measure of locus of control. Each question involves a choice between two alternatives, one reflecting an internal orientation and the other reflecting an external orientation. The subject's score is the sum of all the internal-orientation answers chosen. Mischel et al. (1974) reported that internality was associated with persistence and the ability to delay gratification in a sample of 211 children 3.2 to 5.8 years of age. For subjects over 4 years of age ($n = 38$), test-retest reliability over 4 months was .62. In Israel, Sagi (1982) found that internal locus of control was associated, as predicted, with increased paternal involvement.

California Child Q-Set (CCQ). The CCQ (Block & Block, 1979, 1980) was used to assess the child's ego resiliency and ego control. Ego control was defined by Block and Block (1980) as "the degree of impulse control and modulation" (p. 41) and ego resiliency as "the dynamic capacity of an individual to modify his/her modal level of ego-control, in either direction, as a function of the demand characteristics of the environmental context" (p. 48). In this study, each subject's kindergarten teacher described the child by assigning 100 statements to one of eight 11-item categories and one 12-item category, ranging from *most descriptive* to *most undescriptive* of the child. The subject's profile, consisting of the scores that were assigned to each item by the kindergarten teacher, was then correlated with the profiles for ego resilient and ego undercontrolled children developed by Block and Block (1979). The two correlations were used as scores for analytic purposes.

Preschool Behavior Q-sort (PBQ). This Q-sort was designed to assess interpersonal behavior (Baumrind, 1968). The metapelet described each subject by classifying the 72 statements into nine 8-item categories, ranging from *most descriptive* to *most undescriptive* of the child. Each statement pertained to one of the following dimensions (Baumrind, 1971): hostile-friendly, resistant-cooperative, domineering-tractable, dominant-submissive, goal directed-aimless, achievement oriented-not achievement oriented, and independent-suggestible. The scores on each item (i.e., category ratings ranging from *1* to *9*) were standardized using the means and standard deviations obtained in this sample. Next, each subject's score on each dimension was generated by calculating the mean of the standardized scores of all the items belonging to the dimension. These means were transformed to *t* scores, with a mean of 50 and standard deviation of 10.

RESULTS

Preliminary Analyses

Sagi et al. (1985) reported that it was necessary to curtail 80 of the 251 Strange Situation sessions because the infants were inconsolably distressed. Questions inevitably arise regarding the validity of the attachment classifications that are based on abbreviated Strange Situation sessions. To address this issue, 2 × 2 analyses of variance (ANOVAS) (Attachment Classification × Abbreviated vs. Nonabbreviated Strange Situation Sessions) were conducted on each of the outcome variables. This series of analyses was conducted three times, grouping the subjects according to their attachment classification with mother, father, and metapelet. Interactions would suggest that the pattern of associations between early attachment and later development is different in the abbreviated and nonabbreviated subgroups, which in turn would suggest that the classifications derived from the abbreviated sessions are difficult to interpret and may be invalid. Only a very small number of ANOVAS showed significant interactions, usually when one of the groups compared was very small and thus had an unstable group mean. The implication—that abbreviation of the Strange Situation procedures does not affect the predictive validity of the classifications—is consistent with evidence earlier reported by Sagi, Lamb, and Gardner (1986) concerning the association between Strange Situation classifications and contemporaneous measures of stranger sociability. Therefore, subsequent analyses ignored the difference between subjects whose classifications were based on abbreviated and nonabbreviated Strange Situation sessions.

Thirty-one subjects belonged to kibbutzim that maintained communal sleeping arrangements, whereas the remainder came from kibbutzim that had changed to familial sleeping arrangements during the 4 years between the attachment assessments and the follow-up testing.[2] Following the rationale described above, three sets of 2 × 2 ANOVAS (Attachment Classification × Communal vs. Familial Sleeping Arrangements) were conducted on all the outcome measures to detect interactions suggesting that sleeping arrangements changed the pattern of associations between early attachment and later development. Very few significant interactions were found and these occurred usually when the number of subjects in one of the cells was very small. In subsequent analyses, therefore, no distinction was made between subjects whose sleeping arrangements did or did not change.

Next, t tests comparing the IQ level of B- and C-group subjects were conducted to detect differences between the cognitive level of children in the two attachment groups. Significant differences were found only when the subjects were grouped according to their attachment classification with father: B-group subjects (M = 120.56) scored higher than C-group subjects (M = 108.14), $t(43)$ = 3.51, p < .001. Thus, when subjects were grouped in subsequent analyses according to the attachment classifications with their fathers, IQ differences were controlled using covariance procedures.

---

[2]Sleeping arrangements were unknown in two cases.

Effects of Attachment Classifications

Multivariate analyses of variance (MANOVAS) were used to determine whether subjects classified in the B group with their mothers, fathers, or meta-plot differed from C-group subjects on the peer-play, parent-role perception, empathy, and locus-of-control dependent measures. Multivariate analyses of covariance (MANCOVAS) were used when father-infant attachments were involved. Separate MANOVAS or MANCOVAS considered the two CCQ measures, the five PBQ scales tapping assertiveness (dominance, domineering, goal-direction, independence, and achievement orientation), the two PBQ scales tapping cooperative friendliness (hostility and resistance), and (in the case of parents) the child's perception of the parent concerned using the KPRT. Following established practices, univariate analyses are reported only when there was a significant multivariate effect.

The MANOVAS and MANCOVAS unexpectedly revealed no significant differences between the B and C groups as defined by the infant-mother or infant-father attachments. Such findings preclude examination of univariate effects, although it is worth noting that only 1 of 15 associations with infant-father attachment and 1 of 15 associations with infant-mother attachment were statistically significant. By contrast, all but one of the *manovas* that were based on infant-metapelet attachment revealed significant differences between B- and C-group subjects (see Table 2). Subsequent univariate tests showed that subjects classified in the B-group with their metaplot were more empathic, dominant, purposive, achievement-oriented, and independent than were C-group subjects.

Dimension	Secure (B)		Insecure (C)		F	df*	p
	M	SD	M	SD			
MANOVA					3.91	3, 44	.015
Social play	2.23	.55	2.32	.62	—	—	—
Empathy	12.14	1.40	10.65	1.84	10.13	1, 46	.004
Locus of control	5.14	1.73	5.70	2.02	—	—	—
MANOVA					—	—	—
Hostility–friendliness	49.67	2.81	49.81	7.12	—	—	—
Resistance–cooperativeness	49.60	6.93	49.77	6.89	—	—	—
MANOVA					3.46	5.45	.010
Domineering–tractability	50.77	5.84	49.38	5.92	—	—	—
Dominance–submissiveness	51.52	5.85	48.13	7.23	3.41	1, 49	.070
Goal-directedness–aimlessness	53.44	5.52	47.55	6.39	12.41	1, 49	.002
Achievement–orientation	52.26	4.44	48.15	5.44	8.78	1, 49	.006
Independence–suggestibility	51.57	6.16	47.44	6.74	5.17	1, 49	.028
MANOVA					5.30	2, 47	.008
Ego resilience	.212	.342	.092	.397	—	—	—
Ego undercontrol	.117	.183	−.040	.141	10.63	1, 48	.001

Note. MANOVA = multivariate analysis of variance. * The degrees of freedom vary because there were partially missing data.

Table 2. Means on Developmental Outcome Measures for B and C Groups Defined by Infant-Metapelet Attachment Classifications

They were also significantly more ego-undercontrolled than the C-group subjects.

DISCUSSION

The results of this study confirm an association between Strange Situation behavior and later socioemotional development and shed light on the complexities involved in interpreting patterns of attachment with multiple attachment figures, albeit in a culture different from that in which the procedure originated. By finding essentially no relation between infant-mother or infant-father attachment and later socioemotional development, we failed to replicate the results of many studies conducted in the United States, yet we found several theoretically meaningful associations between infant-metapelet attachment and later socioemotional development. Most surprising, we found attachment status with the metapelet (and not with mother or father) to be the best predictor of various aspects of socioemotional development. Overall, the findings lend further support to the validity of the attachment classifications involving kibbutz-reared Israeli infants (Sagi et al., 1985, 1986) and emphasize the importance of kibbutz infants' relationships with their metaplot. More specifically, infants classified in the B group with their metaplot were later more empathic, dominant, independent, achievement-oriented, ego-undercontrolled, and purposive as kindergartners than were children previously classified in the C group. All of these differences were in the direction predicted on the basis of prior research (Erickson et al., 1985; Sroufe, 1983; van IJzendoorn et al., 1987), and all but one of the multivariate analyses revealed significant group differences, even though several of the individual measures—quality of peer play, locus of control, ego resilience, and ratings of friendliness, cooperativeness, and tractability—failed to reveal the predicted group differences. The finding that attachment status with metapelet was the strongest predictor of aspects of children's socioemotional development suggests that infants' attachment relationships with important attachment figures other than their mothers may be very influential as precursors of later development, especially when the other care-providers are intensively involved in the child-rearing process. Of course, these findings demand independent replication, but the consistency across multiple measures, derived from multiple procedures, underscores the breadth of these associations.

Our failure to replicate prior findings concerning an association between infant-mother attachment and aspects of later child development may be attributable to the fact that the attachment classifications with kibbutz mothers either did not accurately capture the quality of the attachment or else reflected qualities that changed over time. Sagi et al. (1982) suggested that inconsistency in the quality of maternal care could be responsible for the large proportion of C-type infant-mother attachments in their study. Some mothers described difficulties in caring for their infants in the "infant-houses" in the presence of other mothers and metaplot, which may have produced differences between their practices at home and in the infant-houses. Such inconsistency in maternal care may promote C-type attachments (Ainsworth et al., 1978). As infants grow older, mothers typically cease providing care in the infant houses, and this could increase the consistency in caretaking, thus leading some of the C-type attachments to change. Intervening changes in attachment status would decrease the predictive validity of the early attachment classifications (Lamb et al., 1985). This factor probably cannot explain the results concerning predictors from infant-father attachments, however, because fathers seldom care for their infants in the infant-houses and so may have more temporally consistent patterns of interaction.

It may therefore be valuable to consider the integration of influences from multiple attachments. Prior studies confirm that there is no necessary similarity between attachment classifications with mothers and fathers (Grossmann, Grossmann, Huber, & Wartner, 1981; Lamb, 1978; Lamb et al., 1982; Main & Weston, 1981; Sagi et al., 1985) or mothers and careproviders (Krentz, 1983; Sagi et al., 1985). Bretherton (1985) referred to dissimilarity of attachments with mothers and fathers as nonconcordant attachments, noting that attachment theory does not explain clearly how integrated working models of the self are built from children's participation in a number of nonconcordant relationships. A possible interpretation of our results is that relationships with each attachment figure may serve as the precursors of different facets of later development. Attachments with metaplot seem to be related to later social functioning in the children's houses and kindergartens, with B-group status leading to assertiveness and empathy. This is consistent with the fact that metaplot directly socialize children in this out-of-home context on a daily basis. In addition, the relationships between infants and their kibbutz parents may differ from those between urban parents and their infants due to the presence of metaplot, important additional attachment figures who have primary responsibilities for socializing and disciplining young children from early in life. As a result, the correlates of kibbutz infant-parent relationships may be limited, more than in traditional families, to home and family contexts, and, if this were true, the effects of the attachments with kibbutz parents would most easily be detected in the family setting. Such predictions await exploration in future research.

In sum, our findings provide qualified support for the meaningful use of the Strange Situation in Israel. On the one hand, assessments of infant-metapelet attachments in infancy predicted multiple aspects of social and personality development 4 years later, and all associations were in a direction consistent with prior research on the correlates of infant-mother attachment. On the other hand, assessments of attachments between kibbutz infants and their parents were uncorrelated with measures of later child functioning. At the very least, these findings demonstrate the important roles assumed by metaplot on the kibbutz. These findings may underscore the central role of the metaplot in the early lives of kibbutznikim (children who grow up on the kibbutz) or may simply reflect the discordance between the areas in which young kibbutznikim function. Selection between these competing explanations awaits further research.

REFERENCES

Ainsworth, M. D. S., Blehar, M. C., Waters, E., & Wall, S. (1978). *Patterns of attachment*. Hillsdale, NJ: Erlbaum.

Arend, R., Gove, F. L., & Sroufe, L. A. (1979) Continuity of individual adaptation from infancy to kindergarten: A predictive study of ego-resiliency and curiosity in preschoolers. *Child Development, 50,* 950–959.

Baumrind, D. (1968). *Manual for the Preschool Behavior Q-sort*. Department of Psychology, University of California, Berkeley.

Baumrind, D. (1971). Current patterns of parental authority. *Developmental Psychology Monographs, 4*(1, Pt. 2).

Block, J., & Block, J. (1979). *Instructions for the California Child Q-set*. Department of Psychology, University of California, Berkeley.

Block, J H., & Block, J. (1980). The role of ego control and ego resiliency in the organization of behavior. In W. A. Collins (Ed.), *Minnesota Symposia on Child Psychology* (Vol. 13, pp. 39–101). Hillsdale, NJ: Erlbaum.

Borke, H. (1971). Interpersonal perception of young children: Egocentrism or empathy? *Developmental Psychology, 5,* 263–269.

Bretherton, I. (1985). Attachment theory: Retrospect and prospect. In I. Bretherton & E. Waters (Eds.), Growing points in attachment theory and research. *Monographs of the Society for Research in Child Development 50*(1–2, Serial No. 209).

Erickson, M. F., Sroufe, L. A., & Egeland, B. (1985). The relationship between quality of attachment and behavior problems in preschool in a high-risk sample. In I. Bretherton & E. Waters (Eds.), Growing points in attachment theory and research. *Monographs of the Society for Research in Child Development 50*(1–2, Serial No. 209, 147–166).

Grossmann, K. E., Grossmann, K., Huber, F., & Wartner, U. (1981). German children's behavior towards their mothers at 12 months and their fathers at 18 months in Ainsworth's Strange Situation. *International Journal of Behavioral Development, 4,* 157–181.

Grossmann, K., Grossmann, K. E., Spangler, G., Suess, G., & Unzner, L. (1985). Maternal sensitivity and newborn's orientation responses as related to quality of attachment in northern Germany. In I. Bretherton & E. Waters (Eds.), Growing points in attachment theory and research. *Monographs of the Society for Research in Child Development, 50*(1–2, No. 209, 233–256).

Howes, C. (1980). Peer play scale as an index of complexity of peer interaction. *Developmental Psychology, 16,* 371–372.

Kagan, J., & Lemkin, J. (1960). The child's differential perception of parental attributes. *Journal of Abnormal and Social Psychology, 61,* 440–447.

Krentz, M. S. (1983, March). *Qualitative differences between mother-child and caregiver-child attachments and infants in family day care.* Paper presented at a meeting of the Society for Research in Child Development, Detroit, MI.

Lamb, M. E. (1978). Qualitative aspects of mother- and father-infant attachments. *Infant Behavior and Development, 1,* 265–275.

Lamb, M. E. (1987). Predictive implications of individual differences in attachment. *Journal of Consulting and Clinical Psychology, 55,* 817–824.

Lamb, M. E., Hwang, C.-P., Frodi, A., & Frodi, M. (1982). Security of mother- and father-infant attachment and its relation to sociability with strangers in traditional and nontraditional Swedish families. *Infant Behavior and Development, 5,* 335–367.

Lamb, M. E., Thompson, R. A., Gardner, W., & Charnov, E. L. (1985). *Infant-mother attachment: The origins and developmental significance of individual differences in Strange Situation behavior.* Hillsdale, NJ: Erlbaum.

Lieblich, A. (1974) WPPSI *manual.* The Psychological Corporation. The Hebrew University of Jerusalem, Israel. (in Hebrew)

Main, M. B., Kaplan, N., & Cassidy, J. (1985). Security in infancy, childhood, and adulthood: A move to the level of representation. In I. Bretherton & E. Waters (Eds.), Growing points in attachment theory and research. *Monographs of the Society for Research in Child Development, 50*(1–2, Serial No. 209, 66–104).

Main, M., & Weston, D. (1981). The quality of the toddler's relationship to mother and father. Related to conflict behavior and the readiness to establish new relationships. *Child Development, 52,* 932–940.

Mischel, W., Zeiss, R., & Zeiss, H. (1974). Internal-external control and persistence: Validation and implications of the Stanford Preschool Internal-External Scale. *Journal of Personality and Social Psychology, 19,* 265–278.

Miyake, K., Chen, S. J., & Campos, J. J. (1985). Infant temperament, mother's mode of interaction, and attachment in Japan. An interim report. In I. Bretherton & E. Waters (Eds.), Growing points in attachment theory and research. *Monographs of the Society for Research in Child Development, 50*(1–2, Serial No. 209, 276–297).

Pastor, D. L. (1981). The quality of mother-infant attachment and its relationship to toddlers' initial sociability with peers. *Developmental Psychology, 17,* 326–335.

Radin, N. (1982). Primary caregiving and role-sharing fathers. In M. E. Lamb (Ed.), *Nontraditional families: Parenting and child development* (pp. 173–204), Hillsdale, NJ: Erlbaum.

Radin, N., & Sagi, A. (1982). Childrearing fathers in intact families with preschoolers: USA and Israel. *Merrill-Palmer Quarterly, 28,* 111–136.

Sagi, A. (1982). Antecedents and consequences of various degrees of paternal involvement in child rearing: The Israeli project. In M. E. Lamb (Ed.), *Nontraditional families: Parenting and child development* (pp. 205–232). Hillsdale, NJ: Erlbaum.

Sagi, A., Lamb, M. E., Estes, D., Shoham, R., Lewkowicz, K., & Dvir, R. (1982, March). *Security of infant-adult attachment among kibbutz-reared infants.* Paper presented at a meeting of the International Conference on Infant Studies, Austin, TX.

Sagi, A., Lamb, M. E., & Gardner, W. (1986). Relations between Strange Situation behavior and stranger sociability among infants on Israeli kibbutzim. *Infant Behavior and Development, 9,* 271–282.

Sagi, A., Lamb, M. E., Lewkowicz, K., Shoham, R., Dvir, R., & Estes, D. (1985). Security of infant-mother, -father, and -metapelet attachments among kibbutz-reared Israeli children. In I. Bretherton & E. Waters (Eds.), Growing points in attachment theory and research. *Monographs of the Society for Research in Child Development, 50*(1–1, Serial No. 209, 257–275).

Sroufe, L. A. (1983). Infant-caregiver attachment and patterns of adaptation in preschool: The roots of maladaptation and competence. In M. Perlmutter (Ed.), *The Minnesota Symposia on Child Psychology* (Vol. 16, pp. 41–83). Hillsdale, NJ: Erlbaum.

Sroufe, L. A., Fox, N. E., & Pancake, V. R. (1983). Attachment and dependency in developmental perspective. *Child Development, 54,* 1615–1627.

van IJzendoorn, M. H., Goosens, F. A., Kroonenberg, P. M., & Tavecchio, L. W. C. (1984, April). *Dependent attachment: A characterization of B₄ children.* Paper presented at a meeting of the International Conference on Infant Studies, New York.

van IJzendoorn, M. H., & Tavecchio, L. W. C. (1987, September). *Attachment networks in infants: Theoretical perspectives and some data.* Paper presented to the Annual German Meeting of Developmental Psychology, Bern, Switzerland.

van IJzendoorn, M. H., van der Veer, R., & van Vliet-Visser, S. (1987). Attachment three years later: Relationships between quality of mother-infant attachment and emotional/cognitive development in kindergarten. In L. W. C. Tavecchio & M. H. van IJzendoorn (Eds.), *Attachment in social networks* (pp. 185–224). Amsterdam: North Holland.

Waters, E., Wippman, J., & Sroufe, L. A. (1979). Attachment, positive affect, and competence in the peer group. Two studies in construct validation. *Child Development, 50,* 821–829.

PART II: DEVELOPMENTAL STUDIES

8

The Adult Outcome of Early Behavioural Abnormalities

Ann M. Clarke and Alan D. B. Clarke
The University, Hull, United Kingdom

Greater constancies across time are to be expected in seriously deviant conditions compared with less abnormal development. Selective reviews are offered on adult outcomes of severe mental retardation, autism, conduct disorders, mild retardation and adjustment disorders of childhood. In the first category, a highly dependent life path is inevitable. For autism there is a small "escape rate". With conduct disorders, around half have a very poor outcome. An important prospective study of mild retardation, supported by other findings, indicated that two-thirds of those who were administratively classified as retarded in childhood, were as young adults, no longer in need of special services. Finally, adjustment disorders of childhood only rarely show continuities into adult life. Each category is heterogeneous in aetiology, and multifactorial influences commonly operate in individual cases. The presence of an organic component appears to narrow the range of reaction between constitution and environment. It seems probable that, with increasingly common social and familial disruptions, conduct disorders, mild retardation and adjustment problems will become increasingly prevalent, whereas biomedical advances are likely to reduce the incidence of severe retardation.

INTRODUCTION

Major advances in understanding human development have occurred during the last two or three decades (Clarke & Clarke, 1986). The topic of this article

Reprinted with permission from the *International Journal of Behavioral Development*, 1988, Vol. 11, No. 1, 3–19. Copyright 1988 by the International Society for the Study of Behavioral Development.

suggests that two of these should be specifically mentioned. First, the idea that there was a necessary constancy in development has given way to an awareness that there are both constancies and changes during the life path. These may differ for different psychological processes, some being more constant or more variable than others. There are two interacting trajectories during the whole life span, the biological trajectory and the social trajectory. Neither are likely to develop in a linear fashion, hence their interactions are very complex. Sometimes changes represent little more than fluctuations, but quite often reflect long-term trends. They do not arise primarily from errors of measurement, although the extent of these can usually be established. Rather they reside in the nature of development itself (Clarke & Clarke, 1984).

The second major advance in our understanding must also be noted: from the work of Chess and Thomas since the mid-1950s (reviewed by Chess & Thomas, 1984), and from research by Bell (1968), Sameroff and Chandler (1975) and Sameroff (1975), it has become increasingly clear that the individual is not a passive recipient of environmental influences, but reaches out to the environment and receives feedback which tends to modify behaviour. The difficult child is disliked and is thereby reinforced in this behaviour: the bright child seeks and receives more adult attention, while the backward unintelligent child becomes increasingly dispirited by failure experiences. These examples of the transactional model underline the need to be aware that to some extent individuals are agents in their own development, unwittingly but sometimes powerfully. One would expect that these processes would be at their most potent at the extremes of temperament and intellect, simply because the extreme child is likely to have a larger impact upon the surroundings, for good or ill, thus not only altering that environment, but in so doing altering himself. Specifically, greater constancies in development would seem to be more likely where abnormal development already exists, for whatever reason. It would of course be a reasonable hypothesis that organically produced deviance would result in greater constancies than would occur in socially influenced abnormality (Clarke & Clarke, 1984; 1986).

In the space available very brief accounts will be offered of some major early deviant conditions, the nature of these, what is known concerning their aetiologies, and finally their outcome at adulthood. They will be arranged in order of outcome from exceedingly poor to good. The criteria employed for the latter will relate both to adult independence and to freedom from the necessity of treatment or containment. Finally, in an overview, the implications of the summarised data will be examined.

SEVERE MENTAL RETARDATION

Mental retardation is usually defined in terms of an I.Q. below 70 in association with problems of social adaptation (Grossman, 1983). The more severe retardation (sometimes sub-divided into moderate, severe and profound impairment) is taken to describe those below about I.Q. 50. There are a very large number of causes, ranging from genetic (e.g. chromosomal aberrations, the action of recessive or dominant genes) to infective agents (e.g. rubella in early pregnancy, or meningitis in childhood), to toxins (e.g. alcohol, mercury, lead) or complications of the birth process itself. The end-point of these pathologies involves CNS damage or malformation. Even here, however, transactional processes are likely to operate. It would be over-simple to believe that the Down's child functions at a low level simply because of the physical and mental effects of the 47th chromosome; born into a parental, and later wider, environment of disappointment or even outright rejection, such influences are liable to modify even these powerful biological effects. There are obvious methodological problems in comparing the rejected subnormal child with the accepted and stimulated, but differing outcomes are commonly reported. Nevertheless, under varying social conditions such children show either a greater constancy in development, or in some cases a deteriorating condition associated with premature aging (Clarke, Clarke, & Berg, 1986).

Research in the 1950s by such persons as Tizard, O'Connor and the present authors accepted that severely retarded children or adults gave a picture of marked psychological and often physical, impairment. Yet the application of skilled training techniques could transform their functioning in limited areas such as perceptual-motor skills. Particular areas of function could sometimes be substantially increased, with both retention of learning and some transfer. More recently this early work has been replicated by Gold (e.g. 1973; 1978) and the use of prosthetic devices, whether by internalised slogans ("Try another way" aiming to combat the rigidity typical of these persons) or by micro-electronic technology (e.g. Lovett, 1985) has extended the possibilities of amelioration.

At the same time, better medical care has increased the life span of such persons, while there are some indications of a decreasing incidence of severe retardation. Taken together, overall prevalence is probably roughly in balance.

There is a clear correlation between social adaptation and I.Q. below 50. Those persons close to this rather arbitrary borderline may with support achieve a degree of independence. For example, they may travel on their own to sheltered workshops or youth clubs. At the other end of the scale, the more profoundly retarded may fail to achieve speech, may be grossly impaired physically as well as mentally and may die young. Thus the category of severe mental retardation is a wide one. Although functioning at different levels, all members have in common an incapacity to lead independent lives. On this criterion the prognosis is very poor. However, the evolution of behaviour modification techniques has done much to overcome inappropriate behaviour, as well as inducing desirable characteristics. The influence of these methods has been pervasive, and has done much to assist the management of these individuals and to improve the quality of their lives. In only a minority of cases, if identified very early, is there any chance of effective biomedical treatment (e.g. the dietary treatment of phenylketonuria, surgery for hydrocephalus, thyroxin extract for hypothyroidism). An overview of research in this area has been provided by Clarke and Clarke (1987).

AUTISM

Much research on this serious condition has been undertaken since Kanner (1943) published his account of 11 children with an apparently identifiable syndrome common to them all and capable of differentiation from other psychiatric disorders. The most important features are impairment of language, impairment in the ability to form social relationships, an insistence on sameness, and an early age of onset, before 30 months. Despite the prevalence of cognitive and affective problems in autistic persons, it appears valid to differentiate the syndrome from mental retardation and childhood schizophrenia (Rutter, 1978). Causes of autism are not as yet well understood, and indeed remain the subject of controversy. It seems probable that these may be multifactorial, and also that different constellations may lead to the same end-point. For example, autistic features have been identified in cases of lead poisoning and untreated phenylketonuria. There seems to be little doubt that genetic factors are often involved; thus Folstein and Rutter (1977) studied 11 pairs of MZ twins, and 10 pairs of DZ twins, in a group of which at least one twin showed the syndrome of infantile autism. There was a 36 per cent pair-wise concordance rate for autism in MZ twins, with a zero per cent for the DZs. For cognitive abnormalities, MZ concordance was 82 per cent, compared with DZ at 10 per cent. In 12 out of 17 pairs discordant for autism, the autistic twin's condition was associated with a biological hazard likely to result in brain damage. Similarly, Lobascher, Kingerlee and Gabbay (1970) suggested that 56% of their sample exhibited unequivocal evidence of organic cerebral disease. A recent study of concordance in twins is reported by Ritvo, Freeman, Mason-Brothers, Mo and Ritvo (1985).

A long-term study of the outcome in adolescence (Rutter, 1981) showed a large number of differences between autistic children and their controls, selected from the clientele of the same hospital. One quarter had developed epileptic fits during adolescence, with the strong implication that the autistic syndrome had arisen as a result of organic brain dysfunction. Rutter, Greenfield, and Lockyer (1967) have pointed to the preponderence of males, an excess of first borns and of professional backgrounds among parents.

In terms of intellectual and social competence, the later outcome was poor, with very few entering paid employment and about half incapable of leading an independent existence (Rutter et al., 1967). Poor outcome was associated with low I.Q., degree of language impairment and total symptom score in early childhood (Rutter, 1981).

Very little progress has been made in biomedical forms of treatment, so that at present education and social training provide the best means of remediation. Rutter and Bartak (1973) followed up children in three special units with widely differing educational philosophies. Holding constant I.Q. and certain other less powerful predictors of academic achievement, they were able to show a significant effect of a highly structured learning environment and concluded that large amounts of specific teaching in a well controlled classroom are likely to bring the greatest benefits in terms of scholastic attainment and cooperative behaviour in a free play situation. However, there was a marked tendency for children with higher initial I.Q.s to benefit most, and there was no consistent tendency for an improvement in scholastic ability to be associated with social or behavioural improvement. Further, the gains made at school did not transfer to the home situation, and there was no difference between the units on parental measures of behaviour or social responsiveness.

A carefully planned home intervention study was therefore undertaken in which individually constructed programmes based on behavioural techniques were used and the parents were the principal therapists (Howlin, 1980; Rutter, 1981; 1985). Sixteen boys aged 3 to 11 years, without overt neurological or sensory impairment and a non-verbal I.Q. of 60 or above were compared with a short-term matched control group who were receiving no consistent form of treatment. Results after six months showed that the programme was effective in causing parents to modify their behaviour towards their autistic children, and in reducing the level of disturbed behaviour. There was also a significant increase in the children's communication. However, long-term follow-up, while favouring the treatment group on behavioural indices, showed a much less favourable outcome in terms of language use. Initial language capacity rather than the non-verbal I.Q. was related to outcome, and although the children's ability to use language to communicate did not diminish, they failed to make gains in level. In other words the treatment programme appeared to have been useful in modifying their performance but had not affected their competence.[1]

CONDUCT DISORDER

This is defined as "a repetitive and persistent pattern of conduct in which either the basic rights of others or major age-appropriate societal norms or rules are violated. The conduct is more serious than the ordinary mischiefs and pranks of children and adolescents" (*Diagnostic and statistical manual of mental diseases,* 1980). It will be seen that the major element is a persistent violation of societies' rules, and the overlap with the category of delinquency, *particularly recidivism,* is substantial. We offer no apology in a brief section for equating the two for the following reasons:

1. Studies of hidden or self-reported delinquency invariably reveal that although a large number of male juveniles (perhaps all of them) commit at least one indictable offence during their childhood years, those who are caught and convicted on several occasions have committed more and *more serious* offences, either than those who walk free, or than one-time offenders (Gibbons, 1970; West & Farrington, 1973).
2. More controversially, Robins and Ratcliff (1980) offer what seems to the authors very persuasive evidence that there exists a single syndrome made up of a broad variety of antisocial behaviours arising in childhood and continuing into adulthood. The evidence adduced for this view came from three samples with which Robins has been concerned: (a) a thirty-year follow-up of children referred to a child guidance clinic; (b) a follow-up of a sample of inner-city black men aged 30 to 35, with I.Q.s above 85, by means of interview and record searches; (c) a follow-up of Vietnam veterans.

Lack of any recorded anti-social activity in childhood virtually precluded delinquency later, while a wide variety of early misconduct were precursors of adult problems, although in only about half the cases. In other words, the

---

[1]Lovaas (1987) reports the results of intensive behavioural treatment for 19 autistic children below the age of 4 years, who received more than 40 hours of professional one-to-one treatment per week, with parental participation to ensure that every waking hour was accounted for. Compared with two control groups these children made and retained very large gains in I.Q. and scholastic attainment, 47% achieving normal intellectual and educational functioning, in contrast to 2% of the control group subjects. In common with other researches it was found that mental age and degree of language abnormality significantly predicted outcome from pre-intervention measures. Results of this study appear to be so important that, despite the apparent cost, replication would seem mandatory.

overall *level* of childhood deviant behaviour was a better predictor of the level of adult deviance than was any particular childhood behaviour. There was, for example, no evidence that violent offenders were more or less pathological than property offenders, rather a record of violence was associated with the total number of arrests.

Concerning the aetiology of conduct disorders, it has been argued from adoption studies that there is a genetic predisposition for adult criminality (Hutchings & Mednick, 1974), but according to Shields' (1973) careful review, while twin studies of adults show some greater concordance of MZ over DZ pairs, the situation is very different in juvenile delinquency where there was similar MZ/DZ concordance, as would be expected were environmental influences the predominant factor.

One study which has explored these in great depth is that of West and Farrington (1973; 1977) and West (1982) which shows a strong degree of concordance in adult outcome with that by Robins and her associates. The effects of adverse family backgrounds, often coupled with below average intellectual competence were observable by teachers in primary schools whose ratings of "troublesomeness" of children aged 8–10 are significant predictors of future delinquency. West and Farrington's prospective longitudinal study (1973; 1977) is invaluable because it avoids many of the sampling biases which may be found in studies based on clinics or remand homes, and also because it was a planned, prospective longitudinal research.

These investigators chose a crowded working-class area of London in which there were no private schools and where most people did not own their homes; the vast majority were English. They studied all the boys aged 8–9 who were attending six typical primary schools and 12 boys from a school for the educationally subnormal, a total of 411, and then followed them through adolescence and into adult life in order to determine who would become delinquent. Detailed ratings of home backgrounds were made by social workers, and numerous tests were given to the boys.

As noted, the factor which best predicted future delinquency was a measure of "troublesomeness" derived from observations by teachers and classmates at primary school. The 411 boys were then divided into three categories, and of the 92 categorised as most troublesome 44.6% became juvenile delinquents, compared with only 3.5% of the 143 boys in the "least troublesome" category (West, 1982). The author comments that this is somewhat depressing because it implies that deviant behaviour observable at an early age is likely to persist and take a delinquent form as boys grow older. It also seems somewhat mysterious since there is no logical reason why untidiness, poor concentration and similar features at 10 should foreshadow the sort of activities, such as stealing or breaking into shops which are the typical offences of adolescent juvenile delinquents. Moreover, it is unlikely that the teachers' adverse opinions, operating as self-fulfilling prophecies, were the most important causal link in the chain, although this may have been significant in some cases.

West is clear about the limits of prediction on the basis of five adverse background factors: Low family income, large family size, unsatisfactory child rearing practices, parental criminality and low I.Q. in the child. From these it would have been possible to identify a minority of boys who were at risk of becoming delinquents, but it would not be possible to make a confident assertion about the outcome for any given individual. Although the group of 63 boys who had a constellation of several adversities produced as many as 31 juvenile delinquents, they also produced 32 who were to have clean records. Moreover, a majority of the juvenile delinquents, 53 in number, did not belong to the high-risk group as defined by the variables studied in this project.

Could it be that one important factor in the causal sequence by which some children become convicted in adolescence while others do not is the kind of secondary school which they attend? Although West found little evidence to support the view that senior schools differentially affected the outcome for pupils in terms of delinquency, other research bearing upon the problem indicates the likelihood that schools as institutions and individual teachers within them can be important factors in ameliorating anti-social tendencies, or conversely exacerbating them. (See Reynolds, 1976; Rutter et al., 1979; Galloway, Ball, Blomfield, & Seyd, 1982). Rutter and Giller (1983) outline evidence for other protective factors which may tip the balance in individual cases.

Turning now to intervention, West (1982) writes "Most young adult offenders have begun as juvenile delinquents." In his study 68% of the men convicted for offences committed between the 19th and 25th birthdays had been previously convicted. There is general agreement that there are no easy solutions to the problems of treatment and prevention, not surprising in view of the multifactorial nature of the causes which involve a personal predisposition, adverse family influences, the wider social context including the peer group, and also opportunity. West maintains that the question now being asked is whether research has anything at all of practical value to contribute to policy on prevention, treatment and control of delinquency. He offers a summary of the methodologically sound investigations which include either random allocation to treatment and control groups, or carefully matched controls, and both short-term and long-term follow ups. The relatively few systematic evaluations of important projects have on the whole failed to demonstrate a significant decrease in arrests or convictions, although there are exceptions, particularly with programmes including an element of systematic behaviour modification such as that of Seidman, Rappoport, and Davidson (1980). Successful treatment of delinquents by means of counselling has not been statistically validated, and in this connection the long-term outcome of the Cambridge Somerville project (McCord, 1978) stands as a monument to the careful planning of a community treatment project designed to prevent delinquency and its failure to fulfil its promise.

MILD MENTAL RETARDATION

As noted under severe retardation, the criteria involve both low I.Q. and problems of social adaptation, whether already existing or envisaged in the individual child or adult. In practice, mild cases are seldom identified before the age of school entry, and indeed sometimes not at all. Here the distinction must be made between true and administrative prevalence, the latter normally being far smaller than the former. There is clear evidence that many children with I.Q.s between 50 and 70 (the conventional range for these conditions) are never labelled as such. They are likely to be drawn from less deprived circumstances and/or to show less difficult behaviour.

This brings us to a consideration of causes. First, there is no doubt that a proportion of the administratively identified individuals owe their condition to the same range of aetiologies as do the severe. However, by definition the effects have been less damaging; these persons usually comprise about 30% of the whole mildly retarded group. The remainder appear to owe their condition to polygenic inheritance interacting with social adversity, sometimes of extreme degree. There has in the past been some controversy concerning these causes, some arguing for a wholly environmental and some for a wholly genetic explanation. The truth lies between these; there is no doubt that social factors play a part, and often a very significant part, in aetiology but they are not the only factor (Clarke & Clarke, 1986).

An important prospective study in Aberdeen, initiated by the late Herbert Birch, has thrown much light on mild retardation in a number of reports over the last 17 years. All children in the city, born between 1952–1954 were carefully assessed in 1962. Those administratively classified and with I.Q.s less than 70 comprised 9.4 per 1000; all those administratively classified, 12.6 per 1000; and all administratively classified plus those having I.Q.s below 70, 27.4 per 1000. From this it is clear that there were many labelled cases with I.Q.s above 70, and that many children with I.Q.s below 70 were not labelled at all. Hence different criteria yield different estimates. Nevertheless, at the age of 22, two-thirds of the administratively classified were not receiving any special mental retardation services, and of these, 89% of the males were in full-time employment (Richardson & Koller, 1985; and for a summary, see Clarke & Clarke, 1985, pp. 443–444).

There is unanimity in the literature that administrative prevalence declines steeply after school age, during the last few years of which intellectual demands upon the child may be at their greatest. Thereafter, some individuals become "camouflaged" in an undemanding life style. Others slowly learn what society demands of its members; yet others exhibit delayed intellectual maturation as a recovery from severe early adversity (Clarke, Clarke, & Reiman, 1958; Svendsen, 1982). Those whose condition is the result of an organic pathology, however, show a considerable constancy in development and their prognosis is relatively poor. The remainder if removed from conditions of adversity, tend to merge into the duller, unskilled section of the population. Numerous prospective follow-up studies underline this difference; however, current social problems, including unemployment in developed countries may have already altered this otherwise reasonably hopeful picture. Certainly, at all levels of retardation, there is a heightened prevalence of emotional instability, and personality problems as much as intellectual retardation are often the reasons for administrative action.

It has been argued that, since relatively spontaneous improvements occur in many of the mildly retarded, greater assistance might accelerate and increase such changes. To effect these, long-term intervention would be needed.

ADJUSTMENT DISORDERS OF CHILDHOOD

Adjustment disorders have been defined in DSM-III as "a maladaptive reaction to an identifiable psycho-social stressor, that occurs within three months after the onset of the stressor. The maladaptive nature of the reaction is indicated by either impairment in social or occupational functioning or symptoms that are in excess of a normal and expected reaction to the stressor. It is assumed that the disturbance will eventually remit after the stressor ceases or, if the stressor persists, when a new level of adaptation is achieved" (*Diagnostic and statistical manual of mental disorders*, 1980, p. 299). The final section of this statement represents a succinct summary of research findings in this area.

As with other abnormal conditions, adjustment disorders may arise from a variety of different, and sometimes overlapping, causes. There are a number of obvious variables: the family context, especially the quality of parenting; the degree of match or mismatch between parents, and between parents and child; the qualities of individual vulnerability and resilience during or following stress, to which we have drawn attention from time to time since 1959; the enhanced probability of disorder in those with organic brain dysfunction (e.g. Rutter & Sandberg, 1985); the doubled risk of emotional and conduct disorders in Inner London compared with the Isle of Wight (Rutter et al., 1975). Identifying six risk factors, these authors showed that the possession of one yielded no greater risk than occurred in controls. Two had a multiplicative effect resulting in a fourfold increase in risk, while four factors produced a tenfold increase.

Whether the disorder is situation-specific or pervasive is obviously relevant to outcome. Isolated transient emotional or conduct disorders are very common in normal children. What is important is the developmental inappropriateness of the problems (Rutter & Sandberg, 1985, p. 213).

The work of Chess and Thomas (1984) has already been mentioned. Commencing in 1956, they initiated the New York Longitudinal Study, a prospective programme of intensive assessment and follow-up from infancy to early adulthood. As the authors note (Chess & Thomas, 1984, p. 9), it "represents the one study with prospective longitudinal data starting in early infancy and antedating in all cases the onset of behaviour disorder, with a substantial sample size and no loss of subjects over time". As such it provides the main data set for this part of our article.

The sample consisted of 133 middle- to upper-middle class subjects, gathered through personal contact during pregnancy or shortly after birth, with parents who were willing to cooperate in a long-term study of normal child development. Only one parent refused to participate. There was an advantage in using a socioculturally homogeneous group, allowing this powerful variable to be held roughly constant. An important incentive, both in joining the study and remaining within it, lay in the free availability to parents of highly qualified and experienced staff over many years. It is a tribute to this, and to the personal relationships built up, that sample attrition did not occur.

Adjustment disorders represent a wide range of very common behavioural problems which, as the authors note, in many cases represent age-specific behaviours, which though troublesome, are not suggestive of pathological deviation. Sometimes the issue is a simple one involving inappropriateness of the routines employed by parents. Suggestions of alternative ways of handling the child can be effective. When problems do not resolve, psychiatric evaluation and sometimes treatment are necessary (Chess & Thomas, 1984, p. 34).

In childhood, some 40 cases out of the total of 133 children were identified as exhibiting adjustment disorders. Of the former, 25 were mild cases, 10 moderate and 5 were severely disturbed. Onset occurred modally between 3 and 5 years. By adolescence 24 out of 40 had recovered and 2 had improved, with no significant predictive differences arising from the early classification in mild, moderate or severe.

The adjustment of 3 children was unchanged by adolescence, 10 were mildly or moderately worse and 1 was markedly worse. By early adulthood, 29 cases had recovered, with an additional 5 showing improvement. In the vast majority, those who had shown recovery in adolescence maintained this into early adult life. Those, however, who neither recovered nor improved by adolescence tended to grow worse with the years.

Twelve new cases appeared during adolescence, of whom half had recovered, and 2 had improved by early adulthood, that is, over a rather short period.

Not only were qualitative evaluations available, but sophisticated statistical techniques were also employed. These confirmed and elaborated the clinical findings. Age 3 ratings were used as predictors in multiple regression analyses. Maternal attitudes as a set of attributes always showed a significant relationship with adult adjustment. Adjustment at 3 years was almost always a significant predictor; temperament, however, was not so. Using these main dimensions, the multiple correlations with adult adjustment ranged from 0.42 to 0.46, close to what one of the present authors described as "nature's favourite correlation coefficient," that is, the expected relation over lengthy periods for behavioural characteristics (Clarke, 1978). These figures account for between 17 and 21% of common variance, suggesting some continuities but considerable change over time. However, using the set correlation method, the 11 variables representing childhood adjustment, difficult-easy temperament, childhood environment and presence of a clinical diagnosis together accounted for 0.429 of the adult attribute variance. Unbiased estimates reduced this to 0.341, an estimate (34%) of the communality between child and adult sets of data. This is a relatively high figure "considering the 15-year age span involved, and the tremendous physical and psychological changes and social expectations in the transitions from childhood to adolescence to early adulthood. At the same time this leaves over 60% of the variance unaccounted for . . . an interactionist viewpoint would predict that quantitative group measures could not capture the many special features of the child's behaviour and the environmental influences which would affect the sequences of psychological development differently in different youngsters" (Chess & Thomas, 1984, p. 99).

In summary, this important study shows a considerable (but not total) discontinuity between childhood and early adulthood adjustment disorders. The discontinuity is doubtless enhanced by the skilled professional advice available to parents, advice which the authors regarded as moderately or highly successful in about half the cases. The writings of Chess and Thomas emphasise the "goodness of fit" model, and the transactional consequences on both children and their parents when either match or mis-match occur. Chess and Thomas (1984, pp. 20–23) define "Goodness of fit" between parents and children as follows: "When the organism's capacities, motivations and style of behaving and the demands and expectations of the environment are in accord, goodness of fit results . . . (potentiating) . . . optimal positive development. Should there be dissonance . . . there is poorness of fit which leads to maladaptive functioning and distorted development."

Although the sample was exclusively middle class, there is evidence that the findings have much in common with those of other studies. Where social values and parental practices differ markedly, however, one would expect different frequencies and indeed different types of disorder. It would nevertheless be our expectation that the general principles arising from the New York Longitudinal Study would have considerable general application.

The classic 30-year retrospective follow-up study by Robins (1966) of a child guidance clinic sample is entirely consistent with the description noted above. Emotional disorders, such as abnormal anxiety or depression, were in the majority of cases self-limiting, unlike the poor outcome for those exhibiting antisocial disorders. Or again, the Isle of Wight study (Rutter, Tizard, & Whitmore, 1970) showed that in a total population of 10–11 year olds with disorder, more than half were better some 4 or 5 years later.

A study by von Knorring, Andersson, and Magnusson (1987) adds further information to this area of research, for it provided data on a large representative sample, prospectively from 10–24 years, and retrospectively from 0–9 years. In reviewing relevant literature, these authors note the higher incidence of childhood disorders in cities, compared with towns and rural areas, and a higher incidence in boys than girls which, however, is reversed during adolescence. Conduct disorders may, however, be dealt with in other ways than clinically, but the authors underline the poor prognosis for these, with good outcomes for children with emotional disorders.

The criteria for inclusion in the von Knorring *et al.* (1987) sample were different from those of the Chess and Thomas research, for they depended on the rather tough criterion of psychiatric referral during childhood through to early adulthood.

The findings, however, endorse other work; only 3 out of 28 children exhibiting anxiety and emotional disorders before 9 years were still in psychiatric care in early adulthood, while a quarter of a large group with later onset, 10–14 years, and almost half with an onset between 15–19, were still in psychiatric care between 20–24. Males who had attended special classes were at particular risk for disorder.

DISCUSSION

For reasons of space this review has had to be selective. The precursors of schizophrenia, or the hyperkinetic syndrome, for example, have not been considered. Moreover, each condition outlined would justify an article, or indeed a book, on its own. In spite of omissions, and brief summaries of complex issues, the principles which emerge from the present evaluation seem to be well-supported. For those readers who require a more detailed acquaintance with the literature, the book edited by Mednick and Baert (1981) is highly recommended. This covers a very large number of carefully conducted European prospective longitudinal studies, presented as an empirical basis for the primary prevention of psychosocial disorders.

Within each of the categories of abnormality described in this article there are common factors which justify their compartmentalisation. It must be recognised, however, that there is a heterogeneity of aetiology within each; as an extreme example let us recall that there are some 200 or more different causes of severe retardation. Many paths lead to Rome, and outcome, too, can be varied, sometimes minimally and sometimes greatly, depending upon the particular condition. It is also obvious that in an individual child or adult two or more conditions may coexist; for example, a mildly retarded individual with epilepsy and a conduct disorder.

The role of genetic and constitutional factors is often misunderstood. These do not normally dictate a precise outcome, but determine a range of reaction within which the phenotype may be formed, depending on genetic-environment interactions. This range may be narrowed where substantial CNS impairment exists (as in severe retardation where genetic aetiologies are common) or wide where psychosocial causes are primarily involved (as in many adjustment disorders in children). There are also transactions; as noted, to some extent the characteristics of individuals affect their environments, and in so doing through feedback mechanisms modify or reinforce their own development.

A favourite slogan at one time was that "there are no problem children, only problem parents," an attractive over-simplification. While there are, indeed, problem parents (e.g. uncaring, or psychopathic) there are also problem children (e.g. autistic, or temperamentally extreme). Above all there are problem interactions and transactions. Such poorness of fit can set off a chain of events through development. Most transactions, for a variety of reasons (e.g. maturation in the child, changing social environment) are incomplete, and are likely, except in temperamentally extreme children, to attenuate over time. Not only are genetic factors often involved, their programmes unfolding in a non-linear fashion, but equally the child's environment inevitably changes as age increases. To regard these interactions as complex is an understatement.

On many occasions (e.g. Clarke & Clarke, 1976) we have described human development as potentially somewhat open-ended, taking into account both the theoretical motion of ranges of reaction, and empirical studies on changes during development in individuals exposed to changing ecologies. How far do these views fit abnormal early development and its outcome? In cases of severe retardation, not at all, using our criteria of adult independence and freedom from the necessity of treatment or containment. In autism, however, there is a small but significant "escape rate." This seems to be considerably greater in mild retardation, administratively defined, but the prognosis for conduct disorders is generally regarded as poor, although only about half the cases in Robins and Ratcliff's study showed continuity. Adjustment disorders in childhood do not in general lead to continuities, except in extreme cases, so here the outcome for these very common, and sometimes at the time, serious problems, is good.

Throughout we have commented on psychological treatment, indicating that there can be positive though limited improvements in severe retardation and autism. For conduct disorders, which certainly arise in the context of severe stressors, the situation seems poor, unless a drastic change in ecology can be achieved. Mild retardation in many cases improves more or less spontaneously, but active educational and directive counselling techniques can help. Counselling of parents and children with adjustment disorders is also often effective.

In the future, more information is needed on the processes initiated in pathological situations, and on why certain children are highly resistant to stress, while others have a low threshold for stress reactions (e.g. Clarke & Clarke, 1959; Garmezy & Tellegen, 1984). In a wider context, social and familial disruptions, which appear to be increasingly common, are likely to augment the incidence of conduct disorders, mild retardation and adjustment problems of childhood. Psychosocial causes require social and educational solutions which societies will underestimate or ignore at their peril. On the other hand, biomedical advances are probably already reducing the incidence of the pathologies leading to severe mental retardation.

REFERENCES

Bell, R. Q. (1968). A reinterpretation of the direction of effects in studies of socialization. *Psychological Review, 75*, 81–95.

Chess, S. & Thomas, A. (1984). *Origins and evolution of behavior disorders: From infancy to adult life*. New York: Brunner/Mazel.

Clarke, A. D. B. (1978). Presidential address: Predicting human development: problems, evidence, implications. *Bulletin of the British Psychological Society, 31*, 249–258.

Clarke, A. D. B. & Clarke, A. M. (1959). Recovery from the effects of deprivation. *Acta Psychologica, 16*, 137–144.

Clarke, A. D. B. & Clarke, A. M. (1984). Constancy and change in the growth of human characteristics. *Journal of Child Psychology and Psychiatry, 25*, 191–210.

Clarke, A. D. B. & Clarke, A. M. (1986). Etiology update and review: II. Psychosocial factors: correlates or causes? In J. Wortis (Ed.), *Mental retardation and developmental disabilities, 14*, 36–49. New York: Elsevier.

Clarke, A. D. B. & Clarke, A. M. (1987). Research on mental handicap, 1957–1987: a selective review. *Journal of Mental Deficiency Research*, in press.

Clarke, A. D. B., Clarke, A. M., & Reiman, S. (1958). Cognitive and social changes in the feebleminded: three further studies. *British Journal of Psychology, 49,* 144–157.

Clarke, A. M. & Clarke, A. D. B. (1976). *Early experience: Myth and evidence.* London: Open Books.

Clarke, A. M. & Clarke, A. D. B. (1985). Lifespan development and psychosocial intervention. In A. M. Clarke, A. D. B. Clarke & J. M. Berg (Eds), *Mental deficiency: The changing outlook.* 4th edn. London: Methuen.

Clarke, A. M. & Clarke, A. D. B. (1986). Thirty years of child psychology: a selective review. *Journal of Child Psychology and Psychiatry, 27,* 719–759.

Clarke, A. M., Clarke, A. D. B., & Berg, J. M. (1985). (Eds), *Mental deficiency: The changing outlook.* 4th edn. London: Methuen.

Diagnostic and statistical manual of mental diseases, 3rd edn. (DSM-III) (1980). Washington, D.C.: American Psychiatric Association.

Folstein, S. & Rutter, M. (1977). Infantile autism: a genetic study of 21 twin pairs. *Journal of Child Psychology and Psychiatry, 18,* 297–321.

Galloway, D., Ball, T., Blomfield, D., & Seyd, R. (1982). *Schools and disruptive pupils.* London and New York: Longman.

Garmezy, N. & Tellegen, A. (1984). Studies of stress-resistant children: methods, variables and preliminary findings. In F. Morrison, C. Lord & D. Keating (Eds), *Applied Developmental Psychology, 1,* 231–287. New York: Academic Press.

Gibbons, D. C. (1970). *Delinquent behaviour.* Englewood Cliffs, N.J.: Prentice-Hall.

Gold, M. W. (1973). Research on vocational habilitation of the retarded: the present, the future. In N. R. Ellis (Ed.), *International Review of Research in Mental Retardation,* Vol. 6, 97–147. New York: Academic Press.

Gold, M. W. (1978). *Try another way.* Training manual, National Institute of Mental Retardation, Austin: Marc Gold and Assoc.

Grossman, H. J. (1983). *Classification in mental retardation.* Washington, D.C.: American Association on Mental Deficiency.

Howlin, P. (1980). The home treatment of autistic children. In L. A. Hersov & M. Berger (Eds), *Language and language disorders in childhood.* Oxford: Pergamon. (Pp. 115–145.)

Hutchings, B. & Mednick, S. A. (1974). Registered criminality in the adoptive and biological parents of registered male adoptees. In S. A. Mednick, F. Schulsinger, & B. Bell (Eds). *Early detection and prevention of behaviour disorders.* Amsterdam: New Holland Publishing Co.; New York: American Elsevier.

Kanner, L. (1943). Autistic disturbances of affective contact. *The Nervous Child, 2,* 217–250.

Lobascher, M. E., Kingerlee, P. E., & Gabbay, S. S. (1970). Childhood autism: an investigation of aetiological factors in twenty-five cases. *British Journal of Psychiatry, 117,* 525–529.

Lovaas, O. I. (1987). Behavioral treatment and normal educational and intellectual functioning in young autistic children. *Journal of Consulting and Clinical Psychology, 55,* 3–9.

Lovett, S. (1985). Microelectronic and computer-based technology. In A. M. Clarke, A. D. B. Clarke, & J. M. Berg (Eds), *Mental deficiency: The changing outlook,* 4th edn. London: Methuen. (Pp. 549–583.)

Mednick, S. A. & Baert, A. E. (Eds) (1981). *Prospective longitudinal research: An empirical basis for the primary prevention of psychosocial disorders.* Oxford: Oxford University Press on behalf of the W.H.O. Regional Office for Europe.

McCord, J. (1978). A thirty-year follow-up of treatment effects. *American Psychologist, 33,* 284–291.

Reynolds, D. (1976). The delinquent school. In P. Woods (Ed.), *The process of schooling.* London: Routledge and Kegan Paul. (Pp. 1–12.)

Richardson, S. A. & Koller, H. (1985). Epidemiology. In A. M. Clarke, A. D. B. Clarke, & J. M. Berg (Eds), *Mental deficiency: The changing outlook,* 4th edn. London: Methuen. (pp. 356–400.)

Ritvo, E. R., Freeman, B. J., Mason-Brothers, A., Mo, A., Ritvo, A. M. (1985)., Concordance for the syndrome of autism in 40 pairs of afflicted twins. *American Journal of Psychiatry, 142,* 74–77.

Robins, L. (1966). *Deviant children grown up.* Baltimore: Williams & Wilkins.

Robins, L. N. & Ratcliff, K. S. (1980). Childhood conduct disorders and later arrest. In L. N. Robins, P. J. Clayton & J. K. Wing (Eds), *The social consequences of psychiatric illness.* New York: Brunner/Mazel.

Rutter, M. (1978). Diagnosis and definition. In M. Rutter & E. Schopler (Eds), *Autism: A reappraisal of concepts and treatment.* New York: Plenum.

Rutter, M. (1981). Longitudinal studies of autistic children (United Kingdom). In S. A. Menwick & A. E. Baert (Eds), *Prospective longitudinal research: An empirical basis for the primary prevention of psychosocial disorders.* Oxford: Oxford University Press for W.H.O. Regional Office for Europe. (Pp. 267–269.)

Rutter, M. (1985). Psychopathology and development: links between childhood and adult life. In M. Rutter & L. Hersov (Eds), *Child and adolescent psychiatry: Modern approaches,* 2nd edn., Oxford: Blackwell Scientific Publications. (Pp. 720–739.)

Rutter, M. & Bartak, L. (1973). Special educational treatment of autistic children: a comparative study. II. follow-up findings and implications for services. *Journal of Child Psychology and Psychiatry, 14,* 241–270.

Rutter, M. & Giller, H. (1983). *Juvenile delinquency: Trends and perspectives.* Harmondsworth: Penguin Books.

Rutter, M. & Sandberg, S. (1985). Epidemiology of child psychiatric disorder. *Child Psychiatry and Human Development, 15,* 209–233.

Rutter, M., Greenfield, D., & Lockyer, L. (1967). A five to fifteen year follow-up study of infantile psychosis. II. Social and behavioural outcome. *British Journal of Psychiatry, 113,* 1169–1182.

Rutter, M., Tizard, J., & Whitmore, K. (1970). *Education, health and behaviour.* London: Longman.

Rutter, M., Maughan, B., Mortimore, P., Ouston, J., & Smith, A. (1979). *Fifteen thousand hours: Secondary schools and their effects on pupils.* London: Open Books.

Rutter, M., Yule, B., Quinton, D., Rowlands, O., Yule, W. & Berger, M. (1975). Attainment and adjustment in two geographical areas: III. Some factors accounting for area differences. *British Journal of Psychiatry, 126,* 520–533.

Sameroff, A. J. (1975). Early influences on development: fact or fancy: *Merrill-Palmer Quarterly, 21,* 267–294.

Sameroff, A. J. & Chandler, M. J. (1975). Reproductive risk and the continuum of caretaking casualty. In F. D. Horowitz, M. Hetherington, S. Scarr-Salapatek, & G. Siegel (Eds). *Review of child development research, 4,* Chicago: University of Chicago Press. (Pp. 187–244.)

Seidman, E., Rappoport, F., & Davidson, W. S. (1980). Adolescents in legal jeopardy: initial success and replication of an alternative to the criminal justice system. In

R. R. Ross & P. Gendreaux (Eds), *Effective correctional treatment*. Toronto: Butterworths.

Shields, J. (1973). Heredity and psychological abnormality. In H. J. Eysenck (Ed.), *Handbook of abnormal psychology*, 2nd edn., London: Pitman Medical. (Pp. 540–603.)

Svendsen, D. (1982). Changes in IQ, environmental and individual factors: a follow-up study of former slow learners. *Journal of Child Psychology and Psychiatry, 24*, 405–413.

Von Knorring, A-L., Andersson, O., & Magnusson, D. (1987). Psychiatric care and course of psychiatric disorders from childhood to early adulthood in a representative sample. *Journal of Child Psychology and Psychiatry, 28*, 329–341.

West, D. J. (1982). *Delinquency: Its roots, careers and prospects*. London: Heinemann.

West, D. J. & Farrington, D. P. (1973). *Who becomes delinquent?* London: Heinemann.

West, D. J. & Farrington, D. P. (1977). *The delinquent way of life*. London: Heinemann.

Part III
GENDER AND RACE

In the first paper in this section, Eleanor Maccoby observes that all known languages include terms to distinguish boys from girls and men from women, and all known societies differentiate to some degree the roles that are assigned to each sex. Thus, gender is ubiquitous as a social category. A wealth of research data and observation is assembled to explore the proposition that social interactions among children constitute a major milieu in which the development of sex-typing takes place. The review provides the basis for the construction of models for the understanding of the gendered aspects of relationships among children. Noting that any model must employ a developmental perspective, Maccoby finds merit in the currently popular socialization-personality perspective to the understanding of sex typing. From this vantage point, sex typing is understood as resulting from the "shaping" of each new generation of children by previously socialized members of a particular society, who function to reinforce sex appropriate, and to inhibit sex inappropriate, attitudes and behavior. While acknowledging that "shaping" variables can play a large part in the formation of gender-related personality characteristics in individual children, Maccoby augments the model in important respects. She suggests that differentiating biological processes contribute to the development of the different play styles of boys and girls, which, in turn, provide a basis for the experimentally demonstrated preference of even very young children to seek same-sexed playmates. Girls' groups and boys' groups develop distinctive cultures, which provide gender-socializing contexts. Gender segregation is viewed as a group process, one that is not dependent, to any great extent, on the individual sex-typed personality characteristics developed by individual children as a consequence of their reinforcement histories. Children develop cognitive constructs in relation to gender on the basis of the culture-wide information available to them. Maccoby believes that it is likely that human beings almost automatically code the gender of any person with whom they interact. While on some occasions the gender of the social partner is of utmost importance, on others it is irrelevant to the nature and purpose of the interaction. Of critical importance to students of sex role development, as well as those concerned with the problem of altering social stereotypes of what constitutes appropriate sex role behavior, is the elaboration of the developmental processes involved in the development of children's understanding of the implicit rules that govern cross-sex interactions.

By way of contrast, Sandra Scarr approaches the question of research into gender and racial differences from a social and ethical perspective. In this very personal account, Scarr offers a tightly reasoned summary of a number of critical issues. Observing that race and gender are sensitive issues in psychological research, she characterizes as subterfuge the common practice of including samples of blacks and whites, and males and females in the seeming service of conducting a "representative" study. The subsequent analysis of data along racial and gender lines fools no one and, moreover, is potentially detrimental to the very groups many investigators seek to protect from the consequences of potentially unfavorable results. By failing to ask direct questions about the nature and origins of racial and gender differences, one loses the opportunity to investigate the strengths of underrepresented groups, and to acquire information that may provide a basis for developing approaches designed to improve undesirable life circumstances. Nevertheless, the pursuit of race and gender issues cannot be undertaken with impunity. Although Scarr castigates professionals who criticize the motives of colleagues who undertake research, the outcome of which may be politically undesirable, she does indicate that it is incumbent upon investigators to be aware of the values they bring to the framing of research questions. Only by asking fair questions and seeking honest answers can one make a contribution to both science and to one's society. Scarr distinguishes between the question of potential damage to individual participants in research and the potential damage that might accrue to an individual by virtue of his or her membership in a disfavored group, arguing that it is inappropriate to include the possibility of harm to one's valued group in a request for informed consent. In Scarr's view, investigators cannot be held responsible for politically unfavorable outcomes of their research or for the uses that others may make of their findings. While many may well disagree with some or all of Scarr's positions, this thoughtful discussion of ethical issues involved in the design of investigations that do or should involve issues of race and gender is of importance both to researchers and to consumers of research.

PART III: GENDER AND RACE

9

Gender as a Social Category

Eleanor E. Maccoby

Stanford University, California

In the years between preschool and puberty, the free play of children occurs largely in sex-segregated groups. Some differences in the socialization setting provided by all-boy and all-girl playgroups are described, and possible reasons for children's tendency to congregate in same-sex groups are explored. This article suggests that sex-differentiated play styles and modes of exerting peer influence are important factors. Three classes of possible explanatory processes are considered: biological factors, socialization pressures from adults, and gender cognitions. The article claims that "masculinity" and "femininity," as dimensions of individual differences, may not be linked to preference for same-sex playmates, and that these two aspects of sex-typing require different explanations. Segregation is depicted as a group phenomenon, essentially unrelated to the individual attributes of the children who make up all-girl or all-boy groups. Concepts of gender identity and core categorical membership are seen as the primary cognitive underpinnings for segregation.

Gender is ubiquitous as a social category. All known languages include terms to distinguish boys from girls and men from women. All known societies differentiate to some degree the roles that are assigned to the two sexes. Belief systems accrue to gender in the form of stereotypes and culturally coded expectations. Certain cross-cultural universalities may be detected in these patterns, some of them clearly stemming from the different biological roles of the two sexes in reproduction. But interesting though these universals are, the amount of variation within and between social groups is even more so.

Reprinted with permission from *Developmental Psychology,* 1988, Vol. 24, No. 6, 755–765. Copyright 1988 by the American Psychological Association.

The research reported here was supported by grants from the Ford and Spencer Foundations and from the National Institutes of Health (HD 09814).

Status differences between the sexes are great in some societies, small in others. The content of gender stereotypes and role requirements varies among cultures and, to some extent, within them as well. Individuals differ in the degree of their conformity to the sex-linked expectations of others. Moreover, we continue to have evidence of what is perhaps the most important fact of all: Any individual varies greatly, from one situation to another, with respect to how gender-linked his or her behavior is (Deaux & Major, 1987).

Most individuals emerge from childhood into adulthood equipped with the sex-typed characteristics that their societies deem appropriate. It is the thesis of this article that the social interactions among children constitute a major milieu in which the development of sex-typing takes place. A first step will be to examine the degree to which these social interactions occur in sex-segregated social groupings. The nature of the distinctive cultures developed in girls' groups and boys' groups and the way they function as gender-socializing contexts will then be considered. The two following questions are then raised: What is the developmental course of same-sex attraction and cross-sex avoidance? and Why do the attraction and avoidance occur? I will argue that sex-distinctive interactional styles play a mediating role in bringing gender segregation about. The role of three fundamental processes—biological predispositions, socialization pressures, and cognitive categorizing—will be considered. The theme of this analysis is that all three processes must be involved in the development of gender-differentiated social relationships.

A word about terminology: Some writers attempt to distinguish the biological aspects of sex from the social aspects by using the terms *sex* for the one and *gender* for the other. This usage is not adopted here, on the assumption that the two factors interact in any psychological function that we might want to consider. Furthermore, uncovering the biological and social connections to behavior is a major research objective, not something to be assumed at the outset through the choice of terminology. Therefore, the words *sex* and *gender* are used here interchangeably; the word *sexual* is used for behavior that has to do specifically with mate attraction and genital activity.

GENDER AND PEER GROUPINGS

The significance of gender in childhood manifests itself especially clearly in children's social groupings. From the preschool years up to puberty, children congregate mainly in same-sex groups. From this fact alone it is evident that the sex of other children is a salient fact to which children respond. Reviews of studies in which the sex composition of playmate pairs and groups has been reported (Hartup, 1983; Lockheed & Klein, 1985; Maccoby & Jacklin, 1987) find that the proportion of playmate groupings that are homogeneous as to sex varies by setting and age, but that a clear tendency toward same-sex groupings can be seen whenever children have a choice of playmates near their own age. Although the tendency to segregate is clearly present at preschool age, it increases greatly from the preschool to the school-age years and remains strong through middle childhood. In their longitudinal study, Maccoby and Jacklin (1987) found that, among nursery school children 4½ years of age, children spent three times as much time playing with same-sex playmates as they did with cross-sex partners, with some play also occurring in mixed groups. When the children had reached 6½ years, the ratio of same-sex to opposite-sex play had shifted to 11:1.

Similar results are found cross-culturally. In their report of observational studies conducted in 12 communities in widely scattered parts of the world, Edwards and Whiting (1988) found that children tend to congregate with same-sex playmates in all of them to some degree, although the strength of this tendency varies. They found (as U.S. studies have) that gender segregation increases from early to middle childhood. They also report that it is greater when there are many children available as potential playmates and when children are in same-age versus mixed-age groups. (In mixed-age groups, an older child is frequently placed in charge of the younger ones, and this is done without regard to the gender match between the caretaker and the young child who needs supervision.) Edwards and Whiting concluded: "In sum, our findings . . . suggest that the emergence of same-sex preferences in childhood is a cross-culturally universal and robust phenomenon" (p. 81).

There is evidence, at least from American society, that segregation is greatest in situations that have not been structured by adults (Luria & Herzog, 1985; Thorne, 1986). Lockheed and Klein (1985) pointed to greater segregation in lunchrooms than in classrooms. In a 1984 study the same authors also noted more spontaneous cross-sex interaction in classrooms in which teachers have overridden the children's preference for same-sex working partners and formed mixed-sex workgroups than in classrooms where such structuring by the teacher has not taken place.

The preference for same-sex playmates or the avoidance of cross-sex playmates (or both) appears to be strongly motivated, at least in some settings. Both Thorne (1986) and Best (1983) have underscored the intensity of teasing by grade-school peers when a child shows interest in a child of the other sex. Interviews with children of grade-school age reveal that children believe that if they are seen interacting with a child of the other gender, other children will think they are "going with," or that they "like" or "love" that other child (Best, 1983; Schofield, 1981). Gottman (reported in Gottman & Parker, 1987) searched intensively for cross-sex friendship pairs among 7-year-olds and found very few. These rare friendships had been maintained over several years—most commonly since about the age of 3. Of especial interest is the fact that by 7 years of age these children's cross-sex friendships had gone underground; that is, the boys and girls seldom acknowledged one another at school, but continued to play together mainly in the privacy of their own homes.

Why children should be so intensely concerned with the romantic implications of cross-sex contact is a question for which we do not yet have a good answer. It does not seem accurate to characterize the age period of 6 to 12 years as a "latency period," as Freud did. Thorne (1986) and Best (1983) described the "borderwork" that occurs between boys' groups and girls' groups: Chasing is often accompanied by threats to kiss. Taunting about contamination is common (boys can get "cooties" through contact with girls, and to some degree vice versa). Boys and girls of this age are intensely aware of one another as future romantic partners, but they appear to be following a pattern of avoidance of sexuality—one that is monitored through the vigilance and teasing of other children. It is interesting that children of this age are able to be at least moderately comfortable while interacting in mixed-gender groups provided that the structure has been supplied by adults. It is as though adult direction relieves them of the danger that peers will think that they have chosen opposite-sex partners themselves.

Whatever the source of children's strongly motivated cross-sex avoidance, it is worth emphasizing that it need not result in any large degree from adult pressure. Of course in some societies and at some secular periods, boys and girls are sent to separate schools, asked to line up in separate lines, sent to separate summer camps, given chores in different localities, and so forth. Thus, there is a great deal of variation in the degree to which the structures set up by adults support or counteract the segregation of children by gender. Perhaps a more conservative way to describe children's role in the process is this: In some situations there will be adult pressures to segregate, but, in the absence of adult pressure, children of grade-school age are likely to establish a gender-segregation system on their own.

As noted above, the tendency to confine social interaction to same-sex partners is weaker at preschool age than it is a few years later. Nonetheless, it is present at this early time and is surprisingly resistant to modification by adult intervention. Behavior-modification programs designed to increase cross-sex interaction have a temporary effect, but children return to a segregated pattern once adults stop rewarding them for doing otherwise (Serbin, Tonick, & Sternglanz, 1977). How early can the tendency to prefer same-sex playmates be detected? Observations in a large Canadian day-care center (LaFreniere, Strayer, & Gauthier, 1984), which included children ranging from 1 to 6 years of age, indicated that just about the time of the second birthday, girls began to address more of their social approaches to other girls. Boys remained gender-neutral a little longer but by the age of 3 were taking their share of the initiative in producing segregation and by the age of 5 showed stronger same-sex preferences than girls.

In a study with unacquainted same-sex and cross-sex pairs of 33-month-old children, most of whom had had little or no experience in preschool or day-care settings, Jacklin and Maccoby (1978) found considerably higher levels of social interaction in same-sex pairs. Girls exhibited considerably more "passive" behavior (standing quietly and watching the partner play with the toys) when paired with boys than when with female partners and more than seen in boys with partners of either sex. These findings suggest that a foundation for gender segregation exists before children enter group settings.

It is worth noting that this foundation exists at a time when, according to Thompson's work (Thompson, 1975), the children are just on the threshold of being able to label their own gender and that of others accurately and just beginning to know which other children are of the same sex as themselves. Leinbach and Fagot (1986) reported that at this age about half the children in their study were accurate in sorting by gender a set of pictures that has been selected for gender-typicality. Presumably, fewer would have been able to match the gender of other children with their own—a cognitively more complex task. It is doubtful, therefore, whether the same-sex compatibility that Jacklin and Maccoby (1978) observed is based on cognitive coding of another child as being of the same sex as the self, although this possibility cannot be entirely ruled out. It is also doubtful that these very young girls' passivity in interaction with boys was based on any belief that boys in general have higher status than girls and hence a greater right to take control of the toys or on a motive to avoid the appearance of sexual interest—the phenomenon that was pointed to above as operating powerfully in middle childhood.

Role of Play Styles and Modes of Social Influence

A likely explanation of the findings with 33-month-old pairs is that even at this early age the two sexes have somewhat different play styles and that each sex finds its own play style more compatible than the play style of the other sex. Play style differences can be seen somewhat more clearly when the children are a little older. Observations of three cohorts of 4½-year-old children during free play in nursery school are relevant here. The subjects were enrolled in the Maccoby-Jacklin longitudinal study and attended a number of different nursery schools. Each child, along with two familiar same-sex playmates, was brought into a mobile lab that was parked at the nursery school that the target child attended. The lab contained a playroom equipped with a

Behavior	Cohorts 1 and 2			Cohort 3		
	Boys (n = 30)	Girls (n = 22)	t	Boys (n = 25)	Girls (n = 16)	
Aggressive physical assault	.10	.00	1.79	.40	.00	1.66
Rough-and-tumble play*	14.30	4.70	2.97***	20.00	3.30	3.14***
Jumping (trampoline)	9.20	15.20	−1.88*	11.50	19.00	−2.20**

* DiPietro (1981) reported data on rough-and-tumble play and jumping for Cohorts 1 and 2. The remaining data are reported for the first time here.
* $p < .10$. ** $p < .05$. *** $p < .01$.

Table 1. Percentage of Intervals in Which Target Child Engaged in Each Behavior by Sex of Child and Cohort

thick carpet, a child-size trampoline, and a beach ball. Halfway through the session a large inflated Bobo doll was brought in. The play styles of trios of boys and trios of girls are compared in Table 1. As the table shows, girls spent more time jumping on the trampoline than did boys, a finding that was replicated in successive cohorts. Thus, the girls' play style was not a passive, inactive one. However, a girl would almost never throw herself on top of another girl who was jumping on the trampoline, whereas boys, at least in some trios, did so. Boys' encounters with the trampoline and the Bobo doll fairly often ended up in bouts of wrestling or mock fighting, all in high good humor. Rough play of this kind was seldom seen among trios of girls. In the first two cohorts of children in this study, male target children playing with two male playmates displayed more than three times as much rough-and-tumble play as did female target children with two female peers. In the third cohort, the discrepancy was even greater (see Table 1), and the sex difference in both cases was highly significant. The findings on the target children were closely matched by the data on their two partners (data not shown).

The rough, physical, body-contact nature of boys' play may be seen in other contexts. In some recent work by Charlesworth and Dzur (1987), quartets of children were introduced to a movie-viewer with an eyepiece, designed so that only one child at a time could see the movie. Even if a child established dominance of the eyepiece, this did not guarantee seeing the movie: The equipment was designed in such a way that the movie did not run unless two of the other children cooperated—one operating lights, the other turning a crank to keep the projector running. Comparing quartets of boys with quartets of girls, Charlesworth and Dzur found that the level of cooperation was similar for the two kinds of groups, in that total successful viewing time, taking the total for all the children in each group, was about the same. In both boys' groups and girls' groups, a dominant child tended to emerge; that is, there was usually one child who got considerably more than a fair share of the viewing time. But the dominant child's techniques for achieving access to the viewer differed by sex. Dominant boys more often attained their extra time by shouldering other boys out of the way; dominant girls managed it by greater use of verbal persuasion. (This finding is consistent with the observations of Savin-Williams, 1979, concerning sex differences in dominance behavior among older children.) It is worth noting that more positive affect was shown in the boys' groups than in the girls' groups. The boys' rough, body-contact style did not usually involve hostility, and the boys appeared to be having a good deal of fun.

Charlesworth and colleagues (Charlesworth and LaFreniere, 1983) also tried their movie-viewing procedure with mixed-sex groups, each group being composed of two boys and two girls. In these groups, boys generally achieved the dominant positions. Boys, on the average, spent three times as much time in the viewing position as the girls, whereas boys and girls spent equal amounts of time in the helping positions. The implication of the two studies considered jointly is that the techniques adopted by dominant girls for gaining control of resources in all-girl groups do not work very well with boys.

There is other evidence supporting this interpretation. Serbin, Sprafkin, El-man, and Doyle (1984) observed children 3½ to 5½ years of age during their free play at preschools. They found that over this age range there was considerable increase in the frequency with which children attempted to influence their playmates. The two sexes, however, developed different kinds of influence techniques. Among girls, the increase in influence attempts from 3½ to 5½ years was almost entirely in the form of a growing use of polite suggestions. Among boys, the increase took the form of increasing numbers of direct demands. Furthermore, Serbin and colleagues found that, over this age range, boys were becoming less and less responsive to polite suggestions. Thus, girls were developing a style of mutual influence that worked with one another but was progressively more ineffective with boys.

In a study of preschoolers, Fagot (1985) reported that both boys and girls are primarily responsive to "reinforcements" from members of their own sex, being essentially unaffected by the reactions of opposite-sex children. There is reason to believe, however, that the cross-sex influence patterns may not be symmetrical. In a study of mixed-sex math groups in grade school, Webb and Kenderski (1985) reported that among high-achieving children, girls responded to requests for information from either male or female group members, whereas boys responded almost exclusively to other boys. Lockheed (1985), via a meta-analysis of 64 data sets involving mixed-sex working groups of school-age children, showed that boys were fairly consistently more influential over group decisions than were girls. Furthermore, Lockheed and Harris (1984) reported that the more experience children had in mixed-sex groups, the stronger some of their cross-sex stereotypes became. In particular, girls' experiences in mixed-sex groups appeared to confirm and strengthen their (mainly negative) stereotypes about boys.

There were symptoms of gender asymmetry in influence patterns among the 33-month-old children observed in cross-sex pairs (Jacklin & Maccoby, 1978). These children were at a very early point in the development of social skills. In same-sex pairs, when one child issued a vocal prohibition to a partner (perhaps because the partner was trying to take away the possessor's toy) the partner would usually simply back away. In mixed-sex pairs, a boy's vocal prohibit was usually followed by the girl's desisting in her undesired behavior. When the girl issued a vocal prohibit, however, it did not appear to influence her male partner's behavior.

A possible motive for gender segregation appears to have emerged in the work summarized above. It is reasonable to assume that, in any relationship that is freely entered into by both parties, the relationship is more likely to be continued over time and be satisfactory to both parties if each can influence the behavior of the other. If girls develop influence styles that are ineffective with boys, this becomes a reason for avoiding interaction with them. It would also be a reason for girls to seek out situations in which their influence styles *would* work with boys—situations in which they might more easily hold their own in any conflicts over access to desired resources. In a recent study, Powlishta (1987) gave mixed-sex pairs of preschoolers an opportunity to play with a modified version of the Charlesworth et al. movie-viewer. She found that when no partner cooperation was required (i.e., in situations in which a dominant child could gain access to the viewer merely by shouldering the other child away), boys got considerably more than their share of the viewing time *if* no adult was present. In the presence of an adult, however, the girls got somewhat more viewing time than the boys. Coding from videotapes indicated that the adult's presence inhibited the boys in their utilization of their more power-assertive influence techniques. One can see a dynamic here that would bring girls into proximity with adults, and, hence, into proximity with one another. One might expect, moreover, that the girls' avoidance of boys would be less marked in situations where adult monitoring and mediation was available.

The account given above suggests reasons why girls might avoid playing with boys, at least in free play situations distant from adults. It is less clear why boys should avoid playing with girls. Further exploration of the factors affecting their playmate configurations is needed. One possibility is that boys enjoy roughhousing and seek playmates who will respond positively to overtures to rough and noisy play, a response that they elicit more commonly from other boys. Whatever the dynamics, the main claim here is that the two sexes do find same-sex partners more compatible in play styles from an early age. For this reason and no doubt others as well, the two sexes draw apart into gender-segregated groups.

Distinctive Cultures of Boys' and Girls' Groups

The distinctive play styles of the two sexes manifest themselves in the distinctive cultures that develop within boys' groups and girls' groups as the children grow older. Much has been written concerning the kinds of games and other activities that occupy boys' groups and girls' groups, the kinds of friendships that are formed, and so forth. It is clear that the male and female childhood cultures do differ in these respects. Here, the focus will be on the nature of the interactive processes that occur in all-girl and all-boy groups. In boys' groups there is more concern with dominance (Maccoby & Jacklin, 1974, p. 254–265), activities are more hierarchically organized (Goodwin, 1980), and male dominance hierarchies are somewhat more stable than those formed in girls' groups. Several sociolinguists have listened to the verbal exchanges within sex-homogeneous play groups, and Maltz and Borker (1983) have summarized some of the findings as follows: Boys in all-boy groups, compared with girls in all-girls groups, more often interrupt one another, more often use commands, threats, and boasts of authority, more often refuse to comply with another child's demand, more often give information, heckle a speaker, tell jokes or suspenseful stories, "top" someone else's story, or call another child names. Girls in all-girl groups, on the other hand, more often express agreement with what another speaker has just said, pause to give another girl a chance to speak, and acknowledge what another speaker has said when starting a speaking turn. It is clear that speech serves more egoistic functions among boys and more socially binding functions among girls. The research on linguistic styles (mainly involving children of school age) appears to reflect a developmental continuity from the influence patterns that Serbin and colleagues saw unfolding during the preschool period.

If boys' and girls' distinctive play styles and influence techniques do indeed constitute part of the set of forces underlying gender segregation and the formation of somewhat different group cultures in boys' and girls' groups, we need to ask two further questions: Why do boys and girls develop such distinctive styles in the first place? and What other factors, beyond distinctive play styles, might be feeding into gender segregation? In considering further explanations, it is necessary to give explicit consideration to individual differences. So far, boys' groups and girls' groups have been discussed as though each sex were homogeneous. Of course, this is far from being the case. Some boys like rough, body-contact sports, others do not. Some girls like dolls and frilly dresses, others do not. As we turn now to an examination of the possible contributions of adult socialization pressures, biological predispositions, and cognitive processes to the within-sex and cross-sex interaction patterns that we have been discussing, we will consider whether and how individual differences within each sex are implicated in same-sex and cross-sex relationships.

EXPLANATORY MODELS

Socialization-Personality Perspective

It is evident that any attempt to understand the gendered aspects of relationships among children must embody a developmental perspective. One explanatory approach that emphasizes individual childhood histories is what we may call the socialization-personality model. In this model, children's sex-typing is presumed to be a result of the "shaping" of each new generation of children by previously socialized members of a society. The sequence of events is presumed to be as follows: Adult socialization agents and older children treat children of the two sexes somewhat differently, using reinforcement, punishment, and example to foster whatever behaviors and attitudes a social group deems sex-appropriate. Socialization pressures are also applied to inhibit sex-inappropriate attitudes and behavior. The result of this differential socialization is that boys and girls, on the average, develop somewhat different personality traits, skills, and activity preferences.

Within these general trends, however, there is great variation in the amount of sex-typing pressure that is applied to individual children of each sex. Some parents give toy trucks and guns to their sons and dolls to their daughters; other parents make few distinctions of this kind. Whatever initial variations in temperament there may be among children are built upon by parental guidance and pressure so as to produce a range within each sex in terms of how sex-typed individual children become. Reports of the temporal stability of standard measures of sex-typing are rare, but those that are available indicate that stable individual differences in degree of sex-typing have been established by 4 years of age (e.g., Jacklin, DiPietro, & Maccoby, 1984).

A first hypothesis derivable from the socialization-personality perspective would be that children of a given sex, having been similarly shaped, would be more likely to be similar to each other than to cross-sex children in terms of personality characteristics and activity preferences and that this similarity would lead children to find same-sex play partners more compatible. A second hypothesis stemming from this perspective would be that, among children of a given sex, the more sex-typed a child is when entering nursery school or some other group setting, the more likely that child would be to prefer same-sex playmates. That is, the more feminine little girls would be attracted to the doll corner or the kitchen equipment or the dress-up clothes, where they would meet other feminine little girls who would become their playmates. Similarly, the more masculine boys would be drawn together by their mutual interest in trucks or war games. It would be reasonable to expect that delicate or timid little girls, who had been treated gently by their parents, would be especially likely to avoid the rough play of boys and that the robust, active boys—perhaps those who were accustomed to roughhousing with their fathers—would be the ones most strongly attracted to male playmates with similar inclinations.

In the Maccoby-Jacklin (1987) observations of 4½-year-old children during free play in nursery school, both the sex of playmates and the degree of sex-typing of the activities in which the children were involved were coded. There was little relationship between these two measures, although both were coded with high reliability. Boys and girls tended to play with same-sex playmates when engaged in sex-neutral activities to about the same degree as they did when engaged in more sex-stereotypical activities. In some settings, where play equipment was replicated (e.g., where there were two jungle gyms or two swing sets), the boys had established territorial rights to one set, and the girls, to another. Thus, if mutual interest in sex-typed toys and activities was a major factor in drawing same-sex playmates together initially, the playmate preference had generalized beyond such activities by the time that the children were observed halfway through a nursery-school year.

Of greater importance is the fact that same-sex playmate preference was not a variable that provided a stable rank-order of individual children. In other words, it was not a good personality variable. At nursery-school age, there was considerable variability among children on any given day in their degree of same-sex playmate choice. Some children played almost entirely in mixed groups; a few played exclusively with cross-sex partners. Other children played only in same-sex groupings. A small subset of children were observed a second time, a week after the initial observation. On this second occasion, the variation in degree of same-sex partner choice was also wide. But individual stability was low ($r = .39$, *ns*). That is, the children who played exclusively with same-sex others at Time 1 were only slightly (not significantly) more likely than other children to do so at Time 2. There were indications that whatever temporal stability did occur at this age was contributed mainly by girls. Confirming evidence comes from the fact that girls' same-sex preference during outdoor play was moderately but significantly correlated with their preference in indoor play, whereas this was not true for boys. In an unpublished study with a new sample of 20 boys and 20 girls, Laura Williamson (1986) observed preschoolers on four different days to test for the temporal stability of individual children's same-sex playmate scores. For girls, the Kendall's coefficient of concordance was .45 ($p < .05$); for boys, it was .24 (*ns*).

When the children in the Maccoby-Jacklin (1987) longitudinal study had reached the age of 6½, there was little variability among children: On each of

2 days of observation, children's play was strongly segregated by sex. With such highly skewed distributions, stability correlation coefficients are not meaningful; they could be expected to be near zero, and were 30. More interesting is the fact that the few children whose playmate choice was in the more gender-neutral range on one of the occasions were not more likely than other children to be in this range at Time 2. Thus, it was only among girls at nursery-school age that there was enough stable individual variation in playmate choice to justify a search for within-sex factors in children's earlier experience that might lead them to prefer same-sex playmates especially strongly.

Maccoby and Jacklin (1987), from longitudinal data, explored possible antecedents for a girl's being more or less likely than her peers to prefer same-sex playmates at nursery-school age. The hypothesis that it would be the more "feminine" little girls who had the highest scores on same-sex playmate preference was not sustained. Indeed, the significant correlations ran counter to the hypothesis. It was the girls receiving the highest scores on earlier measures of activity and self-assertion who later showed the strongest tendency to play primarily with other girls. Standard measures of sex typing, taken with one cohort of children a year before they entered nursery school, did not correlate with the children's subsequent choice of same-sex playmates. Indeed, same-sex playmate choices were strongest among the girls whose parents had described them as rough and noisy at play the year before. With reference to socialization pressures from parents, the study showed that it was the little girls whose fathers had played most roughly with them when they were 12 and 18 months old who were the ones who spent most time with female playmates in nursery school.

If other studies replicate the finding that it is the more active, assertive girls who are especially likely to play in all-girl groups, we may speculate that these are the very girls who would be least likely to accept domination by boys. Or possibly, their interaction styles are such as to elicit more aggression from boys than the styles of more compliant girls. The main point of interest here, however, is that no continuity has been found between the earlier development of sex-appropriate personality traits (masculinity in boys and femininity in girls) and the tendency to seek same-sex playmates. Of course it is possible that with more and better measures of early characteristics and socialization experiences, such connections would emerge. One cannot prove the null hypothesis. But the contention here is that the absence of individual continuity is part of a larger fact: Individual children of a given sex hardly differ stably from one another in their degree of same-sex preference.

In observational studies of school-age girls, both Thorne (1986, 1987) and Best (1983) described one or two tomboy girls who consistently joined boys' play groups (although they did not necessarily avoid girls). These girls were primarily distinguished by exceptional skill at sports. Green (1987) reported that highly effeminate boys—boys who like to dress in girls' clothing and play with girls' toys and who sometimes express the wish to be girls—also preferred to play with girls. In our samples, however, such boys did not appear, and among first-grade girls we also did not find children who clearly and consistently preferred to play with boys. For the large majority of children, within-sex individual differences in the sex-typing of playmate preferences appear to be minimal by the age of 6 and above, and for boys this was true at an even younger age. At the same time, traditional measures of masculinity and femininity do show significant temporal stability, and these variables thus represent useful personality dimensions. It appears, then, that the frequency with which a child plays with same-sex or cross-sex others may not be part of the within-sex masculinity and femininity personality clusters. This means that a boy who is not good at sports and does not like rough play generally would not seek the company of girls more often than other boys. Rather, he would spend more time alone, unless and until he could find compatible male friends. Gender segregation, in other words, is more a group phenomenon than it is a reflection of the tastes and preferences of individual children.

It should be noted that cross-sex and mixed-sex play does occur at nursery school and even, although more rarely, on the first-grade playground. If children who are highly sex-typed and those who are more androgynous are nearly equal in their tendency to be involved in such play (so that it is not a result of individual children's tastes and preferences), how and why does cross-sex play occur? A possibility is that the occasion-to-occasion variation in children's playmate choice reflects the implicit rules that children understand and follow concerning the conditions under which such play is acceptable. It is as though *any* boy can, and does, interact with girls under some conditions, and *no* boy will do so under others.

If cross-sex avoidance and same-sex preference were based on masculine and feminine personality characteristics developed by individual children through socialization pressures—pressures that vary in strength among children of a given sex and produce concomitant within-sex variation in degree of sex-typing—then it would be plausible that it was these socialization pressures that led children to prefer same-sex playmates with personalities like their own. But because the connection between individual personalities and preference for same-sex playmates is weak at best, we must ask what other foundations are plausible. To explain a phenomenon that varies strongly between sexes and minimally within we need to identify causal factors that impinge on all boys in one way and all girls in another, while affecting all children of a given sex to a similar degree. What could such factors be? As far as pressures from socialization agents are concerned, boys and girls are treated quite differently (and homogeneously within sex) when it comes to gender identifiers. They are given sex-distinctive names and dressed in ways that permit others to know whether they are boys or girls. In general, however, most of the "shaping" variables that have been shown to differ by children's sex (see Huston, 1983, p. 428–431, for a review) do not fit the required pattern, because distributions for the two sexes overlap greatly.

This is not to deny that shaping variables can play a large part in the formation of masculine, feminine, or androgynous personality characteristics in individual children. The contention here is merely that we must cast a wider net in seeking the causes of gendered playmate preferences or any other characteristic for which the variance between sexes is considerably greater than the variance within. Let us now consider two other classes of explanatory variables—biological and cognitive factors—together with their interactions in order to see whether they provide a better fit to the pattern of sex differences that we have described.

Biological factors. Although hermaphrodites exist, the world of human beings can be almost perfectly divided into males and females, with their distinctive primary and secondary sex characteristics and their distinctive reproductive functions. With respect to these attributes, there is vastly more variation between sex groups than within them. It is now well known that the basis for the biological differentiation of the sexes lies in hormonal processes occurring during the first trimester of prenatal life (Money & Ehrhardt, 1972). Although the differentiation of primary sex characteristics occurs at this time, other aspects of sex differentiation (such as the appearance of secondary sex characteristics at puberty) are programmed to occur later according to a developmental timetable laid down prenatally.

Does prenatal programming affect gender segregation or any of the play styles that we have claimed underlie it? Ehrhardt and Baker (1974) reported that a group of prenatally androgenized girls differed from their normal sisters in that they strongly preferred to play with boys. Studies of nonhuman primates have shown that infants and juveniles play mainly with same-sex others (Suomi, Sackett, & Harlow, 1970; and see Meany, Stewart, & Beatty, 1985, for a review). Probably this phenomenon reflects differential sensitivity on the part of males and females to certain social cues and differential responses to certain social behaviors of others. Observations by Meany and colleagues indicate that when a male makes a bid to initiate rough play, males tend to respond with aroused interest and a matching response, and females, with withdrawal. In the language of social learning theory, the two sexes find different partner behaviors to be reinforcing or aversive. Meany et al. (1985) provided substantial evidence for an organizing role of androgens present at or prior to birth in the development of these behavior patterns in primates as well as lower mammals. (What is especially interesting is that the hormonal factors do not function in the same way for rough-and-tumble play as they do for aggression.)

The probabilities are great that, for human children as well, there is a contribution of prenatal androgenization to the play styles that children display in the prepubertal years. Money and Ehrhardt (1972) were among the earliest researchers to call attention to this process and to provide evidence for it. The mediating processes are not yet understood. A number of studies indicate that males show faster rise-times, or higher levels, of emotional arousal under conditions of stress or conflict (e.g., Frankenhauser, 1982; Frankenhauser et al., 1978). In a review article, Gottman and Levenson (in press) amassed considerable evidence (from both animal and human subjects) for the hypothesis that under extreme stress males become more physiologically and behaviorally aroused and are slower to return to prestressor levels than females. Sex differences on the positive side of emotional arousal have not been systematically studied, but there is reason to suspect that males may also be more susceptible to being aroused into states of positive excitement. Marcus, Maccoby, Jacklin, and Doering (1985) have reported higher levels of happy-excited moods in boys than girls in the first 18 months of life, whereas girls' moods could more often be characterized as quiet-calm. Previously I noted the report by Charlesworth and Dzur (1987) that quartets of boys exhibited more positive affect than quartets of girls during group sessions, and similar patterns have been observed in same-sex groups of young adults (Aries, 1976). A sex difference in the lability of both positive and negative emotional responding might contribute to children finding same-sex playmates more compatible—in particular, to girls not finding a boy's rough play pleasantly exciting. We must note, however, that the tendency to engage in rough play varies considerably within sex, and many boys exhibit this behavior in the same range as girls. Furthermore, the within-sex individual differences in rough-and-tumble play are temporally stable. Thus, the pattern of gender differentiation in this behavior does not quite fit the binary pattern that we are looking for. Whatever binary biological underpinnings there may be for sex differences in play styles, they are surely modified in individual children by within-sex variations in temperament, social experience, or other factors.

A different and more distinctive role that can be assigned to biology is simply one of preparedness to learn to distinguish between persons of the two sexes. This readiness may involve low thresholds of response to certain universally available clues to gender. Studies by Fagan and colleagues (Fagan & Shepherd, 1982; Fagan & Singer, 1979) showed that infants as young as 5 months old can distinguish pictured faces according to gender, although they do not show a *preference* for faces of either gender. Clearly, the ability to make the distinction appears well before infants have the linguistic capacity to apply gender labels to themselves and others. The cognitive labeling that comes later, then, is built on a prepared base, although of course in every culture the cues used by the culture to signal gender quickly join whatever cues are species-wide to provide the basis for categorizing. Once the labeling processes are in place they have enormous importance in gender differentiation, and it is to the cognitive processes that I now turn.

Cognitive factors. I have noted that the world of human beings can be almost perfectly divided into males and females on the basis of their biological characteristics. There is a similar binary quality to the categorical distinctions that human beings make in their cognitions of others' gender. In their fourth year, most children appear to be able to apply gender labels correctly to themselves and to other children. As noted above, they can also respond differentially to the gender of others even before they are able to apply the verbal labels *boy, girl, man,* and *woman.* The implication is that any language that did not have gender terms would soon have to invent them. All known languages do have such terms, however, and children learn to apply them accurately in temporal synchrony with their acquisition of an array of sex-typed behaviors.

It has been argued that the primary sex characteristics—specifically, genital differences—are the main basis for our knowledge of our own gender and that of other persons. The developmental data do not bear this out. As noted above, infants in their first year can distinguish gender from still photos; possibly, they could do even better if they had body-movement or voice-quality information to work from as well. There are many households where people do not see one another naked, and children raised in such households are often unaware of genital differences and cannot use genital information as a basis for classifying unclothed dolls as to gender (Thompson & Bentler, 1971). Nevertheless, such children can accurately identify which other children are boys and which are girls. We do not know all the cues whereby human children signal their gender to one another. But it seems clear that the distinction is made at an early age with or without genital knowledge. It is possible that children make gender distinctions with respect to other children at a different age than they make them among adults. There is no reason why the two distinctions need be achieved at the same age, and they may not be initially joined. That is, it is possible for a young child to know that he is a boy and that his father is a man without knowing that they both belong in a larger inclusive category of males.

Once a categorical distinction has been established cognitively, it can become a powerful organizer of social functioning. In order to understand the meaning of gender or any other social category, it may be useful to consider how categories or concepts are formed. In an important article Armstrong, Gleitman, and Gleitman (1983) pointed out that there is probably more than one kind of category and more than one process whereby categories are formed. Some categories, they pointed out, are basic or core categories, and these are binary. Others are prototypical, and these are graded. Let us consider an example that Armstrong et al. offered: the concept *grandmother*. The core concept is simply defined: A grandmother is the mother of a parent. Any individual either is or is not a grandmother. The conceptual distinction is binary, and there are no variations of degree. However, we also have a prototypical definition of *grandmother*. Its cluster of attributes describes a middle-aged woman who has grey hair, is fairly small and perhaps a little plump, wears glasses, has a warm smile, and stands at the doorway with open arms. This is what we now call a fuzzy set; no one of the attributes is either necessary nor sufficient for an individual to be classified as belonging to the category. Indeed, individuals vary according to how closely they fit the prototype, and one may be more or less grandmotherly. Thus, Zsa-Zsa Gabor and Marlene Dietrich are both indubitably grandmothers in terms of their membership in the core binary category. They are not very good exemplars of the prototype, however, and would not rank very high on a scale of grandmotherliness. Lakoff (1987) pointed out that graded information is sometimes used to arrive at a probability that an individual exemplar should be assigned to a binary (core) category, but, once assigned, categorical membership need not be graded.

The suggestion here is that the concepts *male* and *female* are binary core categories, whereas the concepts *masculine* and *feminine* are fuzzy sets. One can be more or less feminine. One cannot be more or less female. Hermaphrodites are socially ascribed one gender or the other and adopt one gender identity or the other. As cognitive psychologists proceed with their work, we will no doubt achieve some better insights than we now have about how these two kinds of concepts can exist side by side and how they function jointly to mediate our reactions to people and events. An experiment on gender inferences (Gelman, Coleman, & Maccoby, 1986) sheds a little light on the issue. The items in this study were sets of three pictures such as those in Figure 1. Distinctive information was given about either familiar or unfamiliar properties of the boy and girl pictured in the top pair. For example, in one unfamiliar item, the experimenter pointed to the boy figure in the top pair and said "This boy has seeds inside"; then, pointing to the girl, "This girl has eggs inside." Then pointing to the third child (dressed like the girl above), the experimenter asked one of two different questions: either "This child has seeds inside. Is this a boy or a girl?" or "This child is a boy. Does he have seeds or eggs inside?"

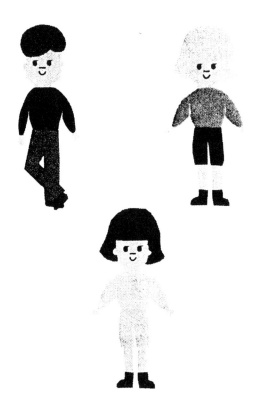

Figure 1. Sample picture set used in the Gelman, Coleman, & Maccoby (1986) study of property or category inferences.

Questions of the second kind proved to be much easier and could be answered confidently by considerably younger children than the first kind. When asked to infer gender from an attribute such as having seeds inside, young children were confused or distracted by the contradictory cues from clothing and hairstyle; when asked to infer an attribute from gender, they were not. These findings held for items with familiar content (e.g., which sex can grow up to be a daddy; which sex urinates sitting down, etc.) as well as for unfamiliar content. We interpret these findings to mean that a gender label functions as a kind of magnet, which attracts new incoming information. Thus, fuzzy sets appear to be organized around core categories, but they do not define the categories. The content of a fuzzy set changes with age and cultural experience, but this does not imply a change in the core category with which it is associated. As children grow older, they accumulate knowledge about the kinds of occupations men and women occupy, the kinds of reactions they are likely to display in a variety of situations, and, perhaps most important, the kind of exceptions there are to the modal trends in sex-linked behavior. These developmental changes can occur at the same time that children are carrying along relatively unchanged their tendency to code other persons in terms of the primitive, binary distinction between male and female persons.

We turn now to a consideration of how these categorizing processes, along with the other processes previously discussed, may affect sex-differentiated social behavior.

OVERVIEW

The socialization-personality model appears to fit children's acquisition of sex-typed attitudes and personality traits quite well. Just as socialization pressures are variable in degree, so are the outcomes in certain aspects of children's perceptions and behavior, and these gradations may be seen within a gender group as well as between the sexes.

The phenomenon of gender segregation appears to be of a different order, however. A child's choice of playmates seems to depend primarily on whether the child is a male or female child. It seems to depend very little on how masculine or feminine the child is. There is some support for the hypothesis that the separation of the sexes into distinct social groupings is based, at least in part, on their different play styles and on some asymmetries in patterns of mutual influence occurring in between-sex encounters. In this article I have suggested that, to some degree, play styles are influenced by differentiating biological processes, some of which are binary and some of which probably are not. It is not clear why play styles and influence patterns—which certainly vary in degree within as well as between sex—should feed into a binary behavior pattern (gendered choice of playmates) rather than a graded one. Perhaps avoidance of sexuality is more powerfully binary. Probably, group membership on the basis of the binary coding of gender identity is the most powerful of all. Children know unequivocally that they belong either to the group of males or the group of females, and their identity is bound up in this group membership. As Tajfel (1982) has shown, membership in a group entails many things, including attraction to in-group members, preferential treatment of them, and beliefs that the out-group is more homogeneous (and less valued) than the in-group. There is little research that compares the power of gender identity with that of other aspects of identity (e.g., race and age) in producing group identification, but one might predict that it would be very powerful between the ages of 6 and 12—perhaps more powerful than at any other time.

We have seen that young children use gender as a social category. They begin to do so at such an early age that one must be skeptical as to whether they are responding to status differences. Doubtless gender does function as a diffuse status characteristic for older children and adults. However, when 2- or 3-year-old boys and girls avoid one another as playmates, it does not seem plausible that they do this because they believe that boys are somehow more important or valued by society. Of course, the children's parents may be responding to the potential status of male children, but we have seen that young children seem to use gender as a basis for social grouping regardless of the existence of adult pressures to do so. An implication is that status characteristics accrue to gender after some of the behavioral foundations have already been laid.

In what way are the socialization pressures from adult society implicated in children's development of sex-typed behavior? The argument in this article has been that, although rewarding children for "sex-appropriate" behavior and punishing them for "inappropriate" behavior no doubt supports their acquisition of the behavioral attributes that we consider masculine or feminine, such differential reinforcement and punishment does not tell the whole story. We have argued that differentiating biological process provides some setting conditions influencing the social behavior of the two sexes. In addition, the claim is made that gender segregation (and probably other aspects of gendered social behavior as well) are *group* processes that do not depend, to any great extent, on the individual sex-typed personality characteristics developed by individual boys and girls as a result of their reinforcement histories.

"Socialization" of each new generation of children by adult society occurs not only through the direct reinforcement and punishment of individual children—the processes traditionally emphasized in psychological analyses—but through providing the raw material from which all children construct gender concepts that they then use to guide their own behavior. Processes of cognitive categorizing are powerful. It would hardly be possible to prevent children or adults from sorting and classifying incoming information on the basis of gender if there is some initial factual basis for the sorting. So long as certain occupations or certain sports, for example, really are predominantly populated by people of one gender, children will construct stereotypes that reflect these social realities. A primary way, then, in which older generations socialize upcoming generations into gender roles is by providing the exemplars that depict the appropriate social behaviors for each sex. Some of the messages transmitted to growing children are fixed by biological universals (e.g., that women give birth and men do not). Some are in a grey area where there are both biological and social elements underlying the behavior, so that societies might not be entirely free to eliminate or reverse an existing pattern but are free to modify it. Others are completely arbitrary and may change over time within a given society (e.g., whether men, women, or both should have jobs as bank tellers). Children make inferences from the culture-wide information available to them. As is well known, once the stereotypes are formed, they tend to become self-perpetuating and resistant to change even on the basis of disconfirming information.

If binary and protypical gender concepts are always available, they are not always activated (see Deaux & Major, 1987, for an analysis of conditions affecting gender salience). They can be overridden or bypassed when other available category systems are called into play. It appears likely that human beings almost automatically code the gender of any other person with whom they interact. This coding is fast and may be unconscious. The question is: How much does it matter? On some occasions and for some social purposes the gender of one's social partners can be ignored even though it has been coded. On other occasions and for other social purposes it is of the greatest importance.

There are two aspects of social cognitive development that now appear to hold some of the most interesting issues for students of sex role development. One has to do with the factors governing the activation or relevance of our gendered social categories. The other concerns children's developing understanding of the implicit rules that govern how, when, and whether cross-sex interactions may be appropriately entered into.

REFERENCES

Aries, E. (1976). Interaction patterns and themes of male, female, and mixed groups. *Small Group Behavior, 7*, 7–18.

Armstrong, S. L., Gleitman, L. R., & Gleitman, H. (1983). What some concepts might not be. *Cognition, 13*, 263–308.

Best, R. (1983). *We've all got scars: What boys and girls learn in elementary schools.* Bloomington: Indiana University Press.

Charlesworth, W. R., & Dzur, C. (1987). Gender comparisons of preschoolers' behavior and resource utilization in group problem-solving. *Child Development, 58*, 191–200.

Charlesworth, W. R., & LaFrenier, P. (1983). Dominance, friendship utilization and resource utilization in preschool children's groups. *Ethology and Sociobiology, 4*, 175–186.

Deaux, K., & Major, B. (1987). Putting gender into context: An interactive model of gender-related behavior. *Psychological Review, 94*, 369–389.

DiPietro, J. (1981). Rough and tumble play: A function of gender. *Developmental Psychology, 17*, 50–58.

Edwards, C. P., & Whiting, B. B. (1988). *Children of different worlds.* Harvard University Press.

Ehrhardt, A. A., & Baker, S. W. (1974). Fetal androgens, human central nervous system differentiation, and behavioral sex differences. In E. C. Friedman, R. M. Richart, & R. L. VandeWiele (Eds.), *Sex differences in behavior.* New York: Wiley.

Fagan, J. F., & Shepherd, P. A. (1982). Theoretical issues in the early development of visual perception. In M. Lewis & L. Taft (Eds.), *Developmental disabilities: Theory, assessment and intervention.* New York: S.P. Medical and Scientific Books.

Fagan, J. F., & Singer, L. T. (1979). The role of single feature differences in infant recognition of faces. *Infant Behavior and Development, 2,* 39–45.

Fagot, B. I. (1985). Beyond the reinforcement principle: Another step toward understanding sex roles. *Developmental Psychology, 21,* 1097–1104.

Frankenhaeuser, M. (1982). Challenge-control interaction as reflected in sympathetic-adrenal and pituitary-adrenal activity: Comparison between the sexes. *Scandinavian Journal of Psychology, 71,* 158–164.

Frankenhaeuser, M., von Wright, M. R., Collins, A., von Wright, J., Sedvall, G., & Swahn, C. G. (1978). Sex differences in psychoneuroendocrine reactions to examination stress. *Psychosomatic Medicine, 40,* 334–343.

Gelman, S. A., Coleman, P., & Maccoby, E. E. (1986). Inferring properties from categories versus inferring categories from properties: The case of gender. *Child Development, 57,* 396–404.

Goodwin, M. H. (1980). Directive-response speech sequences in girls' and boys' task activities. In S. McConnell-Ginet, R. Borker, & N. Furman (Eds.), *Women and language in literature and society* (pp. 157–173). Praeger.

Gottman, J. M., & Levenson, R. W. (in press). The social psycho-physiology of marriage. In P. Noller & M. A. Fitzpatrick (Eds.), *Perspectives on marital interaction* (pp. 182–200). Multi-lingual Matters Press.

Gottman, J. M., & Parker, J. G. (Eds.). (1987). *Conversations of friends: Speculations in affective development.* New York: Cambridge University Press.

Green, R. (1987). *The "sissy boy syndrome" and the development of homosexuality.* New Haven, CT: Yale University Press.

Hartup, W. W. (1983). Peer relations. In P. H. Mussen (Series Ed.) and E. M. Hetherington (Vol. Ed.), *Handbook of child psychology: Vol. 4. Socialization, personality, and social development* (4th ed., pp. 103–196). New York: Wiley.

Huston, A. C. (1983). Sex typing. In P. H. Mussen (Series Ed.) and E. M. Hetherington (Vol. Ed.), *Handbook of child psychology: Vol. 4. Socialization, personality, and social development* (4th ed., pp. 387–467). New York: Wiley.

Jacklin, C. N., DiPietro, J. A., & Maccoby, E. E. (1984). Sex-typing behavior and sex-typing pressure in parent-child interaction. In H. F. L. Meyer-Bahlburg (Ed.), Gender development: Social influences and prenatal hormone effects [Special Issue]. *Archives of Sexual Behavior, 13*(5).

Jacklin, C. N., & Maccoby, E. E. (1978). Social behavior at 33 months in same-sex and mixed-sex dyads. *Child Development, 49,* 557–569.

LaFreniere, P., Strayer, F. F., & Gauthier, R. (1984). The emergence of same-sex preferences among preschool peers: A developmental ethological perspective. *Child Development, 55,* 1958–1965.

Lakoff, G. (1987). *Women, fire and dangerous things.* Chicago: University of Chicago Press.

Leinbach, M. D., & Fagot, B. I. (1986). Acquisition of gender labels: A test for toddlers. *Sex Roles, 15,* 655–666.

Lockheed, M. E., (1985). Sex and social influence: A meta-analysis guided by theory. In J. Berger & M. Zeldich (Eds.), *Status, attributions, and rewards.* San Francisco: Jossey-Bass.

Lockheed, M. E., & Harris, A. M. (1984). Cross-sex collaborative learning in elementary classrooms. *American Educational Research Journal, 21,* 275–294.

Lockheed, M. E., & Klein, S. S. (1985). Sex equity in classroom organization and climate. In S. Klein (Ed.), *Handbook for achieving sex equity through education* (pp. 189–217). Baltimore, MD: John Hopkins University Press.

Luria, Z., & Herzog, E. (1985, April). *Gender segregation across and within settings.* Paper presented at the biennial meetings of the Society for Research in Child Development, Toronto, Ontario, Canada.

Maccoby, E. E., & Jacklin, C. N. (1974). *The psychology of sex differences.* Stanford, CA: Stanford University Press.

Maccoby, E. E., & Jacklin, C. N. (1987). Gender segregation in childhood. In E. H. Reese (Ed.), *Advances in child development and behavior* (Vol. 20, pp. 239–287). New York: Academic Press.

Maltz, D. N., & Borker, R. A. (1983). A cultural approach to male-female miscommunication. In J. A. Gumperz (Ed.), *Language and social identity* (pp. 195–216). New York: Cambridge University Press.

Marcus, J., Maccoby, E. E., Jacklin, C. N., & Doering, C. H. (1985). Individual differences in mood in early childhood: Their relation to gender and neonatal sex steroid. *Developmental Psychobiology, 18,* 327–340.

Meany, M. J., Stewart, J., & Beatty, W. W. (1985). Sex differences in social play: The socialization of sex roles. In J. S. Rosenblatt, C. Bear, C. M. Busnell, and P. Slater (Eds.), *Advances in study of behavior* (Vol. 15, 1–58). New York: Academic Press.

Money, J., & Ehrhardt, A. A. (1972). *Man and woman, boy and girl.* Baltimore, MD: John Hopkins University Press.

Powlishta, K. (1987, April). *The social context of cross-sex interactions.* Paper presented at the biennial meetings of the Society for Research in Child Development, Baltimore, MD.

Savin-Williams, R. C. (1979). Dominance hierarchies in groups of early adolescents. *Child Development, 50,* 923–935.

Schofield, J. W. (1981). Complementary and conflicting identities: Images of interaction in an interracial school. In S. A. Asher & J. M. Gottman (Eds.), *The development of children's friendships* (pp. 53–90). New York: Cambridge University Press.

Serbin, L. A., Sprafkin, C., Elman, M., & Doyle, A-B. (1984). The early development of sex differentiated patterns of social influence. *Canadian Journal of Social Science, 14*(4), 350–363.

Serbin, L. A., Tonick, I. V., & Sternglanz, S. (1977). Shaping cooperative cross-sex play. *Child Development, 48,* 924–929.

Suomi, S. J., Sackett, G. P., & Harlow, H. F. (1970). Development of sex preferences in rhesus monkeys. *Developmental Psychology, 3,* 326–336.

Tajfel, H. (1982). Social psychology of intergroup relations. *Annual Review of Psychology, 33,* 1–39.

Thompson, S. K. (1975). Gender labels and early sex role development. *Child Development, 46,* 339–347.

Thompson, S. K., & Bentler, P. M. (1971). The priority of cues in sex discrimination by children and adults. *Developmental Psychology, 5,* 181–185.

Thorne, B. (1986). Girls and boys together, but mostly apart. In W. W. Hartup & Z. Rubin (Eds.), *Relationship and development* (pp. 167–184). Hillsdale, NJ: Erlbaum.

Thorne, B. (1987, February). *Children and gender: Construction of difference.* Paper presented at conference on Theoretical Perspectives on Sexual Difference, Stanford University, Stanford, CA.

Webb, N. M., & Kenderski, C. M. (1985). Gender differences in small-group interaction and achievement in high- and low-achieving classes. In L. C. Wilkinson & C. B. Marrett (Eds.), *Gender influence in classroom interaction* (pp. 209–236). New York: Academic Press.

Williamson, L. (1986). *Individual differences in preschoolers' gender segregation and sex-typed play.* Unpublished manuscript, Department of Psychology, Stanford University.

10

Race and Gender as Psychological Variables: Social and Ethical Issues

Sandra Scarr

University of Virginia, Charlottesville

No one doubts that race and gender are sensitive issues in psychological research, so sensitive that many investigators try to hide such variation under the general rubric of research on children or social class or parenting practices, all of which are well-known to vary by race and gender. Rare is the investigator who highlights racial or gender variation as a major thrust of the research because the ratio of excess baggage to payoff is very high. If one purposely examines racial or gender variation in psychology, one is likely to be suspected of reactionary politics or malevolence toward socially disadvantaged groups. Such is the social setting for research on gender and racial differences.

On the other hand, many researchers who conduct psychological studies analyze their data by race and gender as a seeming afterthought. By including samples of Blacks and Whites, males and females, one may seem to aim toward representative sampling. As an innocent byproduct of the research, one may inadvertently find that women score lower, are more vulnerable, or are less efficient than men at some behavior, but one is not often blamed for what appears to be serendipity. Or one might find that Blacks are less effective at

Reprinted with permission from *American Psychologist,* 1988, Vol. 43, No. 1, 56–59. Copyright 1988 by the American Psychological Association.

This article is based on a paper presented at the annual meeting of the American Psychological Association, Los Angeles, August 26, 1983. I wish to express my thanks to the following individuals who have shaped my thinking, even if we do not always agree: Richard A. Weinberg, who has shared the dangerous journey into research on racial differences; Arthur R. Jensen, who dared to hypothesize the unacceptable; Wendell R. Garner, who braved teaching and writing on racial issues in psychological testing; Robert J. Sternberg, who has kept his head and his integrity about testing; and Janice Hale-Benson and Melvin Wilson, members of a new generation of Black investigators and colleagues. There are others I would like to derogate for their attempts to suppress scientific inquiry, but that would be unbecoming in so public a forum. Moreover, recriminations recall the many unpleasantnesses that I should perhaps forgive but not forget.

solving some task and report the results without premeditation because one allegedly was not aware that race and gender would be issues in the research results. By just following rigorous research protocol, one happened to find racial or gender differences lurking in the results.

Of course, this is mostly subterfuge because good psychologists are aware of the enormous research literatures on race differences on nearly every behavioral measure and gender differences on many measures. Somehow, by not seeming to be aware, by not planning studies based on these dangerous variables, and by not incorporating them into the design, one may appear to be exonerated from any blame for outcomes that demonstrate racial or gender differences, especially those that seem unfavorable to minorities and women. Unfortunately, I think, just the reverse is true. By not asking direct questions about the nature and origins of racial and gender differences in behavior, researchers have failed to investigate the strengths of underrepresented[1] groups and failed to assess their ways of functioning well. Ignorance of the importance of racial and gender differences in this society has not served those very groups that many investigators believed they were protecting.

In this article, I argue that cowardice about minority and gender differences in research will lead us nowhere. There should be no qualms about the forthright study of racial and gender differences; science is in desperate need of good studies that highlight race and gender variables, unabashedly, to inform us of what we need to do to help underrepresented people to succeed in this society. Unlike the ostrich, we cannot afford to hide our heads for fear of socially uncomfortable discoveries.

A PERSONAL HISTORY

For those of us who have incorporated race into research designs, there is great danger in the outcome. If one deliberately sets out to investigate racial or gender differences that have unfavorable possibilities for the underdog, one is in danger of ostracism and worse from one's socially well-intentioned colleagues. The messenger with the bad news seems to be blamed for having invented the message. Consider the following quote from my own work (Scarr, 1981):

> I acknowledge that questions of genetic differences fascinated me because they loomed at me from the darkness, and I decided not to be afraid to ask them. This was a very personal and political decision.

---

[1]The term *underrepresented* is used here to connote both political powerlessness and sparse representation in scientific inquiry. Both matter.

Once I had decided to study genetic differences in human behavior, however, I tried to frame the questions in ways that could reveal the "true" nature of the human condition. That is, I was prepared to accept whatever results were obtained by the scrupulous exercise of the greatest objectivity I could manage. As my friends know, I was prepared to emigrate if the blood-grouping study had shown a substantial relationship between African ancestry and low intellectual skills. I had decided that I could not endure what Jensen had experienced at the hands of colleagues. (pp. 524–525)

It is doubtless well known that from 1969 to the 1980s Arthur Jensen was harassed, threatened, and driven virtually into protective custody by colleagues, students, and other radicals who resented his hypothesis that Blacks may be genetically inferior to others in intelligence. By marshaling the hundreds of observations that Blacks in the United States do not perform as well as Whites and other ethnic groups on IQ tests, academic achievement tests, and occupational selection measures, Jensen made an interpretation of the results. His hypothesis so inflamed and alarmed some others that he became a prime target for unconscionable abuse in public and in private.

I concluded that the abusive treatment directed toward Jensen would not deter me from asking dangerous questions about the nature of racial differences in intelligence, but I was not naive about the potential reactions of colleagues, students, and others to possible results. To continue my quotation (Scarr, 1981):

> Neither Rich Weinberg nor I was prepared to discover that adolescents at the end of the child-rearing period bear so little resemblance to those with whom they have lived for so many years. We were dismayed by the obvious implications of the adolescent adoption study for the nature of social class differences.
>
> Perhaps even more telling is our experience with the transracial adoption study. In this case we did anticipate the result that black and interracial children reared in the culture of the tests and the schools would perform better on tests and in school than black children reared in the black community.
>
> The major point of all this personal history is to say that I have always tried to frame questions in such ways that my hypotheses could be falsified. . . . The black and interracial children could have had low IQ scores; the adolescent adoptees could (and did) bear little resemblance to their families of rearing; the black twins could have performed worse on more "culture-fair" than "culture-

loaded" tests . . . the black children with more African ancestry
could have performed worse on the intellectual tasks. Surely, I had
personal and political reasons for pursuing such questions, but the
results could have proved me wrong, and did in some cases.
(p. 525)

Before launching the several research studies on racial and social class differences, I was aware that the results could come out "wrong" from a political point of view. This is a risk in all honest research. Only dishonest
investigators can promise that the results of their investigations will hew to
any party line, but I believed then and believe now that only by asking fair
questions and seeking honest answers can one make a contribution to science
and to one's society. Issues of social disadvantage are dangerous questions, but
they are not trivial.

VALUE CONTEXTS FOR RESEARCH

The personal values that investigators bring to their studies and that lead
them to ask questions about race and gender make great differences in how
they will perceive their results. Investigators frame questions based on their
own preconceptions about the world. The positive or negative value attached
to particular observations is often very much in the eye of the beholder (Scarr,
1985). Research investigators must be aware of the values they bring to the
framing of research questions.

If questions about minorities and women are framed in terms of what is
wrong with, deficient about, or needs improvement for these underrepresented
groups, then the research outcomes for such groups are very likely to be negative. If the standard for good behavior is always the white male group, then
the behavior of women and ethnic minorities is likely to seem negative. If
being reared in a single-parent family (whose members also happen to be poor,
badly educated, and housed in slums) is correlated with negative outcomes
for children, then more Black children than White children appear to show
deficits. If being more concerned with primary relationships than with universal principles of morality is called inferior, then women on average appear
deficient.

If, on the other hand, one asks how women actually solve mathematical
problems, how Black males learn to read, or how children of lower socioeconomic status (SES) get jobs, one may actually learn how to help others to use
socially and culturally available means to succeed in the society.

Unfortunately, there is very little research on the strengths of underrepresented groups in the social science literature because mainstream investigators

have either not had the value perspectives to generate the questions or because they have been frightened by the consequences of getting "wrong" answers. Minority investigators who could frame more positive questions about women and racial groups have had little impact until recently.

Even when the answers to research questions turn out to be politically palatable to the majority of social scientists, others object to inferences that investigators draw from the results and call for censorship. In response to the transracial adoption study (Scarr & Weinberg, 1976), which found that Black and interracial children adopted by White, middle-class families performed very well on IQ and school achievement tests, Oden and MacDonald (1978) said that they largely approved of the research questions, design, and methods but objected to the implications of the study. The high achievement of Black children reared in White families, they felt, was derogatory to the Black community. They called for censorship of authors' discussions of their results to protect what they perceived to be minority interests. Both authors and editors are unethical, they implied, if they publish articles that do not take minority perspectives on research results into account.

In our reply (Scarr & Weinberg, 1978), we argued for the competition of ideas in a free press and reminded readers that minorities and advocates for minorities calling for such censorship now were the same groups who had been denied their Constitutional rights just a few years before. Studies of socially sensitive issues often evoke ethical criticism no matter what their outcomes. Ought psychologists then to include group interests as part of their ethical concerns?

INDIVIDUALS AND GROUPS

To protect underrepresented groups in research, a crucial distinction must be made, and has rightly been made, between potential damage to individual participants in research and potential damage to individuals by virtue of their membership in disfavored groups. The former threat to individual participants in research is carefully covered in the many regulations of the Department of Health and Human Services (DHHS) that protect the health, safety, and civil rights of individuals who consent to participate in biobehavioral research. The latter threat to individuals' reputations as members of a disfavored group is *not* protected by such regulations because to do so would require censorship of research proposals and selective reporting of research results.

I will not detail here the extensive protection of individual participants in research, as these regulations apply to everyone. Rather, I will describe the controversy over the lack of protection given the reputations of human subjects to whom research results about ethnicity or gender may bring personal discomfort and even potential personal or professional discredit. A fundamental difference in the nature of the research threat to individuals and group members must be recognized.

One can be physically and psychologically damaged by participation in research that threatens one's health, safety, or welfare, especially if one is not fully informed of the probable consequences of participation. Invasive surgical treatments, experimental drugs, painful shock, and public humiliation are examples of such threats. Procedures that are dangerous to individual participants in research are scrutinized carefully by institutional review boards (IRBs), which are justifiably concerned about the protection of human participants in research. Few today doubt that IRB review is a good and necessary safeguard for individuals.

Potential embarrassment to one's group(s), however, is not protected by IRB regulations for very good reasons. One cannot be said to be *individually* damaged by research that exposes one's group to criticism or derogation however psychologically painful the implications might seem to be. Although many advocated protection of groups in ethical standards under consideration by the American Association for the Advancement of Science (AAAS), the DHHS, and the American Psychological Association (APA), it became very clear that to do so would infringe on investigators' freedom of speech and retard inquiry into pressing social problems. The distinction between individual and group protection is crucial to maintaining the civil liberties of investigators because they cannot determine in advance what outcome the research will yield.

Proximal Responsibility

Investigators cannot be held responsible for politically unfavorable outcomes of their research because only dishonest research can guarantee results that the majority of social scientists will applaud. Some badly kept secrets in psychological research on peer and parent-child relations, for example, concern the pervasive effects of intelligence on many aspects of social life. On the average, bright children have better relations with peers (and teachers and parents) than less bright children, and bright parents are on average less abusive and more supportive of their bright children than less intelligent parents of their less bright children (Scarr, in press). These results lurk in the background of many studies because to report them would be unpopular. Investigators who do report their results in unpopular frameworks are likely to be criticized by colleagues. But whose fault is it if measures of general intelligence better explain social relations than other measures?

Investigators are also not responsible for use of their data for others' political ends. As an AAAS report (Edsall, 1975) on the rights and responsibilities of research investigators concludes, there are many examples of scientists who could not have anticipated the evil uses that were made of their research results. The development of nuclear weapons is only one of many possible examples. Researchers in the area of aversive conditioning did not anticipate its use in physical control of political prisoners in the third world. Sleep researchers did not anticipate the role of their research in brain washing or cult indoctrination. I conclude that unanticipated (and unanticipatable) consequences of research cannot be held against the investigators. But there are predictable consequences of one's research results toward which one should act responsibly.

If an investigator chooses to study race or gender as part of a research design, it is incumbent upon the researcher to consider the most likely, proximal uses of the data and to explain where she or he stands on the major issues. Research on women's math abilities, on racial differences in IQ, and on differences in occupational achievements by race and social class are examples for which investigators have, in my opinion, responsibilities to interpret their data clearly, according to what they believe the results to mean.

This is not to say that the investigator's interpretation must meet any political test: That is, the investigator may choose to interpret the data in a way that is largely unacceptable to the participants and to the larger research community. It takes courage to do so, and in many cases it is justified for the advancement of discussions in science. But I believe that any investigator of socially sensitive issues has the responsibility to spell out what he or she makes of the results. Similarly, others who have different interpretations of the results have the freedom and responsibility to say so. Science must operate with free inquiry, free discussion, and the competition of ideas.

THE APA POSITION

Ethical Principles in the Conduct of Research with Human Participants (APA, 1982) devotes its last page to investigators' responsibilities to protect research participants from harm by virtue of their membership in disfavored groups. In my view, the issue is dealt with badly. According to Point 9 on Confidentiality of Information About the Participant's Valued Groups,

> Sometimes a problem of confidentiality involves the individual participant's valued groups. The concept of betraying confidentiality "by category" arises when research reveals things that may be seen as degrading these groups.

This issue presents the investigator with a severe value conflict. On one side is an obligation to research participants who may not wish to see derogatory information (in whose validity they will probably not believe) published about their valued groups. On the other side is an obligation to publish findings one believes relevant to scientific progress, an objective that in the investigator's view will contribute to the eventual understanding and amelioration of social and personal problems.

Such value conflicts can sometimes be resolved before a problem arises. When the problem may be anticipated before the data are collected, the investigator will be wise to include information about potential uses of the data in the explanation provided to the potential research participants at the time of their recruitment to the study. The participants may then give informed and uncoerced consent to participate, knowing in advance that there may be unpalatable items among the research outcomes. The issue, in fact, is conceived better perhaps as one of informed consent not as one of confidentiality.

To make this suggestion is not to diminish the magnitude of the dilemma under consideration. The investigator must be constantly aware that many potential topics of study are emotionally and politically explosive. Just as investigators are sensitive to their scientific responsibilities, they must also be sensitive to the social, political, and human implications of the interpretations that others might place upon this research once the findings have been published. (p. 74)

In *Ethical Principles in the Conduct of Research* (APA, 1982) the issue of harm to one's valued groups was evidently found to be exceedingly difficult to include in the directives. The issue was left to the very last page and was dealt with ambiguously. It was merely stated that investigators may feel some value conflicts about informed consent that does or does not include statements about the potential of possible results to cause embarrassment to the participants' valued groups.

Although these principles cover the possibility of research that produces embarrassing results about the valued groups to which individuals belong, the placement of this topic under the rubric of confidentiality is misguided. In fact, the statement that "the issue, in fact, is conceived better perhaps as one of informed consent not as one of confidentiality" acknowledges part of the problem. The problem is not really one of individual confidentiality but of having information published that seems to reflect badly on one's valued groups.

What protection is offered? The advice is to inform one's research participants of the possibly unfavorable outcomes for *all* groups to which they may belong. Imagine saying to potential participants in a research study on stress and hypertension that the results of this study may prove embarrassing to them because of their membership in such groups as men, aging adults, Black Americans, New Yorkers, residents in high-rise buildings, gay rights activists, Christian fundamentalists, the Ladies Garment Workers Union, and so forth. Is this realistic? Can we categorize our research participants by every group to which they pay dues or have psychological membership? I think not.

OVERPROTECTION

Protection of research participants by virtue of their membership in disfavored groups is creeping into the IRB system (Ceci, Peters, & Plotkin, 1985) despite explicit instructions to IRBs that such considerations are irrelevant. IRBs' reactions to socially sensitive research that proposed to study positive racial and gender discrimination and reverse discrimination were found to be quixotic and often contrary to DHHS regulations under which IRBs operate. Ceci and his colleagues documented that IRBs disapprove such proposals at a much higher rate than more neutral proposals. More than half were disapproved, although they met ethical guidelines for IRBs.

The reasons given by the IRBs for disapproval were often stunningly candid and openly defiant of DHHS regulations. Even though socially sensitive proposals contained no ethical violations, as defined by the DHHS regulations, their approval rate was lower than that of other proposals with explicit ethical violations. Thus, IRBs seem to be acting *in loco parentis* for disfavored groups, preventing research on socially sensitive issues that they fear may have results that could damage the reputations of such groups.

In my opinion, noblesse oblige has no place in psychology. Misguided protectionism both violates investigators rights and prevents psychology from developing research information that could help members of disadvantaged groups to achieve what they want within this society. We need more research by more investigators on more topics of real social use to disfavored groups, including groups defined explicitly by race and gender.

REFERENCES

American Psychological Association. (1982). *Ethical principles in the conduct of research with human participants.* Washington, DC: Author.

Ceci, S. J., Peters, D., & Plotkin, J. (1985). Human subjects review, personal values, and the regulation of social science research. *American Psychologist, 40,* 994–1002.

Edsall, J. (1975). *Scientific freedom and responsibility: A report of the AAAS Committee on Scientific Freedom and Responsibility.* Washington, DC: American Association for the Advancement of Science.

Oden, C. W., Jr., & MacDonald, W. S. (1978). The RIP in social scientific reporting. *American Psychologist, 33,* 952–957.

Scarr, S. (1981). *Race, social class and individual differences in IQ.* Hillsdale, NJ: Erlbaum.

Scarr, S. (1985). Constructing psychology: Making facts and fables for our times. *American Psychologist, 40,* 499–512.

Scarr, S. (in press). Protecting general intelligence: Constructs and consequences for intervention. In P. R. Laughlin (Ed.), *Intelligence: Measurement, theory, and public policy.* Champagne-Urbana: University of Illinois Press.

Scarr, S., & Weinberg, R. A. (1976). IQ test performance of black children adopted by white families. *American Psychologist, 31,* 726–739.

Scarr, S., & Weinberg, R. A. (1978). The rights and responsibilities of the social scientist. *American Psychologist, 33,* 955–957.

Part IV

SPECIAL STRESS AND COPING

The papers in this section examine the impact of a wide range of adverse circumstances on the development of the children exposed to them. In the first paper, Pynoos and Nader describe the clinical characteristics of 10 children between the ages of 5 and 17 years who have witnessed sexual assaults of their mothers. In the best tradition of clinical research, they include compelling clinical vignettes along with quantitative ratings of interview responses. Although there were differences in severity of reaction, all 10 children met DSM-III criteria for Post-Traumatic Stress Disorder. Symptoms included disturbances in aggression and sexuality, alterations in sense of security and vulnerability, challenged self-esteem, as well as stress in intrafamilial and peer relationships and changes in orientation towards the future. Although the sample was small, the age and sex of witnesses appeared related to the particular constellation of symptom expression in individual children, suggesting that developmental and gender issues need to be considered in the planning of special therapeutic interventions for families with members who have been victims of sexual assault.

In the second paper in this section, the focus shifts from a consideration of the impact of a specific traumatic stressor to the examination of what has been commonly characterized as chronic strain on the developmental course. Monroe Blum, Boyle, and Offord have used survey data deriving from the Ontario Child Health Study, an interview survey of 1,869 families including 3,294 children, to determine the prevalence and epidemiology of mental and physical health problems in Ontario children, to examine the association between single-parent family status and child psychiatric disorder and poor school performance. Children of single-parent families were at a small but statistically significant increased risk for poor outcome. However, a significantly greater number of single-parent families also experienced severe economic and social hardship. When variables indicative of hardship, such as poverty and family dysfunction, are controlled for, the relationship between single-parent family status and childhood psychiatric disorder and poor school performance becomes statistically nonsignificant. The data of this study add an epidemiologic perspective to the results of numerous more fine-grained analyses of the impact of family disruption on children (see sections on divorce in the 1984 and 1986 volumes of *Annual Progress*). However, as the authors are careful to point out, it is not economic disadvantage alone that puts children at increased risk for disorder. Single parents often have major conflicting responsibilities, having to balance care of children with the generation of family income. Nevertheless, it should be realized that given adequate financial support, many single-parent families appear to manage quite well. Efforts directed to insuring adequate financial resources for custodial parents will facilitate the functioning of single-parent families.

The study by Block, Block, and Gjerde examines the impact of divorce from yet another vantage point. This report, which utilized a Q-sort method to assess family functioning, derives from the study of 101 families enrolled when the index child was between 3 and 4 years of age, and followed until he or she reached 14–15 years. The data are analyzed both prospectively and concurrently. Although generalization from the findings of this study is limited somewhat because of curtailment in the size of sub-groups, certain trends are clearly apparent. The subset of intact families in which divorce eventually occurred was characterized by unsupportive parenting of children and interparental tension long before the formal dissolution of the marriage, with strains between parents and sons relatively greater than between parents and daughters. Concurrent analyses indicate that divorced mothers establish relationships that are warm, intimate, even sisterly with their daughters, while they seem to have lost parental authority in their relationships with their sons. Lack of prospective data on families eventually experiencing divorce has resulted in confusion between the causes and consequences of the dissolution of families. This study fills an important gap in our understanding of the complex relationships among divorce, family functioning, and child development.

The next paper in this section considers stress of an entirely different kind. Fritz and Williams have assessed the adjustment of 41 adolescent survivors of childhood cancer who were recruited as part of a larger prospective study of the effects of cancer treatment termination some two to eight years previously. The findings indicate that a majority of adolescents are able to integrate the cancer experience without major distortion in their development. Although the global adjustment of one-fourth of the sample was considered to be marginal or poor, frank depression was uncommon and self-concept scores were higher than normative values. The statistical data is augmented by illustrative case examples. The authors emphasize that the psychosocial impact of cancer survival in the adolescent age group is both complex and unpredictable. However, the finding that serious psychological toll is by no means inevitable, is yet another example of human resiliency in the face of stress, and underscores the limitations of generalizations developed from the study of a psychiatrically referred population.

The impact of chronic disease on children's relationships is the topic of the critical review authored by Lobato, Faust, and Spirito. The authors set the stage with a brief summary of the literature on typical sibling relationships, followed by an examination of studies comparing siblings of healthy and ill children. To date, studies have been confined to a narrow range of issues, the most prominent being the detection of maladjustment. The review summarizes the methodological weakness of available studies which have led to the popular assumption that siblings of handicapped and seriously ill children are at increased risk of psychological disturbance. The authors propose a model for the selection of variables to govern future research in this important area, emphasizing the need for studies which are multifactorial in design in order to capture the complexity of the impact of serious illness on all family members.

The final paper by Fritz, Williams, and Amylon extends the study of the psychosocial sequelae in pediatric cancer survivors discussed above, to the examination of the varied coping strategies employed by the children and their families. Communication patterns during treatment were most predictive of psychosocial outcome, and measures of medical severity were least predictive. The coping patterns of individuals who were rated as well adjusted, free of depression, successful at school, and popular with friends were very different. While some well-adjusted survivors had become experts and advocates, others encapsulated the illness and acknowledged it as little as possible. Assertiveness and argumentativeness were as compatible with good outcome as were compliance and passivity. Some survivors were concrete and nonphilosophical about their illness and its consequences; others attributed a larger meaning or purpose to their experiences. Some used hospital resources extensively; others preferred to avoid all but essential services. The authors emphasize the need for those working with victims of cancer to be aware that there is no common path to health, and that families who express no interest in psychosocial interventions are not necessarily "resistant." The successful conclusion of cancer treatment may be associated with psychological gains in the absence of professional assistance.

11

Children Who Witness the Sexual Assaults of Their Mothers

Robert S. Pynoos and Kathi Nader

Neuropsychiatric Institute, Los Angeles, California

This paper examines the traumatic responses of 10 children who witnessed the sexual assaults of their mothers and presents five case examples. With the use of a specialized parent questionnaire, interview format, and reaction index, researchers found that the children exhibited prominent post-traumatic stress disorder symptoms, disturbances in aggression and sexuality, alterations in their sense of security and vulnerability, challenged self-esteem, stress in intrafamilial and peer relationships, and changes in future orientation. These reactions are similar to those of sexually abused children and indicate that child witnesses need special therapeutic attention.

Clinical research has delineated many traumatic characteristics that develop in children who have been sexually assaulted. Recent clinical studies have noted the similarity between these symptoms and those of post-traumatic stress disorder (PTSD) (Frederick, 1986; Goodwin, 1985; Green, 1985). In addition, disturbances in sexuality have been noted, including repetitive masturbation; compulsive sex play; and sexual knowledge, interests, and behaviors that are not age appropriate (Finkelhor, 1984). Other children have exhibited a set of avoidant-type behaviors (Frederick, 1986). Although the symptoms of assaulted children have been examined extensively, the reactions of those who witness sexual assaults have been overlooked.

The authors have been investigating the reactions of children who witness varying acts of violence. This preliminary study of those who witness sexual assault examines, clinically and statistically, the post-traumatic sequelae of 10

Reprinted with permission from the *Journal of the American Academy of Child and Adolescent Psychiatry*, 1988, Vol. 27, No. 5, 567–572. Copyright 1988 by the American Academy of Child and Adolescent Psychiatry.

children who witnessed the assaults of their mothers. Specific symptomatology, prominent sexual and aggressive behavior, gender and sexual role differences, the influence of intrafamilial and peer relationships, and the postrape milieu are described.

In 1984, there were over 84,000 reported rapes outside of marriage in the United States (Center for Disease Control, 1985), and rape is an underreported crime by as much as a 10 to 1 ratio. In Los Angeles County, the Sheriff's sexual assault investigators estimated that of the rapes that occur in the home (approximately 40%), a child is present as often as 50% of the time and directly views the assault in approximately 10% of reported cases (personal communication, Sgt. Beth Dickerson, Chair, California Association of Sexual Assault Investigators).

The children in this report ranged from 5 to 17 years old, including eight school-age children and two adolescents. There were seven boys and three girls, predominantly from white, middle-class families, with one white and two black families from lower socioeconomic levels. The cases were referred by rape crisis centers or hotlines, victim witness assistance programs, and mental health professionals.

The incidents frequently lasted over an hour and included attempted sexual assault, forced penetration, and oral copulation. In half the cases, the children's mothers were raped at knife-point. In seven cases, they were threatened with harm to their children, and in two, the child was threatened directly. In five cases, the children were made to watch, and in all other cases they were present at some point.

CASE EXAMPLES

Five cases representing seven children, of school, preadolescent, and adolescent ages, are described briefly below, with an emphasis on each child's experience or view of the rape. All described their experiences as profoundly frightening.

Case I: School-Age Girl

A rapist entered through the screen window of an 8-year-old girl's room. In the parent's bedroom, he subdued and bound the father and began to sexually assault the mother. The child awakened and entered the hallway, seeing the rape through the open bedroom door. The rapist then dragged the mother into the hallway where she tried to fight him off, while the child continued to watch.

The child later reported that at a friend's house, a few days before the rape, she had seen part of a pornographic movie showing multiple rapes, which her friend's brother was watching on the VCR. The intrusive images of her mother's rape and the pornographic film combined to give her a continued feeling of vulnerability. She was afraid to let her parents know she had seen this film, especially after the rape, and felt extremely burdened by this secret.

Case II: School-Age Boy

In another case, a 7-year-old boy was awakened by his mother's screams. He found her pinned down by a man who had recently become a friend of his father. The man told him to return to bed, and the frightened boy obeyed. After again hearing his mother scream to him for help, he ran to the kitchen for a knife and attempted to throw it at the rapist, who then picked him up and threw him against the floor. The boy felt for his back, fearing that it was broken. After the rapist threatened him, the boy went back to bed. He came out later and found his mother dead with her hands tied above her head. He ran for the landlord. His eyewitness testimony was critical to the assailant's conviction.

The child focused on the blood on his mother's nose and on the wall but had no recall of seeing her slit throat. Although he remembered that she was naked from the waist down, he did not want to think of what else the rapist might have done to her. He was afraid that the knife that he had thrown at the man had been used to kill her.

Case III: School-Age Boy and Preadolescent Girl

At 3 A.M., a divorced mother was awakened and raped by a stranger. Her seven-year-old son, who earlier had wandered into her room and was sleeping next to her, was awakened when the man began to rape her. The rapist had the mother bring her 11-year-old daughter into the room, threatening to rape the daughter if it wasn't "good enough" for him with the mother. He repeatedly raped the woman over a long period of time. When he demanded fellatio, the mother said that she would throw up if she did it. He threatened her, saying, "If you do [throw up], you don't know what will happen to you."

The mother described the children as shaking and holding her hands. She sang to them during the assault, and tried to calm them by telling them several times that the rapist was their father. On occasions when she screamed, the children cried and loudly begged the man to stop. At other times, the mother tried to entice him in order to keep him away from her daughter. He did force the daughter to touch his genitals, and she asked, "How could my daddy want me to do that? He never wanted me to do it before."

After approximately an hour and a half of raping the mother, the man began to cry, calling himself a coward. The mother said, "You are not a coward only if you go and leave us intact.'' As he moved toward them, the daughter began to scream with panic. He finally tucked them into bed and left. Although the mother could only remember that the man was approximately 6 feet tall and potbellied, the children were able to describe him in detail to the police.

Case IV: Preadolescent and Adolescent Boys

In the very early hours of the morning, while an 11-year-old boy lay half asleep on the couch in his mother's bedroom, a rapist wearing a ski mask (who was later discovered to have committed multiple rapes and murders), entered through the unlocked sliding glass door. He pushed the boy lightly with his foot, then went to the bed where the mother slept, held a knife out as though to strike, put it away and then forcibly penetrated her. The boy observed the man withdraw and ejaculate on the mother.

He continued to watch, dazed, while his mother then kicked her assailant, flinging him across the room. In the ensuing struggle, the rapist threw her into the fireplace. The woman, a nurse, thought he appeared drugged. She ordered him not to use the knife and to leave. She hit him with the fire poker after which the man fled. The boy's 17-year-old brother was awakened by the noise and entered the room just as the assailant was leaving. The boy gave his 17-year-old brother a knife, telling him to chase the rapist, then telephoned neighbors and the police, and ran for a paper bag for his hyperventilating mother. He reportedly vomited later when he found out that the odor persisting in the room was that of semen.

Case V: Adolescent Boy

On a school night, while a 17-year-old boy watched television, a delivery man known to his mother appeared at the door asking to use the phone. Once inside, the man grabbed the mother from behind and hit her with the phone. He then pulled out a knife, severely cutting her several times, and attempted to rape her. Hearing her screams, the boy came running into the study and found the man struggling with her on the floor and yelling demeaning remarks at her. He banged the assailant over the head with a chair but lost his footing. When he saw that the man had a knife, he ran to the kitchen for two knives. He then yelled at his 11-year-old brother to lock himself in the bathroom, returned to the study, and attacked the man. He reported that it took all of his energy to put one knife into the man's back. They began to fight, while his mother escaped, and then the man disarmed the boy and fled. The police arrived and at first drew their guns on the young man, ordering him to "drop the knives" he still held. He froze, dropped them, and then yelled at the police to catch the man, who was driving off in a van. They did, and the man was arrested. The boy was treated for lacerations and bruises. His mother required extensive surgery and rehabilitation to regain the use of one hand that had been seriously cut. She was unable to return to work for months.

Clinical Evaluations

Clinical data were obtained directly from parents and children. The parents were administered a special child post-trauma questionnaire and a behavioral checklist. The children were engaged in a semistructured interview to examine thoroughly their experience of the rape and to identify any resulting symptomatology and efforts at coping (Pynoos and Eth, 1986).

INSTRUMENT

Post-Traumatic Stress Reaction Index

The Post-Traumatic Stress Reaction Index is a 20-item scale patterned after criteria for PTSD, as described in *DSM-III*. It has been used to assess symptoms after exposure to a broad range of traumatic events (Frederick, 1985). An earlier version was employed with children in such samples as the Three Mile Island Nuclear Accident (Tokuhata et al., in press), the San Ysidro Massacre (Lipson and Pubner, 1985), a sniper attack on a school yard in south central Los Angeles (Pynoos et al., 1987), and in cases of child sexual molestation and child physical abuse (Frederick, 1986). In this study, the children's reactions were evaluated based on parent and child interviews, using a revised school-age version of the index, with a new frequency rating scale.

The total number of symptoms a child reported at the time of the interview was recorded as his or her reaction index score. Empirical comparisons of reaction index scores with independent clinical assessments for severity levels of PTSD resulted in these guidelines: a score of 12 to 24 indicates a mild level of PTSD: 25 to 39 a moderate level; 40 to 59, severe; and >60, very severe (Frederick, 1985). With these guidelines, correlation of reaction index scores with confirmed clinical cases of PTSD was reported as 0.95 with adults and 0.91 with children (Frederick, 1985).

In a study of children under sniper fire using the Reaction Index, the authors tested for differences between raters in reaction index scores; no significant differences were found in mean scores, and the same relative differences were

TABLE 1. *Reaction Index Scores for Child Witnesses to Sexual Assault by Age (Ascending Order) and Sex*

Sex[a]	Age	Reaction Index Scores
M	5	48
M	6	51
M	7	48
M	7	50
F	8	48
F	11	55
M	11	40
F	12	52
M	17	45
M	17	37

[a] M = male; F = female.

Table 1. Reaction Index Scores for Child Witnesses to Sexual Assault by Age (Ascending Order) and Sex

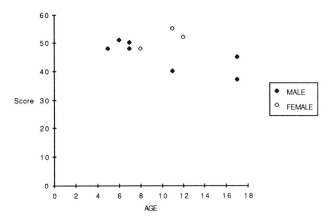

Figure 1. Reaction Index scores by age.

found in reaction index scores between exposure levels. Ten children were re-interviewed within 1 week by a different rater without the prior knowledge of either interviewers or child. For the Reaction Index Items, inter-item agreement for the two raters was 94%. Cohen's kappa was 0.878 (Pynoos et al., 1987).

Analysis

The children were examined for differences in their reaction index scores by age. The Pearson Product Moment Correlation was obtained using BMDP6D. Table 1 lists the percentage endorsing each index item. Although the sample was too small to examine differences by sex satisfactorily, Figure 1 displays the differences in scores by age and sex.

RESULTS

Reaction Index

Reaction index scores ranged from 37 to 55 (Table 1), with a mean score of 47.4. Nine of the 10 children exhibited severe, and one moderate, PTSD. Pearson R was -0.51, indicating that as age increased symptoms decreased. The correlation was not significant, however, for this small a sample.

Examination of the reaction index scores by sex and age suggested the following trends (Fig. 1): (a) For children ages 5 to 8, scores were similar; and (b) For children over 10, scores decreased for males and increased for females.

Table 2 examines individual symptoms. Seventy to one hundred percent of the children reported the following symptoms at least every other day:

	% Endorsing Each Item, at 2 Frequencies		Group Mean[a,b]	SD
	At Least Every Other Day	At Least Once per Week		
Identifies event as extreme stressor	100	100	3.5	0.167
Afraid when thinks of event	90	100	3.4	0.221
Tense or upset in response to reminders	70	100	3.0	0.258
Intrusive images and sounds	70	90	2.8	0.291
Avoids reminders	80	80	2.8	0.359
Decreased interest in activities	80	90	2.7	0.213
Avoids knowing own feelings	60	80	2.7	0.367
Fears repeat of event	60	90	2.6	0.267
Reduced impulse control	70	80	2.6	0.400
Intrusive thoughts	60	90	2.5	0.224
More jumpy or nervous (startles)	50	80	2.3	0.260
Feels alone inside	40	80	2.2	0.360
Dreams of event/other bad dreams	30	80	2.1	0.233
Sleep disturbance	30	70	2.0	0.314
Feels guilty	30	70	2.0	0.365
Regression	40	80	2.0	0.365
Difficulty paying attention	30	70	1.8	0.291
Somatic complaints	10	70	1.7	0.260
Too upset to talk or cry	30	50	1.5	0.401
Thoughts of event interfere with learning	10	30	1.1	0.314

[a] Scale: 4, most of the time; 3, much of the time; 2, some of the time; 1, once in a while; 0, never.
[b] $N = 10$.

Table 2. Responses to Reaction Index Questions

thoughts of the event as extremely upsetting; fear when thinking of it; intrusive thoughts, images, and sounds; a decrease in normal activities; reactions to reminders of the trauma; and reduced impulse control.

Clinical Symptom Description

In this study, the authors focused on post-traumatic stress reactions because of their previous observations of the psychological consequences of witnessing violence (Pynoos and Nader, in press). Children exhibited symptoms from each of the major criteria of PTSD described in *DSM-III*.

Reexperiencing phenomena took several forms. All described recurrent, intrusive images of the rape, vividly recalling seeing the knife at their mother's throat, their mother's screams or cries of pain, the forceful penetration by penis, hand, or dildo, the sight of blood or injury, and their mother's desperate attempt to seek help afterwards.

Certain images became crystallized in each child's memory. After a period of looking dazed as he had during the rape, one 11-year-old boy vividly recalled the assailant's "evil eyes" staring directly at him for four long seconds before the man left the house; he continued to report nausea at recalling the smell of semen. Another boy remained haunted by the image of his half-naked mother lying with her arms tied above her head, her eyes open but not moving.

In five school-age children, traumatic play (Terr, 1981) took the form of self-stimulation or simulated sexual acts. One five-year-old boy, who had witnessed the rapist's use of a dildo, rubbed up and down on his toy baseball bat during the interview, as he talked of the break-in and the knife held at his mother's throat. Some of the children engaged siblings and friends in games of attacker and victim, exhibiting what one parent described as "humping" behavior. Two of the children, in addition to reenacting the assault, began repetitively to play more "happy family" games.

The youngest boys and all three girls became inhibited in their play. Pretend violence such as shooting games served for some as an unwanted reminder of the trauma. All eight school-age children discontinued certain types of play because they were more fearful of leaving home, wanted to stay closer to the parent, or generally became less interested.

All of the children described repetitive traumatic dreams, with the rapist nearly always returning. They dreamed of being threatened or severely physically harmed, of directly confronting the assailant, or of taking revenge. One 11-year-old boy dreamed that he used a 10-foot long samurai sword in an attempt to subdue an attacker. Weeks later, he began to have explicit sexual dreams. One 17-year-old dreamed repeatedly of being in a knife fight with a man-monster who would never die no matter how many times he stabbed him.

Adolescents and school-age children exhibited constricted affect and an inhibited range of emotions. The two adolescent boys complained of inhibition in interpersonal attachment as well as intensified anger. One attributed his social withdrawal and isolation to the continued feeling that no one had ever experienced what he had. The school-age children often described the event in a third person or journalistic fashion and described a fear that they would once again feel overwhelmed if they talked directly about their emotional experience. Parents described them as less animated and spontaneous and more withdrawn. They characterized children with a previous reluctance to express emotions as even more inhibited after the assault.

Even during the event, children attempted to mute their awareness of what was happening. Two boys, 7 and 5-years-old, attempted to go to sleep during the rape. Others, in their recounting, tried to minimize the degree of their exposure. One boy who had been next to his mother during the rape, reported that he had been the one in the other room instead of his sister, and furthermore, that his sister had blocked his view. He stated that he did not think that there was anything sexual happening. Memory distortions such as these appeared to insulate the children from intolerable affect.

The children were hypervigilant about personal safety and all became conscious about the security of their homes; checking the locks became a nightly ritual. One child insisted on having extra locks on her bedroom window, and two kept a knife or sword at their bedsides. One girl kept asking to move back to their former house where their neighbor was a policeman. The same child stayed up every night past 3 A.M., the time the rapist had entered her home. One adolescent, years later, still answers the front door from 10 feet away. Six of the school-age children began to "stay glued to the home" and feared being alone. They worried when their mothers would leave the house just to empty the garbage or when a man came to visit even a next door neighbor who was only being friendly.

New or exaggerated fears extended to objects beyond the house. The 7-year-old boy and his sister felt frightened when it grew dark or when they heard, for instance, a branch move in the wind. Both boys and girls became extremely frightened in the presence of a male stranger. Two children would not go back to a neighborhood restaurant because a "bum" had approached them there. For younger and older children alike, viewing of TV or movie violence intensified their fears and renewed traumatic anxiety.

Six school-age children showed increased somatic complaints. They could vividly describe intense psychophysiologic reactions that occurred during and immediately after the rape, and reminders of the trauma often brought back similar feelings. Three children complained of recurring nausea, while others described just feeling ill more often. School-age children actually appeared to be more susceptible to minor infections (Haggerty, 1980). Parents reported children to be chronically fatigued, which the authors were sometimes able to correlate with a persistent sleep disturbance. The older adolescents both sustained physical injuries; one seemed to become accident prone, and the other had an interval of engaging in physical altercations.

Boys, especially, reported feeling guilty for not successfully intervening during the assault. Two seven-year-old boys wished they had run for a neighbor, while one little boy regretted that he had not grabbed his baseball bat and hit the man. One child who had had martial arts training felt guilty for having remained in an immobilized daze, and the 17-year-old for not having inflicted a fatal knife wound.

Feelings of guilt often led a child continually to reappraise his or her role or ability to provide protection during the rape and in the future. The 17-year-old who engaged in hand-to-hand knife fight with the rapist felt extreme weakness and cowardice for having been overwhelmed. He became more intensely involved with bodybuilding and imagined meeting up with the man and killing him. The 11-year-old boy continued his martial arts training and repeatedly imagined using it against the rapist. Two school-age boys elaborated over time on their attempts to prevent the attack, one 11-year-old boy increasing the amount of contact with the rapist in his storytelling.

Influence on Life Attitudes

The children's affective responses to the event appeared to influence their life attitudes and, sometimes, their behaviors. Children described a sense of threat that an attack could occur unexpectedly at any time. The girls, especially, anticipated again being afraid when they became adults. The 8-year-old girl planned to always have a roommate until she married, stating she would never feel safe living alone. The two adolescent boys described a sense of incomplete resolution regarding their reactions to the event, which confounded their planning for the future. One 17-year-old who had planned to be a lawyer was confused by fantasies about becoming a gun merchant.

Witnessing the sexual assaults appeared to affect children's attitudes toward sex and marriage. Children became precocious in their use of sexually explicit terminology. The 7-year-old boy and his 11-year-old sister asked to be taken to the library to look up how babies were born. The 7-year-old boy who had held his mother's hand during the rape began to speak repeatedly of holding his wife's hand during childbirth and taking good care of his wife and family.

Impulse Control

Witnessing the violence challenged the children's sense of impulse control. The motivations they attributed to the rapist, such as anger or desire, were emotions that they themselves sometimes felt. One 7-year-old boy feared that he might now hurt someone when he was angry. An 11-year-old boy thought that the man "did that" to his mother because he was lonely and had "an urge," and did not know how to get a woman to be with him in any other way. He now considered that if he himself ever had urges like that, he would go and sit alone for a while until the feeling passed.

Irritability and anger were common responses to the trauma, resulting in reduced tolerance of the normal behaviors, demands, or slights of peers and a readiness to respond with aggression. One 11-year-old girl began to snap at her friends, to insult them more readily, and to demand that they answer for irritating her. The 17-year-old boy who had been a model teenager engaged in several barroom fights and was nearly arrested for reckless driving.

Revenge fantasies, in particular, eroded confidence in their impulse control. One 11-year-old boy had thoughts of torturing the rapist, first by poking out his eyes and then by sticking a pen up his penis "so the man could never do it again." Two children became almost transfixed to TV violence, especially those with themes of attack or revenge. One adolescent boy was frightened at becoming enraged as he watched one such show. In contrast to the children who showed increased impulsive behaviors, others became inhibited and wanted to avoid any excitement, loud voices, or hint of conflict. They feared that conflict would escalate into violence or that it would excite them to violence. Four children avoided watching violence on TV or in movies in order, they said, to prevent renewed aggressive fantasies.

Change in Intrafamilial Relationships

Children's intrafamilial relationships changed after the traumatic experience. All 10 children became more protective of their mothers. An 11-year-old girl and her 7-year-old brother both became upset if their mother left their sight or stepped out of the house. An 11-year-old boy took up cooking in order to spend more time with his mother. Five children became more ambivalent towards their mothers. One 7-year-old boy occasionally became angry and screamed, "You wanted that man to do that to you." At other times, he told her, "You must have loved us very much to have saved us that way." Both 17-year-old boys described unwelcomed anger toward their mothers. One boy refused to use the same toilet, towels or drinking glasses that his mother used for fear of contracting venereal disease.

In two cases, the husband was tied up or restrained and forced to watch under the threat of violence. The father's ineffectualness was very difficult for the child to tolerate afterwards. In one instance, the child stopped showing any affection toward her father and refused his efforts to comfort her. Children felt estranged from those family members who were not at home during the rape.

Angry feelings were rekindled about the absence of a divorced father and the loss of his protection. One 11-year-old boy began to "purposely hurt his [absent] father's feelings." The adolescent boy who engaged in hand-to-hand combat with the rapist was intensely angry with his father, who showed no understanding of the boy's severe fright.

DISCUSSION

This paper reports on a preliminary study of a small number of child witnesses to the sexual assaults of their mothers. Because of the sample size, the results of statistical analysis are only suggestive. They pointed out, however, the direction for further hypothesis testing. Children who witness sexual assault are likely to exhibit significant symptoms of a post-traumatic stress disorder, and school-age boys and girls seem to be at equal risk for a severe reaction. Sexual differences may be more critical in preadolescents and adolescents: preadolescent and adolescent girls may be especially traumatized by the witnessing, whereas adolescent boys may appear less overtly affected.

Although there were differences in severity of reaction, all 10 children met the *DSM-III* criteria for PTSD. Nine children had a severe reaction and one a moderate reaction as measured by the PTSD Reaction Index. In Frederick's (1986) study of 15 preadolescent and adolescent boys molested by male mental health professionals, all 15 children met the criteria for PTSD using the Reaction Index. Severity levels were not rated.

Age and Sex Differences

Witnessing these violent sexual assaults markedly increased the sense of vulnerability in all the children. After seeing that a grown woman, especially a parent, can be violated, the child may feel that much more vulnerable. Identification with the mother as victim was especially terrifying to the girls in this study and may help to explain the differences between the older boys and girls.

The girls had repeated dreams of being attacked and became afraid of strangers or of being in their own neighborhoods. Boys, too, felt more vulnerable to being violated. However, six boys also showed signs of identifying with the rapist rather than with their helpless mothers. In their play, and occasionally in dreams, they became the male attacker. These boys appeared visibly frightened by the implication of resembling the assailant in their behavior. Preadolescent boys fantasized about intervention and revenge, and each adolescent boy either physically intervened or actively pursued the assailant. Differences in responding to traumatic helplessness may explain why girls may appear more depressed or fearful while boys may be more likely to exhibit disturbances in conduct.

Age also appeared to be a significant factor in determining the children's reactions. The younger children had greater difficulty processing the event because of cognitive confusions. A 5-year-old boy, confused by the dildo, afterwards worried about his own physical intactness. He anxiously played at having his finger come on and off his hand, later asking if his own penis could come off like that. Awareness of these developmental differences is essential to help the child to clarify what happened and to distinguish the reality of an external threat from internal age-appropriate anxieties.

Differential Handling of the Sexual and Aggressive Components

Initially, the children appeared preoccupied with the aggressive aspects of the assault, the violence, and the mother's vulnerability. The overt sexual aspects, on the other hand, were often omitted, denied, or acutely repressed. These children responded to the event's sexual component through their traumatic play and through an increased interest in sexual issues. Longitudinal study is needed to determine whether cognitive omissions inhibit the affective working through of the experience or, instead, are protective.

The Postrape Milieu

The postrape milieu is typically anxious, affecting the child's course of recovery. Almost all of the mothers felt guilty or responsible for having traumatized their children, which made it difficult for them to tolerate awareness of their children's reactions or hearing their children talk about the event. In their own post-trauma states, they commonly felt less effective as parents. Startle responses to their children's or husband's entering the room, especially at night, were often persistent and disturbing. Fathers who had not been present at the rape often had difficulty appreciating their children's experiences and subsequent anxiety. Therefore, at times, children experienced estrangement from both parents. "Happy family" games may have been some children's attempts to reinstate the united family atmosphere present before the assault.

CONCLUSION

Sexually abused children and child witnesses to sexual assault share in common prominent post-traumatic stress symptoms (Frederick, 1986; Goodwin, 1985; Green 1983), disturbances in impulse control and sexuality (Finklehor, 1984), alterations in their sense of security and vulnerability, challenge to self-esteem, stress in intrafamilial and peer relationships, and changes in future orientation. The cooperative efforts of both child trauma programs and adult rape response programs are needed to ensure the recovery of the total family.

REFERENCES

Center for Disease Control (1985), *Violent Crime: Summary of Morbidity.* Atlanta, GA.: Violence Epidemiology Branch.

Finkelhor, D. (1984), *Child Sexual Abuse: New Theory and Research.* New York: Free Press.

Frederick, C. J. (1985), Selected foci in the spectrum of post-traumatic stress disorders. In: *Perspectives on Disaster Recovery,* ed. J. Laube & S. A. Murphy. Norwalk, Conn.: Appleton-Century-Crofts, pp. 110–130.

—— (1986), Posttraumatic stress disorder and child molestation. In: *Sexual Exploitation of Clients by Mental Health Professionals,* ed. A. Burgess & C. Hartman. New York: Praeger Publishers.

Goodwin, J. (1985), Posttraumatic symptoms in incest victims. In: *Posttraumatic Stress Disorder in Children,* ed. S. Eth & R. S. Pynoos. Washington, D.C.: American Psychiatric Press.

Green, A. (1983), Dimensions of psychological trauma in abused children. *J. Am. Acad. Child Psychiatry,* 22:231–237.

—— (1985), Children traumatized by physical abuse. In: *Posttraumatic Stress Disorder in Children,* ed. S. Eth & R. S. Pynoos. Washington, D.C.: American Psychiatric Press, pp. 133–154.

Haggerty, R. K. (1980), Life stress, illness and social support. *Dev. Med. Child Neurol.,* 22:391–400.

Lipson, G. S. & Pubner, J. S. (1985), *San Ysidro Massacre: Impact on Police and Community* (NIMH Contract (PO-84M29507801D). Bethesda, Md.: National Institute of Mental Health.

Pynoos, R. S. & Eth, S. (1986), Witness to violence: the child interview. *J. Am. Acad. Child Psychiatry,* 25:306–319.

—— Frederick, C., Nader, K. et al. (1987), Life threat and posttraumatic stress in school age children. *Arch. Gen. Psychiatry,* 44:1057–1063.

—— Nader, K, (in press), Children exposed to violence. *Psychiatric Annals.*

Terr, L. (1981), Forbidden games: Post-traumatic child's play. *J. Am. Acad. Child Psychiatry,* 20:741–760.

Tokuhata, G., Bratz, J. & Kim, J. (in press), *Three Mile Island: Mother-Child Mobility Survey.* Pennsylvania Department of Health.

PART IV: SPECIAL STRESS AND COPING

12

Single-Parent Families: Child Psychiatric Disorder and School Performance

Heather Munroe Blum, Michael H. Boyle, and David R. Offord
McMaster University and Child and Family Center, Ontario, Canada

Data from the Ontario Child Health Study were used to examine the association between single-parent family status and child psychiatric disorder and poor school performance. Bivariate results indicate that children of single-parent families are at a small but statistically significant increased risk for poor outcome. These same families, however, experience severe economic and social hardship. When variables indicative of hardship, such as poverty and family dysfunction, are controlled for in a multivariate analysis, the relationship between single-parent family status and childhood psychiatric disorder and poor school performance becomes statistically nonsignificant. The implications of these findings are discussed.

The investigation of correlates of child psychiatric disorder and poor school performance can lead to the identification of high-risk groups of children and suggest strategies for primary prevention and treatment. With the recent dramatic increase in the number of single-parent families in the United States (Weinraub and Wolf, 1983), Canada (Statistics Canada, 1984), and Britain (Wadsworth et al., 1985), exploring the relationship between family structure and child psychiatric disorder and poor school performance becomes increasingly important.

A number of investigators have already begun to research whether children of single-parent families are at increased risk for poor health and other diffi-

Reprinted with permission from the *Journal of the American Academy of Child and Adolescent Psychiatry*, 1988, Vol. 27, No. 2, 214–219. Copyright 1988 by the American Academy of Child and Adolescent Psychiatry.

This study was supported by the Ministry of Community and Social Services, Ontario, Canada.

culties. A British study following almost 80% of a cohort of all children born in the United Kingdom in 1 week (April 5–11, 1970) found that at 5 years of age, children born to single mothers were more neurotic, more antisocial, and had poorer scores on vocabulary and visuomotor coordination than did children of two-parent families (Wadsworth et al., 1985). These relationships persisted even after controlling for income level. A recent random sample of 20% of the households in a poor suburb in Australia found that single mothers reported higher rates of both emotional and physical disorder in their children than did mothers of children from two-parent households (Underwood and Kamien, 1984). These reports were validated by a survey of related medical records.

A Canadian study, comparing children on probation from juvenile court with age, sex, school, school performance, and social-class matched children, found that delinquent children were more likely to be from broken homes than were children who had not had contact with the law (Offord, 1982). An American survey of a national sample of adolescents found increased deviance (law contacts, arrests, school discipline, truancy, runaway, and smoking) among children from single-parent families, and this difference remained when family income was taken into account (Dornbusch et al., 1985).

Although these studies collectively demonstrate that children from single-parent families are at increased risk for disorder and school difficulties, none has looked at both factors in a large community sample reporting psychiatric disorder based on DSM-III criteria. In addition, although most of these studies report that "income was accounted for," in general, they do not provide adequate details of either their definition of income or the procedures that were used to control for the effects of low income on the relationship between single-parent status and childhood morbidity.

The objectives of this paper are twofold. The first aim is to determine the strength of single-parent family status (SPFS) as a marker for child psychiatric disorder and poor school performance in a large community sample of children. The second is to determine the interdependence of SPFS and other conceptually important socio-demographic and family variables as they relate to psychiatric disorder and poor school performance among children. Specifically, this paper will examine the effects of SPFS on child psychiatric disorder and poor school performance when controlling for the confounding influences of other important variables, and it will test for interactions; that is, the extent to which the effects of SPFS on child outcomes are constant across different levels of these other socio-demographic and family variables. It will draw on data from the Ontario Child Health Study (OCHS), a province-wide cross-sectional survey of children's health (Boyle et al., 1987; Offord et al., 1987a).

The variables that will be examined in this paper were selected on the basis of their availability in the OCHS data set as well as on the basis of their theoretical and empirical significance. SPFS was operationally defined as "only one parenting figure in the household currently." Other socio-demographic variables were included because of their close relationship to SPFS and, thus, the possibility that they may confound the effects of family status or interact with family status in the relationship to psychiatric disorder and poor school performance. The socio-demographic variables examined in this study include: age of the child (12 to 16 vs. 6 to 11); sex of the child (male vs. female); residency (urban vs. rural); welfare status (yes vs. no); poverty, operationally defined as family earnings less than $10,000 annually (yes vs. no); and subsidized housing (yes vs. no). Family variables were also included because of reports in the literature that the within-house family environment may be more important in the production of child psychiatric disorder than socio-demographic variables (Robins, 1979). Socio-demographic and family variables were assessed using a parent self-report completed by the female head of household. All variables included in this paper are defined in the Appendix.

METHOD

The Ontario Child Health Study was an interview survey of 1,869 families, including 3,294 children, carried out to determine the prevalence and epidemiology of mental and physical health problems in Ontario children. The survey methodology and measurements have been described elsewhere in detail (Boyle et al., 1987; in press) and are summarized here.

Sampling Design

The target population of the OCHS included all children born from January 1, 1966 through January 1, 1979 whose usual place of residence was in a household dwelling in Ontario. The survey excluded three groups of children representing 3.3% of the population of children aged 4 to 16 years: those children living on Indian Reserves, those in collective dwellings such as institutions, and those residing in dwellings constructed after June 1, 1981 (Census Day). The sampling unit consisted of all household dwellings listed in the 1981 Census of Canada (the sampling frame was the 1981 Census), and the sampling selection was done by stratified, clustered, random sampling from the census file of household dwellings (Statistics Canada, 1982).

The major strata for the survey consisted of the four administrative regions of the Ontario Ministry of Community and Social Services (MCSS) with each region subdivided into three strata based on the 1981 population: large urban areas with more than 25,000 population; small urban areas ranging in population from 3,000 to 25,000; and rural areas of less than 3,000 population. A simple random sample of households was selected from all urban areas within each MCSS region, whereas a two-stage sampling procedure was used in small urban and rural areas. In the first stage, areas or clusters were selected; in the second stage, households were selected—both with a known probability. Statistics Canada interviewers (employed by the federal government to collect data for the Census of Canada, the Canada Labor Force Survey, and other government reports) visited all sampled households to screen for eligibility and conducted home interviews with the female head of eligible households. The survey was carried out during January and February of 1983. Ninety-one percent of all eligible household participated; only 3.9% refused to be interviewed.

Survey Measures

The survey investigated four childhood psychiatric disorders: Conduct Disorder, Hyperactivity and Emotional Disorder (neurosis)—for children aged 4 to 16; and somatization—for adolescents aged 12 to 16. For measuring each of the four disorders, scales were developed comprised of problem behaviors (items) summed to form a score. DSM-III criteria guided the selection of items for each scale. The Child Behavior Checklist (Achenbach and Edelbrock, 1983) furnished the basic pool of items for the scales. When items from the Child Behavior Checklist were felt not to describe adequately a particular criterion, additional items were generated. The resulting checklist was termed the Survey Diagnostic Instrument (SDI) (Boyle et al., in press). Similar checklists were used for three sources: parents, teachers, and adolescents 12 to 16. Checklist items applicable to a particular disorder were grouped to form a scale. Each item could be scored 0, 1, or 2, indicating responses of "never or not true," "sometimes or somewhat true," and "often or very true," respectively.

Threshold scores for the checklist scales for disorders (based on the summed responses from the scale items) were established on the basis of their ability to discriminate best the presence or absence of a diagnosis made by a child psychiatrist (Boyle et al., 1987; in press). Separate thresholds were established for each data source for the two age groups. Children within each age group had to score below the thresholds on both sources to qualify as *not* having a disorder. The completion rate on the teacher form in the older age group was too low for use in measuring disorder. A 4- to 11-year-old child could have a disorder on the basis of one source (i.e., parent or teacher) or both sources (i.e., parent and teacher). Similarly, a 12- to 16-year-old adolescent could have a disorder on the basis of one source (i.e., parent or adolescent) or both sources (i.e., parent and adolescent).

The second outcome variable, poor school performance, was defined as "failed a grade ever" and/or "full-time remedial education ever" (yes vs. no) and was assessed as part of a parent interview-administered questionnaire.

Analysis

All children from among those eligible aged 6 to 16 were included from each of the 1,869 participating households. (Data on 4- and 5-year-olds are not presented in this paper because of the large amounts of missing school performance data for this age group.) The total number of children aged 6 to 16 was 2,852, including 304 children of single-parent families. These single-parent families were almost exclusively headed by females. The age and sex distribution of children was: 1,550 aged 6 to 11; 1,302 aged 12 to 16; 1,443 male, and 1,404 female (five children were missing data on sex).

The strength of association between SPFS and each correlate (bivariate relationship) was estimated using the odds ratio. Statistical significance was determined with chi-square tests with Yates' correction where appropriate. Each multivariate analysis consisted of a forward stepwise logistic regression. The models for the two outcome variables, psychiatric disorder and poor school performance, were specified to control for confounding and to test for interactions between family status and the other independent variables.

Poverty and family dysfunction were treated as confounders in each multivariate analysis and forced into each model. The family dysfunction variable was based on the 12-item Family Assessment Device (Miller et al., 1985) and is defined in the Appendix along with all other study variables. This variable reflects the relationships among the family members residing in the household and is conceptually different from marital discord. The scale upon which it is based demonstrates good test-retest reliability and good construct validity (Byles and Byrne, 1988). Single-parent family status was also forced into each model.

All other variables, including interactions between age and sex and interactions between SPFS and each of the other variables, were allowed to compete for entry into the model. These other variables were welfare status, residence, housing, and maternal education. Weights were generated to reflect each respondent's probability of selection in the sample, but because these weights, when applied to responses, had very little impact on estimates, they were not used for any of the analyses (Boyle et al., 1987; Offord et al., 1987a).

The definition of emotional disorder is based on the correlate rather than the prevalence threshold (Boyle et al., in press). The correlate threshold is higher than the prevalence threshold and increases the likelihood that a child is a "case." The forward stepwise logistic regression procedure used in these analyses came from the BMDP statistical package (Dixon et al., 1983).

RESULTS

Table 1 provides comparative data for single-parent family and two-parent family children on psychiatric disorder and poor school performance. These results are in keeping with the first objective of this investigation; i.e., to assess the strength of SPFS as a marker for psychiatric disorder and poor school performance. The strength of the relationship between SPFS and the

TABLE 1. *A Comparison of Single-Parent Children and Two-Parent Children on Psychiatric Disorder and Poor School Performance*

Variable	%	Relative Odds	Significance
Any psychiatric disorder for			
Single-parent children	22		
		1.7	$p = 0.001$
Two-parent children	14		
Conduct Disorder for			
Single-parent children	10		
		2.2	$p = 0.007$
Two-parent children	5		
Hyperactivity for			
Single-parent children	9		
		1.8	$p = 0.02$
Two-parent children	5		
Emotional Disorder (neurosis) for			
Single-parent children	6		
		1.1	NS[b]
Two-parent children	5		
Somatization[a] for			
Single-parent children	9		
		1.2	NS[b]
Two-parent children	8		
Poor school performance for			
Single-parent children	21		
		1.7	$p = 0.001$
Two-parent children	14		

[a] Measured only among 12- to 16-year-olds.
[b] Not significant.

Table 1. A Comparison of Single-Parent Children and Two-Parent Children on Psychiatric Disorder and Poor School Performance

child morbidity variables is expressed in relative odds; e.g., the relative odds of 1.7 between presence of any psychiatric disorder and SPFS indicates that children with psychiatric disorder are 1.7 times more likely to be from a single-parent family than a two-parent family. There is a small but statistically significant ($p = 0.001$) relationship between child psychiatric disorder and SPFS when no other potential confounding or intervening variables are taken into consideration. When looking at the relationships between SPFS and the four individual psychiatric disorders, SPFS puts children at greatest risk for exhibiting Conduct Disorder, at 2.2 times the rate of children from two-parent families.

Finally, single-parent children are 1.7 times as likely to demonstrate poor school performance as are two-parent children. This, again, indicates that single-parent children are at a small but statistically significant ($p = 0.001$) increased risk for poor school performance when other variables that may help to account for some of this increased risk, e.g., poverty, are not taken into consideration.

Table 2 displays the bivariate relationships between SPFS and other family socio-demographic correlates. These correlates are presented in order of the strength of their relationship with SPFS. Expectations that welfare status and poverty would be strongly associated with single-parent status were confirmed. Roughly 40% of these single-parent households lived on welfare and/or in poverty. The single-parent families were 31 times as likely to live on welfare and 18 times as likely to live in poverty as were two-parent families. SPFS was also strongly and significantly related to living in subsidized housing. Family dysfunction and low maternal education demonstrated a weak but statistically significant relationship with SPFS. SPFS was not related to child age or sex.

TABLE 2. *Bivariate Relationships Between Socio-demographic Correlates, Family Correlates, and Single-Parent Family Status*

Correlate	Single-Parent Children (%)	Relative Odds	Significance
On welfare	41	31.0	$p < 0.0001$
Poverty (income < $10,000)	40	18.0	$p < 0.0001$
Subsidized housing	21	11.2	$p < 0.0001$
Urban	77	2.2	$p < 0.0001$
Family dysfunction	15	1.5	$p < 0.02$
Mother (grade 8 education or less)	18	1.3	$p < 0.02$

Table 2. Bivariate Relationships Between Socio-demographic Correlates, Family Correlates, and Single-Parent Family Status

TABLE 3. *Relative Odds in Logistic Regression Analyses of*
Psychiatric Disorder and Poor School Performance With Selected
Correlates

Variable	Any Psychiatric Disorder Odds Ratio[a]	Poor School Performance Odds Ratio[b]
Main effects		
Single-parent family	NS[c]	NS
Poverty[d]	1.97	1.63
Family dysfunction[d]	3.07	1.01[e]
Welfare	1.74	1.77
Maternal education		
Grade 8 vs. high school[e]	NS	2.63
Some high vs. high school[e]	NS	2.40
Subsidized housing	NS	NS
Interactions		
Male sex by age		
Ages 6–11	2.01	1.12
Ages 12–16	0.85	1.81
Single-parent by residence		
Rural	1.95	NS
Urban	0.74	NS
Single-parent by child age		
6 to 11	1.71	NS
12 to 16	0.84	NS
Single-parent by child sex		
Male	NS	0.71
Female	NS	1.88

[a] Goodness of fit: $\chi^2 = 2.94$; $p = 0.94$.
[b] Goodness of fit: $\chi^2 = 4.44$; $p = 0.82$.
[c] NS, not significant.
[d] Forced in both models as control variables.
[e] Not significant; all other variables statistically significant.

Table 3. Relative Odds in Logistic Regression Analyses of Psychiatric Disorder and Poor School Performance With Selected Correlates

Table 3 presents the results of the logistic regression analyses with psychiatric disorder and poor school performance as the dependent, or outcome, variables. These multivariate analyses address the second major aim of this study; i.e., to examine the relationship between SPFS and child morbidity when controlling for the effects of poverty and family dysfunction and to test for interactions between SPFS and other family and socio-demographic variables.

Table 3 demonstrates that family dysfunction is the variable that makes the strongest independent contribution to child psychiatric disorder. Poverty (a variable forced into the model) and welfare status also have significant independent associations with child psychiatric disorder. Family status does not make an independent main effect contribution to this model. Several interactions enter the model. Sex and age interact such that the relationship between child psychiatric disorder and male sex is stronger in the younger than the older age group. Two single-parent interactions also enter the model. Rural children of single-parents are more likely to experience psychiatric disorder than are urban children, and younger children of single-parents are more likely to experience disorder than are older children. The Hosmer-Lemeshow goodness-of-fit chi-square test was used to assess the "fit" of the model to the data where there were many cells and some small cell sizes (Dixon et al., 1983). The p value for the goodness of fit chi-square is significant when the null hypothesis is supported and nonsignificant when the alternate hypothesis is supported. Thus, the goodness of fit chi-square test applied here indicates that this model provides a good fit for the existing data ($p = 0.94$).

With respect to poor school performance, poverty, being on welfare, and low maternal education contribute to the model as main effects. Two interactions enter the model. Sex and age interact such that older boys are more likely to experience poor school performance than are younger boys. SPFS and gender interact such that girls from single-parent families are more likely to experience poor school performance than are boys. Family dysfunction is not related to poor school performance. This model also provides a good fit for the data ($p = 0.82$).

One additional analysis was carried out to determine whether the relationships between family status and the measures of childhood morbidity are influenced by the recency of parental separation in single-parent families. This analysis demonstrated that recency of separation (defined as "separation in the past 6 months") did not have any statistically significant effect on the relationships of primary interest in this study.

DISCUSSION

Bivariate results indicate that children of single-parent families are at a small but statistically significant increased risk of psychiatric disorder, especially Conduct Disorder, in comparison with their two-parent counterparts. In addition, single-parent children are at a small but significant increased risk for poor school performance.

Bivariate findings also indicate that children of single-parent families experience significant socioeconomic hardship. They are more likely to live in poverty and to live in subsidized housing than are children of two-parent families. Fully 41% of the single-parent families in this study were receiving welfare assistance. Nevertheless, the Ontario finding is somewhat lower than the report of Dornbusch et al. (1985) that, in 1980, the proportion of female-headed families living in poverty in the United States was 54% among non-Hispanic whites.

Given the high prevalence of poverty among single-parent families, it is important to examine whether children of single-parent families are at increased risk of child psychiatric disorder and poor school performance when the effects of increased poverty are removed. This study found that when income is controlled, SPFS does not have a significant independent relationship with either child psychiatric disorder or poor school performance, except in particular subgroups: rural children, girls, and older boys. Family dysfunction, welfare status, and poverty were associated with increased risk for child psychiatric disorder, whereas welfare status and maternal education successfully identified children at risk for poor school performance. Single-parent families in rural areas may be more isolated from protective formal and informal supports than are urban single-parent families, leading to an increased vulnerability to psychiatric disorder in the rural children. Girls from single-parent families may shoulder a disproportionate share of the domestic/child care burden than do their male counterparts, and their greater home responsibilities may interfere with school accomplishments. Alternatively, the girls' poor school performance may be evidence of a nonclinical level of depression in reaction to the single-parent family environment. In boys, older child age was also associated with increased risk for poor school performance. Because the school performance measure covers the child's lifetime and thus allows for the probability of school failure and poor school performance increasing with age, given more time, the now younger boys might also develop problems on school performance measures.

The finding that SPFS is not significantly associated with psychiatric disorder or school problems when income is accounted for is in contrast with the results of the studies cited earlier in this paper. Wadsworth et al. (1985) and Dornbusch et al. (1985) found that even when income was controlled, children of single-parent families were more likely to be antisocial and neurotic and to do poorly on psychological tests or school performance. These earlier studies used various definitions of outcome variables and reported on data collected before 1971. They looked at 5-year-olds and adolescents, respectively, compared with the broad age range (6 to 16 years) studied here; however, this age difference should not explain the contrast in findings, because age was controlled for in the analysis of the OCHS data. It is possible that the difference in findings is largely related to varying definitions of poverty. It is unclear how Wadsworth et al. (1985) defined poverty, whereas Dornbusch et al. (1985) appear to have defined it as income under $5,000 in the time period 1966 to 1970, a somewhat overinclusive estimation of poverty for that time.

The findings of this study arise from data collected cross-sectionally; thus it is unclear whether or not single-family status preceded disorder and poor school performance. Investigating the cause (e.g., divorce, death, no marriage) of SPFS, the degree of preceding stress and the length of any preceding stress might contribute further to understanding the relationships being studied. Secondly, very few of the single-parent children in this study (6 of 304) had access to another nonparent adult who might have ameliorated the effects of socio-economic hardship and parent deprivation. Dornbusch et al. (1985) found that the presence of an additional adult in the home provided a buffering, protective effect that resulted in reduced deviance in adolescents. Although it is known that in the OCHS sample the recency of separation of the parents did not affect the results, a study comparing substantial numbers of single-parent families with and without additional adults in the home would further examine the impact of fragmented family status.

It is clear from this study that when income is controlled, detrimental risk of SPFS is reduced in the areas of psychiatric morbidity and poor school performance. Poverty, welfare status, and family dysfunction differentiate those single-parent families that experience child psychiatric disorder from those that do not; whereas maternal education, poverty, and welfare status differentiate single-parent families that experience poor school performance from those that do not. Other findings from the OCHS sample indicate that low income and welfare status have statistically significant independent relationships with psychiatric disorder (Offord and Boyle, 1987), indicating that it is not economic disadvantage alone that puts children at increased risk for disorder. Single-parents often have the unenviable conflicting responsibilities of being the primary adult shaper of family culture, while at the same time having sole responsibility for generating family income. These factors, among others, may give rise to the significant prevalence of poverty, welfare status, and, to a lesser extent, family dysfunction in single-parent families. The preventive/treatment potential of social interventions that are designed to increase income in single-parent families and provide social support programs and skill development programs for the parents and children of high-risk single-parent families might usefully be explored. Clinicians involved in child custodial disposition should be aware that given adequate financial support, single-parent families appear to manage well. Efforts made by the courts and others to ensure necessary financial resources for the custodial parent will facilitate single-parent family functioning.

APPENDIX

Definition of Variables

1. *Psychiatric disorder:* Child in the past 6 months has one or more of:
   a. *Conduct Disorder:* Characterized by either physical violence against persons or property or a severe violation of social norms;
   b. *Hyperactivity:* Characterized by inattention, impulsivity, and motor activity;
   c. *Emotional Disorder:* Characterized primarily by feelings of anxiety and depression;
   d. *Somatization Disorder:* Characterized by distressing, recurrent somatic symptoms with no known organic cause and perception of oneself as sickly.
2. *Poor school performance:* Child has failed a grade and/or received fulltime remediation or special class placement at some time during his or her school career.
3. *On welfare:* Any portion of the family income in the prior year (1982) was in the form of public assistance, such as welfare or mother's allowance.
4. *Poverty:* Total family income in preceding year was < $10,000.
5. *Urban/rural:* Urban areas are those with a population of < 25,000. Rural area in this definition includes both small urban areas (population 3,000 to 25,000) and rural areas (population < 3,000).
6. *Subsidized housing:* Currently living in a dwelling where the rent is subsidized by the government.
7. *Low mother's education:* Female parent or guardian has completed grade 8 or less; or, some high school vs. high school completion or more.
8. *Family dysfunction:* A score of 27 to 48 (range 12 to 48) on the 12-item general functioning scale derived from the McMaster Family Functioning Assessment Device (Miller et al., 1985). Family functioning is assessed on six dimensions: problem solving, communication, roles, affective responsiveness, affective involvement, and behavior control. Examples of specific items include:
   a. "Planning family activities is difficult because we misunderstand each other."
   b. "In times of crisis we cannot turn to each other for support."
   c. "We cannot talk to each other about the sadness we feel."
   d. "We avoid discussing our fears and concerns."
   e. "Making decisions is a problem for our family."

REFERENCES

Achenbach, T., & Edelbrock, C. (1983), Manual for the Child Behavior Checklist and Revised Child Behavior Profile. Burlington, Vt.

Boyle, M. H., Offord, D. R., Hofmann, H. G., et al. (1987), Ontario child health study: I. methodology. *Arch. Gen. Psychiatry,* 44:826–831.

—— Byles, J. A., Offord, D. R., et al. (in press), Ontario child health study: measurement of psychiatric disorder in children. *J. Child Psychol. Psychiatry.*

Byles, A. & Byrne, C. (1988), The General Functioning Scale of the Family Assessment Device: reliability and validity. *Fam. Process,* 27.

Dixon, W. S., Brown, M. B., Engleman, L., et al. (1983), *BMDP Statistical Software,* Los Angeles, Calif.

Dornbusch, S. M., Carlsmith, J. M., Bushwall, S. J., et al. (1985), Single parents, extended households, and the control of adolescents. *Child Dev.,* 56:326–341.

Miller, I. W., Bishop, D. S., Epstein, N. B. & Keitner, S. I. (1985), The McMaster Family Assessment Device: reliability and validity. *Journal of Mental and Family Therapy,* 11:345–356.

Offord, D. R. (1982). Family backgrounds of male and female delinquents. In: *Abnormal Offenders, Delinquency and the Criminal Justice System,* J. Gunn & D. P. Farrington, New York: Wiley, pp. 129–151.

Offord, D. R. & Boyle, M. H. (1987), Morbidity among welfare children in Ontario. *Can. J. Psychiatry,* 32:518–525.

Offord, D. R., Boyle, M. H., Szatmari, P., et al. (1987a), Ontario Child Health Study: six-month prevalence of disorder and rates of service utilization. *Arch. Gen. Psychiatry,* 44: 832–836.

Robins, L. N. (1979), Longitudinal methods. In: *The Study of Normal and Pathological Development,* Vol. 1, eds. K. P. Kisher, J. E. Meyer, C. Muller & E. Stromgren. Heidelberg: Grundlagen und Methoden der Psychiatrie, pp. 627–684.

Statistics Canada (1982), *1981 Census Directory.* Ottawa, Canada: Minister of Supply and Services.

—— (1984) *Canada's Lone-Parent Families* (Cat. 8-5200-738). Canada: Minister of Supply and Services.

Underwood, P. & Kamien, M. (1984), Health care needs of the children of single mothers in a Perth suburb. *Aust. Paediatr. J.,* 21:203–204.

Wadsworth, J., Burnell, I., Taylor, B. & Butler, T. (1985), The influence of family type on children's behaviour and development at five years. *J. Child Psychol. Psychiatry,* 26:245–254.

Weinraub, M. & Wolf, B. M. (1983), Effects of stress and social supports on mother-child interactions in single- and two-parent families. *Child Dev.,* 54:1297–1311.

13

Parental Functioning and the Home Environment in Families of Divorce: Prospective and Concurrent Analyses

Jack Block, Jeanne H. Block, and Per F. Gjerde

University of California, Berkeley

Relationships between marital status and parental functioning were evaluated both prospectively (years before marriage dissolution) and concurrently (after marriage dissolution). Prospective analyses included only then-intact families and compared parents who subsequently were divorced with parents who subsequently did not divorce. The subset of intact families in which divorce eventually occurred was characterized by unsupportive parenting of children and interparental tension years before the formal dissolution of the marriage. Concurrent analyses compared intact and divorced families. Marital status was shown to be related to parental self-concepts. Mother-daughter and mother-son relations subsequent to divorce are described.

About half of the marriages entered into during the 1970s can be expected to dissolve (Cherlin, 1981) and, according to the Select Committee on Children, Youth, and Families (1983), over one million children each year experience the divorce or separation of their parents. Projections indicate that by 1990, more than one third of American children aged 18 will have lived with a divorced parent (Glick, 1979). This prevalence of divorce has resulted in increasing interest in examining the subsequences of divorce.

Reprinted with permission from the *Journal of the American Academy of Child and Adolescent Psychiatry*, 1988, Vol. 27, No. 2, 207–213. Copyright 1988 by the American Academy of Child and Adolescent Psychiatry.

This study was supported by National Institute of Mental Health Grant MH 16080 to Jack and Jeanne H. Block.

Divorce research has included careful studies of both the physical and the psychological home environment that divorced parents thereafter can provide for their children (cf. Colletta, 1979; Derdeyn, 1976; Emery, 1982; Fine et al., 1983; Hetherington, 1979, 1984; Hingst, 1981; Hoffman, 1977; Jacobson, 1978a, b, c; Kurdek and Siesky, 1980; Nelson, 1981; Rosen, 1979; Rosenthal, 1979; Sorosky, 1977; Spanier and Thompson, 1984; Wallerstein, 1984, 1985; Wallerstein and Kelly, 1980).

The many existing studies of familial environments *after* divorce unfortunately yield no systematic information on family functioning *before* divorce. Lack of prospective data, therefore, makes it impossible to determine which problems in family functioning are antecedent to divorce and which problems are subsequent to divorce. Problems in children's behavior, stress in the family, and hostility between parents are documented occurrences after divorce, but they may be present before divorce as well.

Sole reliance on retrospective data introduces other problematic factors, most notably, response bias. Subjects' differential willingness to discuss painful personal events from the past and their tendency to reconstruct the past so that it makes current sense can result in inaccurate and misleading information.

Sampling problems reflect another major methodological inadequacy in many current studies of divorce. These include preoccupation with special samples, sometimes involving only clinical populations, and sampling narrowly from only one level of socioeconomic status. Such sampling deficiencies may yield results not replicable or generalizable beyond a specific group (Hainline and Feig, 1978). The use of inadequate measuring techniques, such as a single outcome measure of unknown quality or a lack of independence among clinicians in subject evaluations across time, also weakens the results of several divorce studies (Levitin, 1979). The interpretation of earlier studies may be complicated by failure to provide appropriate control groups of intact families for comparison. Finally, as Hetherington (1979) has observed, existent studies of divorce are not always comparable (e.g., Hodges et al., 1979; Wallerstein and Kelly, 1976) because they examine the divorcing families at different periods in the long separation process and thus observe differing levels of emotional disturbance and familial disorganization.

The present analyses attempt to respond to several of the methodological inadequacies present in the existing divorce literature. The authors examined a longitudinally followed, heterogeneous, nonclinical sample using both self-report and observational data collected independently over 10 years. The study

The authors are indebted to Suzanne Manton and Marie Tisak for creating the family status index.

Jeanne H. Block is now deceased.

consists of two sets of analyses: prospective and concurrent. Because of the longitudinal nature of the larger study and the analytical design, the authors can provide a *prospective* view on divorce by relating parental attitudes and perceptions *before* divorce to the subsequent fact of formal dissolution of a marriage. The authors also evaluated parental functioning and the home environment in intact and divorced families after marriage dissolution in order to examine and compare the qualities of parenting both before and after divorce. The present report complements an earlier one (Block et al., 1986) focusing on the personality of children before divorce.

THE Q-SORT METHODOLOGY

The study used the Q-sort method to assess family functioning. The Q-sort is an "ipsative procedure" (Block, 1957, 1961/1978; Cattell, 1944; Stephenson, 1953). The term *ipsative measurement* can best be understood by contrasting it to the more common *normative measurement*. In normative measurement, "there is a scale for every *trait* and a population of individuals is distributed about the mean of that population. In ipsative measurement, there is a scale for every *individual* and a population of an individual's trait scores is distributed about that individual's mean" (Guilford, 1952, p. 30). In other words, in ipsative measurement, a score, or a Q-sort item, reflects the salience of that score, or Q-item, relative to other scores, or Q-items, with reference to the particular subject under study. The Q-sort as an ipsative method has therefore been said to prove "person-centered" rather than "variable-centered" data and is especially suited to express clinical descriptions of individuals (Block, 1961/1978). It is important to note that despite the ipsative nature of the Q-sort, individual Q-items can be employed in a normative manner (Block, 1957).

The procedure of Q-sorting. In Q-sort methodology, the assessor is provided with a set of statements, printed on separate cards, which contains the entire vocabulary that the assessor is permitted to use (Block, 1961/1978). The assessor is required to arrange the Q-sort items according to a predetermined distribution that specifies the number of cards allowed to be included in each pile. The items are arranged by the sorter according to their judged salience and representativeness with reference to the individual, or construct, being evaluated. Those items judged by the Q-judge to be most characteristic of the subject are assigned high scores; those items judged least characteristic of the subject are assigned low scores.

The requirement that different assessors use identical Q-sort distributions confers several advantages: A large number of discriminations can be gained from each Q-sorter or clinical judge, and because all participants use the same scaling metric, comparisons among raters (and averaging of raters) can proceed straightforwardly rather than be befuddled by noncomparable language usage. In addition, the forced distribution reduces response sets and problems associated with the social desirability of ratings. The reader is referred to J. Block (1956, 1961/1978) for a detailed description of the Q-sort rationale.

METHOD

Subjects

The subjects were the parents of children participating in an ongoing longitudinal study of personality and cognitive development (Block and Block, 1980). These children were drawn from the two nursery schools constituting the Harold E. Jones Child Study Center at the University of California, Berkeley, over the 3-year period 1969–1971. The numbers of children participating varied by year, ranging from a high of 128 at age 4 to a low of 104 at age 7. Previous analyses of subject loss showed no differential attrition as a function of socioeconomic level or ethnic origin.

The Harold E. Jones Child Study Center offers two preschool programs to the community. One of the programs is a laboratory school administered by the University of California; the second is a parent cooperative administered by the Berkeley Public Schools. The two programs together enroll children from family backgrounds heterogeneous with respect to education, socioeconomic level, and ethnic origin. Although the sample overrepresents the middle and upper classes, the socioeconomic status (SES) range as measured by the Duncan (1961) index is wide. Sixty-one percent of the children are white, 31% are black, and 8% include other ethnic groups, primarily Asian and Chicano.

Determining Family Status

In order to execute fully *prospective* analyses relating to family dissolution, the divorce or intact status of the subjects' families was established at several times during the course of the project. For each of the 110 subjects at age 14 to 15, family status was determined. Of these 110 families, 60 families had remained intact throughout the study, 8 families were separated, 33 families had been formally divorced, and 9 families had been dissolved for other reasons, such as death of spouse. For the analysis to be reported, the divorced and separated groups were merged ($N = 41$) and compared with the group of intact families ($N = 60$). Within the sample of girls at age 14 to 15, there were 27 (51%) divorced or separated families and 26 (49%) intact families. Within the sample of boys at age 14 to 15, there were 14 (29%) divorced or separated families and 34 (71%) intact families.

Interestingly, within this subject sample, significantly fewer boys than girls experienced divorce ($p < 0.03$). The authors have learned that in several other investigations of family disruption, it was also found that significantly fewer boys than girls were subjected to the experience of divorce (personal communications: Cowan, 1986; Hetherington, 1985; Magnusson, 1986). This observation, although replicated, is nevertheless unusual enough to warrant even further replication and extension before its implications, some of them poignant, can be drawn.

In subsequent references to the "divorced" group, it should be recognized that this group also includes separated parents. Divorced and intact families did not differ in SES or in parental educational level.

By going backward in time and contrasting those children and parents who subsequently experienced divorce with those children and parents who did not, any differences found between these groups are fully prospective and may foretell the later marital dissolution.

To implement this logic, for the 101 families categorized as either separated/divorced or intact when the subjects were at age 14 to 15, family status was determined at earlier ages of the subjects. At the age of 3 to 4, more than a decade earlier, 47 families of girls and 41 families of boys were found to have been fully intact (13 families already had experienced divorce). Of the 47 families intact when the girls were 3 to 4, 26 were still intact at age 14 to 15, whereas 21 had now experienced dissolution. Of the 41 families intact when the boys were 3 to 4, 33 were still intact at age 14 to 15, whereas 8 had now experienced dissolution.

| | Child's Age at the Time of Prospective Analyses | | | |
| | Age 3 to 4 | | Age 6 to 7 | |
	Girls	Boys	Girls	Boys
No. of intact families at the time of prospective analyses	47	41	39	38
No. of these families still intact at age 14 to 15	26	33	26	33
No. of these families having experienced dissolution at age 14 to 15	21	8	13	5

Table 1. Family Status Information: Prospective Analyses

At age 6 to 7, 39 families of girls and 38 families of boys were found to be fully intact. Of the 39 families found intact when the girls were 6 to 7, 26 were still intact at age 14 to 15, whereas 13 had now experienced dissolution. Of the 38 families found intact when the boys were 6 to 7, 33 were still intact at age 14 to 15, whereas 5 families had now experienced dissolution. Table 1 summarizes the information on family status relevant to the prospective analyses.

Although data were obtained also when the children were 11 years old, the authors have not attempted prospective analyses for this age. Too few families experienced divorce between the ages of 11 and 14 to 15 (four families of girls and one family of boys) to permit meaningful prospective analyses.

Measures

Child-rearing Practices Report. When the children were 3 years old, mothers and fathers independently described their child-rearing values via the Q-sort method (Block, 1961) using the Child-rearing Practices Report (CRPR) (Block, 1965), with *specific reference to the child who was a subject in our study.* The CRPR was developed to provide a self-descriptive instrument that would tap both common and uncommon child-rearing dimensions. It consists of 91 items that are arranged by parents in a forced-choice, seven-step, rectangular distribution according to the perceived salience of each item with reference to particular child-rearing orientation. Only parents in intact families provided CRPR descriptions of their child-rearing practices. Hence, the CRPR data are prospective.

Adjective Q-sort. When the children were 6 years old, an interviewer visited their parents in their homes. During the first visit, the mother was asked about the child's physical health and special interests and activities. At this time, the mother was also asked to describe herself, her spouse, and her child, each time using a 43-item Adjective Q-sort (AQ-sort) (Block and Block, 1980). During a second visit by another interviewer, 6 years later when the children were age 12, both parents were asked about their educations, occupations, and daily activities (including family, church, and politics). At this time, each parent provided a self-description, again using the AQ-sort.

Because only intact families were included at age 6, the AQ-sort data collected at this time are prospective with regard to subsequent changes in marital status. At age 12, however, AQ-sort self-descriptions were obtained from parents in both intact and already divorced families.

Environmental Q-sort. An Environmental Q-sort (EQ-sort) (Block, 1971) was used to capture the relative salience of the various features of the familial environment in which a child grows. The EQ-sort taps dimensions regarding physical, social, and psychological aspects of the home and environmental context in which the child grows up. The items of the EQ-sort include such aspects of the familial context as parenting style (level of authoritarianism and attitudes toward punishment), political orientation (liberal versus conservative), psychological characteristics of the mother and of the father, intellectual and cultural interests, degree of investment in the parental role, and the economic status of the family.

In the present study, the EQ was completed by an interviewer after a prolonged visit to the home when the children were 12 years old. These data are concurrent rather than prospective with regard to divorce.

Family Interaction Q-sort. When the child was 13 years old, maternal interactive patterns with the child were compared in intact and divorced families in a laboratory setting. Three separate interaction tasks were devised to obtain a representative sample of interaction patterns: The mother and adolescent child were asked (1) to describe the phenomenology of two emotions using a 16-item adjective Q-sort; (2) to think of possible consequences of three unlikely, hypothetical events; and (3) to create a joint design, using the plastic shapes of the Lowenfeld Mosaic Test (Lowenfeld, 1954).

The videotaped mother-child interaction sessions were assessed using the Family Interaction Q-sort (FIQ) (Gjerde et al., 1981). The FIQ-sort, consisting of 33 widely ranging statements about the interactive behavior of parents, was developed as a macroscopic assessment instrument for objectifying parents' behavior toward children or the other spouse. The judges, mostly graduate students or Ph.D.-level professionals, had extensive experience in working with families in a variety of clinical and/or research settings. They described the mother by arranging the Q-sort items in a forced-choice, nine-step, quasinormal distribution according to the evaluated salience of each item with reference to a particular parental behavior.

Pairs of trained and calibrated judges, selected from a panel of 18 judges, working independently, assessed each mother-child session. Their two Q-sorts were averaged, and this consensus FIQ-sort formulation was used in subsequent analyses.

Data Analysis

Point-biserial correlations were calculated between parental marital status (divorced versus intact)—determined when the children were 14 to 15—and the independently obtained descriptions of parental and home characteristics. In the *prospective* analyses, only families then intact were evaluated. The comparisons made were between those parents subsequently experiencing divorce and those parents who, to date, have remained together. In the *concurrent* analyses, characteristics of intact and divorced families were compared after marriage dissolution of the divorced families.

The reader's attention is called to the perspective with which the authors offer the present findings. Although the total sample size is reasonably large by usual standards, when further subdivided to meet the logical requirements of the analytical design, the subsamples inevitably become small, thus weakening the power of the statistical tests. Although from a clinical perspective, it would have been desirable to further subdivide the divorced group according to the age of the child when divorce occurred, the sample size was simply insufficient to statistically implement this additional inquiry. Furthermore, the reader should recognize that in the present context, the point-biserial correlations used fall on a compressed scale. Because of constraints set by the relative sizes of the two groups (divorce versus intact) being contrasted, point-biserial correlations necessarily have theoretical maximal values appreciably less than ±1.00. Consequently, and separate from the more general and endemic attenuation problem (Block, 1963, 1964), the point-biserial coefficients to be reported here can be said to underestimate the magnitudes of the underlying relationships. This underestimation is greatest for the sample of boys where the divorced group is especially small relative to the intact group. Although these analytical constraints represent facts of life, the unusual opportunity for prospective study warrants the exploratory analyses reported here.

RESULTS

Prospective Analyses

Parental child-rearing orientations before divorce. Parental marital status (divorced versus intact), determined when the children were 14 to 15 years old was correlated with the parents' CRPR-items describing their child-rearing orientations completed 11 years earlier, when the children were 3 years old. To ensure strictly *prospective* relationships, only families intact at the time the CRPR descriptions were completed are included in these analyses. Because parental CRPR Q-sorts were completed with a particular target child in mind (i.e., the child participating in this longitudinal project), the CRPR item analyses were conducted separately for the samples of boys and girls. The differentiating CRPR items and their associated point-biserial correlations are reported.

As much as 11 years before the occurrence of marital disruption, the fathers of boys from families eventually experiencing divorce tended to characterize themselves as *often angry with their sons* (0.69), as *having conflict with their sons* (0.57), as *forgetful of their promises to their sons* (0.50), as *helping of their sons when teased by friends* (0.43), as *uninterested in how well their sons eat* (0.41), as *not using supernatural explanations* (0.40), as *without strict rules for their sons* (0.39), as *without warm and intimate ties to their sons* (0.39), and as *expecting a great deal of their sons* (0.38). The mothers of these boys who later experienced divorce, compared with the mothers of the boys who will not experience divorce, reported *more conflict with their sons* (0.50), *wish their husbands were more interested in their sons* (0.39), are *strict and tense with their sons* (0.35), and are *accepting of the chances their sons must take while growing up* (0.34). All of these correlations reach the 0.05 level of significance.

Evaluating the separate and conjoint implications of these relationships, the authors note that these fathers acknowledged having conflict with their sons and expressing anger toward them. Perhaps as a reaction to these interpersonal difficulties, they seemed disengaged and uninvolved with their boys, forgetful of promises made, uninterested in how the sons were developing, and unconcerned with laying down the behavior-guiding prescriptions and proscriptions their to-be-socialized sons required. The mothers also had problems with their sons, were tense and anxious with them, and wished for more help from their husbands in dealing with their sons who, not surprisingly, were rambunctious and undercontrolled *before* the dissolution of the marriage (Block et al., 1986).

The fathers of girls in families that later dissolve tended to characterize themselves as *prohibiting their daughters to tease and trick others* (0.36), *unhurried with respect to the weaning* (0.36) and the *toilet training* (0.35) of their daughters, and *easy-going and relaxed with their daughters* (0.34). The mothers of daughters who later experienced divorce, more than mothers of daughters who do not experience divorce, *believed it is good for their daughters to play competitive games* (0.34), *encouraged their daughters to do their very best* (0.31), and opted for *physical punishment as the choice discipline for their daughters* (0.33). All of these correlations reach the 0.05 level of significance.

The fathers of these girls characterized themselves as relaxed, tolerant, and unforcing of their daughters, whereas the mothers, in harsh contrast, pressed their daughters toward achievement and competition and were willing to invoke physical punishment to move their girls in desired directions.

Mothers' descriptions of self and of spouse before divorce. Marital status when the children were 14 to 15 years old was related to the mothers' Q-item descriptions of themselves and, separately, of their spouses formulated when their children were 6 years old. To ensure strictly *prospective* relationships, this analysis used only the descriptions offered by mothers whose families still remained intact when their children (whether boys or girls) were age 6.

The mothers in families eventually experiencing divorce tended to describe themselves before the divorce in negative terms. Thus, more than mothers who would remain married, they saw themselves as *likely to get upset easily* (0.38), *unmischievous* (0.38), *restless* (0.33), *not calm and relaxed* (0.31), relatively *unsociable* (0.29), *self-centered* (0.27), *not obedient* (0.26), *ambitious* (0.25), and *not assertive* (0.23), all of these correlations reaching the 0.10 level of significance. (The authors deliberately lowered the threshold of statistical significance here from 0.05 to 0.10 because, with small samples (*N* of 32 through 36) and in an exploratory study such as this one, it is strategically desirable to lessen the likelihood of type II errors even at some risk of making more type I errors.)

In the families subsequently experiencing divorce, the mothers' descriptions of the husbands to whom they still were married were generally negative. The mothers characterized the husbands they would later divorce as relatively *ambitious* (0.30), *not calm or relaxed* (0.27), *not affectionate or loving* (0.25), *not obedient* (0.24), *not helpful* (0.23), and *as assertive* (0.23), *critical* (0.23), *talkative* (0.23), and *stubborn* (0.23), all of these correlations reaching at least the 0.10 level of significance. Note that these characterizations were made sometimes as long as 8 years before divorce.

The mothers characterized themselves as relatively vulnerable, tense, restless, resentful, unplayful, self-preoccupied, and unsociable, a sad and unhappy picture indeed. Their perceptions of their husbands portrayed a failing relationship; a husband who was not affectionate or supportive or flexible or calm but who was dominating, freely critical, and ambitious.

Concurrent Analyses

Mothers' and fathers' self-descriptions in intact and divorced families. Both mothers and fathers described themselves using the AQ-sort when the children were 12 years old. By this time, with only a few exceptions, family dissolution had already occurred in the divorced group. These parental self-descriptions were then related to the marital status index. Hence, these AQ-item analyses compare intact parental pairs with already separated parents. The authors do not report additional fractionation of the results according to whether the child involved is male or female because our analyses suggest this distinction is not relevant here.

Marital status was extensively related to maternal self-descriptions. Relative to mothers still living with their husbands, the divorced mothers viewed themselves critically. They believed themselves to be *distractable* (0.51), *not orderly* (0.48), *easily upset* (0.35), *not creative* (0.34), *not logical* (0.33), *not self-confident* (0.30), *not sensible* (0.30), *not calm* (0.28) but as *affectionate* (0.28). All of these correlations were significant at or beyond the 0.05 level.

Fewer AQ items discriminated between the self-descriptions of fathers in divorced and intact families possibly because the sample of available fathers at this age was appreciably smaller than the sample of mothers (father $N = 44$; mother $N = 61$). Relative to fathers living in intact families, divorced fathers tended to describe themselves as *rebellious* (0.31), *not needing of approval* (0.30), *curious* (0.28), *self-controlled* (0.27), *unhelpful* (0.26), and as *not getting upset easily* (0.25). All of these correlations are significant at or beyond the 0.10 level.

After, as well as before, divorce, the divorced mothers conveyed a sense of low self-esteem. Although affectionate, they tended to characterize themselves as lacking in self-confidence, tense, readily upset, erratic, and not in control of their lives. After divorce, fathers, providing their own characterizations, ascribed largely positive qualities to themselves that in interesting ways are convergent with the largely negative descriptions of them offered 6 years earlier by their then wives. These fathers viewed themselves as independent, even rebellious and unhelpful, self-controlled, not easily disturbed, and curious. Overall, the fathers' self-picture can be seen as the obverse of a personality described earlier by wives as assured but unrelating and unsupportive.

Descriptions of the home environment in intact and divorced families. When the children were approximately 12 years old, the EQ-sort was used to obtain descriptions of the home environment for both divorced and intact families. The results reported derive from the pooled samples of boys and girls.

The differentiating EQ-items (and their correlations) characterizing the single-parent family are as follows: *the family situation is unstable, without a sense of permanence* (0.59); *practicality and function is stressed in the home* (0.43); *the mother is career-oriented* (0.40); *the family is not financially comfortable* (0.40); *the house decorations are not ornate* (0.38); *the house and grounds are ill-tended* (0.38); *the mother does not stress the value of culture and the arts* (0.36); *the mother does not emphasize power, status, or materiality* (0.33); *the child is not in a sophisticated, complex home environment* (0.32); *the mother works outside the home* (0.32); *the house appears messy, dirty, and unkempt* (0.32); *the home is not orderly or predictable* (0.31); *the family is unconcerned with socio-political issues* (0.30); *there are hazards about the house* (0.30); *the family atmosphere is discordant and conflicted* (0.30); *the family atmosphere is constricted and suppressive* (0.30); *many tragedies and misfortunes beset the family* (0.30); *the home situation is child-oriented* (0.30); *the family atmosphere is informal* (0.29); *the mother's needs and limitations are apparent to the child* (0.27); and *the mother does not em-*

phasize an intellectual orientation (0.25). All of these relationships reach the 0.05 level of significance.

The many characteristics distinguishing the single-parent family portray a marginally-maintained home situation. The mother, necessarily off to work for economic reasons, does not appear to have the time, energy, or orientation to establish a stable and supportive family atmosphere for the adolescent child. Pressed by external circumstances, the mother, as the primary and perhaps solitary adult, seems able to invoke only minimal standards for family survival: unembellished practicality is emphasized, the house is not kept up, there is little cultural richness in the surround. Ever present is a sense that the mother is close to being overwhelmed, and her child knows this.

Stresses associated with being a working mother, both in the home and out, both before and after divorce, may account for some of the pre- and postprofile dimensions of the eventually divorced wife found in this study. Future studies controlling for stress-related work factors and the SES variability in this sample might further define the profile of the divorced mother and help to delineate characteristics unique to her.

Descriptions of mother-adolescent interaction in intact and divorced families. Interactive patterns of mothers from intact and divorced families were compared. These FIQ item analyses were conducted separately for girls and boys because rating of maternal interactive behaviors were conducted vis-à-vis a specific child. Because fathers from divorced families had only infrequently retained custody of the child, similar analyses were not attainable for fathers.

The qualities of maternal interactive behaviors in single-parent families differed substantially for the samples of girls and boys. Divorced mothers, more than the married mothers, were seen as *unevaluative* (0.57), *aware of and comfortable with their daughters' sexuality* (0.57), *egalitarian* (0.49), *unenforcing of directives* (0.46), *affectively warm* (0.45), *seductive* (0.42), and *protective* (0.36) with their early adolescent daughters. All of these correlations reached the 0.05 level of significance.

The mother-son relationship was less strongly associated with marital status. In single-parent families, the mother-son relationship was described as less harmonious than the mother-daughter relationship. In particular, mothers from the separated/divorced group, more than married mothers, were described as *competitive* (0.46) and as *not having influence over their sons* (0.35). Both of these correlations were significant beyond the 0.05 level.

The distinguishing FIQ-items add further to the authors' picture of mother-adolescent interactions after divorce. The relationship that mothers establish with their daughters may be characterized as warm, intimate, even sisterly. In contrast, the mothers of sons seem to have lost parental authority; their sons go their own way with the mother trying to keep up.

DISCUSSION

The authors' prospective analyses converge in suggesting that in families eventually experiencing divorce, parental orientations toward child rearing are relatively unsupportive of the child years before the family formally ceases to be intact. As early as 11 years before divorce, parents of boys reported considerable differences in their child-rearing orientations (the father is disengaged and the mother is resentful) and conflict with their sons. This finding is consonant with, and a multifaceted extension of, the finding the authors earlier reported (Block et al., 1981) that a quantitative measure of parental disagreement on child-rearing orientations foretold later divorce.

One of the most common findings in the divorce research literature is that boys appear more reactive than girls to divorce: boys' postdivorce behaviors have consistently been characterized in terms of increased undercontrol of impulse and aggression (Hetherington et al., 1979; Wallerstein and Kelly, 1980). However, other data from the authors' longitudinal study indicate that, long before divorce occurs in a family, sons tend to be impulsive and undercontrolled relative to boys in families that will remain intact (Block et al., 1986). This early-observed personality characteristic of boys who eventually will experience divorce, besides compelling a reinterpretation of research on the affects of divorce in children, helps explain why, in families that will in time dissolve, there is relatively more conflict between parents and sons than between parents and daughters.

Not surprisingly, the strain between spouses is apparent years before the divorce occurs. This tension is revealed, for example, when the subsequently divorcing mothers, long before divorce, characterized their husbands as stubborn, critical, and lacking in affection. There would appear to be some reality to these early characterizations by the wives because years later, after divorce, divorced fathers portray themselves in terms that, although mostly positive or neutral, seem nevertheless in deep correspondence with the early characterizations of them as affectively uninvolved by their then-wives. Both before and after divorce, mothers in families that cease to be intact describe themselves in terms that indicate low self-esteem, suggesting that marital strain and a failing or failed marriage may affect mothers more strongly than fathers. Because the mother is the parent who most often is given custody of the child, the poor self-image of the mother may impose yet another source of strain upon children living in single-parent households.

When the mother-adolescent relationship in already divorced families was evaluated, the mother-son relationship was described as more conflicted and tense than the mother-daughter relationship. Interestingly, even in intact families, the mother-son relationship is described as more conflict-ridden than the mother-daughter relationship *but only when the relationship is assessed in a mother-child dyad (i.e., in the absence of the father)*. When the mother-son dyads from intact families are transformed into a mother-father-son triads, the harmony of the mother-son relationship improves markedly (Dornbush et al., 1985; Gjerde, 1986). That is, we find the presence of the father moderates the degree of conflict between mothers and sons in early adolescence. However, in divorced single-parent families, this positive paternal influence is not available, thus raising the possibility that the mother-son relationship will deteriorate further over time and not manifest the communication improvement commonly seen in intact families as the son grows older (cf. Hill et al., 1985; Steinberg, 1981).

Our findings have implications for decisions regarding child custody in divorce cases. It is still true that mothers generally receive custody of their children, both daughters and sons. Because the mother-daughter relationship tends to be relatively comfortable, warm and egalitarian in comparison to the mother-son relationship in divorced families, there would appear to be no clear indications arguing against mother custody of the daughter. The troublesome nature of the mother-son relationship, however, introduces some additional complexities. If the mother-son difficulties are related to some intrinsic qualities of the mother (as compared with the father or any available adult) then it might be wise to consider father custody of the son or, if feasible, joint custody so as to introduce the *further* structuring provided by the male parent.

The authors suggest that the general lack of prospective data on families eventually experiencing divorce has resulted in confusion between the causes and consequences of the dissolution of families. In order to clearly determine the consequences of divorce for children's lives, we must evaluate home environments, parents' personalities and values, and children's behaviors both before and after divorce. Only if prior "baseline" information is available can we begin to comprehend the complex relationships among divorce, family functioning, and child development.

REFERENCES

Block, J. (1956), A comparison of forced and unforced Q-sorting procedures. *Educational and Psychological Measurements, 16:481–493.*
—— (1957), A comparison between ipsative and normative ratings of personality. *J. Abnorm. Soc. Psychol., 54:50–54.*
—— (1961), *The Q-sort Method in Personality Assessment and Psychiatric Research.* Springfield, Ill.: Charles C Thomas. (Reprinted: (1978), Palo Alto, Cal.: Consulting Psychologists Press.)
—— (1963), The equivalence of measures and the correction for attenuation. *Psychol. Bull., 60:152–156.*

—— (1964), Recognizing attenuation effects in the strategy of research. *Psychol. Bull.*, 62:214–216.

—— (1971), *Lives Through Time*. Berkeley, Calif.: Bancroft Books.

Block, J. H. (1965), *The child-rearing practices report (CRPR)* (in mimeo). University of California, Berkeley: Institute of Human Development.

—— Block, J. (1980), The role of ego-control and ego-resiliency in the organization of behavior. In: *Minnesota Symposia on Child Psychology, Vol 13*, ed. W. A. Collins. New York: Lawrence Erlbaum Associates, pp. 39–101.

—— —— Morrison, A. (1981), Parental agreement-disagreement on child-rearing orientations and gender-related personality correlates in children. *Child Dev.*, 52:965–974.

—— —— Gjerde, P. F. (1986), The personality of children prior to divorce: a prospective study. *Child Dev.*, 57:827–840.

Cattell, R. B. (1944), Psychological measurement: ipsative, normative, and interactive. *Psychological Review*, 51:292–303.

Cherlin, A. J. (1981), *Marriage, Divorce, and Remarriage*. Cambridge, Mass.: Harvard University Press.

Colletta, N. D. (1979), The impact of divorce: father absence or poverty? *Journal of Divorce*, 1:27–38.

Derdeyn, A. P. (1976), A consideration of legal issues in child custody contests. *Arch. Gen. Psychiatry*, 33:165–171.

Dornbush, S. M., Carlsmith, J. M., Bushwall, S. J., et al. (1985), Single parents, extended households, and the control of adolescents. *Child Dev.*, 56:326–341.

Duncan, O. (1961), A socioeconomic index for all occupations. In: *Occupations and Social Status*, ed. A. J. Reiss, Jr. New York: Free Press, pp. 109–138.

Emery, R. E. (1982), Interparental conflict and the children of discord and divorce. *Psychol. Bull.*, 2:310–330.

Fine, M., Moreland, J. & Schwebel, A. (1983), The long-term effects of divorce on parent-child relations. *Developmental Psychology*, 19:703–713.

Gjerde, P. F. (1986), The interpersonal structure of family interaction settings: parent-adolescent relations in dyads and triads. *Developmental Psychology*, 22:297–304.

—— Block, J. & Block, J. H. (1981), *The family interaction Q-sort* (in mimeo). Department of Psychology, University of California, Berkeley.

Glick, P. C. (1979), Children of divorced parents in demographic perspective. *Journal of Social Issues*, 4:170–182.

Guilford, J. P. (1952), When to factor analyze, *Psychol. Bull.*, 49:26–37.

Hainline, L. & Feig, E. (1978), Correlates of childhood father absence in college-aged women. *Child Dev.*, 49:37–42.

Hetherington, E. M. (1979), *Toward a life-course conception of divorce and its effects on children*. Report written under a contract issued by the National Institute of Education.

—— Cox, M. & Cox, R. (1979), Play and social interaction in children following divorce. *Journal of Social Issues*, 4:26–49.

Hill, J. P., Holmbeck, G. N., Maslow, L., Green, T. M. & Lynch, M. E. (1985), Pubertal status and parent-child relations in families of seventh-grade boys. *Journal of Early Adolescence*, 5:31–44.

Hingst, A. G. (1981), Children and divorce: the child's view. *Journal of Clinical Child Psychology*, 3:161–164.

Hodges, F. H., Wechsler, R. C. & Ballantine, C. (1979), Divorce and the pre-school child: cumulative stress. *Journal of Divorce,* 1:55–63.

Hoffmann, S. (1977), Marital instability and the economic status of women. *Demography,* 14:67–77.

Jacobson, D. S. (1978a), The impact of marital separation/divorce on children: I. parent-child separation and child adjustment, *Journal of Divorce,* 4:341–355.

—— (1978b), The impact of marital separation/divorce on children: II. interparent hostility and child adjustment. *Journal of Divorce,* 1:3–19.

—— (1978c), The impact of marital separation/divorce on children: III. parent-child communication and child adjustment, and regression analysis of findings from overall study. *Journal of Divorce,* 2:175–194.

Kurdek, L. A. & Siesky, A. E. (1980), Effects of divorce on children: the relationship between parent and child perspectives. *Journal of Divorce,* 2:85–93.

Levitin, T. E. (1979), Children of divorce: an introduction. *Journal of Social Issues,* 4:1–23.

Lowenfeld, M. (1954), *Lowenfeld Mosaic Test.* London: Newman and Neame.

Nelson, G. (1981), Moderators of women's and children's adjustment following parental divorce. *Journal of Divorce,* 3:71–78.

Rosen, R. (1979), Some crucial issues concerning children of divorce. *Journal of Divorce,* 1:19–25.

Rosenthal, P. A. (1979), Sudden disappearance of one parent with separation and divorce: the grief and treatment of preschool children. *Journal of Divorce,* 1:43–52.

Select Committee on Children, Youth, and Families of the United States House of Representatives. (1983), *U.S. Children and Their Families: Current Conditions and Recent Trends.* Washington, D.C.: Government Printing Office.

Sorosky, A. D. (1977), The psychological effects of divorce on adolescents. *Adolescence,* 45:123–136.

Spanier, G. & Thompson, L. (1984), *Parting: The Aftermath of Separation and Divorce.* Beverly Hills, Cal.: Sage.

Steinberg, L. D. (1981), Transformations in family relations at puberty. *Developmental Psychology,* 17:833–840.

Stephenson, W. (1953), *The Study of Behavior.* Chicago: University of Chicago Press.

Wallerstein, J. S. (1984), Children of divorce: preliminary report of a ten-year followup of young children. *Am. J. Orthopsychiatry,* 54:444–458.

—— (1985), The overburdened child: some long-term consequences of divorce. *Social Work in Health Care,* 30:116–123.

—— Kelly, J. (1976), The effects of parental divorce: experiences of the child in later latency. *Am. J. Orthopsychiatry,* 46:255–269.

—— —— (1980), *Surviving the Breakup: How Children and Parents Cope with Divorce.* New York: Basic Books.

14

Issues of Adolescent Development for Survivors of Childhood Cancer

Gregory K. Fritz and Judith R. Williams

Rhode Island Hospital, Brown University Program in Medicine

The adjustment of 41 adolescent survivors of childhood cancer was assessed. Global functioning was good or excellent for 61% of the group and marginal or poor for 27%. Depression was uncommon and self-concept scores were higher than normative values. Concerns about their bodies were problematic for more than half the group. Over 27% were rated as counterphobic and 26% as hypochondriacal. Subtle concerns about their sexuality, attractiveness to the opposite sex, and reproductive capacity were frequent. Over 60% also identified a positive effect of the illness.

Professionals in a variety of disciplines question whether or not children and adolescents are psychologically damaged by the stresses of a chronic illness. It has been argued that chronic childhood illness in general, and cancer in particular, predisposes patients to psychopathology (Kashani and Hakani, 1982; Maguire, 1983; Obetz et al., 1980). Others have emphasized the patients' psychological normalcy (Kellerman et al., 1980; Orr et al., 1984). Studies dealing specifically with long-term survivors of cancer are few and the findings inconclusive (Li and Stone, 1976; Koocher and O'Malley, 1981; Lansky et al., 1986). Adolescence, with its physical and psychological changes and developmental challenges, may be a particularly vulnerable period in which to grapple with the consequences of cancer. This paper focuses on variables of particular relevance to adolescents in a group of teenage cancer survivors.

Reprinted with permission from the *Journal* of the *American Academy of Child and Adolescent Psychiatry,* 1988, Vol. 27, No. 6, 712–715. Copyright 1988 by the American Academy of Child and Adolescent Psychiatry.

This work was supported by the W. T. Grant Foundation through a Faculty Scholar Award to Dr. Fritz, and by the California Division of the American Cancer Society.

METHOD

The subjects were 41 adolescents who were recruited as part of a larger, prospective study of the effects of cancer treatment termination (Fritz and Williams, 1988). Characteristics of the study group are summarized in Appendix 1. The adolescents had successfully completed treatment for a variety of malignancies (excluding brain tumors) from 2 to 8 years earlier at the Children's Hospital at Stanford. Diagnoses included leukemias (34%), Hodgkins disease (21%), non-Hodgkins lymphomas (22%), and bone sarcomas (10%), with other diagnoses accounting for 13% of the sample. Overall, the group was relatively free from significant physical sequelae of their diseases and treatment. Seventy-seven percent had no visible scars or physical deformities and 95% had no physical impairment that interfered with daily living, as rated by the Physical Impairment Rating Scale (Koocher and O'Malley, 1981). The mean number of years of treatment was 3.7. The study group was almost equally divided between males and females and included adolescents from all social strata and religious backgrounds. Most subjects were Caucasian, with Latinos comprising the only significant minority group. Forty-seven percent of eligible subjects were contacted, of whom only two refused to participate. The group was representative of the institution's adolescent cancer survivors.

The study protocol has been described in detail elsewhere (Fritz and Williams, 1988). It included both standard assessment instruments (described below) and separate, structured interviews with the adolescents and with their parents. These interviews each lasted 60 to 90 minutes and covered a wide range of issues, including those relating to the developmental tasks of adolescence. The interviews were videotaped and independently rated by the two investigators. Interrater reliability was high, with Pearson correlation coefficients for most items ranging between 0.75 and 0.93. Each interviewer dictated extensive case history notes to complete the data set.

RESULTS

Psychopathology and overall functioning were assessed in several ways. The Children's Depression Rating Scale (CDRS) was used to quantify the presence or absence of depressive symptomatology (Poznanski et al., 1984). Three adolescents (7%) were identified as definitely depressed and in need of treatment (CDRS > 40), five (12%) were rated as questionably depressed (CDRS > 30 to 40), and 33 (81%) were rated as not depressed (CDRS < 30). The Piers-Harris Self Concept Scale (Piers, 1983) revealed a high self-image for the survivors as a group, with almost 75% scoring in the upper third on the instrument's normative scale.

A final rating resulted in an index of Global Adjustment. In contrast to other ratings, the Subject's Global Adjustment score was a consensus rating arrived at in a case conference in which the interviews, process notes, and medical record comments (but not the scores on standard ratings or assessment instruments) were reviewed by the three members of the research team. The adolescent was rated by consensus on a five-point scale as to the degree he or she had (1) integrated the illness experience, (2) developed satisfying peer relationships, (3) evolved a sense of purposefulness and direction, and (4) achieved age appropriate separation from the family. These factors were summarized in the index of Global Adjustment, in which 29% of the group was rated as showing excellent adjustment; 32%, good adjustment; 22%, average or satisfactory adjustment; 7%, marginal to poor adjustment; and 10%, very poor adjustment. The four subjects rated very poorly adjusted were among the eight who had completed treatment a second time after a relapse, an association that was highly significant (χ^2 = 10.86 with 2 df; p = 0.004). The global adjustment ratings were also analyzed to see if adolescent survivors whose treatment had ended before adolescence were better adjusted than those who were treated during adolescence. The 20 subjects who had ended treatment prior to age 13 had a mean global adjustment score of 3.75 on the five-point scale while the 21 who had been treated during adolescence had a mean of 3.52; t-test showed this difference to be nonsignificant (F = 1.06; df = 39; p = 0.572).

The standard instruments showed that psychopathology was relatively rare and the ratings indicated that global functioning was satisfactory. However, the extensive interviews suggested subtle but enduring psychological consequences for the adolescent cancer survivors. Although 24% were rated as appropriate and realistic with regard to their attitudes about their bodies, most of the adolescents had persisting concerns about their bodies that were manifested in a variety of ways. Twenty-one percent were rated as counterphobic with regard to their bodies. Included in this group were those who involved themselves in especially challenging, often dangerous physical activity.

> Allan, 21 years old at the time of the interviews, had started treatment for advanced rhabdomyosarcoma of the leg when he was 13. A relapse, after a 1-year remission, necessitated a second round of treatment. Against long odds, he was free of disease and apparently cured five years after the end of his last therapy. Despite his weakened leg, he had become involved in free climbing (without safety ropes) of cliffs and rock faces. He used his mechanic's job to modify a car that he drove fast and recklessly. He acknowledged

his risky behavior, and described himself as fearless: "After all I've been through, I'm not afraid to die anymore."

Others in this group were exhibitionistic and would flaunt a stump or a scar as a matter of pride but also for shock value.

Kathy, a gregarious 17-year-old Hispanic girl, had concluded treatment for an osteogenic sarcoma of the femur three years previously. A high amputation of her leg was followed by chemotherapy. She was the first to dance at a party, often by herself, and enjoyed the amazement of her peers. At the beach she would unstrap her prosthesis and go for a hopping "walk" along the water's edge. Despite the physical arduousness of such a feat, she said the pride she felt was worth the effort.

Twenty-six percent of the adolescent survivors were rated as still extremely preoccupied with their physical condition in a hypochondriacal manner. They continued to scrutinize their bodies and bodily functions, often justifying their preoccupation as preventative surveillance. Illnesses or symptoms that resembled those that preceded the cancer diagnosis were especially worrisome. A 16-year-old who was diagnosed with Hodgkins disease after some weeks of persistent coughing and low grade fevers, became anxious with any cold or flu symptoms. An 18-year-old survivor of leukemia was convinced that his remission depended on a rigid regimen of exercise and dietary control.

Twenty-nine percent were rated as having a low or negative body image. A negative body image could be a consequence of both medical and psychodynamic factors.

Bill, a 14-year-old ninth grader, interviewed three years posttreatment for acute lymphocytic leukemia, described himself as a "sports nut" prior to his diagnosis. During his treatment and subsequently, Bill lost all interest in sports. "Dungeons and Dragons," his collections, and TV now occupied most of his time. He had become passive, ate excessively and was dependent on his mother. Bill's troubled relationship with his father became aggravated by the illness. The father became more involved with Bill's physically active, athletic and popular younger brother. The changes that had taken place during treatment lessened but persisted after its conclusion.

Some of the adolescents were not "negative" about their physical capacities but keenly aware of the ambiguity and unpredictability of their health status. A high school senior commented on the irony of describing her health as excellent on her college application as she worried about her "fatal disease." An 18-year-old commented on the incongruity of learning of his relapse on the evening of the day he played in a football game.

The relationship between ratings of the adolescents' attitudes toward their bodies and the physical residua from the illness and/or treatment, as reflected in the Physical Impairment Rating Scale scores, was not significant ($\chi^2 = 7.31$ with 4 df; $p = 0.12$). Thus, neither greater nor fewer overt signs of the past treatment were associated with particular attitudes toward their bodies. The association between the global adjustment and the body image ratings was not statistically significant ($\chi^2 = 3.30$ with 2 df; $p = 0.19$), suggesting that the adolescents' views of their bodies were subtle and sufficiently encapsulated to be compatible with adequate or better global functioning.

Since the establishment of a sexual identity and development of heterosexual relationships are important tasks of adolescence, the lasting effects, if any, of the cancer experience on these issues were explored. The adolescents' heterosexual relationships were rated as avoidant/extremely uncomfortable, entirely platonic, or age appropriate. It was recognized in the ratings that age appropriate relationships and activities are different for early, middle, and late adolescents. These ratings were analyzed in relation to age in a one way analysis of variance. The mean age of the survivors in each of the rated groups was not significantly different from the other rated groups or from the mean of the sample ($F = 0.867$ with 3 df; $p = 0.47$). Concerns about sexuality were subtle but pervasive. Twenty-seven percent of the survivors were rated as having significant difficulties or discomfort in relationships with the opposite sex. Predictably, a disproportionate number of these had an overall poor global adjustment. However, significant discomfort in this area did not preclude otherwise good adjustment.

> Jim, age 17, had been treated for a sarcoma of the left scapula diagnosed four years earlier. He was an enthusiastic, conscientious student who had maintained his excellent academic standing during and after treatment. His main interests were writing and reading. He was editor of his school newspaper and worked in the family business after school. After his cancer experience he decided to become a physician, and was soon to start the premedical track at a prestigious college. Asked about his social life, he said he'd never dated and "didn't consider it." He viewed any romantic involvement with girls as unrealistic, denied concern about that as-

pect of his life, and was focusing his energies on his studies and career.

An equal number of the adolescents (27%) were socially active and described friendships with peers of both sexes. However, their relationships with the opposite sex were entirely platonic: they didn't go to dances, date, or have a boyfriend or girlfriend. A ninth grader wistfully described herself as a much sought after confidante but never the girl with whom boys flirted or whom they wanted to date. A 16-year-old boy felt his cancer treatment had made him "more mature and able to talk about problems." He had several close but platonic relationships with girls. He was proud of these intimate friendships but acknowledged his lack of typical adolescent heterosexual relationships.

Forty-six percent of the adolescents dated occasionally, had or had had a boyfriend or girlfriend or, if they were young teenagers, were rated as age appropriate in their relationships with the opposite sex. Yet even within this group, it was the rare adolescent who felt comfortable discussing his or her malignancy. The adolescents were unsure of the reaction they would elicit and concerned they might appear unattractive to the opposite sex. Several of the older adolescents had been secretive about their cancer with otherwise close friends.

The interviews elicited concerns about the long term consequences of the malignancy and its treatment on reproductive capacities for those in middle and late adolescence. These concerns were rarely brought up spontaneously. Over two thirds had not discussed the possibility of sterility with their oncologists, and some of these frankly admitted they were delaying a direct confirmation of their possible sterility. Others claimed they had been "meaning to ask, but always forgot."

> Cindy, a 19-year-old survivor of Hodgkins disease, was enjoying a busy and successful first year in college, both socially and academically. Her steady boyfriend knew of her cancer and she described him as supportive. Cindy had not "bothered" to obtain information about her possible sterility because she had decided not to have children. She "would not want to go through what her mother had" with a child of her own, and expected to be too busy with her career.

The survivors were asked if they felt any good had come from their illness. Their responses are summarized in Appendix 2 and listed in order of their frequency. The 61% who said "yes" were firm in their beliefs and often attributed a number of positive changes to the cancer experience. The interview often corroborated the survivors' assertion that they had become more empathetic, confident, mature, and/or goal directed. They did not romanticize the illness. Only one survivor felt that the positive changes compensated for the negative aspects and saw the diagnosis as a critical turning point in her life:

> Karen was 18 years old and had finished treatment for non-Hodgkins lymphoma two years previously. She learned of her likely diagnosis from a physician at an inner-city clinic which she had visited as a teenage runaway. Alienated from her family and failing at school, she had left home and was largely living on the streets. She had used a variety of drugs on a daily basis and been involved in a series of exploitative relationships. After her cancer was diagnosed, she returned home and allowed her mother to care for her. Her bravery and responsibility during treatment "amazed everyone, including myself." At the time of the study, Karen was working full time, active in a structured, fundamentalist church, and about to take her high school equivalency examination.

The ability to identify some personal benefit from the illness and its treatment correlated significantly with global adjustment (Spearman $r = 0.46$; $p = 0.001$) but not with the CDRS depression score (Spearman $r = -0.16$; $p = 0.174$).

DISCUSSION

Two to eight years after their treatment ended, when they were between 13 and 21 years of age, childhood cancer survivors are psychologically more intact than we had assumed, based on our clinical psychiatric experience before the study. Depression was clearly evident for 7% of the group, a rate that corresponds closely to the 8% incidence of clinically significant depression among adolescents in the general population as reported by Kashani et al. (1987). Global adjustment was satisfactory or better for over four-fifths of the sample. Serious adjustment problems were strongly associated with having suffered a relapse and undergone a second course of therapy. Although the Piers Harris instrument showed higher self-concept scores for the group than the normative sample, we found subtle and enduring alterations in self perceptions. There is evidence of changes in perceived physical vigor and capacity: for some a sense of fragility and vulnerability against which they defend with self-imposed restrictions or regimens; for others a sense of invincibility that leads them to physical excesses and dangerous acts of bravado.

Wasserman et al. (1987) reported that 20% of a group of long-term Hodgkins disease survivors described increased risk-taking behavior in relation to their illness, a rate that, given the sample sizes, corresponds closely to the 15% found in the present study. While Wasserman et al. noted that most of the risking-taking behavior had settled down in their subjects over the years, the adolescents in our study rated as engaged in risk-taking behavior were still actively doing so. The difference may be at least partially explained by the fact that the Hodgkins survivors averaged 9 to 10 years off treatment and 26 years of age compared to our adolescents' 3 to 4 years off treatment and 17 years of age. The proneness to risk-taking behavior and the multiple possible meanings of this behavior among healthy adolescents have been discussed by Jessor (1984) and Irwin and Millstein (1986). Risk taking among adolescent cancer survivors is no more prevalent than among their healthy peers; if anything, it is less prevalent. Those who did engage in overt risk taking were motivated by factors directly related to their cancer; invulnerability, inferiority, or a sense of tentativeness regarding their future.

More than half of the adolescents were avoidant, guarded, or cautious in heterosexual relationships. Precisely comparable statistics for a healthy comparison group are not available. However, the near universal discomfort about discussing the cancer with members of the opposite sex and the avoidance of the issue of sterility suggest that developmentally appropriate experimentation with romantic relationships was complicated by the cancer experience. Wasserman et al. (1987) found that more than half of their sample did not know whether they were sterile or not, a rate comparable to that found in the present study. Wasserman et al. also reported overall reluctance to discuss the illness as a general characteristic of their older survivors. Vincent et al. (1975) reported a startling lack of relevant sexual information even among adult women who had been treated for cervical cancer, and 79% of these patients who actively desired more sexual information said they would not request that information from their physicians. The responsibility for conveying the relevant information about sexuality and childbearing must rest with the medical professionals. At the same time, the defensive need for repression or denial among some teenage survivors must be recognized and respected.

Two other areas of comparison with the Wasserman study point to similarities between the two different but related samples. In neither group were significant or obvious physical residua a major problem, although attitudes about their bodies were affected for large numbers of survivors in both groups. Large numbers of survivors in both groups identified some positive benefits of the cancer experience. The higher rate (95%) of adult survivors who did so compared to the adolescents (61%) may be a result of greater maturity, the longer elapsed time since treatment, or their particular experience with Hodgkins disease treatment.

The psychosocial impact of cancer survival for adolescents is complex and unpredictable. Most adolescents in the present study were successful in integrating the cancer experience without major distortion in their development. This study was stimulated by clinical psychiatric experience with children and adolescents on whom the diagnosis and treatment had taken a psychological toll. The results underscore once again the pitfalls of generalizing from a psychiatrically referred population.

APPENDIX 1

Adolescent Cancer Survivors Demographic Data (N = 41)

Sex: 20 males, 21 females
Age: $\bar{X} = 17.3$ yrs, SD = 3.1 yrs
Age at diagnosis: $\bar{X} = 11.0$ yrs, SD = 3.6 yrs
Age off treatment: $\bar{X} = 13.6$ yrs, SD = 3.3 yrs
Relapse
  34: no
  7: yes
Ethnicity
  Caucasian 70%
  Latino 20%
  Asian 5%
  Mixed, other 5%
Religion
  Catholic 43%
  Protestant 20%
  Other 17%
  None 20%
Socioeconomic status
  I - 2%
  II - 20%
  III - 27%
  IV - 32%
  V - 20%

APPENDIX 2

Adolescent Cancer Survivors Identified Good from Illness ($N = 41$)

Yes 61%
Possibly 13%
No 26%
Most common reasons for positive responses:
  More empathetic
  Greater self-confidence
  Appreciate life more
  Maturity
  Values clarified; more accepting
  Religious faith strengthened
  More serious about school
  More popular
  Helped career planning
  More altruistic
  More reflective
  Greater goal orientation
  Family closer
  More bodily aware

REFERENCES

Fritz, G. K. & Williams, J. R. (1988), After treatment ends: psychosocial sequelae in pediatric oncology survivors. *Am. J. Orthopsychiat.*

Irwin, C. E. & Millstein, S. G. (1986), Biopsychosocial correlates of risk-taking behavior during adolescence. *J. Adolesc. Health Care*, 7:82S–96S.

Jessor, R. (1984), Adolescent development and behavioral health. In: *Behavioral Health: A Handbook of Health Enhancement and Disease Promotion*, ed. J. D. Matarazzo, New York: Wiley.

Kashani, J. H., Beck, N. C., Hoeper, E. W. et al. (1987), Psychiatric disorders in a community sample of adolescents. *Am. J. Psychiatry*, 144:584–589.

—— Hakani, N. (1982), Depression in children and adolescents with malignancy. *Can. J. Psychiatry*, 27:474–477.

Kellerman, J., Zeltzer, L., Ellenberg, L. et al. (1980), Psychological effects of illness in adolescence. *J. Pediatr.*, 97:126–131.

Koocher, G. P. & O'Malley, J. E. (1981), *The Damocles Syndrome: Psychosocial Consequences of Surviving Childhood Cancer*. New York: McGraw-Hill.

Lansky, S. B., List, M. A. & Ritter-Sterr, C. (1986), Psychosocial consequences of cure. *Cancer*, 58:529–533.

Li, F. P. & Stone, R. (1976), Survivors of cancer in childhood. *Ann. Intern. Med.*, 84:551–553.

Maguire, G. P. (1983), The psychosocial sequelae of childhood leukemia. In: *Pediatric Oncology,* ed. W. Duncan, Berlin: Springer Verlag, pp. 47–56.

Obetz, S. W., Swenson, W. M., McCarthy, C. A. et al. (1980), Children who survive malignant disease: emotional adaptation of the children and their families. In: *The Child with Cancer,* eds. J. L. Schulman & M. J. Kupst. Springfield: C. C. Thomas.

Orr, D. P., Weller, S. C., Satterwhite, B. & Pless, I. B. (1984), Psychosocial implications of chronic illness in adolescence. *J. Pediatr.,* 104:152–157.

Piers, E. V. (1983), *Manual for the Piers-Harris Children's Self Concept Scale.* Los Angeles: Western Psychological Services.

Poznanski, E. O., Grossman, J. A., Buchsbaum, Y., Banegas, M., Freeman, L. & Gibbons, R. (1984), Preliminary studies of the reliability and validity of the Children's Depression Rating Scale. *J. Am. Acad. Child Adolesc. Psychiatry,* 23:191–197.

Vincent, C. E., Vincent, B., Greiss, F. C. & Linton, E. B. (1975), Some marital-sexual concomitants of carcinoma of the cervix. *South. Med. J.,* 68:5–12.

Wasserman, A. L., Thompson, E. I., Wilimas, J. A. & Fairclough, D. L. (1987), The psychological status of survivors of childhood/adolescent Hodgkins disease. *Am. J. Dis. Child.,* 141:626–631.

15

Examining the Effects of Chronic Disease and Disability on Children's Sibling Relationships

Debra Lobato, David Faust, and Anthony Spirito
Rhode Island Hospital, Brown University Program in Medicine

Research on siblings of children with a variety of developmental disabilities and major chronic illnesses was reviewed within the context of literatures on typical sibling relationships and family adaptation. Assumptions, questions, and methods guiding current research were analyzed and critiqued. To date, studies have addressed a narrow range of variables and issues—the detection of maladjustment being the primary concern. Further, predominant reliance on more subjective and anecdotal research methods and failure to control for confounding factors limit the value of investigations. Certain popular beliefs and perceptions have gained support but others have not, in particular the assumption that siblings of handicapped and ill children experience more frequent psychological disturbance. A variable matrix is proposed that may help investigators identify relevant factors, avoid potential confounds, and generate productive hypotheses and research designs.

Sibling relationships are among the most important precursors to peer and later adult relationships (Hartup, 1979; Lamb & Sutton-Smith, 1982). Siblings function to socialize and educate one another, to mediate parental attention and control, and to provide a peer-like context for intense emotional experience and power negotiation. By 1 year of age, children spend as much time interacting with their siblings as they do with their mothers and *more* time with their siblings than with their fathers (Lawson & Ingleby, 1974). Furthermore, as compared to parents and children, siblings not only spend more time

Reprinted with permission from the *Journal of Pediatric Psychology,* 1988, Vol. 13, No. 3, 389–407. Copyright 1988 by Plenum Publishing Corporation.

together during childhood but their life-spans overlap to a greater extent as well (Brody & Stoneman, 1986).

Given the lifelong significance of sibling relationships, it seems unremarkable to posit that substantial changes in the health or functioning of a sibling will affect the other(s) and that these changes may correspond systematically to characteristics of the children, the family, and the disease or disability itself.

This paper examines how disruption to child health and functioning affects sibling interactions and subsequent development, and how relationships among affected and unaffected siblings are like and unlike relationships among healthy siblings. Shedding light on factors that influence sibling outcome should not only enhance our understanding of family functioning in general but also improve our effectiveness in counseling parents regarding the practical and emotional sequelae of pediatric illness for all family members.

The area is relatively understudied, and thus a brief review of current knowledge is provided within the context of typical sibling relations. Rather than conducting an exhaustive review of published commentaries (for this see Crnic & Leconte, 1986; Drotar & Crawford, 1985; Lobato, 1983; McKeever, 1983; Powell & Ogle, 1985; Seligman, 1983; Simeonsson & McHale, 1981), emphasis is given to research assumptions, methodologies, and implications that seem critical in the plan and design of further studies.

IMPORTANT ISSUES AND RESEARCH QUESTIONS

Typical Sibling Relationships and Research

Most of the earlier research on typical sibling relationships examined the group effects of sibling constellation variables (such as birth order, sex, and family size) on intelligence, achievement, and personality (for reviews see Rosenberg, 1982; Sutton-Smith & Rosenberg, 1970; Wagner, Schubert, & Schubert, 1979, 1985; Zajonc & Markus, 1975). Attempts were made to describe the psychological characteristics and differences between groups of firstborn and later-born children. From these characteristics, the nature of sibling interactions was inferred.

Recent sibling studies have emphasized more direct observational methods that are used to examine the actual dynamic interactions between siblings and parents (Lamb & Sutton-Smith, 1982). Observational studies show that sibling relationships extend beyond the traditional notions of hostile rivalry and jealousy. Even at a very young age, the relationship is an extremely rich one, characterized by high rates of access, imitation, affection, and cooperation, as well as aggression. Varying rates of prosocial and aggressive verbal and non-verbal interactions have been described for young siblings according to sibling status characteristics such as age-spacing and sex composition (Abramovich, Corter, & Lando, 1979; Abramovitch, Corter, & Pepler, 1980; Dunn & Kendrick, 1982).

Reflecting the richness of the sibling relationship is the variety of independent and dependent variables and methods employed in research on normal sibling pairs. The dependent variables cover a wide terrain, including such personal characteristics as educational and occupational attainment, achievement motivation, self-esteem, peer popularity, neuroticism, physical growth, parent-child relations, and rates of psychopathology (Folit & Falbo, 1985; Wagner et al., 1985). Observational studies of sibling interaction also have spanned a considerable range of dependent variables: problem-solving behavior (Cicirelli, 1975), language development (Gibbs, Teti, & Bond, 1985), reactions to pregnancy and the birth of a sibling (Dunn, Kendrick, & MacNamee, 1981), and locomotor development (Samuels, 1980). Traditional sibling issues such as loyalty and rivalry have been approached less rigorously through anecdotal case reports and theoretical position papers (Bank & Kahn, 1982; Ihinger, 1975; Levy, 1937).

In addition to the importance of individual sibling characteristics and constellation variables in the normal child developmental literature is the acknowledged significance of contextual and ecological variables in shaping sibling relationships (Brody & Stoneman, 1986). An ecological (Bronfenbrenner, 1979) and transactional (Belsky, 1981; Sameroff, 1975) family perspective asserts that sibling relationships are best understood within the context of other family relationships, status and resources, beliefs, and values. The family, in turn, is best understood within its broader social and cultural ecology. Research consistent with this dynamic family model has emerged recently. For example, among the strongest predictors of prosocial, nonpunitive sibling interactions are a mother's consistent, nonpunitive child-rearing practices and positive self-concept and attitude about her life outside the family (Brody & Shaffer, 1982; Brody & Stoneman, 1986). Thus, within the normal developmental literature, child development and sibling interactions are not conceptualized as simple by-products of single or static child or family characteristics. "Outcome," with its multitude of definitions, is the evolving result of an interacting system of child, family, situational, and cultural variables.

Comparison of Siblings of Healthy and Ill Children

In contrast to the normal child development research, a narrow focus characterizes the methods and issues of existing research on atypical sibling pairs. For example, the titles of many articles suggest that research has been conducted with families of disabled children, but it is a rare paper that looks beyond the reactions of mothers to fathers, no less to siblings. Given the emergence of family systems theory and the belief that adaptation and dysfunction are shared characteristics of family members, it is interesting to note that most of the current studies of "families" are dismembering; siblings are essentially excluded.

Most of the information on siblings of disabled and ill children remains founded on more subjective and anecdotal forms of clinical investigation, such as clinical interview and case report. Few controlled or "empirical" investigations exist. As discussed below, matching procedures and descriptive subject information among these empirical studies have been less than ideal. Furthermore, the use of systematic, direct observation of sibling interactions by trained observers is rare (Mash & Johnston, 1980; Stoneman & Brody, 1987).

Empirical Research: Focus on Maladjustment

Most empirically based, group comparisons examine maladjustment rate among unaffected siblings and attempt to identify associated sibling and family status variables (Breslau, 1982; Breslau, Weitzman, & Messenger, 1981; Gath, 1973; Grossman, 1972; Spinetta, 1981; Tew & Laurence, 1973). Group research generally does not support the popular belief that siblings of disabled and chronically ill children exhibit more problems in overall psychological adjustment than do siblings of able children. There is no uniform or direct relationship between a child's illness and psychopathology among his or her siblings. In fact, many siblings of disabled children appear to benefit emotionally and psychologically from the experience. Grossman (1972) reported that nearly half of the siblings of retarded children she interviewed were rated, in comparison to their peers, as more compassionate, more sensitive, more appreciative of their own good health, and having greater understanding of people. Similarly, teachers rated young siblings of children with diabetes and pervasive developmental disorder as more socially competent and positive with peers than siblings of unaffected children (Ferrari, 1984).

Group research has also uncovered adverse psychological outcomes, including increases in aggressive behavior, poor peer relations, anxiety, somatization, and depression (Breslau, 1982; Breslau et al., 1981; Ferrari, 1984; Lobato, Barbour, Hall, & Miller, 1987; Tew & Laurence, 1973). These adverse reactions appear to be weakly related to sibling constellation variables, such as sibling sex, birth order, and age spacing (Breslau, 1982; Breslau et al., 1981); and to more general family factors such as socioeconomic status, mother's social support, and parent reaction to the disability or disease (Farber, 1959; Ferrari, 1984; Graliker, Fischler, & Koch, 1962; Tew & Laurence, 1973).

Other adverse sibling results have been related to the amount of time since the diagnosis of the illness or disability (Ferrari, 1984); and to the source of the collected data, that is, mother, teacher, or sibling (Ferrari, 1984; Lobato et al., 1987). Sibling self-report has been used infrequently and appears to yield quite different results (Ferrari, 1984; Lobato et al., 1987).

Information derived from mother interview or questionnaire alone reveals a more negative perspective on sibling functioning. For example, in a project comparing preschool aged siblings of handicapped children to a matched control group of siblings of nonhandicapped children, Lobato et al. (1987) found no statistically significant differences between the two groups on sibling-derived measures of perceived self-competence, attitude towards family members, understanding of developmental disabilities, and empathy. In contrast, mothers of the same children rated siblings of handicapped children as more depressed and aggressive than control children.

We are aware of only a few comparative investigations across groups of siblings that examined issues other than rates of psychological or behavioral problems. These include comparisons of home and child-care routines of siblings of children with hearing impairments (Schwirian, 1976) and other developmental disabilities (Lobato et al., 1987), and perception of sibling health status (Townes & Wold, 1977). Despite the common perception that siblings of handicapped children assume excessive child care and home responsibilities (Powell & Ogle, 1985), Schwirian found that responsibilities actually appear to be assumed more in accordance with the siblings' age and sex than with the hearing status of their brothers and sisters. Lobato et al. (1987) found female siblings of handicapped children to have the greatest degree of responsibility for child care and household tasks, although the difference was not statistically significant. However, compared to their matched controls, sisters of handicapped children received significantly fewer privileges and experienced more restrictions on social routines while brothers of handicapped children experienced the opposite—more privileges and fewer restrictions on social activity. Thus, sex of the nonhandicapped siblings was associated with the shape of daily living routines among families with handicapped children but not among control families.

Townes and Wold (1977) asked the parents of 22 healthy siblings of 8 children with leukemia to rate each sibling's knowledge of the threat to life posed by the patient's illness. The parents also indicated how much information about the disease had been discussed at home and how often the siblings questioned them about the ill child's disease. Each sibling also rated the health status and life expectancy of himself/herself and the patient. Overall adjustment, as rated by a symptom checklist, was positively related to level of communication between parents and siblings. The authors did not state the exact nature of their statistical analysis or specific subject characteristics, thereby limiting interpretive value. Clinician impression does support a positive relation between communication and adjustment among patient populations, for example, those with childhood cancer (Spinetta, 1978), but impressions regarding siblings are lacking.

Interview, Survey, and Observational Data: Examining Broader Issues

Personal testimonies or interviews with siblings of chronically ill or disabled children (without a comparison group of "typical" siblings) have provided rich information on the breadth of issues siblings face. Without well-structured comparison groups, however, it is difficult to know how unique or typical these experience might be. Nevertheless, within such reports, the greatest concerns voiced by siblings do *not* involve their own adjustment directly. Rather, siblings express concerns that cover their parents' feelings and those of their chronically ill brother or sister, family communication, resentment of the added attention the child receives, behavior management and protection of the child in public, and guardianship planning in the case of lifelong conditions (Powell & Ogle, 1985).

Noncomparative interviews and surveys of siblings have also explored correlations between siblings' experiences with their retarded brothers and sisters and their later life and career goals (Cleveland & Miller, 1977; Farber, 1963). Findings include a positive correlation between the amount of time siblings spend with their mentally retarded brothers or sisters and the siblings' endorsement of humanitarian life goals (Farber, 1963). Older female siblings (who, presumably, share greatest child care responsibility with mothers) are the most likely of all siblings to pursue the helping professions (Cleveland & Miller, 1977).

Single-subject behavioral studies have demonstrated that nonhandicapped siblings can serve beneficial functions as therapists for disabled children (e.g., Cash & Evans, 1975; Colletti & Harris, 1977; Lobato & Barrera, 1988; Lobato & Tlaker, 1985; Schreibman, O'Neill, & Koegel, 1983). However, these are somewhat inverted contributions to the literature on siblings of disabled children: The focus typically is on the behavioral improvements of the handicapped child. Possible changes in the behavior and attitudes of the unimpaired siblings have been overlooked or given secondary emphasis.

A MODEL FOR SELECTING AND EVALUATING SIBLING RESEARCH VARIABLES

There is not yet sufficient research to determine empirically the relative importance of a child's disability or disease on sibling development. Regardless of the diagnostic condition involved (e.g., retardation, cystic fibrosis, cancer, diabetes), well-controlled studies have failed to uncover a one-to-one correspondence between disease or disability and adverse psychological outcome among siblings. Thus, the impact of childhood disease or disability on siblings may best be conceptualized as a risk or stress factor, the significance of which is mediated by other individual and family characteristics and resources. Within the general literature on family adaptation and coping with illness and disability (Crnic, Friedrich, & Greenberg, 1983), family characteristics and needs are interactive, change over time, and moods are affected by broader social and cultural contexts. Such a model is consistent with and can build upon the transactional, ecological models of child and family development (Belsky, 1981; Bronfenbrenner, 1979) that have guided more recent research on typical sibling pairs (e.g., Stoneman & Brody, 1987).

We do not yet know which of the many individual, family, or disease/disability characteristics exert an impact on siblings as they develop, and thus we thought it useful to construct a variable matrix. Our aim is to help researchers identify a range of candidates that can be the focus of study, or, alternatively could confound investigations and obscure the meaning of results if not sufficiently controlled.

We started by dividing factors into two types: those comprising the background of family demographic and adaptive characteristics (Table 1) and those

Table I. Family Background Variables Upon Which Disease or Disability Characteristics are Imposed

Sociodemographic characteristics
  Socioeconomic status
  Birth order
  Age spacing
  Gender
  Age of patient and sibling(s)
  Family size
  Marital status
Individual and family adaptive and functional patterns
  Sociocultural influences
  Family social network
  Family coping style and capacity: closeness, flexibility, role differentiation, communication
  Physical health of family members
  Psychological resources of family members
Functional patterns imposed by disease or disability
  Disruption in family routine
  Contact with other families with affected children
  Patient adjustment to and acceptance of the disease or disability
  Parent attitudes and expectations of patient and siblings
  Parent, sibling, patient understanding of the disease and disability

Table 1. Family Background Variables Upon Which Disease or Disability Characteristics Are Imposed

comprising characteristics of the disease or disability (Table 2) that are super-imposed upon the family and its functioning. When designing research, each of these variables can be considered. Depending on the hypotheses, one or more of the variables would need to be controlled. We briefly describe a selection of factors from each group, along with evidence suggesting the factor's potential relevance, as a way of exemplifying their importance.

Background Variables

Sociodemographic Features

Although sociodemographic features of families are often treated by researchers as the static, structural foundation of family life, within our model they have the potential for change as family circumstances and modes of adaptation evolve.

Table II. Disease and Disability Characteristics

Onset
 Sudden
  Traumatic
  Congenital
 Gradual
Etiology
 Unknown
 Genetic
 Sociocultural
Course or phase
 Stable
 Fluctuating
 Improving
 Deteriorating
Prognosis
 Fatal
 Nonfatal
Visibility
 Physical appearance overtly affected
 Physical appearance not affected
Functional implications
 Behavioral/emotional
 Cognitive
 Communicative
 Motor
 Multiple

Table 2. Disease and Disability Characteristics

A family's socioeconomic status (SES) has a well-known association with many developmental and educational characteristics of children (Mueller & Parcel, 1981). Certain disabling or disease conditions occur more commonly among people of lower SES (e.g., prematurity, head injury), whereas other conditions may cause a downward drift in SES due to financial strain (Holroyd & Guthrie, 1979).

The importance of SES in research on families with handicapped and chronically ill children is clear. SES is a better predictor of eventual developmental outcome of children with birth-related injuries than is the severity or nature of the injuries themselves (Bradley, Caldwell, & Elardo, 1977; Sameroff & Chandler, 1975). Furthermore, the quality of parents' reactions to an existing developmental disability often varies with their SES (Farber & Ryckman, 1965). For example, high achieving/high SES parents often have elaborate achievement expectations for their children. These expectations may be shattered by an intellectually impaired child, in possible contrast to low achieving/low SES parents with more modest expectations. Low SES parents may be more immediately concerned with finances and physical health and less concerned with reduced educational potential (Farber, 1960). Insofar as children incorporate their parents' ideals, expectations, and concerns, the siblings' reactions may also be indirectly affected.

If a family has the financial resources to procure stress-reducing professional and domestic help, then the extra responsibilities of siblings may be more manageable. For example, older sisters of ill and disabled children are more often affected negatively by the child's care when the family is of lower SES, presumably because the family cannot afford extrafamilial respite (Farber, 1960; Grossman, 1972). Research has shown that sibling outcome fluctuates with the severity and nature of a child's handicap or physical needs only among older sisters in low SES families (Grossman, 1972). If there are no other normal, healthy siblings, then the burden of the child's care is even more acutely experienced by the older sister (Farber, 1960; Grossman, 1972; Simeonsson & McHale, 1981). The importance of controlling for family SES in the investigation of sibling functioning lies in its correlation with other family adaptive and functional patterns. Certainly, when SES has been identified as an important factor in sibling adaptation, researchers have interpreted its importance by inferring its relationship with more dynamic functions and adaptive characteristics of families. In and of itself, SES is of little theoretical significance; however, insofar as it reflects coping resources, attitudes, and expectations, it must be controlled for or covaried in investigations of group differences.

Sibling Constellation Variables

Birth order, sex of siblings, age spacing, age, and family size have been the most frequently studied contributors to sibling development (Scarr & Grajek, 1982; Wagner et al., 1979). It is assumed that different sibling constellations are associated with different sibling experiences. There exist complex, yet consistent, asymmetries in the roles of firstborn versus later-born siblings based on the relative cognitive and behavioral competencies of the siblings. Specifically, older siblings generally assume roles of teacher, manager, and caregivers when playing with their younger brothers and sisters; the younger sibling balances the interaction with the role of student and follower (Brody & Stoneman, 1986).

Researchers studying siblings of handicapped and chronically ill children rarely describe their subjects according to essential sibling constellation characteristics. Additionally, they have not controlled for possible constellation effects, perhaps because of the low incidence of the conditions under study and difficulties recruiting subjects. In the better controlled studies, only the interaction of birth order and gender has shown a significant association with variations in personality profiles of siblings of physically disabled children (Breslau, 1982; Breslau et al., 1981; Tew & Laurence, 1973). Specifically, older sisters and younger brothers (in relation to the affected child) show higher rates of behavioral problems, as reported by mothers and teachers. Younger brothers tend to have problems related to aggression and delinquency, whereas older sisters have difficulties with depression and anxiety. Some evidence suggests that sibling constellation factors may be more powerful determinants of outcome among siblings of handicapped than nonhandicapped children (Breslau, 1982). The reason for this difference are uncertain. Perhaps the added stressors created by an impaired child result in greater differentiation of roles and responsibilities with the family. When the handicapped child is the younger, an elder sibling's assumption of caretaking responsibility is consistent with common sibling role asymmetries. Greater role tension and confusion would be anticipated among siblings younger than the handicapped or ill child, as they may be expected to assume roles that contradict birth order.

Of interest, closer age spacings are associated with increased aggression among younger brothers of handicapped children but age spacing exerts no obvious influence on sisters (Breslau, 1982; Breslau et al., 1981). Closer age spacings, in the general sibling literature, are associated with higher morbidity and mortality rates and seem to increase risk of depression, anxiety, and poor social and academic adjustment (Wagner et al., 1985). Close spacing appears to affect eldest more than later born, and boys more than girls (Wagner et al.,

1985). Close spacing fosters sibling identification and shared interests, presumably because narrow spacing increases contact and interaction. However, within the increased contact, closely spaced sibships are associated with more intense competition, conflict, and ambivalence, especially within same-sex pairs (Bank & Kahn, 1982). Thus, age spacing, insofar as it reflects the normal process of sibling identification and deidentification, is an important variable to consider, especially in any study of the effect of disease/disability severity and visibility on sibling relationships.

Adaptive and Functional Patterns

Although background factors, as those described above, can undoubtedly influence sibling response to disease and disability in a brother or a sister, reactions are hardly uniform. A primary reason for variation in sibling effects may be the more dynamic aspects of individual and family adaptation and functioning. Some forms of adaptational functioning and interaction are common to families and others occur specifically in reaction to the presence of a disease or disability.

The quality and strength of the parental relationship has permanent effects on every child's development and should be a focus of attention within the sibling context as well. There is considerable professional speculation regarding the impact of chronic childhood illness on parents' marital harmony and divorce rate (Martin, 1975). Unfortunately, this area of study is significantly compromised by methodological limitations similar to those encountered in the sibling research (Sabbeth & Leventhal, 1984).

A common assumption is that chronic childhood illness leads to higher divorce rates but better relationships among intact couples, that is, they are brought "closer together" by the experience (Carr, 1974; McAndrew, 1976). Careful review of more adequately controlled research, however, demonstrates the opposite (Sabbeth & Leventhal, 1984). Divorce rate is similar between couples with healthy versus chronically ill children, but marital quality often suffers among the latter. Thus, parents are no more likely to separate or divorce following a child's illness, but they are more likely to be dissatisfied and argumentative with their spouses.

Differences that have been identified between sibling groups generally involve increases in anxiety, depression, aggression, and acting out, all of which may be affected more significantly by parental discord than by a brother's or sister's condition. Therefore, differences in behavioral profiles between siblings of healthy and ill children may partially mirror the children's reactions to disharmonious or stressed parental relationships, thereby representing second-order effects of the child's disease or disability.

The stress parents feel in the care of a chronically ill child relates to many other variables, for example, increased financial strain (Holroyd, 1974), sex of the disabled child (Bristol, 1979), and disease characteristics (Gallagher, Beckman, & Cross, 1983). The finding that parental stress and disease characteristics covary (Gallagher et al., 1983) suggest that this is an area deserving considerably greater investigatory effort in the sibling literature. Disease characteristics may not only result in second-order effects transmitted through the changes in the parent relationship but also directly affect sibling-sibling experiences.

Many researchers have addressed anecdotally, but not through formal investigations, the impact of parents' adaptation to a disease on normal sibling response (Caldwell & Guze, 1960; Graliker et al., 1962; Grossman, 1972). Tew and Laurence (1973) noted a significant positive correlation between mothers' reports of their own mental and physical health and measures of sibling adjustment. Further, siblings' attitudes toward professional treatment of their retarded brothers and sisters closely parallel their parents' attitudes towards those treatments (Graliker et al., 1982). Additionally, siblings often attribute their own psychological adjustment or reactions to their parents' patterns of communication about and acceptance of the disease (Gogan & Slavin, 1981; Grossman, 1972; Hayden, 1974; Klein, 1972; Lavigne & Ryan, 1979; Townes & Wold, 1977).

Many authors propose that the comprehensibility of a disease or disability to the patient and family will affect siblings' reactions and adjustment (Lobato, 1985; Simeonsson & McHale, 1981). The belief that better sibling understanding of the disease or disability is associated with better psychological adjustment evolves from clinical lore that accurate knowledge, especially of highly emotional events, improves a child's ability to cope with those events. Unfortunately, to the best of our knowledge, no direct data are currently available to support or refute this notion as regards sibling adjustment. Comparisons between the adjustment of parents of children with disabilities that differ in comprehensibility and predictability suggest that the more comprehensible and predictable developmental syndromes, such as Down syndrome, pose fewer stresses than more difficult-to-grasp disorders such as autism (Holroyd & MacArthur, 1976).

Disease and Disability Characteristics

The characteristics of disabilities vary greatly, but few researchers have hypothesized or tested specific relationships between these characteristics and outcome. Of equal or greater importance, in the research we reviewed, disease characteristics at the time of study were rarely specified. If discussed (e.g.,

Vance, Fazan, Satterwhite, & Pless, 1980), the characteristics were not subject to data analysis. Potentially serious methodological problems result, for example, if one lumps together recently diagnosed and terminal patients. We outline below five categories of disease/disability characteristics, represented in Table 2, and adapted from Rolland (1984).

The five categories include onset, etiology, course or phase, prognosis, and functional complications. These divisions do not cover all potentially relevant disease characteristics, and the investigator should examine other factors particular to populations under study. These might entail frequency and intensity of symptoms and treatment regimen, proportion of home versus hospital-based care, predictability of disease progression, patient control over symptoms (if any), etc. When practical constraints (e.g., the typically low numbers of subjects in pediatric samples) restrict the number of disease characteristics that can be controlled, clear documentation can at least be provided in studies comparing siblings of children with different diagnoses. If enough diagnostic groups are examined, then the relative effects of these independent disease characteristics on sibling functioning could be analyzed.

Time of onset likely exerts a strong and direct effect on the sibling relationship. To illustrate, in the case of traumatic injuries and acquired diseases, the siblings will have spent time together developing a relationship before disease or disability onset. The quality of the children's relationship prior to the illness or injury would be likely to affect their adaptation. Based on the literature on stress and coping, one would expect intense emotional and behavioral instability immediately following a diagnosis or loss of function and such disruptions to recur in conjunction with other disease or developmental milestones (Harris, 1983; Wikler, 1986; Wikler, Wasow, & Hatfield, 1981). Ferrari's (1984) comparison of siblings of normal, diabetic, and developmentally disabled children demonstrate the importance of time of onset and time since diagnosis. Siblings of diabetic children received the most negative ratings of self-esteem and behavior; however, when time since diagnosis was controlled, the differences between them and typical siblings disappeared.

Etiology may also mediate impact in important ways. Genetically based diseases or disabilities, such as cystic fibrosis, may have their primary effect via the parents. Parental shame and guilt, stemming from the belief that they have somehow caused their child's disease, may have both subtle and obvious effects on their parenting style. Complex interactions may also occur. When a younger child is diagnosed with a genetic disease, there is usually little concern that a much older sibling will also inherit the disease. An initial diagnosis made on an older sibling, however, may cast the ominous threat that a similar fate will befall the younger siblings. Could the presence, versus absence, of such concerns make no difference?

The course and prognosis of a disease or disability are often overlooked, but are important factors in research on chronic illness. For example, studies commonly examine the effects of a deteriorating fatal disease, such as cystic fibrosis, together with the effects of a stable nonfatal disability, such as cerebral palsy. General conclusions are then drawn on the effects of illness on siblings. Fluctuating and episodic diseases, such as colitis ar asthma, produce demands and stressors that differ widely from steadily progressive or stable diseases. One would expect these contrasts to be expressed in differing psychological effects on siblings. Only some siblings are faced, for example, with the fear of frequent recurrence and another bout of family disruption. The psychological and behavioral adaptability needed by a sibling in such circumstances could be compared to that required of siblings of children with diseases of differing course.

The impact of any disease/disability on day-to-day functioning needs to be closely considered when comparing the effects on siblings. A disease that primarily produces communications deficits will differ in many respects from one that primarily limits physical capabilities. The corresponding effects on the sibling could also vary substantially, as different functional limitations foster different role requirements. Although there is no direct correlation between the presence of a disease or disability and sibling functioning, this does not preclude the possibility that certain diseases and disabilities, with their idiosyncratic functional sequelae, many create common stresses, complaints, or rewards for siblings. One major goal of clinical research should be to separate disease or disability issues from those that are normally expected on the basis of sibling's age, sex, or other family characteristics.

Four areas of disability seem particularly relevant for a psychosocial classification system. These include effects primarily expressed in behavioral/emotional, cognitive, communicative, or motor realms. Multiple involvement is also often seen. These categories illustrate the varied nature of disease/disability characteristics, the need to recognize all spheres of involvement, and the fact that these spheres are so imperfectly defined in the current literature. When multiple limitations are present (e.g., behavioral and communicative deficits in autism), it would be particularly useful to know whether or which specific functional limitations most affect siblings. Do the motor or cognitive impairments of a child with spina bifida have the greatest impact? Is the behavioral or communicative component of autism the most disturbing to the sibling? Or, do the common behavioral components of autism and severe mental retardation account for so much of the effect of these conditions on the sibling that they need not be considered separately? Greater delineation and investigation of the functional implications of disease/disability categories should help to clarify the nature of sibling effects.

INTEGRATION OF THE MODEL AND CONCLUSIONS

Despite the complex matrix of research variables and potential confounds we have constructed, we have done so upon a foundation that reflects more basic and broad assumptions. These assumptions include the following: (a) disease and disability characteristics and consequences are imposed upon and interact with features of family structure and function; (b) the interrelations of individual, family, and community are critical to the study of sibling life; (c) many of the effects of disease or disability on siblings are indirect or secondary rather than primary and, more generally, reflect interactional or "systems" relationships.

That we list and discuss candidate variables separately should not be taken as an argument for a checklist approach to research. Active conceptualization is required. In selecting dependent or outcome variables, one must select a focus, which in turn should determine what is measured and controlled. However, given the range of mediating variables and the interactions among them, studies should attempt to keep all but a few of the variables constant through matching or other forms of experimental control, or significant confounds will compromise interpretive value. At times, the latter will be unavoidable, but awareness of alternate factors (explanations) can help avoid overly narrow interpretations that have too often characterized the literature and can keep investigators alert to alternate possibilities or directions for more refined and definitive investigations. For example, where interest lies in role changes siblings experience as a function of a child's disease or disability, it would be crucial to control for birth order, age spacing, and SES. If one were interested in the effect of the degree of disability and/or its visibility on sibling identification, other characteristics of the disease as well as sex and age spacing between the well and impaired child would have to be controlled; controlling for SES would be less relevant.

Though family demographic variables and disease characteristics are among the easiest to define and quantify, a transactional, family systems view suggests that dynamic adaptive and functional patterns of the family may be the more essential ingredients to understanding sibling functioning. Parents' and siblings' ability to communicate expectations and feelings openly, to flexibly adjust routines to meet individual members' needs, and to problem-solve effectively have been alluded to the most in clinical interviews with siblings but examined the least in empirical research. As these are elements of family functioning clinicians can assist in altering (as opposed to sibling constellation or family SES), identifying their function would be of both theoretical and practical value.

Children will be affected when one of their brothers or sisters is seriously ill or disabled. To argue the point is callous to the realities of family life. What researchers should hope to achieve, however, is an understanding of how siblings are affected and what determines the effects that occur. Family relationships are complex and difficult to capture empirically. Diseases and disabilities fluctuate in their nature and course. The impact of these events on an impaired child's siblings almost certainly are multifactorally determined. Research should build upon the normal sibling literature to encompass the direct study of actual sibling interactions and experiences, but an understanding of these interactions will occur only if their familial context is fully appreciated both conceptually and methodologically.

REFERENCES

Abramovitch, R., Corter, C., & Lando, B. (1979). Sibling interaction in the home. *Child Development, 50,* 997–1003.

Abramovitch, R., Corter, C., & Pepler, D. (1980). Observations of mixed-sex sibling dyads. *Child Development, 51,* 1268–1271.

Bank, S., & Kahn, M. D. (1982). *The sibling bond.* New York: Basic.

Belsky, J. (1981). Early human experience: A family perspective. *Developmental Psychology, 17,* 3–23.

Bradley, R. H., Caldwell, B. M., & Elardo, R. (1977). Home environment, social status, and mental test performance. *Journal of Educational Psychology, 69,* 697–701.

Breslau, N. (1982). Siblings of disabled children: Birth order and age-spacing effects. *Journal of Abnormal Child Psychology, 10,* 85–96.

Breslau, N., Weitzman, M., & Messenger, K. (1981). Psychological functioning of siblings of disabled children. *Pediatrics, 67,* 344–353.

Bristol, M. (1979). *Maternal coping with autistic children: Adequacy of interpersonal support and effects of child characteristics.* Unpublished doctoral dissertation, University of North Carolina.

Brody, G. H., & Shaffer, D. (1982). Contributions of parents and peers to children's moral socialization. *Developmental Review, 2,* 31–75.

Brody, G., & Stoneman, L. (1986). Contextual issues in the study of sibling socialization. In J. J. Gallagher & P. M. Vietze (Eds.), *Families of handicapped persons: Research programs, and policy issues.* Baltimore: Paul H. Brookes.

Bronfenbrenner, V. (1979). *The ecology of human development.* Cambridge MA: Harvard University Press.

Caldwell, B. M., & Guze, G. B. (1960). A study of the adjustment of parents and siblings of institutionalized and noninstitutionalized retarded children. *American Journal of Mental Deficiency, 64,* 849–861.

Carr, J. (1974). The effects of the severely subnormal on their family. In A. M. Clarke & A. D. B. Clarke (Eds.), *Mental deficiency: The changing outlook.* New York: Free Press.

Cash, W. M., & Evans, I. N. (1975). Training preschool children to modify their siblings' behavior. *Journal of Behavior Therapy and Experimental Psychiatry, 6,* 13–16.

Circirelli, V. G. (1975). Effects of mothers and older siblings on the problem-solving behavior of the younger child. *Developmental Psychology, 11,* 749–756.

Cleveland, D. W., & Miller, N. B. (1977). Attitudes and life commitments of older siblings of mentally retarded adults: An exploratory study. *Mental Retardation, 15,* 38–41.

Colletti, G., & Harris, S. L. (1977). Behavior modification in the home: Siblings as behavior modifiers, parents as observers. *Journal of Abnormal Child Psychology, 5,* 21–30.

Crnic, K. A., Friedrich, W. N., & Greenberg, M. T. (1983). Adaptation of families with mentally retarded children. A model of stress, coping, and family ecology. *American Journal of Mental Deficiency, 88,* 125–138.

Crnic, K. A., & Leconte, J. M. (1986). Understanding sibling needs and influences. In R. R. Fewell & P. F. Vadasy (Eds.), *Families of handicapped children: Needs and supports across the life span.* Austin, TX: Pro. Ed.

Drotar, D., & Crawford, P. (1985). Psychological adaptation of siblings of chronically ill children: Research and practice implications. *Developmental and Behavioral Pediatrics, 6,* 355–362.

Dunn, J., & Kendrick, C. (1982). *Siblings: Love, envy, and understanding.* Cambridge, MA: Harvard University Press.

Dunn, J., Kendrick, C., & MacNamee, R. (1981). The reaction of first-born children to the birth of a sibling: Mothers' reports. *Journal of Child Psychology and Psychiatry, 22,* 1–18.

Farber, B. (1959). Effects of a severely mentally retarded child on family integration. *Monographs of the Society for Research in Child Development, 21*(Serial No. 75).

Farber, B. (1960). Family organization and crisis: Maintenance of integration in families with a severely mentally retarded child. *Monographs of the Society for Research in Child Development, 25*(Whole No. 75).

Farber, B. (1963). Interactions with retarded siblings and life goals of children. *Marriage and Family Living, 25,* 96–98.

Farber, B., & Ryckman, D. (1965). Effects of severely mentally retarded children on family relationships. *Mental Retardation Abstracts, 2,* 1–17.

Ferrari, M. (1984). Chronic illness: Psychosocial effects on siblings—1. Chronically ill boys. *Journal of Child Psychology and Psychiatry, 25,* 459–476.

Folit, D. F., & Falbo, T. (1985, April). *Siblings and child development: Evidence from a meta-analysis of the literature on only children.* Paper presented at the biennial meeting of the Society for Research in Child Development, Toronto, Canada.

Gallagher, J. J., Beckman, P., & Cross, A. H. (1983). Families of handicapped children: Sources of stress and its amelioration. *Exceptional Children, 50,* 10–19.

Gath, A. (1973). The mental health of siblings of congenitally abnormal children. *Journal of Child Psychology and Psychiatry, 13,* 211–218.

Gibbs, E. D., Teti, D. M., & Bond, L. A. (1985). *Sibling communication as a function of age-spacing.* Unpublished manuscript.

Gogan, J. L., & Slavin, L. (1981). Interviews with brothers and sisters. In G. P. Koocher & J. E. O'Malley (Eds.) *The Damocles syndrome: Psychosocial consequences of surviving childhood cancer.* New York: McGraw-Hill.

Graliker, B., Fischler, K., & Koch, R. (1962). Teenage reactions to mentally retarded sibling. *American Journal of Mental Deficiency, 66,* 838–843.

Grossman, F. K. (1972). *Brothers and sisters of retarded children.* Syracuse, NY: Syracuse University Press.

Harris, S. L. (1983). *Families of the developmentally disabled: A guide to behavioral intervention.* New York: Pergamon.

Hartup, W. W. (1979). The social worlds of childhood. *American Psychologist, 34,* 944–950.

Hayden, V. (1974). The other children. *Exceptional Parent, 4,* 26–29.

Holroyd, J. (1974). The Questionnaire on Resources and Stress: An instrument to measure family response to a handicapped family member. *Journal of Community Psychology, 2,* 92–94.

Holroyd, J., & Guthrie, D. (1979). Stress in families of children with neuromuscular disease. *Journal of Clinical Psychology, 35,* 734–739.

Holroyd, J., & McArthur, D. (1976). Mental retardation and stress on the parents: A contrast between Down's syndrome and childhood autism. *American Journal of Mental Deficiency, 80,* 431–436.

Ihinger, M. (1975). The referee role and norms of equity: A contribution toward a theory of sibling conflict. *Journal of Marriage and Family, 37,* 515–524.

Klein, S. D. (1972). Brother to sister: Sister to brother. *Exceptional Parent, 2,* 10–15.

Lamb, M. E., & Sutton-Smith, D. (Eds.). (1982). *Sibling relationships: Their nature and significance across the life span.* Hillsdale, NJ: Erlbaum.

Lavigne, J. V., & Ryan, M. (1979). Psychologic adjustment of siblings of children with chronic illness. *Pediatrics, 63,* 616–627.

Lawson, A., & Ingleby, J. D. (1974). Daily routines of preschool children: Effects of age, birth order, sex, social class, and developmental correlates. *Psychological Medicine, 4,* 399–415.

Levy, D. M. (1937). Sibling rivalry. *American Orthopsychiatric Association Research Monograph* (No. 2).

Lobato, D. (1983). Siblings of handicapped children: A review. *Journal of Autism and Developmental Disorders, 13,* 347–364.

Lobato, D. (1985). Preschool siblings of handicapped children—impact of peer support and training. *Journal of Autism and Developmental Disorders, 9,* 287–296.

Lobato, D., Barbour, L., Hall, L. J., & Miller, C. T. (1987). Psychosocial characteristics of preschool siblings of handicapped and nonhandicapped children. *Journal of Abnormal Child Psychology, 15,* 329–338.

Lobato, D., & Barrera, R. D. (1988). Impact of siblings on children with handicaps. In M. D. Powers (Eds.), *Expanding systems of service delivery for persons with developmental disabilities.* Baltimore: Paul H. Brookes.

Lobato, D., & Tlaker, A. (1985). Sibling intervention with a retarded child. *Education and Treatment of Children, 8,* 221–228.

Martin, P. (1975). Marital breakdown in families of patients with spina bifida cystica. *Developmental Medicine and Child Neurology, 17,* 757–764.

Mash, E. J., & Johnston, J. C. (1980, October). *A behavioral assessment of sibling interaction in hyperactive and normal children.* Paper presented at the annual meeting of the Association for the Advancement of Behavior Therapy, Washington, DC.

McAndrew, I. (1976). Children with a handicap and their families. *Child: Care, Health, and Development, 2,* 213–237.

McKeever, P. (1983). Siblings of chronically ill children: A literature review with implications for research and practice. *American Journal of Orthopsychiatry, 53,* 209–218.

Mueller, C. W., & Parcel, T. L. (1981). Measures of socioeconomic status: Alternatives and recommendations. *Child Development, 52,* 13–30.

Powell, T. H., & Ogle, P. A. (1985). *Brothers and sisters—A special part of exceptional families.* Baltimore: Paul H. Brookes.

Rolland, J. S. (1984). Toward a psychosocial typology of chronic and life-threatening illness. *Family Systems Medicine, 2,* 245–262.

Rosenberg, B. G. (1982). Life span personality and stability in sibling status. In M. E. Lamb & B. Sutton-Smith (Eds.), *Sibling relationships: Their nature and significance across the life span.* Hillsdale, NJ: Erlbaum.

Sabbeth, B. F., & Leventhal, J. M. (1984). Marital adjustment to childhood illness: A critique of the literature. *Pediatrics, 73,* 762–768.

Sameroff, A. (1975). Early influences on development: Fact or fancy. *Merrill Palmer Quarterly, 21,* 267–294.

Sameroff, A. J., & Chandler, M. J. (1975). Reproductive risk and the continuum of caretaking causality. In F. D. Horowitz (Ed.), *Review of child development research* (Vol. 4). Chicago: The University of Chicago Press.

Samuels, H. (1980). The effect of an older sibling on infant locomotor exploration in a new environment. *Child Development, 51,* 607–609.

Scarr, S., & Grajek, S. (1982). Similarities and differences among siblings. In M. E. Lamb & B. Sutton-Smith (Eds.), *Sibling relationships: Their nature and significance across the life span.* Hillsdale, NJ: Erlbaum.

Schreibman, L., O'Neill, R. E., & Koegel, R. L. (1983). Behavioral training for siblings of autistic children. *Journal of Applied Behavior Analysis, 16,* 129–138.

Schwirian, P. M. (1976). Effects of the presence of a hearing-impaired preschool child in the family on behavior patterns of older ''normal'' siblings. *American Annals of the Deaf, 121,* 373–380.

Seligman, M. (1983). *The family with a handicapped child: Understanding and treatment.* New York: Grune & Stratton.

Simeonsson, R. J., & McHale, S. M. (1981). Review: Research on handicapped children: Sibling relationships. *Child: Care, Health, and Development, 7,* 153–171.

Spinetta, J. J. (1978). Communication patterns in families dealing with life-threatening illness. In O. J. Z. Sahler (Ed.), *The child and death.* St. Louis: C. V. Mosby.

Spinetta, J. J. (1981). The sibling of the child with cancer. In J. J. Spinetta & P. Deasy-Spinetta (Eds.), *Living with childhood cancer,* St. Louis: C. V. Mosby.

Stoneman, Z., & Brody, G. (1987). Observational research on retarded children, their parents, and their siblings. In S. Landesman-Dwyer & P. Vietze (Eds.), *Living with retarded people.* Washington, DC: American Association on Mental Deficiency.

Sutton-Smith, B., & Rosenberg, R. B. (1970). *The sibling.* New York: Holt, Rinehart & Winston.

Tew, B., & Laurence, K. M. (1973). Mothers, brothers, and sisters of patients with spina bifida. *Developmental Medicine and Child Neurology, 15,* 69–76.

Townes, B. D., & Wold, D. A. (1977). Childhood leukemia. In E. Pattison (Ed.), *The experience of dying.* Englewood Cliffs, NJ: Prentice Hall.

Vance, J. C., Fazan, L. E., Satterwhite, B., & Pless, I. B. (1980). Effects of nephrotic syndrome on the family: A controlled study. *Pediatrics, 165,* 948–955.

Wagner, M. E., Schubert, H. J. P., & Schubert, D. S. P. (1979). Sibships-constellation effects on psychosocial development, creativity, and health. In H. W. Reese & L. P. Lipsitt (Eds.), *Advances in child development and behavior* (Vol. 14). New York: Academic Press.

Wagner, M. E., Schubert, H. J. P., & Schubert, D. S. P. (1985). Effects of sibling spacing on intelligence, interfamilial relations, psychosocial characteristics, and mental and physical health. In H. W. Reese (Ed.), *Advances in child development and behavior* (Vol. 19, pp. 149–206). New York: Academic Press.

Wikler, L. (1986). Periodic stresses in families of children with mental retardation. *American Journal of Mental Deficiency, 90,* 703–706.

Wikler, L., Wasow, M., & Hartfield, E. (1981). Chronic sorrow revisited: Attitudes of patients and professionals about adjustment to mental retardation. *American Journal of Orthopsychiatry, 51,* 63–70.

Zajonc, R. B., & Markus, G. B. (1975). Birth order and intellectual development. *Psychological Review, 82,* 74–88.

16

After Treatment Ends: Psychosocial Sequelae in Pediatric Cancer Survivors

Gregory K. Fritz and Judith R. Williams
Rhode Island Hospital, Brown University Program in Medicine
Michael Amylon
Children's Hospital at Stanford, California

Fifty-two survivors of childhood cancer and their families were assessed by questionnaire and interview to determine survivors' psychosocial status two years or more after treatment. Most were functioning well and serious psychosocial problems were relatively rare. Communication patterns during treatment were most predictive of psychosocial outcome whereas indicators of medical severity were least predictive. The heterogeneity of effective coping styles, appropriate to varied personality types, was noted.

Major advances in treatment over the past decade have dramatically improved the outlook for children with cancer. Malignancy in childhood now implies an arduous course of therapy and the very real possibility of a cure. Increasing numbers of children are successfully completing treatment and entering the period of off-treatment follow-up. Although termination of treatment brings release from years of pain and anxiety for the child and family, the time after treatment may well be a vulnerable period.

Many aspects of childhood cancer are cruelly paradoxical. The beginning symptoms can be innocuous and remain long overlooked, and the grave diagnosis may come without warning. The treatment and its side effects can be

Reprinted with permission from the *American Journal of Orthopsychiatry,* 1987, Vol. 57, No. 11, 552–561. Copyright 1988 by the American Orthopsychiatric Association, Inc.

A revised version of a paper submitted to the Journal in November 1987. Research was supported by the W. T. Grant Foundation, through a Faculty Scholar Award to the first author, and by the American Cancer Society, California Division.

more painful than the disease itself. Children must believe that medications that make them deathly ill will save their lives. Sophisticated as therapeutic techniques have become, they are often still part of an experimental protocol. Survival rates are remarkably improved, but individual outcomes remain uncertain. These facts and our clinical experience with oncology patients at the Children's Hospital at Stanford led to our interest in the period after treatment ends.

The experiences of children who reach the successful conclusion of their treatment have been given little attention so far, primarily because the number of such children has been small. An exception is the recent interest in the late effects of the central nervous system prophylaxis in leukemia: a number of reports have pointed convincingly to decreased intellectual abilities and increased academic difficulties in some children who received such treatment (*Brouwers, Riccardi, Poplack, & Fedio, 1984; Copeland et al., 1985*). Psychosocial factors were assessed by questionnaire in two early studies of childhood cancer (*Holmes & Holmes, 1975; Li & Stone, 1976*). Both reports described the overall satisfactory adjustment of most subjects but the superficiality of the assessment makes the significance of these results questionable.

The most extensive study of long-term pediatric cancer survivors has been carried out at the Sidney Farber Cancer Institute in Boston. The results have been presented in several papers and summarized in a book with the intriguing title, *The Damocles Syndrome (Koocher & O'Malley, 1981)*. The study documented some degree of adjustment problems among 59% of the survivor group, although many were relatively minor. The chief limitation of the study is its questionable applicability to today's pediatric oncology population. Subjects averaged 13 years since diagnosis; for some, treatment ended as long ago as 1947. The majority of the 114 subjects had experiences that differed from those of current cancer patients.

Lansky, List, and Ritter-Sterr (*1986*) summarized the results of a pilot study of 39 young adults diagnosed with cancer five to ten years earlier, during their adolescence. Preliminary comparisons failed to show significant differences on a number of demographic and career variables between survivors and a sibling comparison group. However, 15% of the survivors had received treatment for depression, alcoholism, or suicide attempts (comparable figures were not available for siblings). In interviews with 40 young adults who had completed treatment for Hodgkin's disease at least five years earlier, Wasserman, Thompson, Wilimas, and Fairclough (*1986*) found no increased incidence of depression or other psychiatric disorders, despite the subjects' vivid negative memories of their experiences. The present paper reports the results of a retrospective study of childhood cancer survivors. The study was undertaken to determine the stresses and psychosocial problems of youngsters who are completing treatment for cancer.

METHOD

Subjects

Subjects were approached for the study if they were between seven and 21 years of age, had successfully completed treatment for a childhood malignancy at least two years earlier, and were followed at the Stanford University School of Medicine. A letter and a phone call from a senior project member, prior to the clinic visit, introduced the project to the family and solicited their participation. Close daily contact with members of the oncology service and the involvement of a pediatric oncologist as a co-investigator facilitated the family's participation. To obtain approximately 50 subjects, 57 families (47% or the pool of eligible subjects) were contacted; contact was in order of scheduled follow-up appointments in the oncology clinic to ensure randomization. Fifty-two families ultimately participated in the study. Of the five refusals, two were teenagers reluctant to think about the past, despite parental encouragement; one child was living with new guardians who did not feel they knew enough to participate; and two parents professed lack of interest without further explanation.

A comparison group of healthy children and adolescents was administered some of the instruments used with the cancer survivors and their families. These data are presented elsewhere (*Anholt, Fritz, Williams, & Amylon, 1988*). The present paper focuses on antecedent predictors of outcome among the survivors. Demographic characteristics of the survivor group are summarized in Table 1.

Procedure

A standard assessment protocol was administered in a building separated from the hospital and clinics. After introductions, review of the procedure, and discussion of informed consent, the patient and the parents were interviewed separately by a child psychiatrist or a senior research psychologist. The structured interview with the child covered the history prior to illness, the illness and therapy course, and a detailed review of all aspects of the child's life since treatment ended. The interview with the parents covered essentially the same ground and also explored the personal, social, and occupational changes in their own lives consequent to their child's cancer. (Detailed child and parent interview schedules are available on request). Following the interviews, the patients and their parents completed several standard instruments (described below). The two investigators independently reviewed videotapes of each interview and rated the parents and child on a number of variables. Interrater reliability was high: Pearson correlation coefficients for the individual items

Table 1

DEMOGRAPHIC CHARACTERISTICS (N = 52)

ITEM	N
Age	
Group mean	15.9 yrs
Age at Diagnosis	
Group mean	9.7 yrs
Sex	
Male	26 (50%)
Female	26 (50%)
Family Status	
Nuclear, intact	28 (54%)
Nuclear, blended	6 (12%)
Single-parent	7 (14%)
Other	11 (21%)
Ethnicity/race	
Caucasian	36 (69%)
Latino	9 (17%)
Asian	2 (4%)
Mixed/other	5 (10%)
Religion	
Catholic	21 (41%)
Protestant	13 (25%)
Other	9 (17%)
None	9 (17%)
Socioeconomic Level	
(Hollingshead Index)	
I	2 (4%)
II	8 (15%)
III	15 (29%)
IV	16 (31%)
V	11 (21%)

Table 1. Demographic Characteristics (N = 52)

rated by the two investigators ranged from .75 to .93, with one exception of .60. Significant disagreements (more than one point on a five-point scale, or more than two points on a seven-point scale) were resolved in a case conference. For smaller disagreements, the average of the two raters' values was used. Extensive case history notes by each investigator completed the data set.

Measures

For the survivors, data were collected to serve two purposes: a "thick description" would clarify the experience of survivorhood; and specific antecedent variables were sought to predict outcome status.

Antecedent variables. Antecedent variables were defined as those pertaining to any time before the end of treatment, including the prediagnosis and treatment periods. In the analyses, they were grouped as demographic, illness-related, and psychosocial antecedent variables. Demographic characteristics expected to affect outcome status included *1) age at diagnosis,* and *2) socioeconomic status* derived from Hollingshead's (*1975*) four-factor index.

Four illness-related antecedent variables were defined. The *nature of the diagnostic process* was a single, five-point rating based on parental report and the medical record. The other three illness-related antecedent variables were indices derived from multiple ratings. *Prognostic characteristics* for the survivor included a faculty oncologist's rating of the child's statistical survival chances based on the diagnosis, cell type, symptoms at presentation, extent of invasion, and other contributory factors; the total length of time on treatment; and the presence or absence of a relapse. Cronbach's alpha for this variable was .59. The index defining the *difficulty of the treatment course* consisted of the sum of three ratings by the faculty oncologist: *a)* the relative expected difficulty of the child's treatment protocol; *b)* the closeness of the actual to the expected course; and *c)* the difficulty of the child's treatment course compared to the range for the service as a whole. The last included the number of procedures, the frequency and toxicity of therapy, associated complications, and degree of pain. Cronbach's alpha for this variable was .62. The *residual physical impairment* index was the sum of four ratings by two investigators of current visibility, interference with daily living, amount of medical attention required, and school hindrance due to physical problems (*Koocher & O'Malley, 1981*). Cronbach's alpha for this variable was .86.

Three antecedent psychosocial variables were derived from the ratings of the interviews. *Directness of communication* during treatment was the sum of ratings, on a five-point scale, of the child's and parents' responses to questions about how the child handled the illness in school, and talked about it with peers, family, and strangers. Cronbach's alpha for this variable was .88. *Peer support* during treatment summarized the ratings of the survivors' and parents' description of how actively helpful peers had been, and whether a "best friend" was available during treatment. Cronbach's alpha for this variable was .49. *Discouragement* during treatment was the sum of five-point ratings about how "down," "depressed," and "miserable" the survivors had been, based on their own and their parents' recollections. Cronbach's alpha was .56 for this variable.

Outcome variables. Seven outcome variables assessed the former patients' functioning at the time of the study, i.e., two or more years after their last cancer treatment. The data on self-image are presented elsewhere (*Anholt et al., 1988*). Of the six outcome variables analyzed here, four were indices derived from five-point ratings of specific items in the parents' and subjects' interviews. *School functioning* is a summary index of the subjects' current academic achievement and enjoyment of school compared to the year prior to diagnosis. Cronbach's alpha for this variable was .80. The *activity index* summarizes the subjects' current level of physical activity including involvement in sports, outdoor pursuits, physical exercise, etc., compared to their activity level prior to diagnosis. Cronbach's alpha was .87. The *social/peer interaction* index summarizes the change, if any, in social involvement and friendships from the period prior to diagnosis to the present. Cronbach's alpha for the items comprising this variable was .89. The survivor's level of comfort in talking about the illness was summarized in an index of *current openness,* which included the survivor's own assessment, the parents' description, and the patterns observed during the interview. Cronbach's alpha for this variable was .56. The presence or absence of depressive symptomatology was quantified by two independent ratings of the *Children's Depression Rating Scale (CDRS) (Poznanski et al., 1981).* The raters used direct observation of the survivor and the content of the survivor's and parents' interviews. Agreement between the two raters was high (Pearson $r = .72$). The final outcome variable was a *global adjustment rating,* based on interview data. The rating took into account the extent to which the survivor: *a)* has put the illness into perspective so that it is no longer the uppermost or organizing factor in his or her life; *b)* has an age-appropriate sense of purposefulness and direction, educationally or vocationally, *c)* is able to have or form satisfactory peer relationships; *d)* has integrated the illness and treatment experience into a sense of self (as opposed to having encapsulated or denied it; and *e)* has achieved age-appropriate separation from the family. The global adjustment rating was a consensus rating arrived at in a case conference in which the interviews, process notes, and medical record comments (but not the scores on standard ratings or assessment instruments) were reviewed by the members of the research team.

RESULTS

Descriptive Findings

The subjects were initially diagnosed with cancer at an average age of 9.7 years. Four of the patients who had completed a second course of treatment after a relapse had initially presented as preschoolers. The subjects had finished treatment between two and seven years prior to the interview; the mean length of time since treatment was 3.7 years.

The diagnostic process varied from a rapid, straightforward diagnosis of an acute presentation to a series of misdiagnoses over a year or more before the definitive diagnosis was made. On a five-point scale, 37% received a rating of one or two, indicating that they had been diagnosed quickly and accurately;

Table 2

DIAGNOSES

CATEGORY	N
Acute lymphocytic leukemia	17 (32.7%)
Other leukemias	2 (3.8%)
Hodgkins disease (all stages)	11 (21.1%)
Non-Hodgkins lymphoma	10 (19.2%)
Solid tumors	10 (19.2%)
Other	2 (3.8%)

Table 2. Diagnoses

34% received a rating of four or five, indicating a protracted and difficult diagnostic process.

The malignancies that were treated are summarized in Table 2. Lymphocytic leukemia and Hodgkins disease, both with relatively high cure rates, accounted for half the diagnoses. The solid tumors included Ewings sarcoma, osteogenic sarcoma, rhabdomyosarcoma, and Wilms tumor. Prognosis for the given child was discussed in detail with every family at the beginning of treatment and thus constituted important information that had to be dealt with throughout the treatment period and into survivorhood. The oncologist's composite rating of each patient's prognosis at the outset of treatment revealed that 25% of the survivors had had a good prognosis (> 70% survival expected), 52% had had an average prognosis (40%–70% survival expected), and 23% had had a poor prognosis (< 40% survival expected). Eight survivors had relapsed but had completed a second course of treatment and had been disease-free for two or more years.

Individual treatment protocols were highly variable in terms of predicted problems such as the number, nature, and frequency of chemotherapeutic drugs and surgical and invasive procedures. The actual treatment courses were equally variable in difficulty of achieving remission, number of infections, and drug side effects. The total number of nights that patients spent in the hospital, as obtained from the medical record, varied from zero to 146. Three quarters of the group spent fewer than 40 nights in the hospital; the average was 32.4. Long hospital stays were uncommon: only five of the 52 had had an admission longer than three weeks. The treatment was rated as average for the service for 77% of the survivors, among the worst for 17%, and among the easiest for 6%. The treatment course went largely as expected with few or only minor surprises for 58% of the group, significantly worse than predicted for 38%, and better than expected for 4%.

The residual physical impairment ratings made at the time of the interview assessed the lasting physical scars. Nine (17%) of the 52 subjects
had a physical abnormality that was obvious to a casual observer. Three
were amputees and the other six had other permanent abnormalities
stemming from surgery or radiotherapy. The level of physical disability
associated with their illness was low for the survivors as a group. Three-
fourths had no hindrance at school or at work, and 21% had only minor
limitations. Thirty-one per cent did need to attend to a residual physical
problem at least once a day with medication, exercise, or cosmetic attention; the remaining two-thirds had no physical interference in their daily
living.

The academic achievement of 10% of the subjects still in school was better
as survivors; for 32%, it was worse or much worse than prior to diagnosis; for
the majority (58%) academic achievement had remained essentially unchanged. Twenty per cent of the subjects enjoyed school more as survivors
than they had prior to the diagnosis of cancer, and 30% reported enjoying it
less. School enjoyment was related to, but not synonymous with, achievement:
Pearson r for each of the two school-related ratings was between .50 ($p < .05$)
and .68 ($p < .001$).

Almost half (47%) of the survivors saw themselves and were seen by their
parents as moderately active physically, 25% as relatively sedentary, and 28%
as more active than average for their age. Twenty-eight per cent felt they had
become less active compared to their peers after their illness, while 20% felt
they had become more active. More than half (52%) believed there was no
change in their physical activity level.

The social/peer interaction index revealed that one-fifth of the subjects had
become more gregarious and socially involved as survivors than they had been
prior to diagnosis; 57% were unchanged and 23% were less sociable and more
solitary in their pursuits. The "current openness" index, reflecting the level of
comfort in talking about the experience with cancer, was high overall. The
interviews with both subjects and parents indicated that 80% were able to talk
with their families about issues related to cancer and 72% could do so with at
least a few close friends. Twenty-six subjects (50%) were rated as open both
with their families and their peers.

Data on depressive symptomatology and the global assessment rating were
summarized for the group. Eighty per cent were clearly free of depression,
with scores below 30. Seven subjects (14%) were rated as questionably depressed and three (6%), with scores above 40, were rated as significantly depressed. The global ratings of functioning ranged from excellent to poor, with
the mid-point of the five-point scale defined as average. Thirteen subjects
(25%) received a global adjustment rating of "excellent"; 19 subjects (36%)

were rated "good"; 14 subjects (26%) average; 3 subjects (6%) marginal; and 4 subjects (8%) "poor."

Antecedent Predictors of Outcome

The effects of antecedent variables on each of the outcome variables were analyzed in two ways. Each antecedent variable was considered singly in a linear regression equation with each outcome variable. The antecedent variables were then grouped into three sets and analyzed together for each outcome variable through a series of hierarchical multiple-regression analyses (*Cohen & Cohen, 1983*). The latter approach enables the examination of the effects of a group of variables entered in a regression equation in a planned, stepwise manner. The variance explained on the final step for the particular antecedent variable reflects the relationship between the antecedent and outcome variables after partialing covariates entered on previous steps. In Tables 3, 4, and 5, the direct effect of an antecedent variable on the outcome variables is summarized in the column labeled "First." The effect of that variable, after partialing out the effects of the other antecedent variables in the set, is summarized in the column labeled "Last" (i.e., the variable was entered in the final step of the hierarchical series). The proportion of total variance explained by the antecedent variables is shown in the right-hand column.

The antecedent psychosocial variables were most strongly associated with outcome. There were significant relationships between direct communication during treatment and current school functioning, social/peer interaction, activity level, current openness, and global adjustment. These relationships remained significant after peer support and discouragement during treatment were partialed out. Direct communication during treatment explained 9% of the variance for school functioning, 31% for social/peer interaction, 14% for activity level, 11% for current openness, and 11% for global adjustment. Peer support during treatment was also significantly related to the global adjustment rating, both directly and when entered as the last variable in the set (12% and 6% of variance explained, respectively). The level of discouragement experienced during treatment showed a significant relationship with social/peer interaction, explaining 10% of the variance initially. This significant relationship was not maintained after direct communication and peer support were partialed out. (See Table 3.)

Of the illness-related antecedent variables, only the physical impairment index was significantly related to any of the outcome variables. Greater physical impairment was significantly associated with more depression and a worse global adjustment rating, both directly and after the other illness-related variables were partialed out (11% and 10% of variance explained). The nature of the

Table 3

PSYCHOSOCIAL ANTECEDENT VARIABLES AND OUTCOME VARIABLES

OUTCOME VARIABLE	DIRECT COMMUNICATION		PEER SUPPORT		PEER DIS-COURAGEMENT		TOTAL VARIANCE
	FIRST	LAST	FIRST	LAST	FIRST	LAST	
School Functioning	.114*	.088*	.000	.008	.039	.006	12.7%
Social/Peer Interaction	.429**	.306**	.038	.002	.105*	.007	43.8
Activity Level	.208**	.142**	.030	.004	.052	.004	21.7
Current Openness	.142**	.106*	.001	.003	.046	.006	15.2
Depression	.086	.050	.013	.002	.035	.007	9.5
Global Rating	.224**	.112*	.124*	.060*	.081	.012	29.8

* $p<.05$; ** $p<.005$.
Entry is change in R^2 when the variable is entered in the first or last regression step.

Table 3. Psychosocial Antecedent Variables and Outcome Variables

Table 4

ILLNESS-RELATED ANTECEDENT VARIABLES AND OUTCOME VARIABLES

OUTCOME VARIABLE	DIAGNOSTIC PERIOD		PHYSICAL IMPAIRMENT		TREATMENT DIFFICULTY		PROGNOSIS		TOTAL VARIANCE
	FIRST	LAST	FIRST	LAST	FIRST	LAST	FIRST	LAST	
School Functioning	.002	.001	.012	.008	.019	.002	.044	.029	5.8%
Social/Peer Interaction	.009	.006	.006	.005	.004	.001	.042	.036	5.3
Activity Level	.000	.000	.067	.062	.011	.001	.046	.040	11.0
Current Openness	.013	.007	.001	.000	.001	.012	.053	.060	7.4
Depression	.020	.018	.109*	.099*	.019	.000	.035	.022	15.7
Global Rating	.001	.001	.101*	.081*	.023	.009	.000	.001	11.1

* $p<.05$.
Entry is change in R^2 when the variable is entered in the first or last regression step.

Table 4. Illness-Related Antecedent Variables and Outcome Variables

Table 5

DEMOGRAPHIC ANTECEDENT VARIABLES AND OUTCOME VARIABLES

OUTCOME VARIABLES	SES		AGE AT DIAGNOSIS		TOTAL VARIANCE
	FIRST	LAST	FIRST	LAST	
School Functioning	.048	.049	.003	.004	5.2%
Social/Peer Interaction	.026	.027	.003	.004	3.0
Activity Level	.006	.006	.001	.061	0.7
Current Openness	.005	.005	.000	.000	0.5
Depression	.012	.015	.086*	.090*	10.2
Global Rating	.146**	.148**	.000	.001	14.8

* $p<.05$; ** $p<.005$.
Entry is change in R^2 with the specific regression step.

Table 5. Demographic Antecedent Variables and Outcome Variables

diagnostic period, the difficulty of treatment, and prognostic factors did not significantly predict outcome. (See Table 4.)

Lower socioeconomic status was significantly associated with a lower global rating. A greater age at diagnosis was significantly associated with depression scores both directly and when entered together. Socioeconomic status explained 14.8% of the variances in the global rating. Age at diagnosis accounted for 9% of the variance in depression. Other significant relationships between antecedent demographic and outcome variables were not found. (See Table 5.)

More than half the variance in the survivors' social/peer interaction and global adjustment was predicted by the nine antecedent variables in the three sets. The antecedent variables were less predictive of school functioning (only 23.5% of variance) and least predictive of the survivors' current openness regarding the illness. (See Table 6.)

DISCUSSION

The study findings provide evidence of successful long-term adaptation for children who had a diagnosis of cancer and underwent the intensive, protracted treatment the diagnosis entails. Despite differences in length of time elapsed, diagnosis represented, and the social and medical climates in which the treatment took place, the present study replicates many findings of Koocher and O'Malley's (*1981*) pioneering work. Our study, like the earlier work, found that global adjustment is good for most survivors and that serious problems such as depression and academic or social malfunctioning are relatively rare. Although the number of outright refusals was small, there were survivors who repeatedly failed follow-up appointments in the oncology clinic and whose

Table 6

TOTAL VARIANCE IN OUTCOME VARIABLES EXPLAINED BY ALL NINE ANTECEDENT VARIABLES

OUTCOME VARIABLE	TOTAL	PSYCHOSOCIAL VARIABLES	ILLNESS-RELATED VARIABLES	DEMOGRAPHIC VARIABLES
School Functioning	23.5%	12.7%	5.8%	5.2%
Social/Peer Interaction	50.1	43.8	5.3	3.0
Activity Level	34.6	21.7	11.0	0.5
Current Openness	20.0	15.2	7.4	0.5
Depression	34.5	9.5	15.7	10.2
Global Adjustment Rating	52.5	29.8	11.1	14.8

Table 6. Total Variance in Outcome Variables Explained by All Nine Antecedent Variables

families could not be located. These patients were thus not part of the subject group, and they may well have been experiencing more psychological disturbance. To the degree that this represents a significant selection bias, a psychologically healthier outcome would be overestimated. Nevertheless, even a cautious interpretation of the results shows that the diagnosis of cancer and the demanding treatment it requires are compatible with a subsequent healthy developmental course for many children. The impressions that sparked the project, stemming from our clinical experience with survivors and families referred because of significant psychosocial symptomatology, may now be seen as not generally applicable. Rather, they exemplify the danger in extrapolating findings from a psychiatric group to a whole population.

The descriptive data testify to the variability in the experience of cancer and in the response to the illness. "Diagnosis and treatment of cancer" implies a single entity and course, but diversity in symptomatology, prognosis, treatment course, pain levels, hospitalization, relapses, and related events makes each individual's experience unique. More similarities exist within a diagnostic category, but even there the variation among individuals is significant. The objective stresses associated with cancer and its treatment do not constitute a consistent "given."

The interviews revealed that individuals who were rated as well adjusted, free of depression, successful at school, and popular with friends used different coping styles. Some well-adjusted survivors had embraced their cancer and had become experts and advocates; others had encapsulated the illness and acknowledged it as little as possible. Assertiveness and argumentativeness toward caregivers were associated with good outcome, as were compliance and passivity. A concrete, nonphilosophical approach served some survivors well, while others ascribed a larger purpose or meaning to the illness. Maximal use of hospital resources was adaptive for some; avoidance of all but the most essential services was the preference for others. Both could be associated with a positive outcome.

The present findings underscore the need for understanding and acceptance of individual response styles in the planning of psychosocial interventions. We must not assume a common definition of what constitutes a need for help. Neither is there a common path to health. There are no "cookbook" answers or interventions; helpful programs must be responsive to individual needs. Patients or families who express no interest in psychosocial interventions are not necessarily "resistant." For some, successful conclusion of cancer treatment may be associated with psychological gains without professional assistance.

Change in an individual's developmental trajectory is difficult to gauge from retrospective data, even using multiple sources. In specific areas, however, it did seem reasonable to compare survivors' current and prior diagnostic status.

In both physical activity levels and social/peer interactions, there was a significant change for somewhat less than half the group, equally divided between positive and negative changes. Academic achievement was the only area in which many more survivors were doing more poorly subsequent to the diagnosis of cancer (33% vs 10%). In all these outcome categories, the majority of the survivors were functioning at a level consistent with their status prior to diagnosis.

The hierarchical regression analyses revealed that most illness-related variables were *not* predictive of psychosocial outcome. The length, difficulty, error, or uncertainty in the diagnostic process; the child's prognosis; the severity of the treatment protocol; and the complications encountered during the active stages of the illness were not significant determinants of psychosocial outcome. Only residual physical handicap predicted significant outcome variance, and only in two of six outcome measures. "The worse the course of the illness, the more difficulty with long-term adjustment" is a widely held belief that is not supported by the data from this study.

Psychosocial variables, especially the communication patterns and availability of peer support during treatment, were more predictive of psychosocial outcome. These data suggest that, for many children, the diagnosis and treatment of cancer constitute a protracted stress that elicits preexisting vulnerabilities but also strengths and positive coping patterns. Qualitative changes that do take place are more often subtle than gross, and they may elude standard, quantitative instruments. Further study is needed that focuses on the clarified values, heightened sensitivity to others, increased altruism, and altered perceptions of the vigor and vulnerability of their own bodies that many survivors remarked upon in the interviews.

REFERENCES

Anholt, U., Fritz, G., Williams, J., & Amylon, M. (1988). Self-concept in childhood cancer survivors. Manuscript submitted for publication.

Brouwers, P., Riccardi, R., Poplack, D., & Fedio, P. (1984). Attentional deficits in long-term survivors of childhood acute lymphoblastic leukemia (ALL). *Journal of Clinical Neuropsychology, 6,* 325–336.

Cohen, I., & Cohen, P. (1983). *Applied multiple regressions: Correlation analysis for the behavioral sciences* (2nd ed.). Hillsdale, NJ: Erlbaum.

Copeland, D., Fletcher, J., Pfefferbaum-Levine, B., Jaffe, N., Reid, H., & Major, M. (1985). Neuropsychological sequelae of childhood cancer in long-term survivors. *Pediatrics, 75,* 745–753.

Hollingshead, A. (1975). *Four factor index of social status.* Unpublished manuscript. Yale University, New Haven.

Holmes, H., & Holmes, F. (1975). After ten years, what are the handicaps and life styles of children treated for cancer? *Clinical Pediatrics, 14,* 819–823.

Koocher, G., & O'Malley, J. (1981). *The Damocles Syndrome: Psychosocial consequences of surviving childhood cancer.* New York: McGraw-Hill.

Lansky, S., List, M., & Ritter-Sterr, C. (1986). Psychosocial consequences of cure. *Cancer, 58,* 529–533.

Li, F., & Stone, R. (1976). Survivors of cancer in childhood. *Annals of Internal Medicine, 84,* 551–553.

Poznanski, E., Grossman, J., Buchsbaum, Y., Benegas, M., Freeman, L., & Gibbons, R. (1984). Preliminary studies of the reliability and validity of the Children's Depression Rating Scale. *Journal of the American Academy of Child Psychiatry, 23,* 191–197.

Wasserman, A., Thompson, E., Wilimas, J., & Fairclough, D. (1987). The psychological status of survivors of childhood/adolescent Hodgkins disease. *American Journal of Diseases of Children, 141,* 626–631.

Part V

TEMPERAMENT STUDIES

The four papers in this section are illustrative of different ways in which a consideration of temperamental factors has enriched our understanding of a variety of developmental and clinical circumstances. In a carefully executed study, Keener, Zeanah, and Anders examine relations between aspects of the sleep behavior of infants and mothers' and fathers' ratings of temperament. Objective measures of sleep-wake organization were derived from time-lapse video recordings in 23 infants at 6 months of age, while Infant Temperament Questionnaires were completed by both parents two weeks prior to the recording sessions. All infants were found to wake during the night, but some were able to return themselves to sleep, while others required interventions from parents to fall asleep again. The sleep architecture of the "signaling" and "self-soothing" infants did not differ. Both mothers' and fathers' ratings of infant temperament were correlated with measures of sleep continuity, but the results for fathers were much more striking. Infants who required care during the night were rated as significantly more difficult and arrhythmic by fathers than by mothers. These findings are of particular interest in light of recent debate over the measurement of temperament. Clearly, temperament is not wholly in the eye of the beholder. Both mothers' and fathers' responses were significantly related to objectively measured behaviors. However, differences in ratings require explanation. Rather, it would appear as if parental responses to questionnaires describing the temperamental attributes of their children are both objectively and subjectively determined. Findings such as these suggest the need for further research examining the effects of interpersonal context on parents' ratings of their infants' temperamental attributes.

Caspi, Elder, and Bem focus on a single temperamental attribute in their study of the life-course patterns of shy children. The data derive from the Berkeley Guidance Study, initiated in 1928–1929, and include information on 87 of 102 boys and 95 of 112 girls who were followed into adulthood. While the original data collection did not include measures of temperament, the authors were able to construct indices of both childhood and adult "shyness." Boys who were shy as children were more likely than their peers to delay marriage, parenthood, and stable careers, to attain lower occupational achievement, and to experience more marital instability. Shy girls were more likely than their peers to follow a conventional pattern of marriage, childbearing, and homemaking. The authors suggest that shyness or moving away from the world persist across the life course through progressive accumulation of their own consequences and by their tendency to evoke maintaining responses from others during reciprocal social interaction, and that these consequences are most evident when age-stage expected life transitions are examined. The findings are of interest in light of recent studies of genetic and other biologic influences. However, in this study, although the childhood and adult shyness indices were significantly correlated, childhood shyness accounted for only 6% of the variance. As Clarke and Clarke indicate in their paper, "The Adult Outcome of Early Behavioural Abnormalities," development is characterized by both continuity and change. A full understanding of developmental processes will be achieved only when factors acting to foster variation as well as those that contribute to the maintenance of consistency are the focus of inquiry.

In the next paper in this section, Rosenbaum, Kagan, and their associates report the results of a methodologically sophisticated and carefully conducted study of Behavioral Inhibition in Children of Parents with Panic Disorder and Agoraphobia. In summary, the data indicate that behavioral inhibition to the unfamiliar, as defined in previous work by Kagan (see Annual Progress, 1988) is significantly more frequent among the offspring of adults in treatment for Panic Disorder with Agoraphopia (PDAG) than among children whose parents are in treatment for Major Depressive Disorder or other psychiatric disorders. As the authors indicate, the findings are consistent with the results of studies suggesting a genetic component to AGPD. However, not all inhibited children are maladaptive, and the frequency of occurrence of behavioral inhibition in childhood (10%–15%) is considerably higher than the prevalence of AGPD in adult life (2.5%–5%). Moreover, although inhibition in children appears with roughly equal frequency in boys and girls, adult PD is much more common among women. Other factors, whether biological, like those surrounding puberty, or psychosocial, appear to influence the possible evolution from behavioral inhibition in childhood to disorder in adulthood. Nevertheless, if behavioral inhibition in early childhood does lead to the development of anxiety disorder or other psychopathology in at least some children, the identification of those at risk may well represent a major opportunity for the development of preventive strategies.

Carey, Hegvik, and McDevitt address an issue of growing clinical concern. This report, "Temperamental Factors Associated with Rapid Weight Gain and Obesity in Middle Childhood," derives from data collected in a private pediatric practice. Carey's long-standing interest in the measurement and relevance of temperament led to the establishment of procedures which guaranteed that measures of temperament as well as the more usual measures of height and weight were obtained during regular well-child visits. In this exploratory study, the authors chose to focus on middle childhood because of the importance of this age period for the prediction of adult weight. The findings suggest a small but significant correlation between the rate of weight gain during the period from 4 years to 9 years and the temperamental attributes of the difficult child. The authors suggest that these temperamental characteristics in interaction with metabolic, dietary, and environmental factors may predispose some children to the development of inappropriate eating habits. At the very least, clinicians need to be aware of a possible linkage between excessive weight gain and the difficult child constellation when planning programs of weight reduction for this extremely difficult-to-treat population of children.

17

Infant Temperament, Sleep Organization, and Nighttime Parental Interventions

**Marcia A. Keener, Charles H. Zeanah,
and Thomas F. Anders**
Rhode Island Hospital, Brown University Program in Medicine

Objective measures of sleep-wake organization derived from time-lapse video recordings were compared with parental perceptions of infant temperament in 23 infants 6 months of age. Although both mothers' and fathers' ratings of infant temperament were correlated with variables reflecting sleep continuity, results for fathers were much more striking. Infants who required care giving during the night were rated as significantly more difficult and arrhythmic by fathers than by mothers. All infants awakened during the night. Some of them soothed themselves and returned to sleep; however, others signaled and required care giving interventions from their parents before returning to sleep. No differences in variables reflecting the biology of sleep distinguished "signaling" infants and "self-soothing" infants, although feedings at bedtime (breast or bottle) were more common in the signaling group.

In recent years, there has been controversy about whether infant temperament questionnaire ratings reflect a biologic or constitutional predisposition of the child or reflect parental characteristics and attitudes. This debate has stimulated interest in the relationship between infant behavior and parental perceptions of temperament. In previous studies, we have investigated the development of parental perceptions of temperament in utero and in early infancy and their relationship to observed infant and maternal behaviors.[1-5] We found

Reprinted with permission from *Pediatrics*, 1988, Vol. 81, 762–771. Copyright 1988 by the American Academy of Pediatrics.

This work was supported, in part, by the David and Lucille Packard Foundation, the Henry T. Kaiser Foundation, and grant MH-16744 from the National Institute of Mental Health.

that parental perceptions of temperament were related to infant behaviors but that they were also influenced by other factors such as prenatal fantasies about the infant, labor experiences, parental anxiety, and sex of the parent. Our results converge with those of other investigators that suggest that parental ratings of infant temperament are both objectively and subjectively determined.[6-8]

The organization of sleep-wake states is an important domain of infant behavior that incorporates several dimensions of temperament: rhythmicity, state regulation, activity, arousal, irritability, and soothability. Therefore, a study of the relationship between parental temperament ratings and nighttime infant sleep-wake patterns is of particular interest.

The establishment of diurnal regularity of waking and sleep is an important achievement of the first year of life. According to a survey of maternal reports of infant sleep habits, 83% of infants began sleeping through the night, or "settled," by 6 months of age, although a substantial proportion of them resumed waking again after settling.[9] Similarly, in a study of infant sleep recorded in the home by time-lapse video somnography,[10] we found that 74% of infants had settled by 6 months of age and approximately half of those who had settled before 5 months resumed waking again later in the first year of life.

The factors that influence settling and night waking are poorly understood, however. Some studies have suggested that settling is related to biologic factors such as early perinatal insults or "constitutional sensitivities" that presumably interfere with the normal maturation of CNS mechanisms governing the entrainment of sleep-wake patterns to the light-dark cycle and the consolidation of nighttime sleep.[9,11-13]

Nevertheless, in a longitudinal investigation, we compared nighttime sleep maturation in two groups: normal, full-term infants and a matched cohort of "at-risk" preterm infants. We found no major differences between the groups in the development of diurnal sleep-wake organization during the first year of life.[14] In particular, the biologically compromised premature infants did not demonstrate more difficulties in settling than the full-term group. Apparently, the contribution of perinatal pathology to settling difficulties is modest.

The evidence to date seems to suggest that a variety of factors contribute to early sleep-wake organization and to settling difficulties. Results from our investigations and from other studies suggest that the maturation and temporal organization of early sleep-wake patterns reflect an interaction between biologic maturity, infant temperament, and the parent-infant relationship.[12,14-17]

The purpose of the present study was threefold. First, we were interested in whether parents' reports of temperament were related to aspects of infant sleep-wake organization. Previous studies of temperament and sleep have been based upon parental descriptions of current or past sleep habits. However, in this study, we obtained objective measures of sleep using time-lapse video recording in the home.

Second, we were interested in whether there were differences in temperament between infants who were waking at night and those who had settled. Other investigators have reported certain temperament characteristics in night-waking infants including low sensory threshold,[12] low malleability and rhythmicity,[18] and more difficult temperament.[15]

Finally, we were interested in whether variations in night waking might reflect differing patterns of parent-infant interaction at bedtime and during the night. Home sleep recordings provide an opportunity to assess aspects of nighttime dyadic interaction.

METHODS

Subjects

The subjects were 23 couples and their firstborn infants, 11 boys and 12 girls. The families were recruited from a sample of 38 couples who were participating in a longitudinal study of early parental perceptions of temperament. Detailed characteristics of the group have been described elsewhere.[1] In brief, the families were white, middle to upper middle class, and well educated. Each infant was the product of a full-term, uncomplicated pregnancy and delivery. A total of 25 couples were randomly selected from the larger sample and invited to participate in the current study, of whom 23 agreed to complete the protocol.

Temperament Assessments

When the infants were 6 months of age, two copies of the Revised Infant Temperament Questionnaire[19] were mailed to the families, one for each parent to complete. The Infant Temperament Questionnaire consists of 95 statements describing infant behavior in a variety of everyday situations. Parents rate the frequency with which each infant behavior occurs, using a sixpoint scale ranging from "almost never" to "almost always." The scale yields ratings in nine dimensions of temperament: activity, rhythmicity, approach/withdrawal, adaptability, intensity, mood, persistence, distractibility (or soothability), and sensory threshold. Scores in five of the dimensions are used in determining a clinical temperament designation: easy, intermediate low, intermediate high, and difficult. Infants who are easy are rhythmic in functioning, adaptable, approaching, mild in their responses, and positive in mood. Infants who are difficult are irregular in bodily functioning, slowly adaptable, slow in initial approach, intense in their responses, and negative in mood. Those infants considered to be between these two extremes are termed intermediate low and intermediate high.

Sleep Recordings

After the parents had returned the completed Infant Temperament Questionnaires, they were contacted by phone and the purpose and procedures of the home sleep recordings were explained. If the family expressed interest in participating, a convenient date for the recordings was arranged, generally about 2 weeks after the questionnaires were completed.

The infants were recorded for two consecutive nights at home sleeping in their own cribs. The methodology for home video recording and coding of nighttime sleep-wake states has been described in detail elsewhere.[10] In brief, the portable time-lapse video equipment was brought to the family's home, set in place, and activated by the experimenters. A video camera that was sensitive to infrared light was focused on the infant's crib. A small infrared light placed in a corner of the room provided sufficient illumination so that the infant's typical sleeping conditions were maintained. A microphone was placed near the crib to record fussy and crying vocalizations.

The parents were asked to follow their usual routine in putting their infant to bed and in responding to the infant during the night. In addition, a brief semistructured interview was conducted, usually with the mother. In the interview, current sleep habits were assessed (e.g., typical bedtime and awakening time, whether the infant had settled and age of settling, frequency of night wakings and typical parental responses, frequency and duration of daytime naps), history of sleep difficulties, current status (e.g., feeding; recent stresses or disruptions, such as illness, trips, or teething; general health and developmental milestones), and whether the infant's routine and sleep on the recording nights was typical.

Coding of sleep-wake states. For the coding of sleep-wake states, the time-lapse video recordings, recorded at a time reduction of 18:1, were played back at normal speed. Thus, a 12-hour sleep period can be reviewed in approximately 45 minutes. At this speed, the phasic activity of sleep, i.e., rapid eye movements, twitches of the extremities, grimaces, rapid or irregular respiration, and body movements, is exaggerated. The criteria for scoring sleep-wake states were similar to other behavioral scoring methods.[20] Interrater reliability and validity of video-recorded sleep-wake states compared with polygraphic recordings is substantial.[10,21,22]

Four states were coded from the videotapes: quiet sleep, characterized by an absence of gross body movements except for isolated startles and by regular respiration; active sleep, characterized by frequent body movements, rapid eye movements, twitches, smiles, grimaces, and brief cries; awake, characterized by the infant's eyes being open and alert. The infant may be lying quietly, moving, and/or crying; and out of crib, characterized by the infant's removal from the crib for soothing, feeding, or other interventions.

Sleep-wake state organization. Eight summary variables obtained from the sleep-wake state codings characterize a night's sleep. In the present study, these variables were averaged throughout the two recording nights for each infant. Previous studies have reported that, unlike laboratory polygraph studies, there is no first-night effect in home video recordings of infant sleep.[21,22]

The four state percentages (quiet sleep, active sleep, awake, out of crib) were calculated as proportions of the total recording time (i.e., from the time the infant was first placed into the crib at night until he or she was removed the following morning). The longest sleep period, the longest interval an infant sustains sleep without awakening, is a measure of sleep continuity. The percentage of longest sleep period (midnight to 5 AM) summarizes the degree to which the longest sleep period occurs within the hours of midnight and 5 AM, the conventional definition of "settling." It is a measure of diurnal entrainment and reflects the infant's tendency to "sleep through the night."

Two sleep maturity scores, the holding time index and the transition probability index,* were calculated from the infant's pattern of state durations and state-to-state transitions during the night using a semi-Markov model.[10,23,24] The holding time index is a measure of the organization of quiet sleep and active sleep during the night. The sleep of an infant with a high (mature) holding time index is characterized by long durations of quiet sleep and short durations of active sleep early in the night. The direction of state-to-state transitions, especially transitions to wakefulness, is measured by the transition probability index, a measure of sleep continuity. The sleep of an infant with a mature (high) transition probability index is characterized by few if any awakenings.

Parent-Infant Interaction at Bedtime and During Awakenings

After the video recordings were coded for sleep-wake states, the bedtime intervals and periods of infant wakefulness during the night were reviewed and coded for infant signaling and parental response. We defined "signaling" as 30 seconds or more of continuous fussing and/or crying.

Five infant behaviors were coded at bedtime and during awakenings.

1. Sleep latency was defined as the number of minutes required for the infant to fall asleep after being placed into the crib at bedtime. For awakenings

during the night, sleep latency was defined as the number of minutes to return to sleep; that is, the duration of the awakening.

2. Signal latency was defined as the number of minutes from the onset of an awakening until the infant fussed and/or cried for 30 seconds or longer. For the bedtime intervals, signal latency was measured from the time an awake infant was placed into the crib.

3. Fuss/cry time was defined as the minutes from the onset of signaling until the infant either quieted for 60 seconds or longer or was removed from the crib by the parent. If the infant quieted and then began fussing again, the intervals of signal time were totaled.

4. Fussiness was defined as a global rating of the amount of fussiness at bedtime and during awakenings, made on the four-point scale that follows: 1—none; 2—brief, isolated fusses or cries (< 10 seconds); 3—intermittent episodes of fussing/crying; and 4—continuous fussing/crying.

5. Self-soothing activity during wakefulness was also rated on a four-point scale: 1, no attempts to self-soothe; 2, one or two brief attempts; 3, several repeated attempts to achieve quiescence, and 4, sustained attempts to achieve or maintain quiescence.

Two parental behaviors were coded at bedtime and during infant awakenings.

1. Intervention latency was defined as the number of minutes from the onset of the infant's signal latency until the parent made an intervention or removed the child from the crib.

2. Intervention time was defined as the total number of minutes a parent spent care giving either at bedtime or during an awakening including the time that the infant was removed from the crib.

We also noted which parent(s) put the infant to bed and responded to awakenings and whether any "special" toys or self-soothing objects were given to the infant at bedtime.

Bedtime and night awakening behaviors were averaged separately during the two nights. Awakenings during which the infant did not signal were tallied separately and also averaged throughout nights.

RESULTS

Temperament and Sleep Organization

To assess the relationship between temperament and sleep organization, Spearman rank order correlations were computed between the infant's summary sleep variables and the parental temperament ratings for both mothers and fathers. In Table 1, the results are summarized. Intercorrelations of sleep variables, day-to-day stability of the summary sleep variables, and intercorre-

TABLE 1. Parental Temperament Ratings and Sleep-Wake State Organization*

Infant Temperament Questionnaire Dimension	Fathers	Mothers
Rhythmicity		
TPI	$-.58^a$	
% OOC	$.42^b$	$.43^b$
% LSP	$-.42^b$	
% AS		$-.42^b$
Intensity: LSP	$.56^a$	
Distractibility		
LSP	$-.56^a$	
% LSP	$-.48^b$	
Easy/difficult		
TPI	$-.63^a$	
% OOC		$-.50^b$
LSP	$-.52^a$	
% LSP	$-.58^a$	

* Low score indicates easier temperament. Abbreviations: AS, active sleep; LSP, longest sleep period between midnight and 5 AM; OOC, out of crib; TPI, transition probability index. Spearman rank correlation coefficient: $^a P < .01$; $^b P < .05$.

Table 1. Parental Temperament Ratings and Sleep-Wake State Organization*

lations between mothers' and fathers' temperament ratings were similar to those in our previous reports.[4,10,22]

There were significant correlations between fathers' temperament ratings of rhythmicity, intensity, distractibility, and the easy/difficult designation and four sleep-wake measurements (percentage of time out of crib, longest sleep period, transition probability index, and percentage of longest sleep period from midnight to 5 AM). These measurements all reflect aspects of sleep continuity. Thus, rhythmic, distractible infants who were easy (as rated by fathers) tended to have more mature patterns of state transitions, to sleep for long periods or "sleep through the night," and to spend less time out of the crib for feeding, soothing, or other interventions. In addition, infants whose fathers rated them as intense also tended to sleep for long periods. At first glance, this seems inconsistent with the other findings, because high ratings on intensity suggest a more difficult temperament. On the other hand, this dimension is described as a measure of the energy content of responses regardless of their quality and suggests that infants who are intense in their responses to the environment during the day tend to sleep for longer periods at night.

For mothers' temperament ratings, there were significant correlations between rhythmicity and the easy/difficult designation and two infant sleep parameters, percentage of time out of crib and percentage of active sleep. Thus, infants whose mothers rated them as arrhythmic tended to have a smaller percentage of active sleep. This finding probably reflects the reduced amount of active sleep that is associated with being removed from the crib. In previous studies,[10] we observed that, when infants awaken briefly during the night, they tend to awaken from and return to active sleep. However, if an infant is unable to return to sleep on his or her own and is removed from the crib for care giving, the period of active sleep may occur "off camera," in the mother's arms. Therefore, the overall percentage of active sleep recorded on videotape was somewhat diminished.

Because the Infant Temperament Questionnaire contains eight items about the infant's sleep behavior, we explored the contribution that these items made to the relationship between parent ratings and infant sleep behavior. Four of the eight items concerning sleep counted as one each on the mood, approach/withdrawal, activity, and threshold dimensions of temperament. The other four items all counted as the rhythmicity dimension. We created a sleep score variable (low score means a "good" sleeper) comprising the total ratings of the eight Infant Temperament Questionnaire items and correlated it with the sleep variables in Table 1. Fathers' sleep score ratings were correlated with the transition probability index $r_s = .59$, $P < .01$ but were unrelated to other objective measures of infant sleep. Mothers' sleep score ratings were unrelated to all objective measures of infant sleep. This finding suggests that the correlations we demonstrated between parental temperament ratings and objective measures of infant sleep behavior were not explained solely or even largely by parents' ratings of the infants' sleep behaviors.

Temperament Ratings and Night Waking

To assess the relationship between temperament ratings and nighttime wakefulness we divided our sample into three groups of infants based upon our codings of infant and parental behaviors during awakenings. Previous studies of home-recorded sleep have shown that many infants awaken briefly at night without disturbing their parents' sleep.[25,26] Similarly, when infants awaken and signal, parents are often able to intervene briefly and help the infant return to sleep without removal from the crib. Therefore, we reasoned that any differences in temperament would not be related to the amount of nighttime wakefulness per se but rather to a given infant's propensity to signaling during an awakening. Furthermore, we expected that the time of night of signaling might influence differentially parental perceptions and responses to the awakening. Specifically, parents might interpret and respond differently to an awakening at 9 PM than to one at 3 AM that interrupted their sleep.

Three groups of infants were defined as follows: a "high signaling" group comprised seven infants who signaled and received a parental intervention on both recording nights between the hours of midnight and 5 AM; a "low to moderate signaling" group (n = 9) who received either an intervention on only one night between midnight and 5 AM, or an intervention on one or both nights but not between midnight and 5 AM; and a "self-soothing" group (n = 7) who either did not awaken or did not signal during an awakening on either night.

A Kruskal-Wallis test was computed to assess differences in temperament ratings between groups (Table 2). There were no significant differences in any of the nine temperament dimensions or the easy/difficult designation for mothers' ratings. However, fathers' ratings of rhythmicity and the easy/difficult designation were significantly different between groups ($P < .01$ and .02, respectively). The fathers' mean ratings for rhythmicity were 2.52 for infants who were self-soothers, 2.46 for infants who were low to moderate signalers, and 3.47 for infants who were high signalers. Mean ratings for temperament difficulty were 2.71 for self-soothing infants, 2.67 for low to moderate signaling infants, and 4.0 for high signaling infants. Thus, fathers rated high signaling infants as significantly less rhythmic and more difficult.

TABLE 2. Differences in Sleep Organization Between Signaling and Self-Soothing Infants

	Self-Soothing Infants (n = 7)	Low to Moderate Signaling Infants (n = 9)	High Signaling Infants (n = 7)
Quiet sleep (%)	41.9	42.8	41.2
Active sleep (%)	51.2	48.3	45.5
Total sleep (%)	93.1	91.0	86.7
Awake (%)	6.9	5.6	6.0
Longest sleep period			
Min[a]	426.2	359.6	234.1
%[a]	78.1	77.1	36.4
Sleep maturity scores			
Transition probability index[b]	12.1	10.4	7.5
Holding time index	13.4	14.9	11.8

* Kruskal-Wallis test: [a] $P < .01$; [b] $P < .02$.

Table 2. Differences in Sleep Organization Between Signaling and Self-Soothing Infants

Differences in Sleep Organization Between
Waking and Settled Infants

We were also concerned whether signaling infants were more "immature" in sleep-wake organization other than their obvious tendency to awaken more frequently and require more parental care giving than self-soothing infants. To test this hypothesis, the Kruskal-Wallis test was computed to assess differences in sleep-wake measurements between the groups. Because the percentage out of crib had been used indirectly in defining the two groups, we did not include this variable in the analysis. We added another variable to the analysis, total sleep percentage (active sleep plus quiet sleep), to test whether the groups differed in the overall amount of nighttime sleep. The results are summarized in Table 2.

Three variables differed significantly between groups: transition probability index, longest sleep period, and percentage of longest sleep period between midnight and 5 AM. These variables all measure sleep continuity. Thus, infants who signaled, especially those who were high signalers, had a less mature pattern of state-to-state transitions, a shorter longest sleep period, and less tendency to "sleep through the night" than self-soothing infants. More importantly, percentage of quiet sleep and percentage of active sleep were comparable between groups as was the holding time index, our measure of mature sleep state organization within the night. This finding suggests that, despite frequent awakenings, the emerging diurnal organization of sleep states did not differ between groups.

Infant and Parental Behaviors at Infant's Bedtime

Most of the infants in this sample (21 of 23) slept in their own bedrooms. In more than half of the families (61%), mothers put the infant to bed. In 22% of the families, both mother and father shared putting the infant to bed and, in the remaining couples (17%), mothers and fathers alternated bedtime duties on the two nights. Approximately one third of the infants used a special toy, blanket, pacifier, or some other self-soothing object at bedtime on both nights.

A substantial proportion (39.1%) of the infants were put into the crib already asleep on both nights. This finding compromised comparisons of differential bedtime infant-parent interaction between infants who were self-soothing and infants who signaled. In general, however, infants who signaled during the night were more likely to be put to bed asleep than infants who were self-soothing (43.8% v 28.6%, respectively). Otherwise, there seemed to be little distinction between these groups in bedtime behaviors: some self-soothing infants signaled during bedtime interactions, whereas some signaling infants fell asleep without interventions.

Of all of the infants who were put to bed awake, nearly two thirds (64.3%) received one or more interventions before falling asleep. Fussiness at bedtime was brief or intermittent, and most infants displayed high levels of self-soothing. The median amount of fuss/cry time was slightly less than 2½ minutes. Parents responded rapidly to infant signaling (Table 3), usually within 15 seconds (median 12.3 seconds), and their bedtime interventions were short and effective (1.6 minutes). All of the infants fell asleep quickly, although infants who signaled at bedtime took longer to fall asleep than those who did not: 15.6 minutes *v* 7.2 minutes.

Infant and Parent Interaction During Night Waking

As previously described, our sample of signaling infants consisted of 16 infants (69.6%) who received parental interventions on one or both nights. Nearly all of these infants (81.3%) attempted to soothe themselves upon awakening. Often, self-soothing behavior lasted only for a few seconds, but in some instances, infants were able to soothe themselves for a long time before signaling. The median latency to signaling was slightly less than 20 seconds but ranged from 0 to 24.6 minutes. There seemed to be some differences between the groups of signalers: low to moderate signaling infants had less fuss/cry time, less fussiness, more self-soothing activity, and quicker return to sleep than the high signaling group (Table 4).

Intervention latencies during the night, although longer than at bedtime, were still short: parents usually responded to infant signaling in less than two minutes. The duration of interventions was somewhat longer than at bedtimes

TABLE 3. Infant and Parent Interaction at Bedtime*

	Awake Infants (n = 14)
Infant behaviors	
Sleep latency (min)	8.8 (0.6–32.8)
Signal latency (s)	56.0 (0–1,030.0)
Fuss/cry time (min)	2.3 (0–10.8)
Fussiness (min)	2.3 (1.5–4.0)
Self-soothing activity (min)	4.0 (1.0–4.0)
Parent intervention	
Latency (s)	12.3 (0–408.0)
Time (min)	1.6 (0.1–9.2)

* Values are given as medians (ranges).

Table 3. Infant and Parent Interaction at Bedtime*

	Low to Moderate Signaling Infants (n = 9)	High Signaling Infants (n = 7)
Infant behaviors		
Signal latency (s)	19.2 (0–180.0)	19.5 (8.2–1,474.0)
Fuss/cry time (min)	1.1 (0.5–6.9)	2.9 (1.3–5.8)
Fussiness (min)	2.8 (1.9–4.0)	3.2 (3.0–4.0)
Self-soothing activity (min)	2.5 (1.0–3.5)	1.8 (1.3–3.8)
Sleep latency (min)	14.1 (2.1–59.5)	25.5 (2.9–47.1)
Parent intervention		
Latency (s)	56.0 (22.0–372.0)	104.0 (31.0–265.0)
Time (min)	2.5 (0.4–53.0)	18.4 (0.1–38.0)

* Values are given as medians (ranges).

Table 4. Infant and Parent Interaction During Night Waking*

as well but ranged from 10 seconds to 53 minutes. Parents of infants who were low to moderate signalers seemed to respond more quickly and spent less time care giving than parents of infants who were high signalers. This response may have been a function of the time of night of the interventions: more of the awakenings of high signaling infants occurred between midnight and 5 AM when their parents were asleep. In more than half of the families, both mothers and fathers provided nighttime care giving on one or both nights; sometimes, one parent responded to one awakening and the other to the next. In one other family, the parents alternated care giving on the two nights. Fathers were as involved with infants who were low to moderate signalers as they were with high signaling infants: 36% of interventions with infants who were low to moderate signalers were shared by fathers v 32% of interventions with infants who were high signalers.

Silent Awakenings of Self-Soothing and Signaling Infants

Ten of the signaling infants had "silent" awakenings on at least one of the recording nights, i.e., awakenings during which they did not signal their parents. Five infants had such awakenings on both nights. Both groups of infants who signaled had silent awakenings, although they were slightly more common in the low to moderate group (66.7% v 57.1% of high signaling infants).

We compared these awakenings to those of the self-soothing infants, each of whom had at least one silent awakening on one of the nights (Table 5). In both self-soothing and signaling infants, there was little if any fussiness during these awakenings. Similarly, both groups also showed high levels of self-soothing activity, although the self-soothing infants showed slightly more sus-

TABLE 5. Silent Awakenings in Self-Soothing and Signaling Infants*

Behavior	Self-Soothing Infants (n = 7)	Signaling Infants (n = 16)
Fussiness (min)	1.5 (1.0–3.0)	2.0 (1.0–2.0)
Self-soothing activity (min)	4.0 (3.0–4.0)	3.5 (1.5–4.0)
Sleep latency (min)	4.2 (1.5–39.0)	2.9 (1.0–5.7)

* Values are given as medians (ranges).

Table 5. Silent Awakenings in Self-Soothing and Signaling Infants*

tained soothing activity. Examples of self-soothing behaviors observed included thumb-sucking, playing with toys in the crib, locating and using a pacifier or bottle, and stroking a soft object such as a satin blanket edging or sheepskin pad.

Although silent awakenings were generally brief for both groups, some self-soothing infants were able to sustain quiescence for as long as 39 minutes. In contrast, signaling infants usually returned to sleep within three minutes.

Sleep Habits in Self-Soothing and Signaling Infants

Given the differences we found between the self-soothing and signaling groups, we wondered whether other differences might be evident in the semi-structured status interviews conducted at the time of the time-lapse video recordings. In the interviews, current and past sleep habits were assessed, as well as general health and development, feeding habits, and recent stresses or disruptions in routine.

All of the infants in the sample were developmentally normal and in good health. A total of 13 infants were settled (sleeping through the night). The average age of settling was 9.9 weeks, ranging from 1 to 22 weeks. Four other infants had settled previously but were night waking again at the time of recording. The remaining six infants had never settled. With few exceptions, parents' descriptions of their infants' typical sleep habits matched the time-lapse video recordings.

At the time of the study, nine infants were breast-fed and 14 bottle-fed. Six of the seven self-soothing infants and eight of 16 signaling infants were bottle-fed. However, there was a significant association between nighttime feedings and night waking: infants who were usually nursed (or bottle-fed) at bedtime and/or during night awakenings tended to be in the signaling groups (Table 6).

	Frequency		
	High Signaling Infants	Low to Moderate Signaling Infants	Self-Soothing Infants
No night feeding (n = 12)	0	5	7
Bottle with bed/waking (n = 4)	1	3	0
Breast or bottle with bed/ waking (n = 7)	6	1	0

* Fisher exact test, $P < .005$.

Table 6. Night Feeding and Variations in Night Waking*

DISCUSSION

Our findings indicate that both fathers' and mothers' perceptions of temperament at 6 months are related to objective measures of infant sleep-wake state organization, especially variables that reflect sleep continuity. Infants considered easy have longer sleep periods and spend less time out of the crib for care-taking interventions during the night.

Nevertheless, the most important finding in this investigation was that fathers' ratings were correlated with more infant sleep variables than mothers' ratings. One likely explanation for this surprising finding is that infants' sleep-wake habits represent a larger, more important domain of behavior for fathers in formulating their perceptions of the infants' temperaments than for mothers. Most of the fathers were employed in daytime jobs outside the home. Except for weekends, much of their day-to-day interaction with their young infants would occur in the evenings and at night, times when the infant was being put to bed and, perhaps, night waking. Thus, a father's ratings of rhythmicity, distractibility, and temperamental difficulty might be influenced more by the child's sleep patterns because that is the context in which he is most familiar with his infant. In contrast, mothers in this study were the infants' primary care givers. They either had not returned to work or had returned to work part time. Because they were with their infants more of the day, mothers would have more opportunity to interact with their infants and observe their behavior in a variety of settings and circumstances. Thus, for mothers, the infant's sleep-wake habits represented only one portion of a much larger domain of infant behaviors available to them for use in formulating their perceptions of temperament.

Further evidence for this explanation comes from our comparisons of perceived temperamental differences in the signaling and self-soothing groups of infants. Although we found no significant differences in temperament ratings for mothers, high signaling infants were rated as significantly less rhythmic and more difficult by fathers. In other words, mothers and fathers may interpret the same infant behaviors differently. Further research examining the effects of interpersonal context on parents' ratings of their infants' behaviors is clearly necessary.

Clearly, these results have implications for the recent debate about the measurement of temperament. On the one hand, the differences in ratings by mothers and fathers indicate that Infant Temperament Questionnaire-measured temperament exists in large part in the eyes of the beholder. On the other hand, fathers' differing perceptions appear to derive from observable differences in infant nighttime behavior, namely, signaling. Previously, we suggested several possible explanations for differences in mother-father ratings.[2] The explanation that mothers simply "know" their infants better because they spend more time with them is not supported, because these results provide more evidence of empirical validity of fathers' than mothers' ratings. The possibility that infants behave differently with their mothers and fathers was not addressed in this investigation because the infant behavior we examined was largely independent of differential parental interactional influence.

These results represent one potential way to understand the means by which infant behaviors may influence parental perceptions. Of course, it is not possible to determine the direction of effects in a cross-sectional, correlational design. It is also possible that some third unknown factor explains both the infants' sleep-wake behavior and the fathers' perceptions of difficulty.

Our comparisons of the sleep organization of signaling and self-soothing infants suggest that despite shortened sleep periods and more awakenings in the signaling infants, the diurnal organization of sleep states and the proportions of active sleep and quiet sleep are comparable between groups. Because these variables reflect maturational aspects of sleep, the lack of differences implies biologic comparability in the groups. This finding suggests that the origins of night waking are environmental rather than biologic in healthy 6-month-old infants.

There were interesting contrasts in the nighttime behaviors of signaling and self-soothing infants. Although we were unable to compare differences between the groups at bedtime, signaling infants were more likely to be put to bed asleep. This may be due to the signaling infants' being less able to put themselves to sleep once alone in their cribs. Of the infants who were put to bed awake, those who needed parental interventions took longer to fall asleep.

There were also some differences between low to moderate and high signaling groups during awakenings. Low to moderate signaling infants were less fussy, showed more self-soothing activity, received briefer parental interventions, and returned to sleep more quickly. Most of the signaling infants attempted to soothe themselves during awakenings although less consistently than the self-soothers. During some brief awakenings, they were able to return to sleep without parental intervention, however.

Finally, there was a relationship between signaling during the night and nursing/bottle feeding at bedtime or during awakenings. This finding should be interpreted with some degree of caution: the sample is small and clearly a number of infants who were not fed at bedtime were signalers (Table 6). Nevertheless, it does corroborate other research. Carey[12] reported an association between breast-feeding and night waking. Similarly, Paret[26] found a relationship between breast-feeding, weaning status, and night waking in 9-month-old infants: good sleepers had progressed further in weaning than wakers. Elias et al.[27] described shortened sleep periods in breast-fed infants, especially those who shared a bed with their mother.

Our results suggest, however, that breast-feeding per se may not be causal. Rather, the timing and function of feeding may be more relevant than the method of feeding. Our results are congruent with previous explanations of an association between night feeding and night waking. Schmitt[28] suggested that, after 4 months of age, middle of the night feedings should be considered conditioned behavior. In other words, if the infant becomes accustomed to a 3 AM feeding, he or she will learn to feel hungry at that time and will awaken in anticipation of being fed. Along similar lines, Ferber[29] suggested that night feedings may result in increased levels of arousal as a result of gastrointestinal or hormonal changes associated with caloric intake.

We agree with the emphasis on early experience in understanding the relationship between night feedings and night wakings. In the neonatal period, the rhythms of feeding and sleeping are tightly coupled: infants awaken hungry and often return to sleep near the end of a feeding. During the early months, as feedings become more substantial and less frequent and the intervals of wakefulness and sleeping are consolidated into a diurnal rhythm, there is a gradual "uncoupling" of the feeding and sleep rhythms. If infants continue to be fed at bedtime and especially if they are nursed (or fed) to sleep, the neonatal coupling of feeding with sleep onset is maintained and reinforced. Then, when the infants awaken during the night, they are unable to return to sleep without their familiar bedtime associations. Thus, feeding becomes complexly incorporated into the emerging bedtime ritual. We suspect that the higher prevalence of nightwaking in breast-fed infants may be attributable to the habit of nursing the infant to sleep: in this instance, the mother herself as well as the feeding becomes an integral element in the process of going to sleep.

SUMMARY AND CONCLUSIONS

In this investigation, we found that both mothers' and fathers' perceptions of temperament were related to objective measures of infant sleep-wake organization, especially to summary variables that reflect sleep continuity. Fathers' ratings were correlated with more sleep-wake variables than mothers'. When we assessed differences in parental temperament ratings for infants who varied in night waking behaviors, we found that infants who required frequent care giving during the night were rated as significantly more difficult and arrhythmic by their fathers. These findings suggest that infant sleep habits are a more potent determinant of fathers' than mothers' perceptions of their 6-month-old infants' temperaments. These results support our previous assertions that parents may interpret certain infant behaviors differently.[2,30] The results also extend the growing literature about the interaction of infant behavior and parents' perceptions of temperament.

When we compared the sleep-wake organization of infants who varied in night waking behaviors, we found no differences in variables that reflect sleep biology. However, we did find that variations in night waking were associated with differing patterns of infant signaling and self-soothing and with parental care giving at bedtime and during the night. The findings confirmed that nighttime feedings exert an important environmental influence upon sleep habits. An explanation of how this effect may develop is adduced.

Finally, given the variations in night waking we observed both throughout the entire sample and for individual infants from one night to the next, in our results a continuum of sleep-wake habits is suggested rather than distinct groups of "wakers" and "sleepers." It seems likely that these variations represent developmental stages in the process of settling. In any case, it seems that these variations differentially shape parental perceptions of the infant and may affect the parent-infant relationship as well. Further understanding of environmental factors that mediate settling may provide insights into the origins of nighttime parent-child interactions that may predispose the child to other sleep disorders later in childhood or the dyad to relational difficulties.

REFERENCES

1. Zeanah CH, Keener MA, Stewart L, et al: Prenatal perception of infant personality: A preliminary investigation. *J Am Acad Child Psychiatry* 1985;24:204–210
2. Zeanah CH, Keener MA, Anders TF, et al: Measuring difficult temperament in infancy. *J Dev Behav Pediatr* 1986;7:114–119
3. Zeanah CH, Keener MA, Anders TF: Adolescent mothers' prenatal fantasies and working models of their infants. *Psychiatry* 1986;49:193–203
4. Zeanah CH, Keener MA, Anders TF: Developing perceptions of temperament and their relation to mother and infant behavior. *J Child Psychol Psychiatry* 1986;27:449–512
5. Zeanah CH, Keener, MA, Anders, TF, et al: Adolescent mothers' perceptions of their infants before and after birth. *Am J Orthopsychiatry* 1987;57:351–360
6. Bates J: Issues in the assessment of difficult temperament: A reply to Thomas, Chess and Korn. *Merrill-Palmer Q* 1983;29:89–97

7. Bates J, Bayles K: Objective and subjective components in mothers' perceptions of their children from age 6 months to 3 years. *Merrill-Palmer Q* 1984;30:111–129

8. St James-Roberts I, Wolke D: Comparison of mothers' with trained observers' reports of neonatal behavioral style. *Infant Behav Dev* 1984;7:299–310

9. Moore T, Ucko L: Night waking in early infancy. *Arch Dis Child* 1957;32:333–342

10. Anders T, Keener M, Bowe, T, et al: A longitudinal study of nighttime sleep-wake patterns in infants from birth to one year, in Call J, Galenson E, Tyson R (eds): *Frontiers of Infant Psychiatry.* New York, Basic Books, 1983, pp 150–166

11. Bernal J: Night-waking in infants during the first 14 months. *Dev Med Child Neurol* 1973;15:760–769

12. Carey W: Night waking and temperament in infancy. *J Pediatr* 1974;84:756–758

13. Richards M: An ecological study of infant development in an urban setting in Britain, in Leiderman PH, Tulkin S, Rosenfeld A (eds): *Culture and Infancy.* New York, Academic Press Inc, 1977, pp 469–493

14. Anders T, Keener M: Developmental course of nighttime sleep-wake patterns in full-term and premature infants during the first year of life. *Sleep* 1985;8:173–192

15. Hertzig M, Beltramini A: Individual differences in the longitudinal course of sleep and bedtime behaviors in preschool children. Presented at the annual meeting of the American Academy of Child Psychiatry, Dallas, TX, Oct 17, 1981

16. Ungerer J, Sigman M, Beckwith L, et al: Sleep behavior of preterm children at three years of age. *Dev Med Child Neurol* 1983;25:297–304

17. Carey W: Breast feeding and night waking. *J Pediatr* 1975;18:327–329

18. Richman N: Sleep problems in young children. *Arch Dis Child* 1981;56:491–493

19. Carey W, McDevitt SC: Revision of the infant temperament questionnaire. *Pediatrics* 1978;61:735–739

20. Anders TF, Emde R, Parmelee A: *A Manual of Standardized Terminology, Techniques, and Criteria for the Scoring of States of Sleep and Wakefulness in Newborn Infants.* Los Angeles, University of California Los Angeles, 1971

21. Anders TF, Sostek AM: The use of time lapse video recording of sleep-wake behavior in human infants. *Psychophysiology* 1975;13:155–158

22. Keener MA: *Time-lapse Video Recording of Infant Sleep-Wake States in Infants at Home and in the Laboratory,* doctoral dissertation. University of Florida, Gainesville, 1983

23. Bowe T, Anders TF: The use of the semi-Markov model in the study of the development of sleep-wake states in infants. *Psychophysiology* 1979;17:41–48

24. Bowe T: *A Systems Analysis of the Maturation of Sleep Using a Semi-Markov Model,* doctoral dissertation. Stanford University, Stanford, CA, 1981

25. Anders T: Night waking in infants during the first year of life. *Pediatrics* 1979;63:860–864

26. Paret I: Night waking and its relation to mother-infant interaction in nine-month-old infants, in Call J, Galenson E, Tyson R (eds): *Frontiers of Infant Psychiatry.* New York, Basic Books, 1983, pp 171–177

27. Elias MF, Nicolson NA, Bora C, et al: Sleep/wake patterns of breast-fed infants in the first 2 years of life. *Pediatrics* 1986;77:322–329

28. Schmitt B: When baby just won't sleep. *Contemp Pediatrics* 1985;2:38–52

29. Ferber R: *Solve Your Child's Sleep Problems.* New York, Simon & Schuster, 1985

30. Zeanah CH, Keener MA, Anders TF, et al: Explorations of difficult temperament. *J Dev Behav Pediatr* 1986;7:122–123

18

Moving Away From the World: Life-Course Patterns of Shy Children

Avshalom Caspi

Harvard University

Glen H. Elder, Jr.

University of North Carolina at Chapel Hill

Daryl J. Bem

Cornell University

What are the life-course sequelae of childhood shyness? Using archival data from the Berkeley Guidance Study (Macfarlane, Allen, & Honzik, 1954), we identified individuals who were shy and reserved in late childhood and traced the continuities and consequences of this behavioral style across the subsequent 30 years of their lives. Shy boys were more likely than their peers to delay entry into marriage, parenthood, and stable careers; to attain less occupational achievement and stability; and—when late in establishing stable careers—to experience marital instability. Shy girls were more likely than their peers to follow a conventional pattern of marriage, childbearing, and homemaking. Results are compared with those from our parallel study of childhood ill-temperedness (Caspi, Elder, & Bem, 1987). Despite differences between shyness ("moving away from the world") and ill-temperedness ("moving against the world"), both persist across the life course through the

Reprinted with permission from *Developmental Psychology*, 1988, Vol. 24, No. 6, 824–831. Copyright 1988 by the American Psychological Association.

This research was supported in part by grants from the National Institute of Mental Health (MH-34172 and MH-41827). Glen H. Elder, Jr. was supported by a Senior Research Scientist Award fellowship from NIMH (MH-00567).

We are indebted to the Institute of Human Development at the University of California, Berkeley, for permission to use archival data from the Berkeley Guidance Study, and to Ricky Ezell, Marjorie Honzik, Guy Swanson, Catherine Cross, and Ellen Herbener for their assistance. Several anonymous reviewers also provided helpful ideas and suggestions.

*progressive accumulation of their own consequences (cumulative
continuity) and by their tendency to evoke maintaining responses
from others during reciprocal social interaction (interactional
continuity).*

Interactional styles established in childhood can shape the course of life in
profound ways. For example, men with histories of ill-temperedness in late
childhood have lower occupational status, more erratic worklives, and less stable marriages than men without such histories. Women with such histories
marry men of lower occupational status, have less stable marriages, and are
more ill-tempered as mothers than other women (Caspi, Elder, & Bem, 1987).

In interpreting these findings, we proposed that we were seeing two kinds of
continuity across the life course. The first results from a person's dispositionally guided selection and construction of environments. An individual's dispositions can lead him or her to select or construct environments that, in turn,
reinforce and sustain those dispositions (e.g., Scarr & McCartney, 1983;
Wachtel, 1977a). For example, when gregarious individuals preferentially seek
out social situations, they thereby select themselves into environments that further nourish and sustain their gregariousness.

This same dispositionally guided process also operates in more far-reaching
ways to influence the life course itself. For example, the boy whose ill-temper
leads him to drop out of school thereby limits his future career opportunities
and selects himself into frustrating life circumstances that further evoke a pattern of striking out explosively against the world. In such cases, behaviors are
sustained across time by the progressive accumulation of their own consequences, producing what we have called *cumulative continuity.* Because the
process of cumulative continuity can amplify and elaborate diverging trajectories of individuals across time, we believe it is responsible for many of the
most striking and enduring individual differences across the life course.

The second kind of continuity results from the reciprocal, dynamic transac-
tion between the person and the environment: The person acts, the environment reacts, and the person reacts back. This very general process can
promote continuity through both behavioral and cognitive mechanisms. At the
behavioral level, Patterson's (1982) work with aggressive boys has shown in
detail how family interactions can create and sustain destructive and aversive
patterns of behavior. By extension, we suggested that a child whose ill-
temperedness coerces others into providing short-term payoffs in the immediate situation may thereby learn a behavioral style that continues to "work" in
similar ways in later years. The immediate reinforcement short-circuits the
learning of more controlled interactional styles that might have greater adaptability in the long run (cf. Wachtel, 1977b).

At a more cognitive level, continuity may arise through self-confirming expectations that are evoked in new situations. For example, because aggressive children expect others to be hostile (Dodge, 1986), they may behave in ways that elicit hostility from others, thereby sustaining their aggression. Expectation-confirming interactions have also been demonstrated in other behavioral domains, such as extraversion-introversion (Snyder & Swann, 1978). We have called continuity of this general kind *interactional continuity* and have proposed that it is most likely to be observed in situations with interactional properties similar to those of the original evoking environment.

Our previous study of ill-tempered children revealed evidence for both kinds of continuity. In the present study, we continue our exploration of life-course continuities in personality by examining individuals with childhood histories of shyness—thereby shifting our focus from children who "move against the world" to those who "move away from the world" (Horney, 1945).

Shyness is not inherently problematic. For example, the shyness of a young child thrust into a novel situation is not only normal (Bronson, 1972) but may be highly functional for avoiding potential dangers in development (Izard, 1984). Beyond the first years of life, dispositional shyness may develop in quite nonpathological ways through the interaction of temperamental qualities with socialization and cognitive factors. Thus, the quality of a child's experiences with adults, siblings, and peers, the labeling of a child as *shy*, and the child's subsequent internalization of this label may aid and abet the development of dispositional shyness (Bronson, 1978; Kagan, 1981; Zimbardo, 1977). And, as shyness in middle and late childhood becomes associated with diffidence about entering social situations (Gottman, 1977; Kagan, Reznick, & Snidman, 1987), with discomfort and inhibition in the presence of others (Cheek, Carpentieri, Smith, Rierdan, & Koff, 1985), and with exaggerated self-concern (Buss, 1980; Fenigstein, Scheier, & Buss, 1975), the stage is set for both cumulative and interactional continuities in this behavioral style across the life course.

Cumulative continuity could arise because shy children may not experience many of the role and rule negotiations important to the growth of social knowledge and social skills (Putallaz & Gottman, 1981). They may thus become increasingly unlikely to initiate or to respond appropriately to social overtures, thereby selecting themselves into further isolation. Even if they do acquire the necessary social skills, their anxious inhibition in novel situations can deter them from initiating new contacts and thereby select them into further isolation (Jones, Freemon, & Goswick, 1981).

Interactional continuity could arise through their lack of assertiveness in ongoing interactions (Cheek & Buss, 1981; Coie, Dodge, & Coppotelli, 1982). Passivity may increase their risk of being ignored or overlooked, thereby sustaining their passivity even when they do expose themselves to social interaction. At a more cognitive level, research on the attributional process suggests that shy persons are more likely than others to make internal and stable attributions for their social distress and are more self-derogating in judging their own interpersonal performance (Arkin, Appelman, & Burger, 1980; Girodo, Dotzenroth, & Stein, 1981). Such cognitions tend to guide new experiences in line with expectancies and may thereby promote the stability of self-conceptions in new situations across the life course—just as the *shy* label may have done for them earlier in childhood.

As we noted above, continuities in personality are most likely to appear in later life when circumstances recreate environments with similar interactional properties. For example, the individuals in our earlier study, who reacted with temper tantrums to frustration and adult authority as children, became undercontrolled, irritable adults when they again faced frustration and controlling authority (as in school, the armed services, and low-level jobs) or were immersed in life situations requiring the frequent negotiation of interpersonal conflicts (as in marriage and child rearing). In contrast, shy individuals seem particularly disadvantaged when they are thrust into unfamiliar settings in which the interpersonal or role requirements are new and ambiguous (Jones & Carpenter, 1986; Pilkonis, 1977a). Indeed, the most frequent and important situational cause of shyness is novelty (Buss, 1980), which includes physical novelty (e.g., moving to a new locale), social novelty (e.g., meeting strangers), and role novelty (e.g., assuming a new job). Each source of novelty is hypothesized to evoke shyness in predisposed individuals.

Accordingly, we have focused in the present study on those points in our subjects' lives when they would have to abandon familiar roles and enter new and unfamiliar social settings, paying special attention to the transition from youth to adulthood when they would have to contend with major sources of novelty surrounding new demands and opportunities caused by changing roles and relationships. In particular, we expected shy children to encounter difficulties during late adolescence and young adulthood when called on by society to initiate those actions and social contacts required for assuming the adult roles of marriage, parenthood, and career. In the present study, then, we set out to examine the implications of childhood shyness for the transition to adulthood and to document the cumulative consequences of this transitional period for subsequent outcomes in the life course.

METHOD

Subjects

Data for this study were obtained from the archives of the Institute of Human Development (IHD) at the University of California, Berkeley. The subjects are members of the Berkeley Guidance Study (Eichorn, 1981), a study initiated in 1928–1929 with every third birth in the city of Berkeley over a period of 18 months. The original sample included an intensively studied group of 113 subjects and a less intensively studied group of 101 subjects matched on social and economic characteristics. Both samples are combined in the present study. Most of the subjects came from White, Protestant, native-born families. Slightly more than 60% were born into middle-class homes.

The original sample contained 102 boys, of which a maximum of 87 have been followed up into adulthood. There are no significant differences between those who were followed up and those who were not in childhood shyness ($t <$ 1), adolescent measures of intelligence ($t < 1$), or family social class at the time of their births ($t = 1.23$). Respondents were slightly better educated than nonrespondents, however ($t = 1.77$, $p = .08$).

Of the 112 girls in the sample, a maximum of 95 have been followed up into adulthood. There are no significant differences between those who were followed up and those who were not in childhood shyness ($t < 1$). Respondents did, however, score significantly higher than nonrespondents on adolescent measures of intelligence ($t = 3.44$, $p < .001$), educational level ($t = 3.84$, $p < .001$), and social class at the time of their births ($t = 2.99$, $p < .01$).

Shyness

Childhood data on the Berkeley subjects were obtained from clinical interviews with their mothers and subsequently organized into ratings on 5-point behavior scales (see Macfarlane, 1938; Macfarlane, Allen, & Honzik, 1954). We have used two of these scales in the present study: shyness and excessive reserve (scale intercorrelations are .68 and .70 for boys and girls, respectively). The shyness scale ranges from 1 *(exceptionally easy and quick social contacts, enjoys meeting new people)* to 5 *(acute discomfort to the point of panic in social situations)*. The reserved scale ranges from 1 *(spontaneous and uninhibited expression of integrated feelings)* to 5 *(emotional inhibition that produces feelings of strain and awkwardness in others)*. For the analyses presented here, we have combined these two ratings into a single 5-point scale and averaged the combined scale scores across the annual assessments at ages 8, 9, and 10 (1936–1938). (Scale reliabilities—alphas—are .91 and .89, for boys and girls, respectively.) Thus, these two scales define shyness as a combination of both social anxiety and inhibited social behavior (Leary, 1983).

For several of our analyses, we have dichotomized our measure, designating any child with a score above 3 on the combined 5-point scale as having had a history of childhood shyness. On the shyness scale, a rating of 3 corresponds to *easy with certain types, not with others;* on the reserve scale, it corresponds to *reserved around some, not around others.* This classification procedure defines 28% of the boys and 32% of the girls as having had a history of childhood shyness.[1] Childhood shyness is not significantly correlated with adolescent IQ (rs = $-.08$ and .05, for boys and girls, respectively). Nor is it significantly correlated with the measure of ill-temperedness from our previous study (rs = .08 and $-.10$, for boys and girls, respectively).

Teacher Reports

To assess the generality and consistency of shyness in late childhood, we turned to teachers' reports of the subjects' behavior. Teachers rated the subjects on six 7-point scales that on a priori grounds appeared to tap shy and reserved behaviors: unfriendly-friendly, unsociable-sociable, reserved-expressive, somber-gay, leader-follower, shows off-withdraws. Each scale, available during fifth and sixth grades (ages 10–12), was summed across the two time periods into a single score for the boys and girls, respectively.

Adult Assessment

The Berkeley subjects were interviewed when they were about 30 years of age (1960) and again when they were about 40 (1968–1971). These interviews provide a detailed record of each subject's education, work, marriage, and parenthood. In addition, at least two professional clinicians read each interview from the 1960 follow-up and provided a Q-sort description of the subject using the 100-item California Q-Set (see Block, 1971). In order to assess the phenotypic continuity of childhood shyness we constructed an index of adult shyness by summing seven of these items: withdraws when frustrated, reluctant to act, aloof, talkative (reflected), bothered by demands, gregarious (reflected), and socially poised (reflected). These items were combined into a single index of adult shyness. This index has reliabilities (alphas) of .76 and .82 for men and women, respectively. (All other measurements are discussed at appropriate points in the article.)

---

[1]This definition is comparable with those used by other researchers in the domain of shyness. Thus, Pilkonis (1977a, 1977b) defined those who score *4* or above (moderately shy) on a 7-point scale as shy; Zimbardo (1977) reported that 37%–43% of the normal adult population are dispositionally shy; and Snyder, Smith, Augelli, & Ingram (1985) used the highest 20% for their cutoff. Kagan, Reznick, & Snidman (1987, 1988) suggested that 15% of the normal population are *extremely* shy and inhibited, and developmental psychopathologists who are interested in extreme populations (e.g., Moskowitz, Schwartzman, & Ledingham, 1985) focused on the top 5%. Elsewhere (Caspi & Elder, 1988), we have presented additional information on the most extreme boys drawn from the current sample (n = 7). The data from their records simply accentuate the results presented here.

RESULTS AND DISCUSSION

Male Subjects

Shyness in late childhood is correlated with a coherent cluster of attributes in preadolescence. Thus, teacher ratings when the boys were 10 to 12 years old revealed that shy boys were significantly less friendly, $r(86) = -.25$, $p < .05$, and sociable, $r(86) = -.26$, $p < .05$, than their male peers. They were also rated as more reserved, $r(86) = .46$, $p < .05$, and somber, $r(86) = .40$, $p < .05$. In addition, teachers believed them to be somewhat more withdrawn, $r(86) = .22$, $p < .05$, and more likely to be followers than leaders, $r(86) = .17$, $p < .10$. (Our measure of childhood ill-temperedness has been partialed out of these correlations.)

The childhood shyness scale was also significantly correlated with the composite shyness index derived from the adult Q-sorts, $r(54) = .26$, $p = .05$, a correlation that is only slightly reduced when controlled for ill-temperedness in childhood, $r = .24$, $p = .07$. As we shall now see, this continuity of shyness into adulthood has consequences for men in their transitions to new roles and life settings.

Timing of role transitions. Our most striking discovery about men who were shy as children is their delay in marrying, becoming fathers, and establishing stable careers. As shown in Figure 1, men with a history of childhood shyness were significantly older than others in their cohort when they married (25.5 vs. 22.5 years), $t(75) = 3.80$, $p < .001$, when they first became fathers (28.2 vs. 24.1 years), $t(67) = 3.25$, $p < .01$, and when they first entered stable careers, that is, careers in which they held a functionally related job for at least 6 years (28.2 vs. 25.3 years), $t(75) = 2.35$, $p < .05$ (see Elder, 1974; Elder & Rockwell, 1979). Moreover, regression analyses showed that childhood shyness remained a significant predictor of these several role-transition ages even with statistical controls for class origin, educational level, age at completion of formal education, age at entry into the labor market, military service, and physical attractiveness.

Because recent longitudinal studies have suggested that children characterized by *both* emotional volatility/aggression and shyness/withdrawal are at greater risk for later difficulties than children with only one of these styles (Moskowitz, Schwartzman, & Ledingham, 1985), we further examined the timing of life-course transitions for men with a history of childhood shyness stratified by their childhood ill-temperedness. The results confirmed that it is uniquely childhood shyness that affects the timing of role transitions. Childhood shyness significantly predicted age at first marriage, $F(1, 72) = 13.54$, $p < .001$, with no significant effect of ill-temperedness and no significant

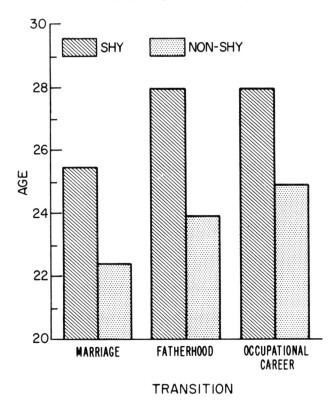

Figure 1. Timing of life transitions as a function of shyness in late childhood.

interaction between these two variables, $F(1, 72) = .05$, *ns*, and $F(1, 72) = .04$, *ns*, respectively. Similarly, childhood shyness significantly predicted delayed fatherhood, $F(1, 64) = 13.71$, $p < .001$, with no significant effect of ill-temperedness and no significant interaction effect, $F(1, 64) = .64$, *ns*, and $F(1, 64) = 1.70$, *ns*, respectively. Finally, childhood shyness significantly predicted age at entry into a stable career, $F(1, 72) = 5.73$, $p < .05$, with no significant main effect of ill-temperedness and no significant interaction effect, $F(1, 72) = 2.35$, $p = .12$, and $F(1, 72) = .01$, *ns*, respectively.

In all, men who were reluctant to enter social settings as children appear to have become adults who are more generally reluctant to enter the new and unfamiliar social settings required by the important life-course transitions into marriage, parenthood, and career. Indeed, it is known that in the domain of heterosexual relations shy men often find it difficult to initiate courtship (Curran, 1977), an interactional difficulty that could itself delay the transition into marriage and parenthood. In the domain of work, shyness may preclude the

American ideal of male self-assertion and conspire to delay men's transition into stable career lines (cf. Super, 1957). It appears, then, that the childhood interactional style is carried across the life course, expressing itself in phenotypically diverse situations that require men to take initiative in exchanging familiar roles for unfamiliar ones. It will be recalled that this is what we have called interactional continuity.

In sociological terms—in terms of life trajectories embedded in the larger social structure—men with a history of childhood shyness can be said to be normatively "off time" in their transitions to age-graded roles (Elder, 1975; Foner & Kertzer, 1978; LeVine, 1980; Neugarten, 1979). If we define *off-time* as at least 1 year above the median age for the cohort as a whole, then 44% of these men are off-time in marrying compared with only 17% of the other men in the cohort; 60% are off-time in becoming fathers compared with only 30% of other men; and 54% are off-time in entering a stable career compared with 30% of other men.

The timing of role transitions into adulthood is consequential and represents an important contingency in the life course that has critical implications for achievements and subsequent behavior (Hogan, 1980). In particular, delays in social transitions often generate conflicting obligations and options that may enhance later difficulties, in part because individuals who are off-time must cope with the demands of their multiple roles without the benefit of those social and institutional structures that support and smooth the way for those persons who are "on time" (Elder, 1975; Goode, 1960). As we shall see below, evidence for this progressive accumulation of consequences is provided by an examination of the occupational careers of men with a childhood history of shyness.

Occupational achievement and stability. In order to assess each subject's occupational history, we constructed three indices of occupational achievement and stability from the 1970 record. The first was simply a 7-point rating of occupational status at midlife, ranging from 1 *(unskilled employee)* to 7 *(higher executive).*

The second was an ipsatized classification of occupational achievement. For subjects who had completed some college but not gone on to postgraduate work, we regressed occupational status at midlife on educational level, adolescent IQ, senior-high GPA, and a measure of adolescent career aspirations (see Elder & Rockwell, 1979). Subjects were classified as low achievers if they fell below their predicted occupational status by 1.0 or more on the 7-point occupational status scale; all others were defined as high achievers. To obtain greater discriminability at the lower and upper ends of the educational spectrum, two judges classified subjects who had either less than a college education or had gone on to postgraduate work into achievement categories on the basis of the detailed life-history records. (Interjudge agreement was .80.)

Finally, we constructed an index of occupational stability by examining the subject's work history during middle adulthood (ages 30 to 40), calculating the number of months of unemployment, the number of jobs held, the number of employers served, and the number of career switches made between functionally unrelated lines of work. These were converted to z scores and averaged into a single index of occupational (in)stability.

As shown in Figure 2, childhood shyness has significant effects on two of these three indices, occupational achievement and occupational stability. There is no *direct* link between childhood shyness and the occupational outcomes. Instead, we see evidence of cumulative continuity: Childhood shyness predicts delayed entry into a stable career ($\beta = .27$, $p < .05$), which, in turn, predicts both lower achievement ($\beta = -.29$, $p < .05$) and occupational stability ($\beta = -.30$, $p < .05$). (Again, any confounding effects of childhood ill-temperedness have been partialed out.)

In our earlier study (Caspi et al., 1987) we found that childhood ill-temperedness also led to greater work instability in the adult years. In that study, however, there was a direct link between the childhood style and the occupational outcome, implying interactional continuity. Men with a childhood history of ill-temperedness continued to carry a distinctive interactional style with them that adversely affected their worklife—especially when they were employed in low-status jobs. In the present study, we see that the child-

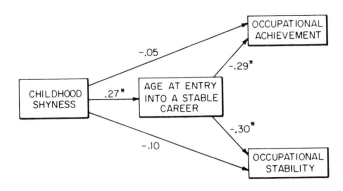

Figure 2. Occupational stability and achievement in adulthood as a function of childhood shyness ($N = 73$). (Class origins, educational level, age at entry into the labor force, and childhood ill-temperedness are included as exogenous variables in estimating this model.)

hood style affects occupational outcomes through the progressive accumulation of its own consequences. By entering an occupational career at an older age, men with a childhood history of shyness may have forgone investments in skills and benefits and thus sacrificed higher achievements and increased their vulnerability to career instability.

Marital stability. In our earlier study (Caspi et al., 1987), we found that men with a history of childhood ill-temperedness experienced significantly more marital instability than other men. Overall, men with a history of shyness do not. To the extent that some do, however, it is again because they are late in entering stable careers: A logistic regression analysis revealed that having a history of shyness *and* entering a stable career late significantly raises the probability of being divorced or separated by midlife ($t = 2.10, p < .05$). Almost half of the men with this cumulative history (42.8%) were divorced or separated by midlife compared with only 20.3% of the other men.

Female Subjects

Shy girls also show phenotypic continuity. According to teacher reports, shy girls, like shy boys, were rated as significantly less friendly, $r(83) = -.28, p < .05$, and less sociable, $r(83) = -.29, p < .05$, when they were 10 to 12 years old. They were also perceived by teachers as more reserved, $r(83) = .36, p < .05$, somber, $r(83) = .39, p < .05$, withdrawn, $r(83) = .20, p < .05$, and to be followers rather than leaders, $r(83) = .26, p < .05$. (Ill-temperedness was again partialed out.)

The correlation between childhood shyness and the composite scale derived from the adult Q-sorts was also significant, $r(71) = .32, p < .01$, and remained unaltered by partialing out the effects of ill-tempered behavior in childhood ($r = .31, p < .01$). But even though this childhood style manifests some persistence in the lives of women, its life-course consequences show little resemblance to those observed for men.

Timing of role transitions. Unlike their male counterparts, women with a childhood history of shy and reserved behavior were not delayed or off-time in entering marriage or starting families compared with the other women in their cohort. This is not surprising. The men and women in this study reached the age of majority during the late 1940s, a time of quite traditional sex roles in American history, and traditional sex roles dictate that men take the most active role in courtship.

Work and family patterns. Women with a childhood history of shyness were also more likely to lead a prototypical feminine life of marriage and homemaking. Although the majority of women in the Berkeley study worked at some point in their lives, there was little variation in their occupational status and, for most of them, no point at which they established stable careers outside the home. Accordingly, we assessed women's career patterns by examining the timing and duration of periods in and out of the labor force from before marriage through midlife in relation to the timing and duration of family events like marriage and childbearing (Helson, Mitchell, & Moane, 1984).

The central finding was that the majority (56%) of women with a childhood history of shyness were more likely either to have no work history at all or to terminate employment at marriage or childbirth with no later reentry into the labor force. In contrast, only 36% of their more outgoing counterparts followed this more traditional pattern ($\tau_b = -.19$, $p < .05$). This pattern was further confirmed by an examination of adult laborforce participation for women with a history of childhood shyness stratified by their childhood ill-temperedness. The results showed that childhood shyness significantly predicted the number of years that women spent in the labor force, $F(1, 85) = 5.25$, $p < .05$, with no significant effect of childhood ill-temperedness and no significant interaction between these two variables, $F(1, 85) = .01$, ns, and $F(1, 85) = .08$, ns, respectively. In all, women with a childhood history of shyness accumulated only 6.25 years in the labor force from ages 18 to 40 compared with 9.41 years for their more outgoing counterparts. Moreover, this effect of childhood shyness remained significant when the women's social class origins, educational attainment, and adolescent IQ were partialed out. It appears, then, that their childhood shyness continues into adulthood where it prompts them to select a more domestic life-style than their peers and to avoid venturing into employment outside the home. This again illustrates what we have called interactional continuity.

The second major finding is that women with a childhood history of shyness were married to men who had higher occupational status at midlife than husbands of other women, $F(1, 70) = 3.87$, $p < .05$. This conclusion emerges from an analysis of variance in which both childhood shyness and ill-temperedness were used as the independent variables. As reported in our earlier study, women with a childhood history of ill-temperedness were married to men who had *lower* occupational status at midlife than husbands of other women, $F(1, 70) = 4.12$, $p < .05$. (There was no significant interaction effect between these variables, $F[1, 70] = .08$, ns.)

Of particular interest here is that the ill-tempered women married men who already held lower occupational status at the time of marriage, $F(1, 79) = 3.92$, $p < .05$ (Caspi et al., 1987), but the shy women married men who did not differ from their peers in occupational status at that point, $F(1, 79) = 1.84$, $p = .18$. (Again, there was no significant interaction effect between these variables, $F[1, 79] = .61$, ns.) This suggests that shy women may actually have aided their husbands' careers by fulfilling the traditional homemaker role. And indeed, when we partialed out the time that these women spent out of the labor force, the correlation between their childhood shyness and their husbands' occupational status at midlife was reduced to nonsignificance (from .23, $p < .05$, to .12, *ns*, in a multiple regression analysis). Alternatively, of course, it may be that more ambitious or capable men marry shy or more domestically inclined women (cf. Winter, Stewart, & McClelland, 1977). The available data do not enable us to choose between these alternatives or among them and several other plausible scenarios.

In any case, these findings contrast sharply not only with those from the women with childhood histories of ill-temperedness, but also with those of the shy men in our sample, a poignant reminder of how the life-course consequences of a personality attribute can be determined by the culture's sex role prescriptions. The women of this cohort who as children moved "away from the world" were dispositionally suited to adhere to the female social clock (Helson et al., 1984) and were thus fortunate to be able to enter an adult environment in which they could successfully "move with the world."

GENERAL DISCUSSION

Clinical and applied developmental psychologists have long suggested that extremely shy and withdrawn children may be "at-risk" for later difficulties, but the evidence is equivocal (Rubin, 1982, 1986; Wanlass & Prinz, 1982). Whereas follow-back studies of disordered adults reveal that many of them have experienced earlier periods of social withdrawal, follow-up studies of such children fail to reveal a causal link with later pathology (Cowen, Pederson, Babigian, Izzo, & Trost, 1973; Kohlberg, LaCross, & Ricks, 1972; Parker & Asher, 1987; Robins, 1966). And psychopathology aside, very little is known about the general, nonpathological consequences of childhood shyness in a normal population.

In this study, childhood shyness did not produce pathological or extreme outcomes, but it did have significant consequences for later adult development independent of childhood ill-temperedness. For example, men with childhood histories of shyness were older than their male peers when they married, became fathers, and entered stable careers. Moreover, these "off-time" transitions to age-graded roles served as the mediating link between their childhood shyness and lesser occupational achievement and stability in adulthood. Tardiness in entering a stable career also appeared to affect marital stability adversely.

Thus, it appears that childhood shyness was evoked again in new settings that required these men to initiate action and social contacts. Their shy interactional style affected them most at precisely those transition points during which young adults are called on to make critical choices about work and family. This suggests that ongoing longitudinal studies of shy/withdrawn children might benefit from examining transitions to work and family roles in late adolescence and young adulthood. For men, in particular, such behavior may prove somewhat problematic in their efforts to negotiate traditional masculine roles involving mate selection and vocational decision making. Indeed, recent evidence from follow-up studies of children identified as withdrawn during the elementary-school years suggests that by adolescence these children consistently underestimate their performance and exaggerate their poor achievement (Moskowitz & Schwartzman, 1988). It is likely that such low expectancies for achievement among withdrawn children may inhibit them from pursuing opportunities in the labor market and create difficulties for them in their efforts to establish opposite-sex relationships.

In contrast to the men, women characterized by shyness and reserve in late childhood manifested no distinctive problems through midlife. Not only did they appear to move through early adulthood with little difficulty, they were more likely than other women in their cohort to follow a conventional pattern of marriage, childbearing, and homemaking. Clearly sex differences in the continuity and consequences of early personality are moderated by cultural and historical prescriptions of gender-appropriate behavior. For this cohort, shy and reserved behavior seemed to be more compatible—if not desirable—for women than for men. It is not clear, however, that sex role changes in our society have altered the patterns observed here. A recent study of shyness and interpersonal relationships found that the correlations were stronger for male than for female respondents, suggesting that the inhibitory effects of shyness on the development of relationships may still be greater for men than women (Jones & Briggs, 1984).

The present study, along with other birth-to-maturity studies (e.g., Kagan & Moss, 1962), suggests that individual differences in shyness can persist into adulthood. Although the cross-time effects are modest, continuity is clearly discernible. What accounts for the preservation of individual differences in this behavior?

Observational studies of twins (Plomin & Rowe, 1979) as well as adoption studies (Daniels & Plomin, 1985) have provided evidence for genetic influences on shyness. It is possible, in addition, that genetic factors may mediate continuity and change in development and contribute to the phenotypic stability of individual differences across time (Plomin, 1986). Indeed, Kagan, Reznick, and Snidman (1988) have suggested that inherited variations in threshold of arousal in selected limbic sites may make a contribution to shyness in childhood as well as to extreme degrees of social avoidance later in the life span.

The observed continuities and consequences of childhood shyness may also be mediated by individual differences in social problem-solving skills. Research on neglected and socially withdrawn groups suggests that shy children may lack certain social skills and display "wait and hover" behaviors during entry into a new group of peers (Dodge, Schlundt, Schocken, & Delugach, 1983). Moreover, socially withdrawn children offer fewer and less flexible solutions to presented problems and are more likely to suggest adult intervention strategies as appropriate for solving social difficulties (Rubin, Daniels-Beirness, & Bream, 1984). It remains unclear, however, whether shy children lack appropriate social skills because they do not have sufficient social knowledge or whether they cannot apply their skill and knowledge because of anxious inhibition. For example, research on young adults suggests that, although shy people are likely to make more self-defeating attributions in response to situations that involve initiating new relationships in a group, they do not do so in task-oriented groups (Hoffman & Teglasi, 1982). Given such situational specificity it may prove more useful to conceive of shyness as an approach-avoidance conflict in social situations and to inquire into the motivational basis of this disposition, specifying the needs, interests, and fears of shy children and adults in relation to their more sociable counterparts.

A self-presentational model of personality may also help to account for the continuities and consequences of childhood shyness (Baumeister, 1982; Snyder, Higgins, & Stucky, 1983). This model proposes that people are motivated to create a favorable impression on others and that when they doubt their ability to achieve this outcome a state of anxiety results. Shyness, in this scenario, is a joint result of wanting to create a favorable impression but doubting one's ability to do so.

According to this model shyness can also serve a strategic self-presentational purpose: When the person cannot create a favorable impression, shyness can become an excuse or self-handicap to preserve some degree of positive self-image. Being labeled as shy is less aversive than being seen as unattractive or incompetent.

Indeed, the differences we have observed between men and women in this study might be caused by sex differences in self-handicapping. Experimental studies suggest that men are more likely to use their shyness as a self-handicapping strategy in response to social-evaluative threat than are women, who become more passively accommodating (Snyder, Smith, Augelli, & Ingram, 1985; also see Pilkonis, 1977b). Moreover, the social norms that still assign males the major responsibility for active roles in social interaction continue, of course, to reinforce these sex differences.

It is clear that life-course continuities and consequences of shyness are mediated by several processes and their interactions—only some of which we have addressed here. Shyness is a phenomenon that requires collaborative attention across the domains of social, clinical, and developmental psychology (Buss, 1980; Hartman, 1983; Kagan, Reznick, & Snidman, 1988).

Finally, we believe that this study illustrates a more general point about personality in the life course. A review of personality and social psychological research indicates that dispositional factors exert their strongest influence in settings that require individuals to master new tasks and negotiate new demands (Snyder & Ickes, 1985). Accordingly, we believe that studying individual differences at those points in the life course at which the individual must make transitions to new roles and relationships provides a unique opportunity for discerning general principles that govern the functions and processes of personality.

Thus, ill-temperedness ("moving against the world") and shyness ("moving away from the world") are very different interactional styles, yet the general mechanisms producing their continuity and consequences appear to be the same: Long-term continuities of personality are to be found in interactional styles that are sustained by the progressive accumulation of their own consequences (cumulative continuity) and by their tendency to evoke maintaining responses from others during social interaction (interactional continuity).

REFERENCES

Arkin, R. M., Appelman, A. J., & Burger, J. M. (1980). Social anxiety, self-presentation, and the self-serving bias in causal attribution. *Journal of Personality and Social Psychology, 38,* 23–35.

Baumeister, R. F. (1982). A self-presentational view of social phenomena. *Psychological Bulletin, 91,* 3–26.

Block, J. (1971). *Lives through time.* Berkeley, CA: Bancroft.

Bronson, G. W. (1972). Infants' reactions to unfamiliar persons and novel objects. *Monographs of the Society for Research in Child Development, 37* (3, Serial No. 148).

Bronson, G. W. (1978). Aversive reactions to strangers: A dual process interpretation. *Child Development, 49,* 495–499.

Buss, A. H. (1980). *Self-consciousness and social anxiety.* San Francisco: Freeman.

Caspi, A., & Elder, G. H., Jr. (1988). Childhood precursors of the life course: Early personality and life disadvantage. In E. M. Hetherington, R. M. Lerner, & M. Perlmutter (Eds.), *Child development in a life-span perspective* (pp. 115–142). Hillsdale, NJ: Erlbaum.

Caspi, A., Elder, G. H., Jr., & Bem, D. J. (1987). Moving against the world: Life-course patterns of explosive children. *Developmental Psychology, 22,* 303–308.

Cheek, J. M. & Buss, A. H. (1981). Shyness and sociability. *Journal of Personality and Social Psychology, 41,* 330–339.

Cheek, J. M., Carpentieri, A. M., Smith, G. M., Rierdan, J., & Koff, E. (1985). Adolescent shyness. In W. H. Jones, J. M. Cheek, & S. R. Briggs (Eds.), *Shyness: Perspectives on theory and research* (pp. 105–115). New York: Plenum.

Coie, J. D., Dodge, K. A., & Coppotelli, H. (1982). Dimensions and types of social status: A cross-age perspective. *Developmental Psychology, 18,* 557–570.

Cowen, E. L., Pederson, A., Babigian, H., Izzo, L. D., Trost, M. A. (1973). Long-term follow-up of early detected vulnerable children. *Journal of Consulting and Clinical Psychology, 41,* 438–446.

Curran, J. P. (1977). Skills training as an approach to the treatment of heterosexual-social anxiety: A review. *Psychological Bulletin, 84,* 140–157.

Daniels, D., & Plomin, R. (1985). Origins of individual differences in infant shyness. *Developmental Psychology, 21,* 118–121.

Dodge, K. A. (1986). A social information processing model of social competence in children. In M. Perlmutter (Ed.), *Minnesota Symposia on Child Psychology* (Vol. 18, pp. 77–125). Hillsdale, NJ: Erlbaum.

Dodge, K. A., Schlundt, D. C., Schocken, I., & Delugach, I. D. (1983). Social competence and children's sociometric status: The role of peer group entry strategies. *Merrill-Palmer Quarterly, 29,* 309–336.

Eichorn, D. H. (1981). Samples and procedures. In D. H. Eichorn, J. A. Clausen, N. Haan, M. P. Honzik, & P. H. Mussen (Eds.), *Present and past in middle life* (pp. 33–51). New York: Academic Press.

Elder, G. H., Jr. (1974). *Children of the Great Depression.* Chicago: University of Chicago Press.

Elder, G. H., Jr. (1975). Age differentiation and the life course. *Annual Review of Sociology* (Vol. 1). Palo Alto: Annual Reviews.

Elder, G. H., Jr., & Rockwell, R. C. (1979). Economic depression and postwar opportunity in men's lives: A study of life patterns and health. In R. G. Simmons (Ed.), *Research in community and mental health* (pp. 249–303). Greenwich, CT: JAI Press.

Fenigstein, A., Scheier, M., & Buss, A. H. (1975). Public and private self-consciousness: Assessment and theory. *Journal of Consulting and Clinical Psychology, 43,* 522–527.

Foner, A., & Kertzer, D. I. (1978). Transitions over the life course: Lessons from age-set societies. *American Journal of Sociology, 83,* 1081–1104.

Girodo, M., Dotzenroth, S. E., & Stein, J. (1981). Causal attribution bias in shy males: Implications for self-esteem and self-confidence. *Cognitive Therapy and Research, 6,* 37–55.

Goode, W. J. (1960). A theory of role strain. *American Sociological Review, 25,* 483–496.

Gottman, J. M. (1977). Toward a definition of social isolation in children. *Child Development, 48,* 513–517.

Hartman, L. M. (1983). A metacognitive model of social anxiety: Implications for treatment. *Clinical Psychology Review, 3,* 435–456.

Helson, R., Mitchell, V., & Moane, G. (1984). Personality and patterns of adherence and nonadherence to the social clock. *Journal of Personality and Social Psychology, 46,* 1079–1096.

Hoffman, M. A., & Teglasi, H. (1982). The role of causal attribution in counseling shy subjects. *Journal of Counseling Psychology, 29,* 132–139.

Hogan, D. P. (1980). The transition to adulthood as a career contingency. *American Sociological Review, 45,* 261–276.

Horney, K. (1945). *Our inner conflicts.* New York: Norton.

Izard, C. E. (1984). Emotion-cognition relationships and human development. In C. Izard, J. Kagan, & R. Zajonc (Eds.), *Emotions, cognition, and behavior* (pp. 17–37). New York: Cambridge University Press.

Jones, W. H., & Briggs, S. R. (1984). The self-other discrepancy in social shyness. In R. Schwarzer (Ed.), *The self in anxiety, stress, and depression* (pp. 93–108). Amsterdam: North Holland.

Jones, W. H., & Carpenter, B. N. (1986). Shyness, social behavior, and relationships. In W. H. Jones, J. M. Cheek, & S. R. Briggs (Eds.), *Shyness: Perspectives on research and treatment* (pp. 227–238). New York: Plenum.

Jones, W. H., Freemon, J. E., & Goswick, R. A. (1981). The persistence of loneliness: Self and other determinants. *Journal of Personality, 49,* 27–48.

Kagan, J. (1981). *The second year.* Cambridge: Harvard University Press.

Kagan, J., & Moss, H. A. (1962). *Birth to maturity.* New York: Wiley.

Kagan, J., Reznick, J. S., & Snidman, N. (1987). The physiology and psychology of behavioral inhibition in children. *Child Development, 58,* 1459–1473.

Kagan, J., Reznick, J. S., & Snidman, N. (1988). Biological bases of childhood shyness. *Science, 240,* 167–171.

Kohlberg, L., LaCross, I., & Ricks, D. (1972). The predictability of adult mental health from childhood behavior. In B. B. Wolman (Ed.), *Manual of child psychopathology* (pp. 217–284). New York: McGraw-Hill.

Leary, M. R. (1983). *Understanding social anxiety: Social, personality, and clinical perspectives.* Beverly Hills, CA: Sage.

LeVine, R. A. (1980). Adulthood among the Gusii of Kenya. In N. J. Smelser & E. Erikson (Eds.), *Themes of work and love in adulthood* (pp. 77–104). Cambridge: Harvard University Press.

Macfarlane, J. W. (1938). Studies in child guidance: I. Methodology of data collection and organization. *Monographs of the Society for Research in Child Development, 3* (Serial No. 6).

Macfarlane, J. W., Allen, L., & Honzik, M. P. (1954). *A developmental study of the behavioral problems of children between twenty-one months and fourteen years.* Berkeley: University of California Press.

Moskowitz, D. S., & Schwartzman, A. E. (1988). *Painting group portraits: Assessing life outcomes for aggressive and withdrawn children.* Manuscript submitted for publication.

Moskowitz, D. S., Schwartzman, A. E., & Ledingham, J. E. (1985). Stability and change in aggression and withdrawal in middle childhood and early adolescence. *Journal of Abnormal Psychology, 94,* 30–41.

Neugarten, B. (1979). Time, age, and the life cycle. *American Journal of Psychiatry, 136,* 887–894.

Parker, J. G., & Asher, S. R. (1987). Peer relations and later personal adjustment: Are low-accepted children at risk? *Psychological Bulletin, 102,* 357–389.

Patterson, G. R. (1982). *Coercive family process.* Eugene, OR: Castalia.

Pilkonis, P. A. (1977a). Shyness, public and private, and its relationship to other measures of social behavior. *Journal of Personality, 45,* 585–595.

Pilkonis, P. A. (1977b). The behavioral consequences of shyness. *Journal of Personality, 45,* 596–611.

Plomin, R. (1986). Multivariate analysis and developmental behavior genetics: Developmental change as well as continuity. *Behavior Genetics, 16,* 25–43.

Plomin, R., & Rowe, D. C. (1979). Genetic and environmental etiology of social behavior in infancy. *Developmental Psychology, 15,* 62–72.

Putallaz, M., & Gottman, J. M. (1981). Social skills and group acceptance. In S. R. Asher & J. M. Gottman (Eds.), *The development of children's friendships* (pp. 116–149). New York: Cambridge University Press.

Robins, L. N. (1966). *Deviant children grown up.* Baltimore, MD: Williams & Wilkins.

Rubin, K. H. (1982). Social and social-cognitive developmental characteristics of young isolated, normal, and sociable children. In K. H. Rubin & H. S. Ross (Eds.), *Peer relationships and social skills in childhood* (pp. 353–374). New York: Springer.

Rubin, K. H. (1986). Socially withdrawn children: An "at risk" population? In B. Schneider, K. H. Rubin, & J. E. Ledingham (Eds.), *Peer relationships and social skills in childhood: Vol. 2. Issues in assessment and training* (pp. 125–139). New York: Springer.

Rubin, K. H., Daniels-Beirness, T., & Bream, L. (1984). Social isolation and social problem solving: A longitudinal study. *Journal of Consulting and Clinical Psychology, 50,* 226–233.

Scarr, S., & McCartney, K. (1983). How people make their own environments: A theory of genotype-environment correlations. *Child Development, 54,* 424–435.

Snyder, C. R., Higgins, R. L., & Stucky, R. J. (1983). *Excuses: Masquerades in search of grace.* New York: Wiley.

Snyder, C. R., Smith, T. W., Augelli, R., & Ingram, R. E. (1985). On the self-serving function of social anxiety: Shyness as a self-handicapping strategy. *Journal of Personality and Social Psychology, 48,* 970–980.

Snyder, M., & Ickes, W. (1985). Personality and social behavior. In E. Aronson & G. Lindzey (Eds.), *Handbook of social psychology* (Vol. 2, pp. 883–947). New York: Random House.

Snyder, M., & Swann, W. B., Jr. (1978). Hypothesis testing processes in social interaction. *Journal of Personality and Social Psychology, 36,* 1202–1212.

Super, D. E. (1957). *The psychology of careers.* New York: Harper.

Wachtel, P. L. (1977a). *Psychoanalysis and behavior therapy.* New York: Basic.

Wachtel, P. L. (1977b). Interaction cycles, unconscious processes, and the person-situation issue. In D. Magnusson & N. S. Endler (Eds.), *Personality at the crossroads: Current issues in interactional psychology* (pp. 317–331). Hillsdale, NJ: Erlbaum.

Wanlass, R. L., & Prinz, R. J. (1982). Methodological issues in conceptualizing and treating childhood social isolation. *Psychological Bulletin, 92,* 39–55.

Winter, D. G., Stewart, A. J., & McCleland, D. C. (1977). Husband's motives and wife's career level. *Journal of Personality and Social Psychology, 35,* 159–166.

Zimbardo, P. G. (1977). *Shyness: What it is, what to do about it.* Reading, MA: Addison-Wesley.

19

Behavioral Inhibition in Children of Parents with Panic Disorder and Agoraphobia: A Controlled Study

Jerrold F. Rosenbaum, Joseph Biederman, Michelle Gersten, Dina R. Hirshfeld, Susan R. Meminger, and John B. Herman
Massachusetts General Hospital, Harvard Medical School, Boston
Jerome Kagan, Steven Reznick, and Nancy Snidman
Harvard University, Cambridge, Massachusetts

To investigate the role of "behavioral inhibition to the unfamiliar" as an early temperamental characteristic of children at risk for adult panic disorder and agoraphobia (PDAG), we compared children of parents with PDAG with those from psychiatric comparison groups. Fifty-six children aged 2 to 7 years, matched for age, socioeconomic status, ethnic background, and ordinal position, were blindly evaluated at the Harvard Infant Study laboratory, Cambridge, Mass. The rates of behavioral inhibition in children of probands with PDAG, with or without comorbid major depressive disorder (MDD), were significantly higher than for our comparison group without PDAG. Further, the data suggest a progression of increasing rates of inhibition from the comparison group without MDD (15.4%), to MDD (50.0%), and to comorbid PDAG and

Reprinted with permission from *Archives of General Psychiatry*, 1988, Vol. 45, 463–470. Copyright 1988 by the American Medical Association.

Read in part at the Annual Meeting of the American Psychiatric Association (New Research Section), Chicago, May 14, 1987.

This study was supported in part by the National Institute of Mental Health grant MH-40619 and by a grant from the John D. and Catherine T. MacArthur Foundation (Dr. Kagan).

Sharon Mrakovich assisted with the manuscript's preparation. Josefina Rotman coordinated the subjects. Maureen Johnson and Jane Gibbons performed the laboratory assessments. The staff of the Clinical Psychopharmacology and Psychosomatic Medicine Units assisted with the research project.

MDD (70%) and PDAG (84.6%). In contrast, the rate of behavioral inhibition in children of probands with MDD did not meaningfully differ from the comparison group without MDD. Behavioral inhibition to the unfamiliar, as defined and measured in the previous work of the Harvard Infant Study program, is highly prevalent in the offspring of adults in treatment for PDAG. These children appear to be at risk for distress and disability in childhood and also perhaps for development of psychiatric disorder in later childhood and adulthood.

Panic disorder with agoraphobia (PDAG) is estimated to afflict between 1% and 6% of the adult population.[1,2] Although the disorder begins most often in early adulthood, with typical onset in the third decade, reports indicate an association with antecedent childhood distress in the form of excessive fearfulness and separation anxiety.[3-6]

Klein[6] reported that half of one series of female adults with agoraphobia (AG) experienced marked degrees of separation anxiety and school adjustment difficulties, including "school phobia," in childhood. Further, those patients with a history of school phobia had an earlier age of onset of AG compared with patients without this history. Others have also observed high rates of a history of school avoidance in adults with AG.[7,8] Although these observations suggest that vulnerability to adult panic disorder (PD) may be manifest in childhood, the nature of the association between childhood behavioral symptoms or disorders and adult disorder is unclear. Childhood symptoms may predispose to the adult condition, may be early manifestations of the same disorder, or reflect common environmental or biological underpinnings.

Several authors[9-12] suggested that the optimal approach to exploring the relation between child and adult psychopathology is the scrutiny and longitudinal follow-up of "children at risk" by systematic study of children of adults with psychopathology. In a cross-sectional study of children at risk for anxiety disorders, Berg[13] reported a 7% overall prevalence of school phobia in children 7 to 11 years old and a 14% prevalence in 11- to 15-year-old children of AG mothers. Although this study did not include a normal comparison group, the prevalence of school phobia in the children at risk exceeded expected population rates. Weissman and coworkers[14] examined the prevalence of separation anxiety disorder in children, aged 6 to 18 years, of depressed and normal adults identified in community surveys. With the use of formal diagnostic criteria and structured clinical interviews for diagnosis, the study reported separation anxiety disorder in 11% of children whose parents had a diagnosis of both major depressive disorder (MDD) and AG and in 37% of those whose parents had depression and PD. In contrast, children of adults with pure MDD and children of normal controls had no (0%) separation anxiety disorder. These results suggest that parental PD or AG was specifically associated with separation anxiety disorder in the offspring.

Although these findings indicate that children of AG parents are more likely to have separation anxiety or other anxiety disorders, as compared with other children, the possibility remains that a precursor of disorder may be manifest in more subtle measures of childhood behavior derived from temperamental characteristics. Thus, separation anxiety disorder may be one particularly severe reflection of a temperamental quality that predisposes a child to school avoidance and an adult to PD and AG. This suggestion implies that developmental research offers an opportunity to observe crucial developmental transformations in the path from predisposition to manifest disorder and to infer both ameliorating and harmful factors in individual experience.

Questions concerning the origins and stability of temperamental characteristics have captured the attention of a number of investigators for more than a decade.[15-21] Temperamental characteristics can be viewed as inherited response dispositions[22,23] that appear early in life, are displayed across situations, are stable, and may have residual impact on later personality. One temperamental dimension involves differences in initial reactions to unfamiliar people or situations.[15-21] In later life it is described as *sociability, introversion-extroversion, approach/withdrawal,* or *social responsiveness.* Although the terms used to describe this source of individual differences vary, the behaviors that operationally define this temperamental dimension at each stage of development are more similar. Following exposure to unfamiliar people, objects, or events, children called *sociable, uninhibited, outgoing, extroverted,* or *fearless* exhibit minimal visible change in their ongoing behavior. Some may vocalize, smile, and spontaneously interact with or approach the unfamiliar object or setting. By contrast, children described as *shy, inhibited,* or *introverted* show quiet restraint and withdrawal when confronted with novelty. They typically stop their ongoing behavior, cease vocalizing, seek comfort from a familiar figure, or withdraw from the unfamiliar event. The literature suggests that social withdrawal in infancy is associated with later anxiety. For example, Chess and Thomas[24-27] found that infants with predominant withdrawal tendencies were at risk for developing avoidant or overanxious disorder in childhood. Moreover, data from the New York Longitudinal Study[26,27] indicated that the tendency to approach or to withdraw from novelty is a relatively enduring temperamental dimension. Rubin[28] suggested that children who show few socially interactive behaviors in school are predisposed by a lower threshold for arousal when confronted with novelty.

The most extensive research on behavioral inhibition to the unfamiliar comes from ongoing longitudinal projects conducted at the Harvard Infant Study laboratory, Cambridge, Mass.[29] This program was designed without a focus on "disorder" or psychopathology per se. The findings from this work suggested that approximately 10% to 15% of American white children are born with the predisposition to be irritable as infants, shy and fearful as toddlers, and cautious, quiet, and introverted when they reach school age. The Harvard group has been following two independent cohorts of white children, selected at 21 or 31 months of age to be either behaviorally inhibited or uninhibited when exposed to unfamiliar rooms, people, and objects. The classification into one of these two groups required a child to manifest consistent withdrawal or approach to a variety of stimuli, such as meeting unfamiliar female examiners and encounters with unfamiliar toys. The major behavioral signs of inhibition were long latencies to interact with the unfamiliar adults, retreat from the unfamiliar object or person, cessation of play and vocalization, clinging to the mother, and crying. In addition, a number of physiological variables correlated with behavioral inhibition, including salivary cortisol level, laryngeal muscle tension (as measured by decreased variability of phonatory cycles), pupillary dilation, a high and stable heart rate, and urinary catecholamine levels.[30]

Follow-up assessments of the two cohorts of children in contexts designed to evaluate social behavior with an unfamiliar peer, school behavior, as well as heart rate and heart rate variability under mild cognitive stress revealed that the differences in behavioral inhibition were preserved to a significant degree from the original assessment in infancy to the later assessments at 4, 5, and 7½ years of age.[29] Many of the children classified as inhibited at 21 months of age continued to be vigilant and cautious in uncertain situations, while the formerly uninhibited children displayed bold and sociable behavior in the same laboratory contexts. The preservation of inhibited and uninhibited behavior also generalized to the school setting. School observations of the inhibited children during their first days of kindergarten and several months later revealed that the majority of inhibited children showed restraint and social avoidance, including behavior reminiscent of the separation anxiety and school avoidance noted in the histories of patients with adult PD and AG.[31]

We hypothesized, therefore, that the temperamental quality of behavioral inhibition to the unfamiliar might be a predisposing characteristic in children at risk for PD and AG in later years. If this were true, the apparent familial[32-38] and probably genetic patterns of transmission of PD[39-44] would imply a higher prevalence of behavioral inhibition in the children of adult patients with PD and AG, as compared with controls from families without this disorder. To our knowledge, no such study has been reported.

METHODS

Subjects

Subjects were children of adult patients treated for PD at the Department of Psychiatry, Massachusetts General Hospital, Boston, and children who had parents without PD but had a family member in treatment at the same outpatient setting. All children were between the ages of 2 and 7 years; this age group was selected because of available normative data for the variables used to assess inhibition in children of this age range.[29,45]

Subjects were identified through their parents. Eligible parents met the following inclusion criteria: (1) psychiatric outpatient attending the Clinical Psychopharmacology Unit at Massachusetts General Hospital, including patients in treatment or recently referred for treatment; (2) white; (3) resident of the greater Boston area; and (4) parent of a child between 2 and 7 years old not known to be psychiatrically ill. There were three main diagnostic groups. The group with PD consisted of parents with diagnosed and treated PD with or without AG. The two comparison groups consisted of parents with MDD and parents without MDD, PD, or AG (non-MDD). The latter was a heterogeneous group of parents treated for other problems (e.g., generalized anxiety disorder, obesity, and tobacco dependence) at the same setting as the parents with PD; to these were added a group of subjects with parents not in treatment, who were identified through having a sibling in treatment for attention deficit disorder (ADD) at the same outpatient hospital setting as the other probands. The latter group was selected to extend comparisons to children without likely genetic loading for or exposure to a parent with PD or MDD but identified at the same clinical setting.

All eligible parents were informed by their clinician of the study and then approached by research staff who were blind to the SES significantly differed from the mean SES of the non-MDD comparison group ($P < .05$). The rates of separation and divorce were lowest in the proband groups with PDAG (7.7%) and MDD (10.0%), were intermediate in the non-MDD comparison group (23.1%), and highest in the group with mixed PDAG/MDD (40%). However, none of these differences reached statistical significance.

Analysis of Continuous Data

The sample sizes of the three groups of children (younger, middle, and older) only permitted analyses of pooled data for all children and separate analysis of the older group. In all children and older children, respectively, mean latencies to speak (in seconds) were as follows: (1) PDAG, 1030 ± 1159 and 1586 ± 1360; (2) PDAG/MDD, 1108 ± 1221 and 1633 ± 1361; (3) MDD, 931 ± 1429 and 545 ± 1204; and (4) non-MDD, 134 ± 162 and 147 ± 176. In all children and older children, respectively, mean number of spontaneous comments were as follows: (1) PDAG, 7.4 ± 7.8 and 2.1 ± 2.5; (2) PDAG/MDD, 15.8 ± 21.8 and 6.1 ± 10.1; (3) MDD, 26.3 ± 47.2 and 40.8 ± 57.9; and (4) non-MDD comparison, 41.6 ± 63.8 and 54.8 ± 79.8 (Figs 1 and 2).

The overall differences between groups were significant in all children and older children, respectively, both for latency to speak (Kruskal-Wallis H = 13.4, df = 3, n = 56, P < .01 and H = 12.2, df = 3, n = 32, P < .01) and for number of spontaneous comments (H = 10.7, df = 3, n = 56, P < .05 and H = 13.5, df = 3, n = 32, P < .01). Pairwise comparisons of the data revealed that children of parents with PDAG, either alone (Mann-Whitney U = 21.0, P ≤ .01) or with comorbid MDD (U = 48.5, P ≤ .01), had a significantly longer latency to speak and emitted substantially fewer spontaneous comments than the non-MDD comparison group (U = 19.0, P ≤ .01, and U = 62, P ≤ .05, respectively). In contrast, the group with MDD did not differ significantly on either measure from any of the other groups (Figs 1 and 2).

Data were also examined after stratifying the children into two mutually exclusive groups based on the presence or absence of difficulties in the children. All participating parents signed informed consent.

Diagnostic Assessments

Consenting parents were further evaluated using the National Institute of Mental Health (NIMH) Diagnostic Interview Schedule[46] and the anxiety module of the Structured Clinical Interview for *DSM-III*[47] to evaluate comorbidity and to confirm the clinical diagnosis. The spouses were also evaluated using the same protocol. All diagnostic information was reviewed by the senior investigators (J.F.R. and J.B.) before proband assignment to a diagnostic group and prior to assessment of the child. The diagnostic groups included PDAG, comorbid PDAG/MDD, MDD, and non-MDD. Diagnostic assignments were made using the diagnosis of the parent (or sibling) patient's case based on all the information available including the clinical records and structured interview data. However, three families were classified based on findings derived from structured interview with the nonpatient spouse. Two families where the proband patient had a diagnosis of MDD had spouses with comorbid PDAG and MDD and were therefore classified as having comorbid PDAG/MDD. One parent of a sibling with ADD was found to have MDD, and her child was reclassified into the proband group with MDD.

Children were thus stratified into subgroups based on the diagnosis of their family member's condition: (1) 13 had a parent with PDAG alone. (One patient with PD did not have sufficient avoidance for a diagnosis of AG but is included in this group.) These patients had to satisfy all three criteria (clinical diagnosis, NIMH Diagnostic Interview Schedule, and Structured Clinical Interview for *DSM-III*), and PDAG had to be the main focus of treatment; (2) ten children had a parent with MDD alone (nine nonbipolar, one bipolar); (3) 20 children had a parent with PDAG and MDD, classified as either primary PDAG/secondary MDD (n = 11) or primary MDD/secondary PDAG (n = 9) depending on age at onset, course, and main focus of treatment; (4) 13 children were without PD, AG, or MDD (non-MDD comparison group) in a parent. This group consisted of siblings of patients with ADD (n = 9) and children of parents with generalized anxiety disorder (n = 2) or seeking behavioral treatment for obesity (n = 1) or tobacco dependence (n = 1); none of these parents or spouses had either PDAG or MDD.

Procedures

Eligible children from the experimental and control groups were matched for age, socioeconomic status (SES), and ordinal position prior to referral to the Harvard University Infant Study laboratory for behavioral evaluation. Laboratory staff were blind to the clinical status of the parents. Mothers remained with their children throughout the testing. Study procedures were explained to the mothers, who attended but did not participate in the session; while the child faced the examiner, the mother sat in a chair about a meter to the right of the child and quietly observed the examination but did not intervene. Electrodes for recording heart rate and respiration were taped to the child's chest and back.

Children were divided into three age groups based on previous research data.[48] Children from 2 to 2½ years were classified as the "younger" group (n = 8), those from 2½ to 4 years were classified as the "middle" group (n = 16), and those from 4 to 7 years were classified as the "older" group (n = 32). The protocols were designed for each of the three age groups and consisted of a series of age-appropriate cognitive tasks. These protocols were developed and used in other studies on behavioral inhibition.[20,29,45] These procedures were designed to obtain an index of each child's behavior under mild cognitive stress with an unfamiliar examiner and included the perceptual and recognition memory tests. The observations of the protocol sessions were videotaped and scored by coders who had no knowledge of parental diagnosis. Videotapes were coded for (1) latency to the first, second, and third spontaneous comments made by the child, (2) spontaneous comments during the testing sessions, and (3) frequency of (*a*) smiles, (*b*), small movement of the fingers, (*c*) movements of the mouth or lips, and (*d*) gross bodily movements of the trunk. A random sample of 12 videotapes were coded by a second rater for reliability assessment. The reliabilities ranged from .91 to .97 for each of the variables measured.

Because we were interested in evaluating the frequency of behavioral inhibition in high-risk children of parents with PDAG, children were dichotomized into two mutually exclusive categories: behaviorally inhibited and not inhibited. Previous data on longitudinal samples in the Harvard study have shown that a long latency to begin to speak spontaneously to the examiner and total frequency of spontaneous comments to the examiner were the most sensitive indexes of inhibition, and differentiated the inhibited from the uninhibited groups.[48]

Therefore, a dichotomous classification of a child as inhibited or not inhibited was made blindly, without knowledge of parental disorder, from videotape scores of frequency of spontaneous comments to the examiner, the child's latency to talk, and the age of the child. As expected, there was a high negative correlation between the two measures of vocal restraint. Older children (aged 4 to 7 years) were classified as inhibited if they took longer than the median value for their group (five minutes) for their first spontaneous comment and had the median value or fewer number of comments (five comments). Nine of the 32 older children did not fall into the expected quadrants of long latency and few comments or short latency and many comments. Because the number of spontaneous comments is considered to be more sensitive in differentiating behaviorally inhibited from not inhibited older children, these atypical children were classified only by number of spontaneous comments.

The median number of comments for the younger and middle groups was 13.5, with a median latency to speak of five minutes. These younger children were classified as inhibited if they spoke 13 or fewer comments and waited five minutes or more to utter their first comment. Eight of the 24 children did not fall into the expected quadrants of low number of comments and long latency to speak or high number of comments and short latency to speak. Younger children have been observed to vocalize more often in the laboratory setting, with latency to speak deemed more sensitive an indicator of inhibition. Thus, with two exceptions, these remaining children were classified based only on latency to speak. Two very young children, aged 2.3 and 2.7 years, were classified by the senior laboratory rater (J.K.) as inhibited because of a small number of spontaneous comments, despite their short latencies to the first comment, which on review of the videotapes were believed to misrepresent their overall behavioral responses. All childhood assignments to the behaviorally inhibited and not inhibited group were done at the Harvard laboratory, blind to the clinical data.

Data Analysis

Because of the nonparametric distribution of our data (see Figs 1 and 2), nonparametric statistics were used. Data were first analyzed by four group comparisons, followed by pairwise comparisons. Kruskal-Wallis analysis of variance (*H* values, corrected for ties) was used for continuous data and 4 × 2 χ^2 analysis was used for nominal data, followed by Mann-Whitney *U* test and χ^2 test with Yates' continuity correction as indicated. Probabilities associated with Kruskal-Wallis *H* values were determined using a χ^2 approximation to the

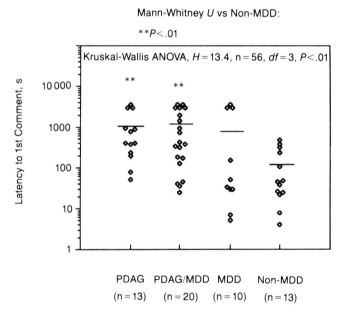

Figure 1. Distribution of latency to first spontaneous comment in children of agoraphobic and comparison probands. PDAG indicates panic disorder alone or with agoraphobia; PDAG/MDD, primary PDAG/secondary depression or primary depression/secondary PDAG; MDD, pure major depressive disorder or primary depression/secondary generalized anxiety disorder; non-MDD, attention deficit disorder in sibling, generalized anxiety disorder, tobacco dependence, or obesity; ANOVA, analysis of variance. Horizontal lines indicate mean values for each group. To facilitate display of data, *y* axis is presented in logarithmic scale; however, data did not undergo any conversion.

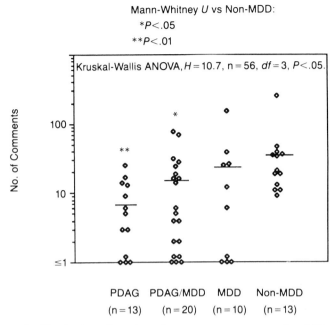

Figure 2. Distribution of number of spontaneous comments for children of agoraphobic and comparison probands. See Fig 1 for key to abbreviations. Horizontal lines indicate mean values for each group. To facilitate display of data, *y* axis is presented in logarithmic scale; however, data did not undergo any conversion.

H distribution.[49(pp 184–193)] Where number of cases in groups being compared by Mann-Whitney *U* test exceeded 20, associated two-tailed probabilities were determined using a normal approximation to the distribution of *U* (*z* value, corrected for ties).[49(pp 116–127)] Spearman's rank correlations (ρ corrected for ties) were performed on continuous measures.

RESULTS

Clinical and Demographic
Characteristics of Sample

Table 1 shows the clinical and demographic characteristics of the proband groups. Although we attempted to match diagnostic groups for ordinal position, age, and sex of child, some unexpected statistically significant differences in demographic characteristics emerged. Small but significant differences were detected in mean ordinal position of children of parents with PDAG compared with the non-MDD comparison group ($P < .05$). Mothers with PDAG (alone and comorbid) were significantly younger than mothers in the non-MDD comparison group ($P < .05$). The group with mixed PDAG/MDD had the lowest mean SES (3.4) of all groups, and this PDAG in the parent, either alone or comorbid (any PDAG). For comparison, data were also analyzed after stratification of the children into mutually exclusive groups based on the presence or absence of MDD in a parent, either alone or comorbid (any MDD). While children of parents with any PDAG had significantly higher latencies to speak ($z = -3.53$, $P \leq .001$) and fewer spontaneous comments ($z = 2.48$, $P \leq .05$), there were no differences in those values between children of parents with any MDD and all others without MDD (Tables 2 and 3).

Analysis of Categorical Data

Significant overall differences were detected in the rate of behavioral inhibition in all children among the four groups ($\chi^2 = 14.8$, $df = 3$, n = 56, $P = .002$). Pairwise comparison of those data revealed that the rates of behavioral inhibition in children of probands with PDAG alone ($\chi^2 = 9.8$, $df = 1$, n = 26, $P = .0017$) or with comorbid MDD ($\chi^2 = 7.4$, $df = 1$, n = 33, $P = .0067$) were significantly higher than the non-MDD comparison group. In contrast, the rate of inhibition in the MDD comparison group did not differ significantly from either group. It is noteworthy that among older children only, the difference in the rate of behavioral inhibition between PDAG and

				Mean (SD)				
Proband Diagnosis	n	Age of Child, y	Ordinal Position	Age of Mother, y	Age of Father, y	No. of Children in Family	SES	Rate of Divorce or Separation, No. (%)
PDAG	13	4.3 (1.6)	1.5†(0.5)	31.2‡(3.6)	36.8 (10.6)	2.2 (0.9)	2.2 (1.5)	1 (7.7)
Comorbid PDAG and MDD	20	4.4 (1.6)	2.0 (1.4)	31.7 (5.8)	35.7 (7.7)	2.2 (1.3)	3.4‡(0.9)	8 (40.0)
MDD	10	4.5 (1.7)	1.8 (.79)	34.9 (4.8)	36.9 (5.1)	2.0 (0.8)	2.4 (0.8)	1 (10.0)
Non-MDD Comparison Group	13	3.9 (1.1)	2.6 (1.2)	35.5 (4.8)	38.7 (4.9)	2.8 (1.3)	2.5 (1.3)	3 (23.1)
Total sample	**56**	4.3 (1.5)	2.0 (1.1)	33.0 (5.2)	36.9 (7.5)	2.3 (1.2)	2.7 (1.2)	13 (23.2)

Table 1.—Demographic Characteristics*

*PDAG indicates panic disorder alone or with agoraphobia; comorbid PDAG and MDD, primary PDAG/secondary depression or primary depression/secondary PDAG; MDD, pure depression or primary depression/secondary generalized anxiety disorder; non-MDD, attention deficit disorder in a sibling, generalized anxiety disorder, tobacco dependence, or obesity; SES, socioeconomic status.
†Unpaired *t* test, two-tailed, vs comparison group with non-MDD: $P<.01$.
‡Unpaired *t* test, two-tailed, vs comparison group with non-MDD: $P<.05$.

Table 1. Demographic Characteristics*

Table 2.—Latency to First Spontaneous Comment in Children of Parents With Any PDAG or Any MDD Compared With Children of All Other Parents*

	n	Mean Latency, s	Mean Rank	Mann-Whitney U Test	
				z Score†	P Values‡
Any PDAG					
Any PDAG	33	1077 ± 1179	34.9	− 3.53	≤.001
All others	23	480 ± 1006	19.3		
Any MDD					
Any MDD	30	1049 ± 1272	30.2	− .825	>.1
All others	26	581 ± 931	26.6		

*PDAG indicates panic disorder alone or with agoraphobia; MDD, major depressive disorder; Any PDAG, PDAG alone, primary PDAG/secondary MDD, and primary MDD/secondary PDAG; Any MDD, MDD alone, MDD with generalized anxiety, primary MDD/secondary PDAG, and primary PDAG/secondary MDD.

†z score is corrected for ties and is used as an approximation to the U distribution for large sample sizes (n>20), as described in "Methods" section.

‡Probabilities are two-tailed.

Table 2. Latency to First Spontaneous Comment in Children of Parents with Any PDAG or Any MDD Compared with Children of All Other Parents*

Table 3.—Total Spontaneous Comments in Children of Parents With Any PDAG or Any MDD Compared With Children of All Other Parents*

	n	Mean No. of Comments	Mean Rank	Mann-Whitney U Test	
				z Score†	P Value‡
Any PDAG					
Any PDAG	33	12.5 ± 18.0	24.0	− 2.48	≤.05
All others	23	35.0 ± 56.5	35.0		
Any MDD					
Any MDD	30	19.3 ± 32.1	26.4	− 1.04	>.1
All others	26	24.5 ± 47.8	30.9		

*PDAG indicates panic disorder alone or with agoraphobia; MDD, major depressive disorder; Any PDAG, PDAG alone, primary PDAG/secondary MDD, and primary MDD/secondary PDAG; Any MDD, MDD alone, MDD with generalized anxiety, primary MDD/secondary PDAG, and primary PDAG/secondary MDD.

†z score is corrected for ties and is used as an approximation to the U distribution for large sample sizes (n>20), as described in "Methods" section.

‡Probabilities are two-tailed.

Table 3. Total Spontaneous Comments in Children of Parents with Any PDAG or Any MDD Compared with Children of All Other Parents*

MDD attained statistical significance (χ^2 = 4.0, df = 1, n = 13, P = .046). Within the comorbid group, there was no significant difference between the rate of inhibition in children of parents with primary PDAG/secondary MDD and those of parents with primary MDD/secondary PDAG. Furthermore, the data suggest a progression of increasing rates of inhibition from non-MDD (15.4%), to MDD (50.0%), and comorbid PDAG/MDD (70%), and PDAG (84.6%) (Fig 3).

When children were stratified into mutually exclusive groups based on the presence or absence of PDAG, either alone or comorbid, in a parent (any PDAG) and, for comparison, into groups based on the presence or absence of MDD, alone or comorbid, in a parent (any MDD), findings supported those for continuous data. While children of parents with any PDAG had significantly higher rates of behavioral inhibition (75.8%) compared with children of all parents with non-PDAG (30.4%) (χ^2 = 9.6, df = 1, n = 56, P = .002),

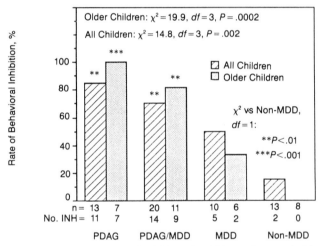

Fig 3.—Rates of behavioral inhibition in children of agoraphobic and comparison probands. See Fig 1 for key to abbreviations. "All Children" includes children aged 2 to 7 years (n = 56); "Older Children" includes children aged 4 to 7 years (n = 32). INH indicates inhibited.

Figure 3. Rates of behavioral inhibition in children of agoraphobic and comparison probands. See Fig 1 for key to abbreviations. "All Children" includes children aged 2 to 7 years (n = 56); "Older Children" includes children aged 4 to 7 years (n = 32). INH indicates inhibited.

there was no difference in the rate of behavioral inhibition between children of parents with any MDD (63.3%) and children of all other parents (50.0%) (χ^2 = 0.54, df = 1, n = 56, P = .46).

The two atypical young children who had been more difficult to dichotomize into behaviorally inhibited and not inhibited groups and who had been classified as behaviorally inhibited based on their number of comments and overall behaviors (see "Methods" section) fell in the group with pure MDD (n = 1) and in the non-MDD comparison group (n = 1). Thus, if they had been classified as not inhibited, our findings would have been even stronger.

Findings regarding behavioral inhibition were more robust for the older group in all analyses. Overall differences in rate of behavioral inhibition among the four diagnostic groups were highly significant (χ^2 = 19.9, df = 3, n = 32, P = .0002), as was the higher rate of behavioral inhibition in the group with PDAG alone (χ^2 = 11.2, df = 1, n = 15, P = .0008) or in the group with comorbid PDAG (χ^2 = 9.4, df = 1, n = 19, P = .0022) compared with the non-MDD comparison group. In the group with any PDAG, the rate of behavioral inhibition in older children was significantly higher (88.9%) than the rate in older children of all parents with non-PDAG (14.3%) (χ^2 = 14.9, df = 1, n = 32, P = .0001); in contrast, there was no significant difference between the rate of behavioral inhibition in older children of any MDD parents (64.7%) compared with older children of all parents without MDD (46.7%) (χ^2 = 0.45, df = 1, n = 32, P = .5).

Correlation and Relative Risk

Correlations of the continuous measures revealed a significant association between latency to speak and number of spontaneous comments in all children (p = −.68, P < .001) and in older ones (p = −.74, P < .001). To further evaluate the strength of the association between behavioral inhibition and diagnosis, relative risk (RR) was computed and found to be significantly higher for children of parents with any PDAG (RR = 2.5, P < .01) but not for children of parents with any MDD (RR = 1.3, P > .4).

COMMENT

Children of parents with PDAG, whether or not "secondary" to depression, were more likely to be behaviorally inhibited to the unfamiliar than children of parents without AG or PD, as manifested by high latency to speak and small number of spontaneous comments. These behavioral characteristics in this sample of high-risk children were consistent with those found in nonclinical populations. In the two longitudinal cohorts followed up by Kagan and colleagues,[50] for the groups originally selected as extremely inhibited, the mean latency to speak and total number of spontaneous comments at age 5.5 years during a session comparable with the one used in our protocol was 360 s and 20 comments, respectively. In a normal population of 70 unselected children, at age 4 years the mean latency to the first comment was 120 s and the mean number of comments was 50 (J.K., unpublished data, 1987). Thus, children of parents with PDAG alone or comorbid in our sample had mean values on both measures consistent with those for the inhibited children in Kagan and colleagues' longitudinal samples, while children in our non-MDD comparison group had means close to the mean latencies and number of comments found in the group of normal 4-year-old volunteer subjects.

The frequency of behavioral inhibition in the children of probands with primary MDD or MDD alone, however, was not significantly different from children of parents with PDAG or primary PDAG. This finding may suggest (1) that behavioral inhibition is a precursor of or marker for later affective or anxiety disorder, (2) that, in some cases, MDD and PD share a common, underlying diathesis,[41,48,51-54] or (3) that behavioral inhibition is a nonspecific early precursor of later psychopathology. Other reports[55,56] have also linked withdrawal behavior in early childhood with later depressive disorders, and families of both anxious and depressed children appear to have similar loading for affective illness.[52]

Family studies have shown that PD and AG aggregate in the pedigrees of probands with these disorders.[36-41] These reports and the higher concordance of anxiety disorders in monozygotic than dizygotic twins[39] suggest a genetic component in this disorder. This finding is underscored by the prevalence of anxiety disorders in children of AG probands.[14] Thus, it is possible that the high prevalence of behavioral inhibition in this sample of children of AG parents may reflect a biological diathesis present in these children.

Although we favor the idea of a biological underpinning to the profile of behavioral inhibition and vulnerability to anxiety disorder, there will be a contribution of environmental forces;[57] our data, however, did not contain indexes of environmental influences. Exposure to an AG parent may predispose a child to develop a more anxious stance by offering a model of caution and fearfulness. Some reports, for example, indicate that AGs were often raised in overprotective families.[58,59] Solyom and colleagues[60-62] noted that mothers of AG patients scored significantly higher than controls on measures of maternal control and concern than the overprotective mothers on whom the scale norms were based. Thus, an AG parent may foster anxious attachment in the child.

If learning to respond to a stimulus with fear is enhanced in children who witness their mother react to events with fear, behavioral inhibition to the unfamiliar in children could correlate with the extent or intensity of exposure to parental fearfulness. Parents with AG in this study, however, were generally in remission or minimally symptomatic for most of their children's lives. Early exposure during critical periods, however, may have been sufficient or the asymptomatic parents with anxiety disorder may have continued to manifest more fearfulness, caution, avoidance, or overprotectiveness than the control parents. Future study should attempt to address the severity and chronicity of parental psychopathology in understanding its contribution to behavioral inhibition in the child.

It is unclear whether behavioral inhibition in a young child is a necessary or sufficient precursor of childhood or adult psychopathology. Onset of panic attacks in adult life may reflect dysfunction unrelated to the expression and extension of this preexisting diathesis. The behaviors that had previously characterized inhibited and uninhibited children were, however, preserved to a significant degree from original assessments at 21 or 31 months to later evaluations at 4, 5, and 7 years of age, suggesting that this temperamental trait may be enduring.[29] Additionally, children identified as inhibited at 21 months of age were more often extremely shy, withdrawn, and restrained in their kindergarten classroom compared with the uninhibited cohort. School observations and teacher interviews suggest that approximately one-third of the inhibited children manifested clinical symptoms of anxiety or social isolation.[31] In many of these cases, the withdrawal from social contact was of sufficient intensity to interfere with everyday social functioning and the formation of peer relations. Thus, the greater frequency of behavioral inhibition observed in children of AG parents indicates, at least, that these children may be at risk for school maladjustment, social dysfunction, and distress in later childhood.

Many children identified as inhibited in previous studies, however, were not maladapted. Depending on setting, an inhibited child might be viewed as "polite," "quiet," "cooperative," or "shy." Furthermore, inhibited behavior in a child is only evident with appropriate stressors, such as separation or novelty. Severe or sustained stress may be necessary for the diathesis to be manifest for some. Nonetheless, the tendency to excessive arousal and withdrawal may be an early marker of later anxiety disorder. As noted above, some of the more extremely inhibited children observed naturalistically already appear to suffer an anxiety syndrome.

If behavioral inhibition to unfamiliar events is, for some children, a precursor of adult PD, the link between early and later diathesis may lie in a lower threshold of limbic arousal to unfamiliar events and challenge that leads to vigilance, withdrawal, and decreased exploratory behavior. Limbic system arousal[63,64] and increased central noradrenergic activity[65-67] have been implicated in inhibition, fear, and anxiety symptoms. Thus, arousal thresholds in the limbic system, particularly the amygdala and hippocampus, and their locus ceruleus-noradrenergic connections, may be implicated in the pathophysiology of behavioral inhibition. This hypothesis finds support in the work of Kagan et al.,[30] who found increased activity in target organs activated by limbic structures (high and stable heart rates, larger pupillary dilation, increased laryngeal muscle tension, higher levels of salivary cortisol, and increased urinary 3-methoxy-4-hydroxyphenylglycol and catecholamine levels) in inhibited, compared with uninhibited, children.

The distinctions between "behavioral inhibition to the unfamiliar" and "separation anxiety" deserve further scrutiny. The responses elicited by a mild stressor in a setting unfamiliar to the child could be viewed as response to a separation threat. However, all children were examined under the same experimental conditions, and they remained in contact with their mothers throughout the testing. Unless one were to posit that any experience with novelty aroused a threat of separation from a parent, we would conclude that separation anxiety was not evoked in our setting. While subtle maternal behaviors could have influenced the behavior of the child during the assessment, no quantifiable evidence to support this assertion was obtained. Furthermore, in an earlier naturalistic observation of inhibited and uninhibited children at school, after six months in school the inhibited children continued to be shy and timid, at a time when separation from the parent was not an apparent provocation.[31] Rather than separation fear generating inhibited behavior, we view a diathesis of excessive limbic arousal to novelty and challenge as the basic dysfunction, with separation being one potential provocative challenge. Further, it is a cross-species characteristic for young mammals, in a state of arousal and uncertainty, to seek safety and protection from the mother. Thus, in those predisposed, a lower threshold to limbic arousal heightens the intensity of attachment. In primate models, for example, while "anxiety" in a monkey can be generated by repeated separation threats,[68,69] Suomi et al.[69] and Suomi[70] reported that the most important predictor of developing persistent anxietylike behavior is genetic loading for the trait of being "high reactive."

The estimated 10% to 15% prevalence of behavioral inhibition in children[29,30,48] is an indication that not all inhibited children develop anxiety disorders in later childhood or adult life. Epidemiologic studies, for example, reported a prevalence rate of anxiety disorders of 2.5% of children in a rural population and 5% in an urban population in England.[71] Inhibition in children, furthermore, appears with roughly equal frequency in boys and girls, as opposed to adult PD, which is clearly more common in women. Thus, other factors, whether biological (e.g., puberty) or psychosocial (e.g., socialization and learning) appear to influence the possible evolution from behavioral inhibition in childhood to disorder in adulthood. Longitudinal study of such modifying variables is a central task to aid in the development of preventive strategies. A few children in the Harvard Infant Study cohort changed from inhibited to uninhibited over time, suggesting that early intervention could have prophylactic effects. Moreover, the relationship between behavioral inhibition and psychopathology is unknown and requires further investigation.

The findings in this study should be viewed in light of their methodologic limitations. First, we combined data from three different protocols for children of different age groups. Unfortunately, the small sample sizes of the younger and middle groups did not permit separate meaningful analysis in these groups. However, examination of the data from the two younger groups indicates that while findings in the middle group followed the direction of the older group, this was not the case in the younger group. Thus, our findings suggest that behavioral inhibition may be more clearly ascertained by these measures in children older than 2.5 years. Second, we did not use normal controls. The mean values for the continuous variables we examined in our non-MDD comparison group, however, were comparable with values observed by one of us (J.K.) in other normal controls. We would expect, therefore, that comparisons with normal controls would have yielded similar differences. Furthermore, the rate of inhibition in the non-MDD group was comparable with the 10% to 15% general population estimates,[29,30,48] suggesting that this comparison group may have been a good contrast for this study. The most important methodologic function of our controls, however, was to preserve the blindness of the ratings.

In sum, the data indicate that behavioral inhibition to the unfamiliar, as defined in the previous work of Kagan and colleagues,[29,30,45] is prevalent in the offspring of adults in treatment for PDAG. It is not clear whether this behavioral characteristic is partly biological or the sole product of experience. If behavioral inhibition in early childhood leads to anxiety disorder or other psychopathology, the identification of young children at risk with this temperamental trait would represent a major opportunity for the development of preventive strategies.

REFERENCES

1. Reich J: The epidemiology of anxiety. *J Nerv Ment Dis* 1986;174:129–136.

2. Robins H, Helzer JE, Weissman MM, Orvaschel H, Gruenberg E, Burke JD, Regier DA: Lifetime prevalence of specific psychiatric disorders in three sites. *Arch Gen Psychiatry* 1984;41:949–958.
3. Gittelman R, Klein DF: Relationship between separation anxiety and panic and agoraphobic disorders. *Psychopathology* 1984;17(suppl 1):56–65.
4. Gittelman-Klein R, Klein DF: Controlled imipramine treatment of school phobia. *Arch Gen Psychiatry* 1971;25:204–207.
5. Gittelman-Klein R: Pharmacotherapy and management of pathological separation anxiety. *Intl J Ment Health* 1975;4:255–271.
6. Klein D: Delineation of two-drug-responsive anxiety syndromes. *Psychopharmacologia* 1964;5:397–408.
7. Deltito JA, Perugi G, Maremmani I, Mignani V, Cassano GB: The importance of separation anxiety in the differentiation of panic disorder from agoraphobia. *Psychiatr Dev* 1986;4:227–236.
8. Berg I, Marks I, McGuire R, Lipsedge M: School phobia and agoraphobia. *Psychol Med* 1974;4:428–434.
9. Philips I: Opportunities for prevention in the practice of psychiatry. *Am J Psychiatry* 1983;140:389–395.
10. McDermott JF: Anxiety disorder in children and adults: Coincidence or consequence? *Integr Psychiatry* 1985;3:158–167.
11. Sameroff A, Seifer R, Zax M: *Early Development of Children at Risk for Emotional Disorder.* Chicago, University of Chicago Press, 1982.
12. Weissman MM, Merikangas KR, John K, Wickramaratne P, Prusoff BA, Kidd KK: Family-genetic studies of psychiatry disorders. *Arch Gen Psychiatry* 1986;43:1104–1116.
13. Berg I: School phobia in the children of agoraphobic women. *Br J Psychiatry* 1976;128:86–89.
14. Weissman MM, Leckman JF, Merikangas KR, Gammon GD, Prusoff BA: Depression and anxiety disorders in parents and children: Results from the Yale family study. *Arch Gen Psychiatry* 1984;41:845–852.
15. Buss AH, Plomin R: *A Temperament Theory of Personality Development.* New York, John Wiley & Sons Inc, 1975.
16. Bronson GW, Pankey WB: On the distinction between fear and wariness. *Child Dev* 1977;48:1167–1187.
17. Carey WB, McDevitt SC: Stability and change in individual temperament diagnoses from infancy to early childhood. *J Am Acad Child Psychiatry* 1978;17:331–337.
18. Hinde RA, Stevenson-Hinde J, Tamplin A: Characteristics of 3- to 4-year-olds assessed at home and their interactions in preschool. *Dev Psychol* 1985;21:130–140.
19. Plomin R, Rowe DC: Genetic and environmental etiology of social behavior in infancy. *Dev Psychol* 1979;15:62–72.
20. Garcia-Coll C, Kagan J, Reznick JS: Behavioral inhibition in young children. *Child Dev* 1984;55:1005–1019.
21. Goldsmith HH, Gottesman II: Origins of variation in behavioral style: A longitudinal study of temperament in young twins. *Child Dev* 1981;52:91–103.
22. Goldsmith HH: Genetic influences on personality from infancy to childhood. *Child Dev* 1983;54:331–355.

23. Daniels D, Plomin R: Origins of individual differences in shyness. *Dev Psychol* 1985;21:118–121.
24. Chess S, Thomas A: Temperamental individuality from childhood to adolescence. *J Am Acad Child Psychiatry* 1977;16:218–226.
25. Chess S, Thomas A: *Origins and Evolution of Behavior Disorders.* New York, Brunner/Mazel Inc, 1984.
26. Thomas A, Chess S: *Temperament and Development.* New York, Brunner/Mazel Inc, 1977.
27. Thomas A, Chess S: Genesis and evolution of behavioral disorders: From infancy to early adult life. *Am J Psychiatry* 1984;141:1–9.
28. Rubin KH: Socially withdrawn children: An 'at risk population,' in Schneider B, Rubin KH, Ledingham J (eds): *Children's Peer Relations: Issues in Assessment and Intervention.* New York, Springer-Verlag NY Inc, 1985.
29. Reznick JS, Kagan J, Snidman N: Inhibited and uninhibited behavior: A follow-up study. *Child Dev* 1986;51:660–680.
30. Kagan J, Reznick JS, Snidman N: The physiology and psychology of behavioral inhibition in young children. *Child Dev* 1987;58:1459–1473.
31. Gersten M: *The Contribution of Temperament to Behavior in Natural Contexts,* doctoral dissertation. Harvard Graduate School of Education, 1986.
32. Noyes R, Clancy J, Crowe R, Hoenk PR, Slymen DJ: The family prevalence of anxiety neurosis. *Arch Gen Psychiatry* 1978;35:1057–1074.
33. Dealy RS, Ishiki DM, Avery DH, Wilson LG, Dunner DL: Secondary depression in anxiety disorders. *Comp Psychiatry* 1981;22:612–618.
34. Pauls DL, Crowe RR, Noyes RR: Distribution of ancestral secondary cases in anxiety neurosis (panic disorder). *J Affective Disord* 1979;1:287–290.
35. Slater E, Shields J: Genetical aspects of anxiety. *Br J Psychiatry* 1969;3:62–71.
36. Crowe RR, Pauls DL, Slymen DJ, Noyes R: A family study of anxiety neurosis: Morbidity risk in family of patients with and without mitral valve prolapse. *Arch Gen Psychiatry* 1980;37:77–79.
37. Harris EL, Noyes R, Crowe RR, Chaudhry DR: Family study of agoraphobia. *Arch Gen Psychiatry* 1983;40:1061–1064.
38. Crowe RR, Noyes R, Pauls DL, Slymen DJ: A family study of panic disorder. *Arch Gen Psychiatry* 1983;40:1065–1069.
39. Torgeson S: Genetic factors in anxiety disorders. *Arch Gen Psychiatry* 1983;40:1085–1089.
40. Moran C, Andrews G: The familial occurrence of agoraphobia. *Br J Psychiatry* 1985;146:262–267.
41. Crowe RR: The genetics of panic disorder and agoraphobia. *Psychiatr Dev* 1985;2:171–186.
42. Kendler KS, Heath A, Martin NG, Eaves LJ: Symptoms of anxiety and depression in a volunteer twin population. *Arch Gen Psychiatry* 1986;43:213–221.
43. Pauls DL, Bucker KD, Crowe RR, Noyes R: A genetic study of panic disorder pedigrees. *Am J Hum Genet* 1980;32:639–644.
44. Carey G, Gottesman II: Twin and family studies of anxiety, phobic, and obsessive disorders, in Klein DF, Rabkin J (eds): *Anxiety: New Research and Changing Concepts.* New York, Raven Press, 1981, pp 117–136.
45. Kagan J, Reznick JS, Clarke C, Snidman N, Garcia-Coll C: Behavioral inhibition to the unfamiliar. *Child Dev* 1984;55:2212–2225.

46. Robins LN, Helzer JE, Croughan J, Ratcliff KS: National Institute of Mental Health Diagnostic Interview Schedule. *Arch Gen Psychiatry* 1981;38:381–389.
47. Spitzer RL, Williams JBW: Structured Clinical Interview for *DSM-III*-Upjohn Version (SCID-UP). New York State Psychiatric Institute, Dec 15, 1983.
48. Kagan J, Reznick JS, Snidman N, Johnson MO, Gibbons J, Gersten M, Biederman J, Rosenbaum JF: Origins of panic disorder, in Ballenger J (ed): *Clinical Aspects of Panic Disorder.* New York, Alan R Liss Inc, in press.
49. Siegel S: *Nonparametric Statistics for the Behavioral Sciences.* New York, McGraw-Hill International Book Co, 1956.
50. Kagan J, Reznick S, Snidman N, Gibbons J, Johnson MO: Preservation of temperamental inhibition. *Child Dev,* in press.
51. Torgersen S: Childhood and family characteristics in panic and generalized anxiety disorders. *Am J Psychiatry* 1986;143:630–632.
52. Livingston R, Nugent H, Rader L, et al.: Family histories of depressed and severely anxious children. *Am J Psychiatry* 1985;142:1497–1499.
53. Klerman GL: Anxiety and depression, in Burrows GD, Davies B (eds): *Handbook of Studies on Anxiety.* New York, Elsevier Science Publishing Co Inc, 1980, pp 145–164.
54. Klein DF: Anxiety reconceptualized, in Klein DF, Rabkin J (eds): *Anxiety: New Research and Concepts.* New York, Raven Press, 1981, pp 235–262.
55. Rubin KH, Cohen J: Predicting peer ratings of aggression and withdrawal in the middle childhood years, in Prinz RJ (ed): *Advances in Behavioral Assessment of Children and Families.* Greenwich, Conn, JAI Press Inc, 1986.
56. Achenbach TM, Edelbrock CS: Behavioral problems and competencies reported by parents of normal and disturbed children aged four through sixteen. *Monogr Soc Res Child Dev* 1981;46:1–82.
57. Raskin M, Peeke HVS, Dickman W, Pinsker H: Panic and generalized anxiety disorders. *Arch Gen Psychiatry* 1982;39:687–689.
58. Roth M: The phobic anxiety-depersonalization syndrome. *Proc R Soc Med* 1959;52:587–595.
59. Terhune W: The phobic syndrome: A study of 86 patients with phobic reactions. *Arch Neurol Psychiatry* 1949;62:162–172.
60. Solyom L, Beck P, Solyom C, Hugel R: Some etiological factors in phobic neurosis. *Can Psychiatr Assoc J* 1974;19:69–78.
61. Solyom L, Heseltine CFO, McClure DV, Solyom C, Ledwige B, Steinberg G: Behavior therapy versus drug therapy in the treatment of phobic neurosis. *Can Psychiatr Assoc J* 1973;18:25–31.
62. Solyom L, Silberfeld M, Solyom C: Maternal overprotection in the etiology of agoraphobia. *Can Psychiatr Assoc J* 1976;21:109–113.
63. Gray JA: Issues in the neuropsychology of anxiety, in Tuma AH, Maser JD (eds): *Anxiety and the Anxiety Disorders.* Hillside, NJ, Lawrence Erlbaum Associates Inc Publishers, 1985, pp 5–27.
64. Insel TR, Ninan PT, Aloi J: A benzodiazepine receptor medicated model of anxiety: Studies in non-human primates and clinical implications. *Arch Gen Psychiatry* 1984;41:741–750.
65. Charney DS, Redmond DE Jr: Neurobiological mechanisms in human anxiety: Evidence supporting noradrenergic hyperactivity. *Neuropharmacology* 1983;22:1531–1536.

66. Huang YH, Redmond DE Jr, Snyder DR, Maas JW: Loss of fear following bilateral lesions of the locus coeruleus in the monkey. *Neurosci Abst* 1976;2:573.

67. Charney DS, Heninger GR: Noradrenergic function and the mechanism of action of antianxiety treatment. *Arch Gen Psychiatry* 1985;42:458–481.

68. Coe CL, Levine S: Normal responses to mother-infant separation in nonhuman primates, in Klein DF, Rabkin J (eds): *Anxiety: New Research and Changing Concepts.* New York, Raven Press, 1981, pp 155–178.

69. Suomi SJ, Kraemer GW, Baysinger CM, DeLizio RD: Inherited and experiential factors associated with individual differences in anxious behavior displayed by Rhesus monkeys, in Klein DF, Rabkin J (eds): *Anxiety: New Research and Changing Concepts.* New York, Raven Press, 1981, pp 179–200.

70. Suomi S: Genetic and environmental factors affecting individual differences in behavioral inhibition in Rhesus monkeys. Read before the Conference on Behavioral Inhibition, Boston, Nov 21, 1986.

71. Graham P: Epidemiological studies, in Quay HC, Werry JS (eds): *Psychopathological Disorders of Childhood.* New York, John Wiley & Sons Inc, 1979, pp 185–209.

20

Temperamental Factors Associated with Rapid Weight Gain and Obesity in Middle Childhood

William B. Carey

Department of Pediatrics, University of Pennsylvania School of Medicine, and Division of General Pediatrics, Children's Hospital of Philadelphia, Philadelphia, Pennsylvania

Robin L. Hegvik

Wayne, Pennsylvania

Sean C. McDevitt

Westbridge Center for Children, Phoenix, Arizona

Studies of the perplexing problem of childhood obesity have considered etiological factors in the child and environment, but have largely ignored the child's temperament or style of interaction with the environment. In this report, a significant relationship is demonstrated between temperament and both rapid weight gain and actual obesity in middle childhood. In a longitudinal study of 138 children, weight-for-height percentile gains between 4 to 5 years and 8 to 9 years were significantly correlated with eight of nine difficult temperament characteristics and with a cumulative "index of difficulty." A separate cross-sectional study of 21 obese (≥ the 95th percentile weight for height) 6- to 12-year-old children found them to be significantly less rhythmical/predictable and lower in persistence/attention span than matched controls. These normal behavioral style characteristics, interacting with metabolic, dietary, and environmental factors, may predispose some children to inappropriate eating habits or make it harder to maintain a dietary plan to remedy the problem.

Reprinted with permission from *Developmental and Behavioral Pediatrics*, 1988, Vol. 9, No. 4, 194–198. Copyright 1988 by Williams and Wilkins Co.

Recent reviews of childhood obesity[1-4] concur that its etiology is multifactorial and complex, and that management is difficult and, usually, unsuccessful. Some report that it is becoming more prevalent.[5] Although the basic mechanism of an excess of caloric intake over expenditure seems evident, the varying interplay of elements in the child and the environment awaits clarification.

In the first year of life, factors reportedly predisposing a child to adiposity have included larger birth weight, bottle feeding, and male sex.[6] Recently, however, the possibility that the child's behavioral style contributes to the problem was suggested by the demonstration of a significant association of difficult temperament (in particular, fussiness) with obesity in the second 6 months of life.[7]

Despite the earlier demonstration of a small but significant relationship between obesity in infancy and the same problem in adulthood,[8] it now appears that onset in middle childhood is a better predictor of adult status. The Hagerstown study[9] reported that 60% of moderately overweight and 85% of markedly overweight children *remained* overweight 30 years later. Therefore, middle childhood, rather than infancy, may be a better time to look for the role of temperament in chronic obesity.

In older children, host metabolic characteristics interact with environmental factors that include ethnicity, and the physical, family, and social milieu.[2] Aspects of behavioral adjustment (relationships with people, tasks and oneself) that reportedly have meaningful associations with obesity fall into three groups: (1) possibly etiological, such as low activity output,[10] an example of which is extended watching of television,[11] (2) correlates or consequences (obese children being less liked,[12] having more social withdrawal or somatic complaints,[13] lower self-esteem,[14] or more negative peer interactions[15]), or (3) problems in management, such as noncompliance and dropping out of treatment plans.[16]

Whereas the child's behavioral adjustment or relationships may be related to obesity in middle childhood, it is a separate issue as to whether the child's behavioral style or temperament is involved. No study dealing with this question can be found. In 1942, Sheldon[17] described his heavy adult endomorph type as good-natured, relaxed, sociable, and communicative, but his scheme has few adherents today, and did not apply to children. However, a link between temperament and obesity is suggested by the associated behavioral adjustment problems (which may have temperamental components),[12-15] the well-known noncompliance with treatment plans,[16] and the previous documentation of the role of difficult temperament in obesity in young infants.[7]

We began this study with the hypothesis that rapid weight gain or actual obesity in middle childhood would be related in some degree to difficult temperament. Furthermore, clinical experience with poor compliance in treatment regimens led us to expect obese children to be generally lower in persistence or attention span.[16] Activity ratings for them should be low.[10,11] The private practice setting of the senior author offered a unique opportunity for a preliminary exploration of temperament characteristics associated with rapid weight gain and established obesity.

SUBJECTS AND METHODS

Background

After many years of neglect, temperament differences in infants and children are again the subject of scientific study. There are several modern conceptualizations of temperament, but the best known and most widely studied is the one introduced by Thomas et al.[18] Defining it as behavioral style, as distinguished from capacities, motivations and behavioral adjustment, they have described nine characteristics: activity, rhythmicity, initial approach/withdrawal, adaptability, intensity, mood, persistence/attention span, distractibility, and sensory threshold (Table 1). The difficult child is one who is low in rhythmicity, approach, and adaptability, and high in intensity and predominantly negative in mood, whereas the easy child has the opposite charac-

---

Activity: The amount of physical motion during sleep, eating, play, dressing, bathing, etc.

Rhythmicity: The regularity of physiologic functions such as hunger, sleep, and elimination.[a]

Approach/withdrawal: The nature of initial responses to new stimuli—people, situations, places, foods, toys, procedures.

Adaptability: The ease or difficulty with which reactions to stimuli can be modified in a desired way.

Intensity: The energy level of responses, regardless of quality or direction.

Mood: Amount of pleasant and friendly or unpleasant and unfriendly behavior in various situations.

Persistence/attention span: The length of time particular activities are pursued by the child, with or without obstacles.

Distractibility: The effectiveness of extraneous environmental stimuli in interfering with ongoing behaviors.

Sensory threshold: The amount of stimulation, such as sounds or light, necessary to evoke discernible responses in the child.

---

[a]In the Middle Childhood Temperament Questionnaire, rhythmicity is replaced by predictability/quality of organization.[20]

Table 1. Temperament Characteristics[18,25]

teristics. Parents also usually rate high activity, low persistence, high distractibility, and low threshold as difficult.[19,20]

Thus, a child's temperament is the way in which he or she typically experiences the internal and external environments and responds to them. These behavioral characteristics all are normal variables, not clinical problems in themselves, but they may generate various clinical conditions by stressful interactions with the environment.

The study of temperament has been greatly facilitated by the development of questionnaires for collecting behavioral data from parents. Two of these, the Behavioral Style Questionnaire (BSQ)[19] for 3- to 7-year-old children and the Middle Childhood Temperament Questionnaire (MCTQ)[20] for 8- to 12-year-old children, were used in this report. These questionnaires have, respectively, 100 and 99 behavioral descriptions which the parent rates as to frequency on a scale of 1–6, from "almost never" to "almost always." An example of predictability (which replaces rhythmicity in the MCTQ) is "has difficulty doing things on time (homework, keeping appointments, etc.)." One of the persistence/attention span items is "leaves projects unfinished (drawings, models, crafts, etc.)." By means of scoring sheets, the questionnaire responses are converted into scores for the nine categories of temperament. These category scores can then be compared with means and standard deviations established in the standardization of the scales.

Longitudinal Study

Since both the BSQ and MCTQ were standardized in the senior author's pediatric practice, for a substantial number of children these two tests had already been performed, as well as weight and height data from routine physical examinations. Of 189 children with results on both the BSQ and MCTQ, 138 had sufficient growth data to be included in this study. This practice is predominantly middle class. The sample consisted of 67 males and 71 females. Although the two temperament determinations were always 4½ years apart, they ranged from 3 to over 7 years for the BSQ and from under 8 to 11 for the MCTQ (Table 2).

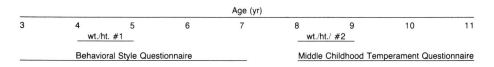

Table 2. Longitudinal Study: Timing of Growth and Temperament Determinations

Since the two questionnaires have different means and standard deviations for the nine categories, and since the MCTQ does not have a recommended scheme for establishing the difficult and easy clusters as the BSQ does, a new summary scoring system was devised. An "index of difficulty" was computed separately for results from the two questionnaires. Each child's score on the six categories of rhythmicity (or predictability on the MCTQ), approach, adaptability, intensity, mood, and persistence, was assigned a value of 1 if the score was on the difficult side of the mean, and 2 if more than one standard deviation in that direction. Low persistence was added to the original five because of indications that this is appropriate for schoolage children.[20] Thus, in addition to the nine category scores, each child received a total "index of difficulty" on both the BSQ and MCTQ. Ratings on the index ranged from 0 to 12.

The two times for growth determinations were chosen so as to include the most likely period of excessive weight gain in middle childhood. The "adiposity rebound"[21] or the typical time of onset of childhood obesity[22] is around 6 years of age. The variable of onset of puberty[23] and the upper age limit of the United States Public Health Service weight-for-height (wt./ht.) percentiles compelled the establishment of the end point at about 9 years. Therefore, change in nutritional state was determined in this study by comparing wt./ht. percentiles at 4 or 5 years (using the mean if both were available) with wt./ht. percentiles at 8–9 years.

Although parents are generally advised to have their children examined at 1- to 2-year intervals during this period, 51 had to be excluded because growth data were insufficient at one of the two times. No consistent factors seemed responsible for this irregular visitation by some; the reasons included joining or leaving the practice, economic hardships, or other factors.

The analysis of these data was a comparison of the increase or decrease in wt./ht. percentiles from 4–5 to 8–9 years, with the index of difficulty and with the nine individual categories on both the BSQ at 3–7 years and the MCTQ at 8–11 years. The correlations also were computed separately for the 45 who gained the most (the top third) and the 41 oldest (BSQ at 6–7 and MCTQ at 10–11 years) on the assumption that the heavier and older ones might show the relationship more strongly.

Cross-Sectional Study

The longitudinal study just described contained only 10 children who reached the 95th percentile or greater in wt./ht. Therefore, an entirely new group was selected to determine the temperament characteristics of a larger sample of obese children. The office files of the pediatric practice of the senior author were examined to find all individuals between the ages of 6 and 12 presently at or above the 95th percentile in wt./ht. This selection process yielded a sample of 22 obese children.

For comparison with these overweight children, a matched control sample was used. Proceeding alphabetically in the office file, individuals available with matching age and sex were selected until 22 were obtained.

The same temperament questionnaire could not be sent to the parents of all children because the range for the BSQ ends and that of the MCTQ begins between 7 and 8 years. Therefore, the parents of the five youngest children received the BSQ and the 16 oldest, the MCTQ. Of the 44 questionnaires sent, 42 were returned properly completed. Fortunately, the one missing obese subject was the match for one missing control. The final sample of children consisted of eight males and 13 females. The age distribution was 6 years, 4; 7 years, 4; 8 years, 1; 10 years, 4; 11 years, 5; and 12 years, 3.

So that the five younger and 16 older children rated on the two different questionnaires could be grouped together for analysis, the category scores were converted to T values (mean $\pm$ 1 SD = 50 $\pm$ 10). For data analysis, t-tests of obese and control group means on the nine temperament characteristics were used. No attempt was made to compare the two groups as to a cumulative score or index of difficulty, as was done in the longitudinal study.

RESULTS

Longitudinal Study

1. Index of difficulty. Correlating the index of difficulty with increase or decrease in wt./ht. percentile points between ages 4–5 and 8–9 yielded several significant values. For the index derived from the Behavioral Style Questionnaire (BSQ), done at 3–7 years, the correlations were $r = 0.22$ ($p = 0.005$) for the whole sample, $r = 0.41$ ($p = 0.003$) for the 45 who gained the most, and $r = 0.39$ ($p = 0.006$) for the 41 oldest children. For the Middle Childhood Temperament Questionnaire (MCTQ), done at 8–11 years, the correlations were $r = 0.15$ ($p = 0.035$) for the whole sample, $r = 0.33$ ($p = 0.013$) for the biggest gainers, and $r = 0.30$ ($p = 0.027$) for the oldest children. In other words, a significant relationship was found between greater temperamental difficulty and greater wt./ht. gain. The correlations were stronger for those who gained the most and for those who were older. However, an increase in the value of the index of difficulty from the BSQ to the MCTQ 4½ years later was not related to an increase in wt./ht. status ($r = -0.03$, $p = 0.36$).

2. Individual category scores. Table 3 shows that the difficult dimensions of all six of the individual temperament categories of which the index of diffi-

Temperament Categories		Total Sample (n = 138)	
Activity—high	BSQ		
	MCTQ	0.16	(0.032)[a]
Rhythmicity/Predictability—low	BSQ		
	MCTQ	0.26	(0.001)
Withdrawal—more	BSQ	0.24	(0.002)
	MCTQ		
Adaptaptability—low	BSQ	0.18	(0.019)
	MCTQ	0.16	(0.031)
Intensity—high	BSQ	0.19	(0.012)
	MCTQ		
Mood—negative	BSQ		
	MCTQ	0.16	(0.034)
Persistence/Attention span—low	BSQ		
	MCTQ	0.20	(0.009)
Distractibility—high	BSQ		
	MCTQ	0.17	(0.024)
Threshold	BSQ		
	MCTQ		

[a]Numbers in parentheses are p values. Blank spaces indicate non-signficant relationships. BSQ, Behavioral Style Questionnaire; MCTQ, Middle Childhood Temperament Questionnaire.

Table 3. Longitudinal Study: Correlations of Temperamental Difficulty with Weight/Height Percentile Increase

culty was composed (e.g., low adaptability, negative mood), and also high activity and low distractibility, were related on the BSQ, the MCTQ, or both, to more rapid wt./ht. gain. A larger number of significant relationships were found at the later time with the MCTQ than with the earlier BSQ, six as compared to three, but they were of about the same magnitude. As with the index of difficulty, these correlations rose (with the exception of distractibility) when just the bigger gainers or the older children were considered, from a median of 0.18 to a median of 0.32 and 0.29, respectively (figures omitted from table).

3. Weight-for-height status at 8–9 years. Predictability was the only temperament category on the MCTQ that correlated with wt./ht. percentile status (rather than increase or decrease) for the whole sample of 138 at the 8- to 9-year end point ($r = 0.22$, $p = 0.004$). Neither the index of difficulty nor any of the other eight characteristics was related. In other words, the heavier the child for his or her height at 9 years, the less predictable he or she was rated by the parent at the time.

Although some of the children who gained considerably from lower to higher wt./ht. percentiles did not become overweight, 10 did reach the 95th percentile in wt./ht. The outstanding characteristics of these 10 on the MCTQ were low predictability, low adaptability, negative mood, and low persistence, all of the mean values for this subgroup being greater than one standard deviation above the standardization sample means.

Cross-Sectional Study

The obese children were less rhythmical/predictable than the controls ($t = 1.71$, $p = 0.05$ for all 21; $t = 2.02$, $p < 0.05$ for the older 16). The obese children were also lower in persistence/attention span ($t = 1.81$, $p < 0.05$). Contrary to expectations, the obese children were more approaching ($t = 1.98$, $p < 0.05$). Thus, the longitudinal and cross-sectional studies are in agreement in finding obese children low in predictability and persistence.

DISCUSSION

These findings demonstrate a weak to moderately significant association between both a rapid wt./ht. gain and established obesity in middle childhood and the more abrasive or "difficult" dimensions of several of the temperament characteristics. In the longitudinal study, greater difficulty on eight of the nine characteristics and a summary index of difficulty all were related to more rapid wt./ht. gain. Lower predictability was associated with greater wt./ht. status at 9 years. The cross-sectional study found that obese children were less predictable and less persistent, but also were more approaching, than matched controls. The simplest statement summarizing these findings is that the obese child in this period may be more disorganized and nonpersistent than his or her peers. It is stressed that these are normal temperamental differences that reveal nothing about these children's behavioral or emotional adjustment.

Predictions

In the longitudinal study, three significant temperament correlations (withdrawing, low adaptability, and high intensity) from the Behavioral Style Questionnaire (BSQ) administered between ages 3 and 7 were clearly predictive of rapid weight gain. All of the BSQs were completed before or during the 4- to 9-year period of growth assessment (Table 2). Only for the youngest of the children were the Middle Childhood Temperament Questionnaire (MCTQ) determinations done during the 4- to 9-year period. Therefore, for the MCTQ correlations, one cannot be certain whether a difficult temperament predicted weight gain or merely accompanied it. However, the possibility that a greater gain somehow induced the behavioral style differences seems unlikely, since an increase in wt./ht. over this time span was not correlated with an increase in the index of difficulty.

Temperament and Clinical Conditions

To understand how temperament may be related to obesity, it is useful to recall the role that has been found for temperament in other clinical conditions. Specific temperament patterns do not inevitably lead to certain clinical problems.[18] Neither do specific care-taking practices produce uniform results in children.[21] Thomas and Chess[18] have suggested that a "poor fit," or incompatible relationship, between the child's temperament and the expectations and values of the caretakers may lead to excessive stress and to reactive clinical conditions in the child. Certain characteristics or groups of them, called "temperament risk factors,"[25] may make children more likely to develop problems, as with the difficult child who is susceptible to deviations of behavioral adjustment.

Temperament and Obesity

A standard contemporary view of the parent-child interaction in obesity is that the parents are having trouble setting limits and must reestablish their authority for management to be effective.[2] However, if the child has a behavioral style predisposing to obesity, the interaction is more complex than has been imagined.

The disorganized, nonpersistent child found in the cross-sectional study may have disorderly eating habits and be less resistant to unnecessary food. The child may lack sufficient persistence to stay on a diet, whether overweight is just beginning, or is an established state. It may be that the only "good fit" for avoiding or overcoming obesity for a child with these behavioral traits, genetic background, and social milieu would be a highly organized environment with limited access to food, such as is found in some summer camps devoted to weight loss.

These characteristics seem similar to Gesell's type C temperament, "uneven and irregular." Although not studied in children or adults with obesity, this pattern was associated with an increased rate of major illness and early death in physicians.[26]

The difficult child characteristics, as determined in the longitudinal study, may predispose to more rapid weight gain in children in two ways. Because of their reaction styles, these children probably experience more stress in their social interactions and may use eating as a technique for comforting themselves. Also, they may be less flexible about changing eating patterns when it is necessary to overcome an established problem of excessive weight gain. This interaction of difficult temperament in middle childhood is, therefore, probably only partially similar to that in infancy, when the irritable child is likely to be fed more by the parent as a soothing technique.[7]

The finding of more approaching behavior in the obese children in the cross-sectional study was not expected, and is not easily accounted for. One speculation is that the obese child is less inhibited about eating unfamiliar or unaccustomed foods. Such children are sometimes described as being "willing to eat anything."

One would expect to find lower activity in overweight children,[2,10] but that was not the case here. One must conclude either that the temperament questionnaires measure only the vigor of a specific set of responses, rather than the total activity and caloric expenditure, or that low activity is not an important factor in the acquisition of obesity in middle childhood. Increased exercise may, nevertheless, be a useful part of a weight control program.[27]

Genetic Basis?

Two recent studies have made a strong case for a significant genetic factor in obesity,[28,29] although the exact nature of this predisposition was not uncovered. Temperament has also been demonstrated to have a major genetic determination.[30] It is tempting to speculate that the child's temperament may be one of the ways in which the genetic tendency to obesity may be expressed. Twin studies of growth and temperament should help to improve our understanding of these possible interrelationships.

Further Investigation

This study has some of the advantages and disadvantages of a clinical investigation in a private practice. Parental compliance and follow-up are extremely high. However, the convenient sample may not be of ideal size, composition, and timing; in addition, detailed simultaneous measurements of other ingredients in the development of obesity, such as choice of foods and parental stature, were not possible. This exploratory study found preliminary support for the hypothesis that, among other factors, aspects of difficult temperament may be related to the onset of obesity in middle childhood. More ideally structured investigations in academic settings should clarify these matters further.

REFERENCES

1. Faust IM: Adipose tissue growth and obesity, in Falkner F, Tanner J (eds): *Human Growth: A Comprehensive Treatise*, 2nd ed, vol 2. New York, Plenum Press, 1986, pp 61–75
2. Dietz WH Jr: Childhood obesity: Susceptibility, cause and management. J Pediatr 103:676–686, 1986
3. Neumann CG: Obesity in childhood, in Levine MD, Carey WB, Crocker AC, Gross RT (eds): *Developmental-Behavioral Pediatrics.* Philadelphia, PA, WB Saunders Co, 1983, pp 536–551
4. Woolston JL: Obesity in infancy and early childhood. J Am Acad Child Adolesc Psychiatry 26:123–126, 1987
5. Gortmaker SL, Dietz WH Jr, Sobol AM, et al: Increasing pediatric obesity in the United States. Am J Dis Child 141:535–540, 1987
6. Kramer MS, Barr RG, Leduc DG, et al: Determinants of weight and adiposity in the first year of life. J Pediatr 106:10–14, 1985
7. Carey WB: Temperament and increased weight gain in infants. J Dev Behav Pediatr 6:128–131, 1985
8. Charney E, Goodman HC, McBride M, et al: Childhood antecedents of adult obesity. N Engl J Med 295:6–9, 1976
9. Abraham S, Collins G, Nordsieck M: Relationship of childhood weight status to morbidity in adults. Public Health Rep 86:272–284, 1971
10. Berkowitz RI, Agras WS, Korner AF, et al: Physical activity and adiposity: A longitudinal study from birth to childhood. J Pediatr 106:734–738, 1985
11. Dietz WH Jr, Gortmaker SL: Do we fatten our children at the television set? Obesity and television viewing in children and adolescents. Pediatrics 75:807–812, 1985
12. Strauss CC, Smith K, Frame C, et al: Personal and interpersonal characteristics associated with childhood obesity. J Pediatr Psychol 10:337–343, 1985
13. Israel AC, Shapiro LS: Behavior problems in obese children enrolling in a weight reduction program. J Pediatr Psychol 10:449–460, 1985
14. Kaplan KM, Wadden TA: Childhood obesity and self-esteem. J Pediatr 109:367–370, 1986
15. Baum CG, Forehand R: Social factors associated with adolescent obesity. J Pediatr Psychol 9:293–302, 1984
16. Spence SH: Behavioral treatment of childhood obesity. J Child Psychol Psychiatry 27:447–453, 1986
17. Sheldon WH: *The Varieties of Temperament: A Psychology of Constitutional Differences.* New York, Harper, 1942
18. Thomas A, Chess S: *Temperament and Development,* New York, Brunner/Mazel, 1977
19. McDevitt SC, Carey WB: The measurement of temperament in 3- to 7-year-old children. J Child Psychol Psychiatry 19:245–253, 1978
20. Hegvik RL, McDevitt SC, Carey WB: The Middle Childhood Temperament Questionnaire. J Dev Behav Pediatr 3:197–200, 1982
21. Rolland-Cachera MF, Deheeger M, Bellisle F, et al: Adiposity rebound in children: A simple indicator for predicting obesity. Am J Clin Nutr 39:129–135, 1984

22. Shapiro LR, Crawford PB, Clark MJ, et al: Obesity prognosis: A longitudinal study of children from the age of 6 months to 9 years. Am J Public Health 74:968–972, 1984
23. Tanner JM, Davies PSW: Clinical longitudinal standards for height and weight velocity for North American children. J Pediatr 107:317–329, 1985
24. Caldwell BM: The effects of infant care, in Hoffman ML, Hoffman LW (eds): *Review of Child Development Research*, vol 1. New York, Russell Sage Foundation, 1964, pp 9–87
25. Carey WB: The difficult child. Pediatr Rev 8:39–45, 1986
26. Betz BJ, Thomas CB: Individual temperament as a predictor of health or premature disease. Johns Hopkins Med J 144:81–89, 1979
27. Epstein LH, Wing RR, Penner BC, et al: Effect of diet and controlled exercise on weight loss in children. J Pediatr 107:358–361, 1985
28. Stunkard AJ, Sørensen TIA, Hanis C, et al: An adoption study of human obesity. N Engl J Med 314:193–198, 1986
29. Stunkard AJ, Foch TT, Hrubec Z: A twin study of human obesity. JAMA 256:51–54, 1986
30. Wilson RS, Matheny AP Jr: Behavioral-genetics research in infant temperament: The Louisville Twin Study, in Plomin R, Dunn J (eds): The Study of Temperament: Changes, Continuities, and Challenges. Hillsdale, NJ, Erlbaum Associates, 1986, pp 81–97

Part VI
DEPRESSION AND SUICIDE

The papers in this section attest to the ever-growing clinical and research interest in depression and suicidal behavior among children and adolescents. Perhaps one of the reasons for this increasing interest lies in Klerman's paper summarizing the evidence pointing to increased rates of depression in the years following World War II. As Klerman has observed, during the 1970s psychiatrists began to speculate that rates of depression might have greatly increased, particularly because depression was being reported with increased frequency in children, and because suicide attempts and death by suicide had increased dramatically among adolescents and young adults. It is often difficult to determine whether such an increase is apparent, deriving from increased clinical and research attention to depression and other affective disorders, or a real reflection of changes in the distribution of depression in the population. The paper provides a very useful review of the epidemiologic concepts of temporal or secular trends, the differences between age, period, and cohort effects and the statistical models that have been developed to distinguish among them. Application of these concepts and models to data deriving from large-sample family studies and community epidemiological surveys has led to the documentation of a marked increase in depression among those in cohorts born after World War II, and an earlier age of onset of depression through the twentieth century. Verification of these changes in rates of depression would have important clinical, public health, and theoretical implications. Data such as these suggest that clinical child psychiatrists will continue to see increasing numbers of children and youth who require treatment for depression.

In contrast to Klerman's focus on secular trends in the prevalence of depression, the review by Angold summarizes research on childhood and adolescent depression in clinical populations. The paper traces the recent development of the concept of depression in children and youth from a period when it was felt that depression was extremely rare or perhaps even nonexistent during childhood, through a period when the concept of masked depression was advanced in an attempt to account for the possibility that depression might have different presentations at different ages, to the DSM-III era in which similar criteria are used to diagnose depression in children, adolescents, and adults. Angold then summarizes studies on developmental changes in psychopathology and biological manifestations of depressive disorder in childhood, bipolar disorder, comorbidity, outcome and treatment, concluding with a discussion on issues of differential diagnosis—with particular reference to the task that confronts the practicing child psychiatrist—that of distinguishing between a child who is depressed and one who is miserable.

Cynthia Pfeffer and her co-workers have added to our knowledge of the prevalence and course of suicidal behavior in the general population of children and adolescents with a two-year follow-up of suicidal behavior in a sample of non-patient school children who were initially studied when they were between 6 and 12 years of age. The children were selected by stratified random sampling from a computerized roster of pupils in a large urban community. The authors conclude that the point prevalence of suicidal ideas for normal preadolescents is between 8.9% and 17.9%. Among 67 children evaluated over the two-year study period, approximately 85% had no suicidal tendencies initially or at follow-up, but approximately 15% of the children who were not suicidal initially were suicidal at follow-up. Furthermore, 50% who had suicidal tendencies at the initial assessment had suicidal tendencies at follow-up. No particular psychiatric diagnosis was associated with suicidal tendencies either initially or at follow-up. For the clinician, who is with increasing frequency asked to evaluate individual children who express suicidal tendencies, the findings of this study suggest that children who warrant close follow-up and monitoring are those with a history of suicidal tendencies, depressive symptoms, past violent behavior, and more recent preoccupations with death.

State of the art programmatic efforts directed toward the prevention of teenage suicide are critically reviewed in the paper by David Shaffer and his colleagues. Strategies include hotlines and crisis services, school-based educational and screening procedures, effective treatment of suicidal attempters, minimizing opportunities for suicide imitation, and controlling access to the methods most often used to commit suicide. The evidence for the efficacy of any existing intervention is limited. Shaffer notes that although concern about teen suicide has increased in recent years, in association with a number of highly publicized outbreaks of suicide in teenagers, and with evidence that suicide rates among young males have increased markedly since 1960, adolescent suicide is uncommon; the rate in 1984 for all 15–19 year olds was nine deaths per 100,000. Efforts directed to the general population, even if completely successful, would reach relatively few teenagers who would eventually commit suicide. The authors suggest that a more efficient strategy may be to target available resources to high-risk groups. Most suicides among teenagers occur in those with identifiable mental or character disorders. Further delineation of both risk factors and effective treatment approaches is clearly needed.

The paper by Hoberman and Garfinkel adds to our understanding of risk factors in adolescent suicide through the examination of the medical examiner's records of 229 youths, 19 years or younger, whose deaths had occurred in two Minnesota counties over a 10-year period. In summary, children and adolescents who committed suicide were most likely to be older males with a current psychiatric disorder, usually an affective disorder or alcohol or drug abuse. Suicides appeared to be impulsive and triggered by age-normative precipitants. In a thoughtful discussion, the authors note that stressors, in and of themselves, do not likely pose a risk for the average adolescent. Instead it appears that risk is heightened when stressors occur in particular individuals with pre-existing psychiatric conditions. While some stressors may be a consequence of depression and/or substance abuse, and may not be independently occurring traumatic events, boys appear to be more affected by arguments in significant relationships and relationship breakups. Girls' suicides are associated with assaults. Relatively few suicides showed evidence of advance planning, and many were associated with a degree of intoxication before death, suggesting a mental state of significantly impaired judgment. The authors relate these findings to the issue of suicide prevention. They suggest that a focus on precipitants, signs of premeditation or planning is likely to be unproductive, given the normative nature of the stresses experienced by young suicides and the apparently impulsive nature of the actual suicidal act. They are especially critical of the tendency of many school-based programs (see paper by Shaffer et al. in this volume) to deemphasize the relationship between psychopathology and suicide, suggesting rather that the emphasis in youth suicide prevention programs be directed towards the early identification and appropriate treatment of the episodes of psychopathology that underlie and precede most instances of adolescent suicide.

21

The Current Age of Youthful Melancholia: Evidence for Increase in Depression Among Adolescents and Young Adults*

Gerald L. Klerman

New York Hospital—Cornell Westchester Division, White Plains

The possibility of a rise in rates of depression among adolescents and young adults was first reported in the 1970s. Particular note was taken of the emergence of childhood depression and the increase in suicide attempts and death among adolescents and young adults. Data from large-sample family studies and community epidemiological surveys have been reviewed and reanalyzed, using life-table statistical methodology. Evidence for secular trends are presented, and the problems of disentangling period and cohort effect are discussed. It appears that the 'baby boomers'—those born in the years after World War II—have had increased rates of depression and other related illnesses, including drug abuse and alcoholism. The theoretical aspects of this are discussed, particularly for gene-environment interactions.

In the 1970s, a number of psychiatrists in the USA speculated that rates of depression might have greatly increased (Schwab, 1974; Klerman, 1976, 1979, 1980b). This speculation was based on a number of observations.

Reprinted with permission from the *British Journal of Psychiatry,* 1988, Vol. 152, 4–14. Copyright 1988 by the Royal College of Psychiatrists.

This work was supported in part by grant MH-6-21724 from the National Institute of Mental Health; Alcohol, Drug Abuse and Mental Health Administration; Public Health Service; U.S. Department of Health and Human Services, Washington, DC.

*Presented in part as the third Eli Lilly Lecture to the Royal College of Psychiatrists, London, 27 January 1987.

(a) Treatment settings, particularly out-patient clinics and psychiatric units in general hospitals, were experiencing an increase in patients being diagnosed as depressed.

(b) Patients diagnosed as depressed were younger than the textbook description of depressed patients as being in middle-aged and involutional periods.

(c) Involutional melancholia, which had been a major admission diagnosis in many in-patient facilities, was being seen with decreased frequency (Weismann, 1979).

(d) Childhood depressions became the focus of considerable clinical and research attention (Kovacs *et al*, 1984).

(e) Increased attention was being given to depression in the lay press, particularly in women's magazines (Scarf, 1980).

(f) A dramatic increase was recorded in suicide attempts and in death by suicide among adolescents and young adults through the 1970s (Holinger & Offer, 1982; Klerman, 1986b).

These observations occurred during a period of increased professional and research attention to depression and affective disorders. New knowledge was being generated from investigations in genetics, psychopathology, and biological psychiatry, and from the experience with new forms of psychotherapy and new psychopharmacological agents for the treatment of depression.

The National Institute of Mental Health (NIMH) (Katz & Klerman, 1979; Katz *et al*, 1979) and the World Health Organization Division of Mental Health (Sartorius *et al*, 1983) initiated large multicentre studies to investigate the symptomatology, diagnosis, and classification of depression and to document its clinical course and natural history.

Changes in the official diagnostic and classification systems were also under way. In 1980 the American Psychiatric Association issued the third edition of its *Diagnostic and Statistical Manual* (DSM-III), which abandoned the major classification division between psychotic and neurotic conditions and created a separate category for affective disorders. Similarly, the draft of the tenth edition of the World Health Organization *International Classification of Diseases* (ICD-10) proposes a new category for mood disorders.

In retrospect, these professional and scientific activities, while valid in their own right, probably reflected changes in the frequency of depression, particularly among adolescents and young adults. This paper will review the theoretical and methodological problems encountered in testing hypotheses about changes in rates of mental illness, and in assessing the evidence, showing that there have been recent changes in the rates of depression and in its age distribution.

TEMPORAL OR SECULAR TRENDS:
AGE, PERIOD, AND COHORT EFFECTS

Documenting and explaining possible temporal trends is usually considered within the province of epidemiology—the medical science concerned with the distribution of disease in populations, and the variations in those distributions by factors of time, place, and person. Variations in rates over time are usually referred to as temporal or secular trends or changes (MacMahon & Pugh, 1970; Susser *et al*, 1985). Temporal trends are well established in the epidemiology of many medical disorders, such as Parkinson's disease, coronary artery disease, and forms of cancer (Frost, 1939; Case, 1956; Day & Charnay, 1982; Magnus, 1982).

Changes in the rates of mental illness may have also occurred (Hafner, 1985). During the first half of the twentieth century, there were decreases in the frequency of general paresis caused by CNS syphilis and in the psychiatric complications of pellagra, changes due to effective treatments of the infectious and nutritional causes of these disorders. In the past decade, the frequency of Acquired Immune Deficiency Syndrome (AIDS) has been increasing dramatically in North America and Africa, along with increases in its major psychiatric complication, the AIDS dementia syndrome.

Temporal trends are usually divided into three types—age, period, and cohort effects—and their interactions (Holford, 1983; Susser *et al*, 1985).

Age effect refers to the frequency of a disorder varying with age. An example of age effect would be Alzheimer's disease, which is rare below the age of 50, and which increases in rates after the age of 60, with further increases in the "old old," those over age 75. As changes occur in the age distribution of the general population—which is the case in most industrialized nations—the prevalence of Alzheimer's disease may increase, but that does not necessarily mean there has been a change in the age-specific incidence.

Cohort effect refers to effects among individuals defined by some temporal experience, effects which are usually sustained over the life of the cohort. The most common cohorts are those defined by year or decade of birth. An example would be the experience of the "baby boom" population cohorts showing increased rates of suicide as they entered adolescence and young adulthood (Offer *et al*, 1984).

Period effect refers to changes in rates of a disease during a particular time period, usually defined in terms of months or years, seldom more than a decade. Period effects are the basis for the popular term "epidemics." The epidemic may be due to an infectious agent, as in the bubonic plague, which decimated the population of Western Europe in the fourteenth century. Another period effect was the large number of deaths due to radiation after the dropping of atomic bombs to Hiroshima and Nagasaki by U.S. aircraft in the summer of 1945. Psychiatric examples would include the increase in Parkinson's disease due to CNS viral infections after World War I, and the impact of episodes of unemployment on suicide rates (MacMahon et al, 1963; Cormier & Klerman, 1985).

Age-period interactions occur if the impact of the period effect varies with age-related vulnerability, as reflected in recent increases in substance abuse in adolescents (O'Malley et al, 1984).

There are complex statistical problems associated with making independent estimates of age, period, and cohort effects. Distinguishing birth cohort effects from age-period interactions can be conceptually and statistically difficult (Holford, 1983; Feinberg & Mason, 1983); however, a number of investigators are working on this problem. Lavori has extended Feinberg's mathematical model to data on depression (Lavori et al, 1987). Feinberg's model has recently been applied to data on anorexia nervosa (Williams & King, 1987). Reich et al (1987) and Rice et al (1984) have incorporated these temporal effects into mathematical models of genetic transmission using information from pedigrees, and Weissman and Wickramaratne are collaborating with Holford on analyses of temporal trends in data from the NIMH Epidemiologic Catchment Area (ECA) Study (Wickramaratne et al, 1987).

DEPRESSION AND AGEING

In applying these epidemiological concepts and statistical methods to depression, it is useful at this point to examine the age distribution of rates of depression. The conventional wisdom has been that depression increases with age. If this were true, it would be reflected in the hypothetical data depicted in Fig. 1. In this figure, three rates of depression are depicted: current (or point) prevalence; incidence (new cases appearing in a finite time, such as per year); and lifetime prevalence (or cumulative incidence), an estimate of all individuals who would have experienced an episode of depression up to the age of assessment. These data are based on a hypothetical survey of a sample of the population in which rates of depression are plotted against current age.

The expected increase of depression with ageing has intuitive "face validity." As individuals grow older, they experience more losses due to deaths of relatives, friends, and other important persons; children grow up, become independent and move away; with age there is increased likelihood of medical illness and limitation of activity, and of infirmity and disability; with retirement there is often a decrease in economic resources and income, as well as a loss of social status; and, perhaps more significantly, the elderly individuals anticipate their own death and the awareness of human mortality increases.

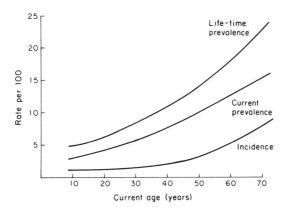

FIG. 1   Risk factors for depression: expected age effect.

Figure 1. Risk factors for depression: expected age effect.

The expected increase in depression among the elderly in response to these biological and social changes is often explained by reference to psychodynamic concepts of object loss and narcissism. Social/psychological interpretations have focused upon lessening of attachment bonds through 'disengagements' (Neugarten, 1975).

Depending on the measure of frequency of depression used, the conventional wisdom is supported by the data. Current prevalence can be assessed either by symptom scales or by categorical diagnosis. When current prevalence is assessed by symptom scales, such as the Zung Scale or the CES-D in community surveys, there is an ageing effect: the elderly report more current depressive symptoms. However, when clinical diagnostic categories are assessed using structured interviews, such as the Diagnostic Interview Schedule (DIS) (Robins *et al*, 1984), Present State Examination (PSE) (Wing *et al*, 1974) or the Schedule for Affective Disorders and Schizophrenia (SADS) (Endicott & Spitzer, 1978), coupled with diagnostic algorithms, such as CATEGO Research Diagnostic Criteria (RDC) or the DSM-III, then, surprisingly, there is no increase of prevalence with age. In fact, the highest prevalence of depression disorder is found to occur among young adults: the elderly population actually shows a falling off in rates of current disorder (Weissman *et al*, 1986).

Also, surprisingly, when the age distribution of lifetime prevalence depression from large samples was analyzed, the data did not behave according to expectations of ageing effect. Fig. 2 depicts data from a sample of over 2500 relatives of probands in the NIMH Collaborative Program on the Psychobiology of Depression Study. The SADS-L interview was used and diagnosis of major depression was made according to the RDC. The subjects were assessed as to whether they had ever had an episode meeting the RDC criteria for major depressive disorder at any time in their life up to the time of the interview; if so, age of onset was determined. Fig. 2 shows the distribution of those ever having experienced major depression by age of individuals at the time of interview. Were an uncomplicated age effect operating, the curve should have shown increased lifetime prevalence depression in the elderly. However, on the contrary, there was less lifetime prevalence depression reported by the elderly than by younger subjects.

It could be argued that these data are from a biased sample, since they derive from interviews with relatives of probands who are patients with major affective disorders. However, almost identical age trends were reported in 1975 in New Haven (Weissman & Myers, 1978) and have also been observed in the NIMH-ECA study (Robins *et al*, 1984). Similar trends have also been reported by Hagnell from the Lundby Study (Hagnell *et al*, 1982). The lifetime prevalence rates of depression are higher in relatives of patients than in the general population; the age distributions are comparable whether the data derive from community surveys or from high-risk family samples.

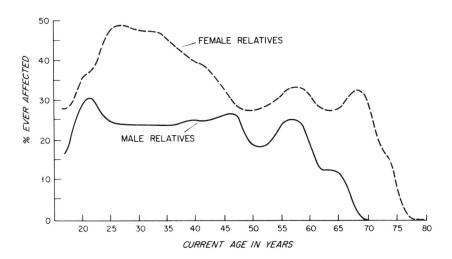

Figure 2. Percentage of probands' relatives affected with major depressive disorder (MDD), bipolar I (BPI), or bipolar II (BPII), for probands with MDD, BPI, or BPII.

TESTING HYPOTHESES REGARDING INCREASED
RATES OF DEPRESSION

These findings are incompatible with an uncomplicated ageing effect. Therefore, some form of period or cohort effect must be operating.

Ideal Designs: Successive Birth
Cohorts Studied Prospectively

Longitudinal follow-up is far superior to conventional cross-sectional design, whether of a community population or of a high-rate family sample. However, even longitudinal designs have some limitations for the detection of secular trends.

The ideal design would involve multiple samples of successive cohorts defined either at birth, after puberty, or in mid-adolescence (before the period of risk for depression), who would be followed up and assessed periodically, using systematic assessments which allowed for the detection of age of onset and of case criteria for selective disorders, particularly depression, and also for those conditions with high degrees of co-morbidity, including alcoholism, drug abuse, and anxiety disorders.

The conduct of prospective multiple cohort studies would, obviously, be expensive and time-consuming. However, the methodologies for sampling the survey techniques and for establishing psychiatric diagnosis by standardized interview have improved considerably, so that it is not unreasonable to imagine such undertakings in the near future. Just as modern nations currently maintain ongoing data collection and report statistical analyses for population change (births, deaths, fertility), and for economic indicators (unemployment, GNP, inflation), in the not-too-distant future, ongoing collections of indices of general health and of mental health, including rates of specific disorders (such as alcoholism, drug abuse, and depression) and related phenomena (such as suicide) will become standard. With such designs, it would be possible to generate a series of curves depicting the cumulative probability of reaching criteria for a given disorder up to an established time point.

As shown in Fig. 3, if there were an uncomplicated age effect, it would be manifested in data presented. If the temporal trends, as suggested earlier, included earlier age of onset, then the evidence from samples of multiple birth cohorts would show no increase in rate and an earlier age of onset. Alternatively, there could be temporal trends in which the age of onset remained constant, but the total rates of depression increased across cohorts.

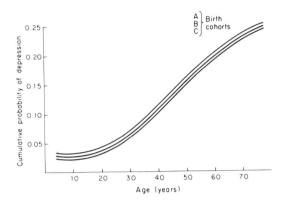

FIG. 3   Risk factors for depression: pure age effect.

Figure 3.   Risk factors for depression: pure age effect.

Approximations of Ideal Designs

While the ideal design of multiple successive birth cohorts followed longitudinally through life is not feasible at the current time, it is possible to approximate this design by use of appropriately analyzed data from currently available cross-sectional surveys, which have established lifetime prevalence and age of onset of community survey samples or family study samples.

In order to approximate designs to test hypotheses regarding temporal trends, the following characteristics are required:

(a) large samples (over 2000 subjects), including subjects from different birth cohorts; these samples could be from three sources—clinically treated patients, families of patients, and community surveys

(b) a reliable and valid assessment system which results in categorical diagnoses which are applied uniformly to all subjects in the sample

(c) information as to the age of onset, essential for reconstructing cumulative probability curves, allowing for an approximation of a prospective incidence study; reliable age of onset data is also required to test various population models for detecting possible genetic modes of transmission

(d) the technical capacity to store, process, and manage large data sets; the availability of high speed electronic computers makes this feasible

(e) statistical techniques to analyze data while controlling for variable sample size; the use of life-table statistical methods is a powerful tool in this effort

(f) appropriate statistical methods to disentangle interactions among age, period, and cohort effects.

Research Programmes which Approximate These Requirements

These requirements have been met by a number of research programmes conducted over the past few decades, utilizing samples derived from community surveys and high-risk samples derived from families of probands without affective disorders.

The community surveys include the NIMH-ECA study conducted in five areas—New Haven, St. Louis, Baltimore, North Carolina, and Los Angeles (Regier *et al,* 1984): the 25-year follow-up study from Lundby, Sweden (Hagnell *et al,* 1982); the epidemiological study of mental disorder in females in Gothenburg, Sweden (Hallstrom, 1984); and the Stirling County Study in Nova Scotia, Canada, initiated by Leighton *et al* (1963) and now being analyzed by Murphy *et al* (1986b).

The family studies include the clinical studies of the NIMH Collaborative Program on the Psychobiology of Depression (Katz & Klerman, 1979); and the Yale-NIMH Family Study, which studied large numbers of family members of patients with bipolar and unipolar disorder (Gershon *et al,* 1982).

Other studies may also be capable of being utilized in testing these hypotheses. This would include the Zurich Study of youthful cohorts now being undertaken by Angst, and the Camberwell Study in London. However, the types of analyses discussed in this paper, especially life-table statistical methods, have not been applied to the data from these samples.

EVIDENCE FOR PERIOD AND/OR COHORT EFFECTS

The evidence thus far presented indicates that the data cannot be explained by an unsophisticated age effect, and that some form of period or cohort effect must be operating. Let us now examine findings from a number of studies which are attempting to establish period and cohort effects contributing to increased rates of depression among young adults.

Evidence from Family Study of NIMH Collaborative Program on Psychobiology of Depression

The family studies of the NIMH Collaborative Program approximate the prospective multiple cohorts design. A large sample of relatives were interviewed directly using the SADS technique, and, in addition to diagnostic information, information was collected about age of onset. The findings for cumulative prevalence for males and females have already been shown in Fig. 2.

Further analyses of data presented in Fig. 2 indicated that both earlier age of onset and increased lifetime rates were present. When one compares the age of onset distributions of two birth cohorts with respect to the first episode of primary major depression, there are two significant differences: the overall prevalence is higher for the sample born in 1956 compared with that born in 1938, and there is a significant earlier age of onset for the younger cohort compared with the age of onset for the 1938 sample. The median age of onset for the 1938 sample was in the mid-to-late 30s, whereas in the 1956 sample it was in the early 20s (Reich et al, 1987).

Moreover, the sample was stratified by decade of birth cohort. Since information on date of onset was available, it was possible to compute rates of cumulative probability that individuals in given birth cohorts would have an episode meeting RDC criteria for major depressive disorder. For each successive birth cohort in the twentieth century, there are increasing cumulative rates of illness and, particularly, earlier age of onset (Klerman et al, 1985; Klerman, 1986a). The samples were further stratified by gender. The same trends are seen, but the rates for females are higher than for males.

Data from the NIMH-ECA Study

The data from the NIMH-ECA study are derived from relatives who, by virtue of familial aggregation, are at greater risk for depression (Fig. 4). Subsequent to the publication of these data in 1984, further analyses have been done on other samples. Using data from the New Haven sample of ECA, and applying life-table methodology, the results are shown in Fig. 5.

The results of the New Haven sample by birth cohort indicate increasing rates of depression for DSM-III major depression assessed by the DIS interview. Cohorts born after 1936, who reached their adulthood after World War II, have early age of onset and higher rates of depression than the cohorts born earlier in the century. In every birth cohort the rates are higher in women than in men. Since this is a community survey, the possible bias introduced by the sample of relatives from the NIMH Collaborative Study is eliminated.

Subsequently, Weissman and associates have reported data from the five U.S. communities participating in the ECA Study and found identical trends from all five sites: New Haven, Iowa City, St. Louis, Baltimore, and Chicago (Weissman et al, 1987).

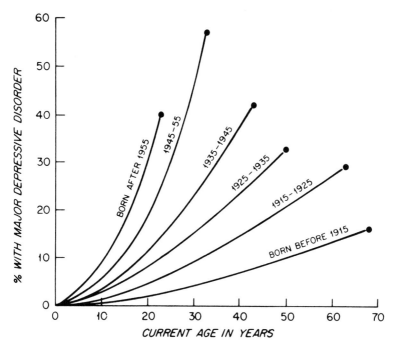

Figure 4. Cumulative probability of diagnosable major affective disorder for relatives and controls by birth cohort (life-table method).

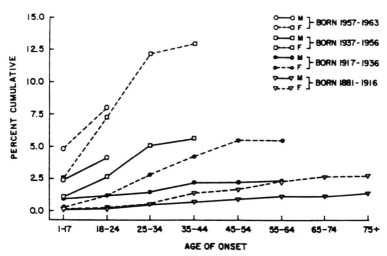

Figure 5. The affective disorders—age of first onset of major depression: results from the ECA study (reprinted from Weissman *et al* [1984]).

Gender Differences

The data on lifetime prevalence from the NIMH Collaborative Depression Study and from the NIMH-ECA study show gender difference; females show higher lifetime prevalence than males. Similarly, the life-table analyses of the data stratified by birth cohorts for both the family studies reported from the NIMH Collaborative Study and from the NIMH-ECA study (Klerman, 1986c) also show higher rates for females. Thus, the previous reports of female predominance in rates of depression (Weissman & Klerman, 1977) are substantiated by these new analyses, whether or not the data are from family samples or from community surveys. There is some suggestion that the male/female differences have narrowed in recent decades (Murphy & Wetzel, 1980; Rice *et al*, 1984).

Distinguishing Period from Cohort Effects

Having established that there has been an overall increase in depression and that there is earlier age of onset, some form of period or cohort effect must be operating.

If a period effect were operating, as has been suggested, a rise in age-specific incidence of depression during the period 1960–1980 would be evident. An age-period interaction is operating and the magnitude of a period effect is greater for the younger cohorts and less for the elder cohorts.

For the purposes of separating cohort from period effects, Lavori *et al* (1987) have analyzed the data from the siblings of probands who were under the age of 50. Temporal trends are strongly operating, especially in the younger age cohorts. Moreover, by the use of appropriate modification of Feinberg's statistical methods, a significant period effect is evident. The age-specific rates for depression were greatest in the late 1960s and 1970s. Wickramaratne *et al* (1987) also report a period effect (increase in new onsets: incidence) during the 1970s using data from the ECA community sample.

DISCUSSION

Coming to maturity in the period 1960–1975 seems to have had an adverse impact on the likelihood of depressive illness. Before discussing the possible explanations for this period effect and its implications, attention must be given to the possible artifacts which would invalidate these conclusions.

Firstly, the findings could be a consequence of selective mortality: clinically depressed persons may die at a younger age. Depressives are more likely than other persons to commit suicide; they may be more prone to other forms of selective mortality. This would mean fewer depressives still alive at the age of 60 or 70 to report current or past major episodes of depression. Moreover, depression-prone individuals could also be subject to differential mortality: they could die before becoming clinically depressed, which would further deflate the rates of depression in the elderly, particularly those with late onset (over the age of 60 or 65).

Secondly, the decline in rates among the elderly could be due to selective migration. For instance, younger individuals who have had depression, or who are prone to depression, may be more likely to have previously migrated into large cities like Boston or St. Louis, whereas less depressive-prone individuals may remain in smaller cities and in rural areas.

Thirdly, the criteria used for depression have changed. Possibly, it has been argued, RDC and DSM-III criteria are too broad. Differences in diagnostic criteria are well described, particularly differences in use between the USA and the UK, as documented in the US-UK Diagnostic Study (Kramer *et al*, 1969). Thus, use of 'major depression' as the basis for the rates reported in this set of studies from either the NIMH Collaborative Psychobiology Study or from the NIMH-ECA study may be considered to include too broad a category, particularly of cases otherwise considered 'neurotic depression', or 'situational depression', or 'demoralization'. Some researchers use more stringent diagnostic criteria based on degree of disability, hospitalization status, or treatment with biological intervention, such as drugs or ECT.

A fourth artifact is related to changes in professional attitudes, particularly the changing theoretical basis of psychiatric practice in both the UK and the USA. Psychiatrists who have worked with adolescents and young adults have, for the most part, been heavily influenced by psychoanalytic thinking and were, in the past, likely to describe depressive and anxious symptoms, but rather than consider them a nosological disorder, explain the distress in terms of psychoanalytic conflicts and dynamics. More recently, with increasing emphasis on psychopathology and the use of structured interviews for the examination of mental state, it has become apparent that conditions which previously were considered adolescent turmoil are now being diagnosed as depressive disorder. Thus, the changes in psychiatric practice could have given rise to an artificial period effect related to the decades immediately following World War II, when psychoanalytic thinking was strongest.

Fifthly, there may have been changes in the cultural or societal meaning of depression among the subjects. Such an artifact is different from the third point raised, which refers to the criteria used by the investigators. Individuals now over the age of 65, who were born before the 1920s, were raised at a time when society was not as psychologically minded as in the era since World War II, and many emotional experiences which today are considered worthy of psychiatric or medical attention were considered in earlier times the vicissitudes of human condition, God's destiny, or below the threshold for professional attention.

Sixthly, the most serious possible artifact would arise from limitations of recall and memory in the elderly. Subjects aged 65 or older may have difficulty recalling events earlier in life and may not be reliable sources of information regarding either the occurrence or age of onset of depressive phenomena, or the degree of impact of such phenomena on their social performance and personal well-being.

To test the possible artifacts created by the RDC criteria for the category 'major depressive disorders' as perhaps being too broad, Endicott has undertaken similar analyses, varying the severity of criteria for depression. Whatever criteria were chosen—hospitalization, 8-week or 12-week duration of symptoms, treated with drugs or ECT—similar trends emerged. Therefore, the findings of secular trends cannot be accounted for by overly inclusive criteria for depression in the RDC.

To circumvent the roles possibly played by selective mortality and recall and memory in the elderly, data derived only from siblings under the age of 50 were analyzed (Lavori *et al*, 1987). By restricting the sample to subjects below the age of 50, it is possible to bypass the complicated issues of differential recall, selective mortality, and problems related to different cultural attitudes toward mental illness across age cohorts.

The evidence from these and other sources indicates that these trends are not due to artifacts. While the issues of memory and recall may influence interpretation of the data for samples of individuals over the age of 50–60, the focus of this paper, on younger adults, is not called into question by memory or recall. Thus, the findings in younger adults, particularly those born since World War II, can be regarded as valid.

Gene-Environment Interactions

Just as these data cannot be explained by an uncomplicated ageing effect, they cannot be explained by a simple factor genetic theory of the aetiology of affective disorders. The evidence for a genetic factor is strong, particularly for bipolar illness, derived as it is from twin studies and cross-rearing studies in addition to familial aggregation studies. In this respect it is noteworthy that Gershon (unpublished) has recently reported evidence for a temporal effect among bipolar patients. Consequently, one must conclude that some complex form of gene-environment interaction is operating. If there is a distribution of liability to depression based on genetic determination, environmental factors must be operating to make that liability manifest in clinical illness. Whatever those environmental factors are, they have shifted, such that there are overall increases, particularly at earlier years of onset.

Most genetic models of transmission presuppose constant age of onset. The demonstration of changing age of onset in the prevalence data, both from family samples and from population surveys, requires recalculation of the appropriate statistical models. These have recently been completed and preliminary reports have been offered by Reich *et al* (1987).

In this respect, it is of note that Crow (1986) has attempted to reinterpret the evidence in secular trends with an exclusively genetic interpretation.

The findings of progressive increases in the rate of depression and earlier age of onset cannot be explained by a single-factor theory that effective illness is due only to genetic predisposition. Although depression is familial and may be genetically determined in part, current evidence does not support a specific mode of genetic transmission, whether the mode of transmission is a single major locus or is polygenic. The demonstration of temporal trends does not rule out genetic vulnerability, as demonstrated for diabetes, phenylketonuria, and other genetic disorders.

Environmental Factors: The Search for "Agent Blue"

Some complex form of gene-environment interaction is likely operating in the pathogenesis of clinical depression. The overall increase in rates, and shifts in age of onset require a multifactorial model that incorporates environmental risk factors along with genetic determinants.

A period effect has been operating since World War II to increase rates of depression. The nature of possible environmental risk factors ('Agent Blue') is not established. While most discussions of possible environmental influences focus on psychosocial factors, the possibility that depression might be caused by biological factors, such as viral agents, or by some environmental substance or nutritional change should also be considered.

The environmental risk factors could be biological, including changes in nutrition, the possible role of viruses, or the effects of an unknown depressogenic chemical agent in the water or air. Other environmental risk factors could be non-biological: historical, cultural, and economic factors have been suggested. These include urbanization, demographic fluctuation, changes in family structure, alterations in the roles of women, an increased role of women in the labour force, and shifts in occupational patterns (Easterlin, 1980; Hagnell, 1982; Murphy *et al*, 1984).

A number of hypotheses have been offered as to this 'Agent Blue'. These hypotheses include (a) demographic shifts, such as the 'baby boom' and its impact on expectations and economic labour force participation and fertility

(Easterlin, 1980), (b) changes in the ratio of males to females in the population, as stressed by Guttentag & Secord (1983), (c) increasing urbanization, (d) greater geographic mobility, with resultant loss of attachments and participation in primary face-to-face groups, and (e) increasing social anomy (Srole & Fischer, 1980).

The Mental Health Problem of
the 'Baby Boom' Generation

If the evidence for increased rates of depression among the more recent birth cohorts were exclusively for depression, it would allow for a focus search, albeit a complex one, about those social, biological, and environmental risk factors ('Agent Blue'), which might be interacting with familial factors, changes related to year of birth and gender.

Similar trends have been reported for suicide (Murphy & Wetzel, 1980; Solomon & Hellon, 1980; Holinger & Offer, 1982; Goldney & Katsikitis, 1983; Klerman, 1986b), homicide among black men (Klerman, 1980a), automobile accidents and other forms of violent death (Holinger *et al*, 1987) and substance abuse (O'Malley *et al*, 1984).

Along parallel lines, secular trends have been described for a number of important social and economic events possibly related to depression, including the age of entrance into the labour force (Easterlin, 1980; Hogan, 1981), economic earnings (Easterlin, 1980), age of marriage (Hogan, 1981), fertility (Easterlin, 1980), and age of termination of maternal child-rearing function (the 'empty nest') (Borland, 1982; Goldman *et al*, 1984).

In contrast to the apparent improvement in the economic, health, and mental health status of the elderly are the contrasting trends among the youth. This finding is of major importance, since the 'baby boom' generation now comprises almost one-third of the population.

Demographers and economists have documented the consequences of large birth cohort size and, in particular, the relationship between the size of a birth cohort and the total population (Easterlin, 1980, 1985, 1986).

Recently, attention has been given to the mental health problems encountered by the 'baby boom' generation, in addition to their economic problems and their reduction in fertility. The best documented changes are those related to suicide. In addition, there are important cohort effects with regard to drug abuse (Fowler *et al*, 1986; Murphy *et al*, 1986a).

However, in as much as the changes in rates are not specific to depression, but also involve drug abuse, suicide attempts, and suicide deaths, a comprehensive explanation would have to account not only for the increased rates among young adults of the 'baby boom' generation from the period 1960–1980, but also for the degree of diagnostic differentiation, to explain why some individuals exposed to the pathogenic factors yet to be determined manifest their clinical picture in depression, whereas others develop drug abuse or substance abuse. To further complicate matters, there are high levels of co-morbidity among many of these disorders, and a comprehensive model would have to take into effect the general increase in psychiatric morbidity for the younger population during this period, as well as the differentiated specific rates of drug abuse, eating disorder, suicide, and affective disorders.

The 'baby boom' generation has experienced increased rates of suicide, drug abuse, and depression. There are important gender and ethnic differences in these rates: females are more prone to depression, whereas males are more prone to suicide, drug abuse, and alcohol; black males are more prone to homicide, particularly with firearms; an epidemic of mental health problems has occurred in young people since 1960, with important age-period effects.

Prospects for the Future

The 'baby boom' generation is now approaching its maturity. The first 'wave' of the 'baby boom' generation is in its early 40s. It is instructive to anticipate what might be the future trends. There are a number of possibilities. One is that the current high rates of depression, suicide, and drug abuse will continue, in which case the cumulative probabilities of mental illness will rise. At this point it is important to distinguish between a specific incidence and prevalence. The prevalence of depression in this cohort may continue to increase because of chronicity and recurrences, even though the peak of insets may have already occurred.

On the other hand, it is possible that if a period effect is operative, the peak of the exposure to 'Agent Blue' has passed and there will be a decline in age-specific incidence. This seems to be the case for suicide, since the suicide rates among young adults and adolescents peaked in 1978–1980 and have been declining steadily.

In addition to tracking suicide rates, incidence of new episodes, recurrence and lifetime prevalence in the 'baby boom' generation, it will be desirable to document the comparable processes among the next generation, those individuals born subsequent to 1970. These individuals are now entering their adolescence, and if the analysis of the period effect is true, the rates of suicide attempts, death by suicide, and depression should be lower in adolescence and young adulthood. These cohorts compare with the 'baby boom' cohort. These possibilities make all the more cogent the need to maintain ongoing sampling of multiple cohorts for detection of future trends.

CONCLUSION

There are seven trends which have been documented:

(a) an increase in prevalence of depression, particularly since World War II
(b) a marked increase in depression among those in the cohorts born after World War II, adults now in their 30s and 40s
(c) an earlier age of onset of depression through the twentieth century
(d) relative to previous older cohorts, an apparent decrease in depression among adults in cohorts born before 1920, individuals now in their 60s and 70s
(e) an effect for family aggregation resulting in increased risk of depression in the first-degree relatives of ill patients, suggestive of, but not conclusively, establishing genetic transmission for certain forms of depression
(f) an increase in risk for females in rates of depression across all cohorts
(g) evidence of a period effect interacting with gender and age, such that young females were greatest at risk during the 1960s and 1970s.

The demonstration of these secular trends in depression requires that any theory of depression take into account environmental as well as genetic factors. These changes cannot be explained by an exclusively genetic theory of the origin of depression. The finding of temporal effects indicates that some complex gene-environmental interactions are under way in the pathogenesis of depression.

The possibility of a change in the rates of depression would have important clinical, public health, and theoretical implications. Clinically, demonstration of temporal trends would be of importance in helping to understand the changes in the patients coming to treatment and the need for modification of diagnostic expectations and treatment decisions. From the public health point of view, changes in rates of a disease, and in the characteristics of those afflicted, influence the techniques used for the monitoring of the aggregate health of the population, the types of data and modes of statistical reporting, plans for deployment of existing resources, and a possible search for new resources to treat the increased numbers of depressed individuals, particularly among the youthful segments of the population. Theoretically, were these temporal trends to be verified, it would raise important issues about the role of various risk factors, especially the balance of genetic and environmental processes in the genesis and perpetuation of affective disorders.

REFERENCES

American Psychiatric Association (1980) *Diagnostic and Statistical Manual of Mental Disorders* (3rd edn) (DSM-III). Washington, DC: American Psychiatric Association.

Borland, D. C. (1982) A cohort analysis approach to the 'empty nest' syndrome among three ethnic groups of women: a theoretical position. *Journal of Marriage and Family,* 117–129.

Case, R. A. M. (1956) Cohort analysis of mortality rates as an historical or narrative technique. *British Journal of Preventive Social Medicine,* **10,** 159–171.

Cormier, H. J. & Klerman, G. L. (1985) Unemployment and male-female labor force participation as determinants of changing suicide rates of males and females in Quebec. *Social Psychiatry,* **20,** 109–114.

Crow, T. J. (1986) Secular changes in affective disorder and variations in the psychosis gene. *Archives of General Psychiatry,* **43,** 1013–1014.

Day, N. E. & Charnay, B. (1982) Time trends, cohort effects and aging as influence on cancer incidence. In *Trends in Cancer Incidence* (ed. K. Magnus). New York, Washington, DC: Hemisphere.

Easterlin, R. A. (1980) *Birth and Fortune.* New York: Basic Books.

—— (1985) The struggle for economic status. Presented at the conference on Non-Replacement Fertility, Hoover Institution, Stanford University, CA, 1985.

—— (1986) "Easterlin Hypothesis." *New Palgrave.* London: Macmillan Press.

Endicott, J. & Spitzer, R. (1978) A diagnostic interview: the Schedule for Affective Disorders and Schizophrenia. *Archives of General Psychiatry,* **35,** 773–782.

Feinberg, S. E. & Mason, W. M. (1983) Discrete archival data: age period cohort effects for vital rates. *Biometrics,* **39,** 311–324.

Fowler, R. C., Rich, C. L. & Young, D. (1986) San Diego Suicide Study: II. Substance abuse in young cases. *Archives of General Psychiatry,* **43,** 962–968.

Frost, W. H. (1939) The age selection of mortality from tuberculosis in successive decades. *American Journal of Hygiene,* **30,** 91–96.

Gershon, E. S., Hamovit, J. & Guroff, J. (1982) A family study of schizophrenia, bipolar I, bipolar II, unipolar and normal controls. *Archives of General Psychiatry,* **39,** 1157–1167.

Goldman, N., Westoff, C. F. & Hammerslough, C. (1984) Demography of the marriage market in the United States. *Population Index,* **50,** 5–25.

Goldney, R. D. & Katsikitis, M. (1983) Cohort analysis of suicide rates in Australia. *Archives of General Psychiatry,* **40,** 71–74.

Guttentag, M. & Secord, P. F. (1983) *Too Many Women: The Sex Ratio Question.* Beverly Hills: Sage Publications.

Hafner, H. (1985) Are mental disorders increasing over time? *Psychobiology,* **18,** 66–81.

Hagnell, O. (1982) The 25 year follow-up of the Lundby Study: incidence and risk of alcoholism, depression and disorders of the senium. In *Mental Disorders in the Community* (eds J. Barrett & R. M. Rose). New York: Guilford Press.

——, Lanke, J., Rorsman, B. & Ojesjo, L. (1982) Are we entering an age of melancholy? Depressive illnesses in a prospective epidemiological study over 25 years: the Lundby Study, Sweden. *Psychological Medicine,* **12,** 279–289.

Hallstrom, T. (1984) Point prevalence of major depressive disorder in a Swedish urban female population. *Acta Psychiatrica Scandinavica,* **69,** 52–59.

Hogan, D. P. (1981) *Transition and Social Change: the Early Lives of American Men.* New York: Academic Press.

Holford, T. R. (1983) The estimation of age, period and cohort effects for vital rates. *Biometrics,* **39,** 311–324.

Holinger, P. C. & Offer, D. (1982) Prediction of adolescent suicide: a population model. *American Journal of Psychiatry,* **139,** 302–306.

——, —— & Zola, M. A. (1987) A prediction model of suicide among youth. *Science* (in press).

Katz, M. M. & Klerman, G. L. (1979) Introduction overview of the Clinical Studies Program of the NIMH Clinical Research Branch Collaborative Study on the Psychobiology of Depression. *American Journal of Psychiatry,* **136,** 49–51.

——, Secunda, S. K., Hirschfield, R. M. A. & Koslow, S. H. (1979) NIMH Clinical Research Branch Collaborative Program on the psychobiology of depression. *Archives of General Psychiatry,* **36,** 765–771.

Klerman, G. L. (1976) Age and clinical depression: today's youth in the 21st century. *Journal of Gerontology,* **31,** 318–323.

—— (1979) The age of melancholy. *Psychology Today,* **12,** 36–42, 88.

—— (1980a) Homicide among black males: concluding remarks. *Public Health Reports No. 6,* **95,** 549–550.

—— (1980b) Adaptation, depression and transitional life events. In *Adolescent Psychiatry* (eds S. C. Feinstein, P. L. Govacchini, P. L. J. Golooney and A. Z. Schwartzberg). Chicago, Illinois: Chicago University Press.

—— (1986a) Evidence for increases in rates of depression in North America and Western Europe in recent decades. In *New Results in Depression Research* (eds H. Hippius, G. L. Klerman and N. Matussek). Berlin/Heidelberg/New York: Springer.

—— (ed.) (1986b) *Suicide and Depression Among Adolescents and Young Adults.* Washington, DC: American Psychiatric Press.

—— (1986c) The National Institute of Mental Health—Epidemiologic Catchment Area (NIMH-ECA) Program. *Social Psychiatry,* **21,** 159–166.

——, Lavori, P. W., Rice, J., Reich, T., Endicott, J., Andreasen, N. C., Keller, M. B. & Hirschfeld, R. M. A. (1985) Birth cohort trends in rates of major depressive disorder among relatives of patients with affective disorder. *Archives of General Psychiatry,* **42,** 689–695.

Kovaks, M., Feinberg, T. L., Crouse-Novak, M. A., Paulauskas, S. L. & Finkelstein, R. (1984) *Archives of General Psychiatry,* **41,** 229–237.

Kramer, M., Zubin, J. & Cooper, J. E. (1969) Cross-national study of diagnosis of the mental disorders. *American Journal of Psychiatry,* **125, Suppl.,** 1–46.

Lavori, P., Klerman, G. L., Keller, M., Reich, T., Rice, J. & Endicott, J. (1987) Age period cohort analyses of secular trends in onset of major depression: findings in siblings of patients with major affective disorder. *Journal of Psychiatric Research,* **21,** 23–35.

Leighton, D., Harding, J. *et al* (1963) Psychiatric findings of the Stirling County study. *American Journal of Psychiatry,* **119,** 1021–1031.

MacMahon, B., Johnson, S. & Pugh, T. F. (1963) Relationship of suicide rates to social conditions. *Public Health Report,* **78,** 285–293.

——, B. & Pugh, T. F. (1970) *Epidemiology: Principles and Methods.* Boston: Little Brown.

Magnus, K. (ed.) (1982) *Trends in Cancer Incidence.* New York, Washington, DC: Hemisphere.

Murphy, G. E. & Wetzel, R. D. (1980) Suicide risk by birth cohort in the United States. *Archives of General Psychiatry,* **37,** 519–523.

——, J. M., Sobol, A. M., Neff, R. K., Olivier, D. C. & Leighton, A. H. (1984) Stability of prevalence. *Archives of General Psychiatry,* **41,** 990–997.

——, E., Lindesay, J. & Grundy, E. (1986a) 60 years of suicide in England and Wales. *Archives of General Psychiatry,* **43,** 969–977.

——, J. M., Olivier, D. C., Sobol, A. M., Monson, R. R. & Leighton, A. H. (1986b) Diagnosis and outcome: depression and anxiety in a general population. *Psychological Medicine,* **16,** 117–126.

Neugarten, B. L. (1975) Adult personality: toward a psychology of the life cycle. In *Human Life Cycle* (ed. W. C. Sze). New York: James Aronson.

Offer, D., Ostrov, E. & Howard, K. I. (1984) Epidemiology of mental health illness among adolescents. In *Significant Advances in Child Psychiatry* (ed. J. Call). New York: Basic Books.

O'Malley, P. M., Bachman, J. G. & Johnston, L. D. (1984) Period, age and cohort effects on substance use among American youth, 1976–82. *American Journal of Public Health,* **74,** 682–688.

Regier, D. A., Myers, J. K., Kramer, M., Robins, L. N., Blazer, D. G., Hough, R. L., Eaton, W. W. & Locke, B. Z. (1984) The NIMH epidemiologic catchment area program. *Archives of General Psychiatry,* **41,** 934–941.

Reich, T., Van Eerdewegh, P., Rice, J. & Mullaney, J. (1987) The familial transmission of primary major depressive disorder. *Journal of Psychiatric Review* (in press).

Rice, J., Reich, T. & Andreasen, N. C. (1984) Sex-related differences in depression: familial evidence. *Journal of Affective Disorders,* **7,** 199–210.

Robins, L. N., Helzer, J. E., Weissman, M. M., Orvaschel, H., Gruenberg, E., Burke, J. D. & Regier, D. A. (1984) Lifetime prevalence of specific psychiatric disorders in three sites. *Archives of General Psychiatry,* **41,** 949–958.

Sartorius, N., Davidian, H., Ernberg, G., Fenton, F. R., Fujii, I. *et al* (1983) *Depressive Disorders in Different Cultures: Report on the WHO Collaborative Study on Standardized Assessment of Depressive Disorders.* Geneva: World Health Organization.

Scarf, M. (1980) *Unfinished Business.* New York: Basic Books.

Schwab, J. J. (1974) Perception of social change and depressive symptomatology. In *Social Psychiatry,* Vol. 1 (eds J. H. Masserman & J. J. Schwab). New York: Grune and Stratton.

Solomon, M. I. & Hellon, C. P. (1980) Suicide and age in Alberta, Canada, 1951–1977. *Archives of General Psychiatry,* **37,** 511–513.

Srole, L. & Fischer, A. K. (1980) The Midtown Manhattan longitudinal study vs the Mental Paradise Lost Doctrine. *Archives of General Psychiatry,* **37,** 209–221.

Susser, M., Watson, W. & Hopper, K. (1985) *Sociology in Medicine* (3rd edn). New York/Oxford: Oxford University Press.

Weissman, M. M. (1979) Myth of involutional melancholia. *Journal of American Medical Association,* **242,** 742–744.

—— & Klerman, G. L. (1977) Sex differences and the epidemiology of depression. *Archives of General Psychiatry,* **34,** 98–111.

—— & Myers, J. K. (1978) Affective disorders in a United States urban community: the use of Research Diagnostic Criteria in an epidemiologic survey. *Archives of General Psychiatry,* **35,** 1304–1311.

——, Leaf, P. J., Holzer, III, C. E., Myers, J. K. & Tischler, G. L. (1984) The epidemiology of depression: an update on sex differences in rates. *Journal of Affective Disorders,* **7,** 179–188.

——, Myers, J. K., Leaf, P. J., Tischler, G. L. & Holzer, C. E. (1986) The affective disorders: results from the Epidemiologic Catchment Area (ECA). In *New Results in Depression Research* (eds. H. Hippius, G. L. Klerman & N. Matussek). Berlin/Heidelberg: Springer.

——, Leaf, P. J., Tischler, G. L. *et al* (1987) Affective disorders in 5 United States communities. *Psychological Medicine* (in press).

Wickramaratne, P. J., Weissman, M. M., Leaf, P. J. & Holford, T. R. (1987) Age, period cohort effects on the risk of major depression: results from 5 United States communities (in press).

Williams, P. & King, M. (1987) The epidemic of anorexia nervosa: another medical myth? *The Lancet, i,* 205–207.

Wing, J. K., Cooper, J. E. & Sartorius, N. (1974) *The Measurement and Classification of Psychiatric Symptoms.* London: Cambridge University Press.

22

Childhood and Adolescent Depression II: Research in Clinical Populations

Adrian Angold
Institute of Psychiatry, London

The tremendous increase in interest in childhood and adolescent depression that has occurred since the early 1970s has resulted in a large and contradictory literature. Development of the concept of childhood depression, and the many clinical studies of depression and its concomitants, both psychosocial and biological, are critically reviewed. A number of methodological and theoretical problems are discussed.

The ICD-9 classification of child psychiatric disorders (Rutter *et al*, 1975) includes no less than 14 diagnoses that require the presence of depressive symptoms, but in 1982 Puig-Antich & Gittelman noted a telling absence of references to depression in textbooks of child psychiatry until recently. Furthermore, despite the sizeable literature that now exists on the subject (Cantwell & Carlson, 1983; Rutter *et al*, 1986), childhood depression is far from being firmly established as a diagnosis as far as many clinicians are concerned. Indeed, there is evidence that the diagnosis is often not made even in the presence of severe depressive symptoms (Friedman *et al*, 1982; Gammon *et al*, 1983). However, it is also true that there are very marked deficiencies in our knowledge, and the adoption of unmodified adult criteria for depression in young people begs a number of important developmental questions (Eisenberg, 1986; Rutter, 1986a,b). This paper reviews the present state of our knowledge in this rapidly changing field.

Reprinted with permission from the *British Journal of Psychiatry*, 1988, Vol. 153, 476–492. Copyright 1988 by the Royal College of Psychiatrists.

The author would like to thank Professor M. Rutter and Dr. Dale Hay. This work was undertaken during an MRC Training Fellowship held in the MRC Child Psychiatry Unit at the Institute of Psychiatry, London.

THE RECENT DEVELOPMENT OF THE
CONCEPT OF DEPRESSION IN YOUNG PEOPLE

Notwithstanding Thomas Hardy's terrifying portrayal of little Jude in *Jude the Obscure* (1896), until recently it was generally held that depression was extremely rare, and possibly non-existent, in childhood. The latter position was developed by psychoanalytical theorists who held that since depression was the product of a persecutory superego, it could not occur in pre-adolescents, who were supposed to lack mature superego structures (Rie, 1966). Depression was said to emerge as a discrete phenomenon only during adolescence, and to be relatively uncommon even then.

This position was maintained even in the face of some empirical evidence to the contrary and clinical descriptions of manic-depressive illness in children (Sadler, 1952; Campbell, 1952; Harms, 1952; Anthony & Scott, 1960). Furthermore, even some psychoanalytic formulations recognized a capacity for depression in children of 'latency age' (Anthony & Scott, 1960; Sandler & Joffe, 1965; Anthony, 1967; Glaser, 1967) and before. Abraham (1911, 1949) referred to a form of pre-Oedipal infantile depression as 'primal parathymia', and Fenichel (1945) suggested that equivalent disturbances could arise in the first year of life. Spitz's description of 'anaclitic depression' (Spitz, 1946) drew on these theoretical positions and described several features as being characteristic of depression arising after separation from the mother during the first year or so of life, these being: 1. apprehension, sadness, weepiness; 2. lack of contact, rejection of the environment, withdrawal; 3. retardation of development, retardation of reaction to stimuli, slowness of movement, dejection, stupor; 4. loss of appetite, refusal to eat, loss of weight; 5. insomnia; and 6. depressed physiognomic expression.

Spitz suggested that very severe developmental delays could result from unrelieved separations, but his assessment techniques left a good deal to be desired in the way of rigour, especially in that such effects might not have been due to the object loss directly but to secondary phenomena springing from the loss, or its concomitant features, such as poverty, a reduced standard of care, or physical illness (Pinneau, 1955; Rutter, 1980, 1986a). He also took pains to distinguish his descriptions of anaclitic depression from Klein's (1975) concept of the 'depressive position', which, far from being a pathological phenomenon, is a cornerstone of human development according to Kleinian thinking. Related approaches, among which Bowlby's (1969) has been the most influential, have led to a considerable debate about the relationships between attachment, separation, and depression, which is still far from being settled as far as either adult or childhood depressions are concerned. Although his and Robertson & Robertson's (1971) descriptions of young children's reactions to separations from their parents have influenced hospital admission policies very considerably, the final separation stage of 'despair' need by no means be interpreted as being a manifestation of depression as it is usually understood in adult psychiatry (Rutter, 1986a).

By the end of the 1960s, studies were documenting the presence of marked levels of 'depressive' symptoms in clinically referred young people. These observations led to the suggestion that if children had symptoms that resembled those of adult depressive patients, then it was reasonable to diagnose them accordingly as being depressed (Frommer, 1968; Poznanski & Zrull, 1970; Annell, 1969a,b; Cytryn & McKnew, 1972). We might note that Kraepelin himself had described such patients and reported that 4% of his manic-depressive cases had first episodes before the age of 10 (Kraepelin, 1921). However, it was also observed that miserable children often had symptoms that would not be regarded as depressive symptoms in adulthood, such as enuresis or refusal to attend school. In fact, an extremely wide range of associated pathology was described in relation to depression (Murray, 1970), and the suggestion arose that depression in children might not be manifested exactly as it was in adulthood, but instead be represented by a variety of *formes frustes* which masked their true depressive origins (Toolan, 1962; Glaser, 1967; Frommer, 1968; Cytryn & McKnew, 1972).

Cytryn & McKnew (1972) proposed a tripartite classification of childhood neurotic depressions as 'acute', 'chronic' or 'masked', with the last of these being the most common. They suggested that masked depressive reactions were most commonly seen in children with severe personality and family psychopathology, while acutely and chronically depressed children were differentiated from each other by the poor premorbid adjustment and histories of recurrent parental depression found in the latter. The concept of masked depression represented an attempt to encompass the possibility that types of depression might have different presentations and psychopathological correlates at different ages, and to provide a theoretical framework for understanding co-morbidity in relation to depression. However, it soon became apparent that there were fatal flaws in the reasoning underlying its formulation. Firstly, the boundaries of masked depression gradually became extended to the point where almost any form of childhood disorder could be considered as a mask. Anorexia nervosa, obesity, enuresis, hyperactivity, and even neurological soft signs were implicated (Malmquist, 1972; Lachenmeyer, 1982; Ossofsky, 1974). Furthermore, in order to make this diagnosis, some depressive symptoms had to be observed, in which case the depression could not really be said to be masked at all (Kovacs & Beck, 1977). Thus the real issue was not one of masking, but of the association of unhappiness with a wide range of disorders, and the problem was to identify specific depressive disorders from this poorly differentiated morass. However, as we shall see, the problems of comorbidity and the possibility of age-dependent phenomenological differences in the presentation of types of depression have tended to be shelved rather than solved by later work (Lefkowitz & Burton, 1978).

PHENOMENOLOGY AND PREVALENCE
IN REFERRED POPULATIONS

Table 1 presents some details of those studies that report rates of depression in clinically referred populations. As might be expected, the majority of reports are based on children referred specifically for psychiatric evaluation, and here the reported rates vary from 0 to 61%. The four studies reporting rates under 5% are atypical, however. Three of them are among the earliest studies considered here, and they do not employ clearly defined diagnostic criteria (Poznanski & Zrull, 1970; Cebiroglu *et al*, 1972; Makita, 1973). Kashani *et al* (1984) report that 4% of their sample were at least possibly depressed, but they were assessing only pre-school children.

On the whole, since the mid-1970s, diagnostic criteria have been more carefully specified and put into operation. This has led to the adoption of unmodified DSM-III (American Psychiatric Association, 1980) criteria by many workers. Lobovits & Handal (1985) found that the DSM-III criteria resulted in lower rates of depression being diagnosed than did the Weinberg criteria (Ling *et al*, 1970), which include such items as school phobia, poor school performance, and aggressive behaviour in addition to more 'adult'-type depressive symptoms. The use of more stringent criteria, such as the Research Diagnostic Criteria (RDC) of Spitzer *et al* (1978), not surprisingly results in lower overall rates of depression being reported (see Poznanski *et al*, 1985, for a detailed comparison of the DSM-III, RDC, Weinberg, and Poznanski criteria). In general, considering the more recent studies, based on direct research interviews and using specified diagnostic criteria, the rates for severe and quite longlasting types of depression seem to be around 5–15%, while unmodified DSM-III criteria yield rates around 15–30%. Studies reporting higher rates than this have usually used either the Weinberg criteria or have not been based on direct interviews, but have used self-report symptom scales instead. However, the problem remains that we do not know which are the best criteria for use with children and adolescents, or which best describe phenomena that are either persistent or directly linked to adult depression.

It is worth noting at this stage that high levels of depressive symptoms have been noted in children referred to an educational diagnostic unit (Weinberg *et al*, 1973), and Kolvin *et al* (1984) considered that 45% of their 51 cases of school phobia showed significant depression. Thus the possibility of depression should be borne in mind in children who present with other behavioural

Author	n	Unit[1]	Age	Assessment	Diagnostic system	Percentage depressed
Frommer (1968)	About 760	O/P	2–16 years	Unspecified clinical	Not stated	~ 10[2]
Poznanski & Zrull (1970)	1788	O/P	3–12 years	Case-note assessments of cases selected by item sheet evidence of marked 'depression'	Evidence of chronic 'affective depression'	0.8 (much greater percentage thought probably depressed)
Ling et al (1970)	25	Neurology clinic with headache and no neurological illness	4–16 years	Record review ± interviews with family	Weinberg criteria	40
Cebiroglu et al (1972)	10 661	O/P	3–16 years	Unspecified clinical assessment	Not stated	0.8
Stack (1972)	About 4500	O/P	Preschool and adolescent	Unspecified clinical assessment	Not stated	11
Makita (1973)	About 3000	O/P	Children to adolescents	Unspecified clinical assessment	Not stated	0
Weinberg et al (1973)	72	Educational diagnostic centre	6–13 years	Paediatric neurologist's assessment	Weinberg	58 49 current 9 past
McConville et al (1973)	141	I/P	6–13 years	Case-note assessment of first 6 weeks of admission	Children described as 'depressed' on symptom list	53
Hudgens (1974)	110	I/P	'Older adolescents', mean age = 16	Clinical assessment	Feigner criteria for manic–depressive psychosis (Feigner et al, 1972)	12
Pearce (1977)	547	O/P	3–17 years	Case-note item-sheet ratings	Symptom of 'morbid depression' empirical syndrome	23
Petti (1978)	73	I/P	6–12.5 years	Clinician's impressions, Bellevue index of depression, Weinberg Index of Depression	Clinician ratings Unspecified BID[3]	61 (clinician's ratings) 59 (BID)
Puig-Antich et al (1978)	—	I/P and O/P	6–12 years	Parent interview about child supplemented by CPRS[3]	RDC	13 children; base population size not stated
Kuperman & Stewart (1979)	372 175	I/P and O/P	7–16 years	Half of group diagnosed by chart and half (175) consecutive O/P or ward admissions diagnosed by structured interviews with parents	Feigner (adapted)	6 (girls = 13) (boys = 5)
Carlson & Cantwell (1980)	210	I/P and O/P	11.6 s.d.2.9	102 = semistructured interview with parent and child	DSM–III	16, O/Ps 36, I/Ps
Strober et al (1981)	150	I/P	12–17 years	SADS and review of all available records	DSM–III	27
Kashani et al (1981)	100	Chronic physical disability admitted for orthopaedic procedures	7–12 years	Semi-structured interview with parent and child. Chart review	DSM–III	23
Friedman et al (1982)	76	I/P	13–19 years	Chart review	DSM–III	59
Kashani et al (1982)	100	Paediatric cardiology O/P	6–18 years	Semistructured interviews with parent and child	DSM–III	13 (100% of lone chest pain)
Gammon et al (1983)	17	I/P	13–18 years	K-SADS-E	DSM–III, and Bipolar I and II	29
Kazdin et al (1983a,b)	104	I/P	5–13 years	Psychiatric interviews with parent and child	DSM–III	19
Weller et al (1983)	100	I/P and O/P psychiatric and paediatric referrals	12–15 years	Structured interviews with mother and child	Feighner criteria	9
Feinstein et al (1984)	224	O/P	4–16 years	Semi-structured clinical evaluation with parents and child	DSM–III	21
Kashani et al (1984)	100	Child development unit	1–6 years	Extensive 2 day clinical evaluation	DSM–III	1–4
Kolvin et al (1984)	51	School phobics presenting at child psychiatry clinic	9–14 years	Clinical assessment	'Significant depression'	45
Kazdin et al (1985)	79	I/P	6–13 years	Interview with parents and child and I/P evaluation	DSM–III	9
Lobovits & Handal (1985)	50	O/P	8–12 years	Unspecified clinical assessment, PIC-D, CDI[3]	DSM–III Weinberg criteria	22 (parent) 34 (child) 50 (Weinberg)

1. O/P = out-patients, I/P = in-patients.
2. Frommer reports on "enuretic depressives", "phobic depressives", and "uncomplicated depressives". This value refers only to the last of these groups.
3. BID = Belleview Index of Depression; CPRS = Children's Psychiatric Rating Scale; PIC-D = Personality Inventory for Children – Depression Scale; CDI = Children's Depression Inventory.

Table 1. Summary of Studies Reporting Rates of Depression in Referred Populations

or educational difficulties, and specific questioning aimed at eliciting affective disturbance should be part of the assessment of every child psychiatric patient.

It might have been expected that older children and psychiatric in-patients would show higher rates of depression than younger children and out-patients, but the studies considered here do not, in general, provide support for these suggestions. On the other hand, neither were they usually designed to test them. However, Pearce (1977, 1978) found that the 23% of children rated as having the symptom of depression were older than the non-depressive group. Furthermore, depressed mood was more common in the pre-pubertal boys than the pre-pubertal girls, but the opposite was the case in the post-pubertal group (Rutter, 1986a).

PROBLEMS WITH STUDIES OF PHENOMENOLOGY AND PREVALENCE IN REFERRED POPULATIONS

Questions of phenomenology and prevalence are inextricably linked, since the rate of occurrence of a disorder will depend directly on how it is defined. The sources of the phenomenological information employed in making the diagnosis also affect the rates obtained (Orvaschel *et al*, 1982; Angold *et al*, 1987). A number of studies have looked at teacher, parent, and child reporting of psychiatric symptoms and found that, in general, teachers and parents report more 'externalizing' or conduct problems than their children report about themselves, while the opposite is true as far as 'internalizing' or emotional symptoms are concerned (Leon *et al*, 1980; Cytryn *et al*, 1980; Weissman *et al*, 1980; Orvaschel *et al*, 1981; Reich *et al*, 1982; Herjanic & Reich, 1982; Moretti *et al*, 1985; Lobovits & Handal, 1985; Edelbrock *et al*, 1985, 1986). It has also been shown that a pattern of low sensitivity and high specificity is characteristic of parental reports of their children's depressive symptoms (Orvaschel *et al*, 1982; Angold *et al*, 1987). In these respects, the pattern of reporting for emotional disorders in children parallels that found for the reporting of similar disorders in adults, in that secondary informants report less symptoms than the patients themselves, but relatively rarely report the presence of affective disorders that are not present according to the subjects themselves. This pattern has proved quite highly consistent and I am aware of only two dissenting studies: Kazdin *et al* (1983a,b) found that parents reported more depressive symptoms in their severely disturbed, inpatient children than the children reported about themselves, and Mokros *et al* (1987) found that parents reported more severe depression in children referred to an affective-disorders clinic than the children did themselves. However, the latter authors found a non-significant trend in the opposite direction in a group of unreferred 6–12-year-old schoolchildren. So it may be that very severely disturbed children tend to underrate their depression, but that the opposite is true with normal or moderately disturbed children (see Angold *et al,* 1987, for a fuller discussion of this issue).

The message of most of these studies is that if parents' or teachers' reports are relied upon as the major source of diagnostic information, then the rates of depression found in the children will, in most circumstances, be lower than if children's self-reports are more heavily weighted. In fact, very considerable misery may be ignored if parent reports are taken as the criterion for the presence of affective symptoms. On the other hand, if the parents say that their child is depressed, then the clinician should take their opinion very seriously, because the child is very likely to agree, although perhaps to underreport the degree of misery when most disturbed.

A number of studies have employed diagnostic instruments such as the Kiddie-SADS (Puig-Antich & Chambers, 1978) (see Table I), which require that summary ratings of the presence of symptoms based on information from both parent and child be made, and it seems at least possible that the process of integration of information from these two sources might vary from study to study, which would again mean that the rates of depression found would be expected to vary because of this factor alone. It may also be that children and parents have different 'schemas' or definitions for the words used in interviews and questionnaires. For instance, an adult may guess rapidly from the content of a questionnaire that we are interested in 'depression' and respond according to his or her idea of whether he or she suffers from 'depression' and what being such a sufferer entails. A young child may not take such a syndromic view, but answer each question individually as it comes along. Clearly, any such differences in the way questions and responses are processed will affect the nature of the responses obtained.

It is also certain that referral processes have differed from study to study, in ways that depended upon the characteristics of the professionals involved and the children's parents, as well as the nature of the children's problems themselves (Shepherd *et al,* 1966, 1971; Taylor & Stansfeld, 1984a,b). We also know that a considerable majority of children with behavioural or emotional disturbances are never referred to any professional agency (Shepherd *et al,* 1966; Rutter *et al,* 1970). So there is little reason to suppose that the clinical samples discussed in this review are representative of depressed or miserable children in the population as a whole. We shall see later than these clinically referred 'depressed' children very often qualify for other diagnoses as well, and it may well be that in the referral process, Berkson's (1946) bias is operating. He pointed out that because the presence of more than one disorder leads to an increased probability of referral, clinical studies tend to find inflated rates of co-morbidity.

THE PHENOMENOLOGY OF
DEPRESSION IN YOUNG PEOPLE

The confusion associated with the diagnosis of depression in adults outlined by Kendell (1976) has not been, by any means, resolved in the last 10 years, and a variety of different nosological systems remain in existence, in the absence of clear criteria for judging between them (Davidson *et al*, 1984). It is therefore hardly surprising that the borders of childhood depression are not clearly drawn. In a companion paper (Angold, 1988) I have discussed the problem of the variable usage of the term 'depression' in the epidemiological literature. The studies reported here deal with depressive syndromes, which their authors have generally regarded as being disorders or illnesses, and which are usually defined by operational criteria that have largely been derived from adult work. But it remains quite unclear how much of the affective disturbance they document is appropriately viewed as part of a disease process (Graham, 1974; Rutter, 1986b). Many of the children seen in these studies have multiple problems and come from families with multiple problems. A good example is found in Kazdin *et al's* (1985) paper documenting higher levels of depressive symptoms in children on their psychiatric in-patient unit who had been subjected to physical abuse than in those who had not. It is clear that, clinically, there is much more than just depression to consider in such cases, and it may be that some children are showing simple unhappiness or misery in the face of difficult circumstances. Calling the manifestations of this unhappiness 'depression' may be drawing an inappropriate parallel with the adult disorder.

The demise of the idea of masked depression represents a victory for the idea that overt mood disturbance must be a central feature of depressive disorders. However, as in adulthood, low mood is a feature of many childhood disorders, and is even quite common in normal children, especially adolescents (Rutter *et al*, 1970; Angold, 1988). Graham (1974) has pointed out that sad mood is nonspecific and therefore a very imperfect marker of depression. We may agree that sad mood alone is insufficient for the diagnosis of depression, but depression is conceptually a disorder of mood, and there is little reason to deny the centrality of low mood in depression just because it is not highly specific to depressive disorders. On the other hand, it is theoretically possible that an underlying 'depressive diathesis' (or maybe even a gene) might manifest itself in childhood in ways that bear no phenomenological resemblance at all to adult depression. It would be a moot point whether such a relationship should lead to the disorder being called 'depression' in the children, but there is enough evidence from family studies to suggest that, at present, it is worth following up on depressed mood as a marker of possible depression.

Poznanski (1982) has emphasized the importance of the duration of "downcast" mood as an indicator of depression as opposed to the misery accompanying a wide range of diagnoses. Her diagnostic criteria require the depressed affect to have been present for a month or more. She also points out that verbal reports of low mood may be difficult to obtain clearly from some children (as indeed that may be difficult to obtain from some adults) and suggests that non-verbal expressions of affect, such as a consistently sad facial expression and the absence of smiles, may be substituted for verbal self-reports of low mood. On the other hand, Inamdar *et al* (1979) found that depressed adolescents who had suffered from depressed moods over periods ranging from months to years usually looked sad only when talking about their depression, and were not continuously depressed, but episodically intensely affected and disabled. The duration of the mood disorder is also of importance in attempting to distinguish between depressive disorders and adjustment disorders with depressed mood. The validity of this distinction has been tested very little, but the findings of Kovacs *et al* (1984a) suggest that the distinction may be important in that children with an adjustment reaction may have a much better prognosis than those with major depression.

Gittelman-Klein (1977) suggested that it might be best to regard the "pervasive and autonomous loss of hedonic experience" as the central feature of depression. However, some degree of anhedonia seems to be very common in the depressions of childhood and a complete loss of hedonic capacity might better be regarded as a marker of severity in the presence of other depressive symptoms. Furthermore, Feinstein *et al* (1984), in their extensive study of 224 child psychiatric clinic cases, found that dysphoric symptoms were common in all diagnostic groups, but that the combination of dysphoria and self-deprecatory ideation discriminated highly between depressed and conduct-disordered subjects. On the basis of this finding, they suggest that self-deprecatory ideation should be regarded as a core feature of childhood depression.

Angold *et al* (1987, unpubl.) found that a core group of self- and parent-reported items from their Mood and Feelings Questionnaire (MFQ) proved to be a good predictor of depression scores obtained from independent interviews using the Diagnostic Interview Schedule for Children (DISC) (Edelbrock *et al*, 1985). This core group consisted mostly of items probing low affect *per se*, anhedonia, and self-deprecation, so perhaps all of the above suggestions have been correct. However, we found that tiredness, restlessness, and poor concentration also seemed to belong to this core group, and, in line with Feinstein *et al* (1984), that marked depressive symptoms were associated with other diagnoses besides depression.

Some workers have assumed (with DSM-III) that depression cannot be said to be present unless low mood or anhedonia are reported, and have therefore adopted a strategy of not asking about other depressive symptoms unless sad mood and/or anhedonia are present (e.g. the studies employing the K-SADS and ISC; see Table I). This approach restricts the information that can be obtained about the specificity of other symptoms for depression, such as pathological guilt or self-deprecation. To establish that a real syndromic association is present among putative depressive symptoms, it is necessary to demonstrate that the observed rate of association among the symptoms is greater than that expected by the chance association of those symptoms, given their individual rates of occurrence in the population (this requirement would not be necessary if there were a clear marker for depression, but since there is not, we have to rely on phenomenological associations for diagnostic purposes). To demonstrate such a specific association, it is necessary to measure the rates of all the relevant symptoms in the whole sample. Unfortunately, this issue has not been adequately considered, and many studies rest upon an unsupported assumption that other 'depressive' symptoms will be rare, or of no psychopathological significance, in the absence of low mood or anhedonia, and that certain 'depressive symptoms' are syndromically related to one another in children and adolescents just because they are in adults (Lefkowitz & Burton, 1978). However, despite the problems, this approach has demonstrated without doubt that all of the symptoms of adult depression can and do occur in childhood and adolescence, and that they occur quite commonly. Children of 7 or 8 seem to be quite capable of convincingly describing pathological guilt or hopelessness, and indeed the whole range of affective and cognitive symptoms of depression in clinical interviews or on self-report instruments (Poznanski, 1982; Kovacs, 1986; Costello, 1986).

DEVELOPMENTAL CHANGES IN PSYCHOPATHOLOGY

The epidemiological evidence suggests that depressive symptoms become much more common after puberty, and that the female preponderance of depressive disorders is not apparent until then (Rutter *et al*, 1970, 1976; Rutter, 1986a; Angold, 1988). Further evidence of the need to consider developmental progressions is found in Puig-Antich's studies of sleep in depressed children, which suggest that sleep disturbance only emerges in relation to depression in later adolescence. We should recognize that if the base rates of symptoms in the population change with age in relation to each other, then their relative weights in contributing to the diagnosis of depression may also change. As yet we are very short of data on such changes (Kovacs, 1986), but there is evidence that they occur and that such developmental progressions need to be incorporated into our diagnostic schemes (Digdon & Gotlib, 1985). For instance, McConville *et al* (1973) have described three forms of depression characterized by 'affectual symptoms', guilt, and low self-esteem respectively. The first of these appeared to be more common in 6–8-year-olds, while the low self-esteem type became more frequent at later ages. The guilt type, which seemed to resemble adult psychotic depression in a number of ways, emerged principally after the age of 11, although it remained relatively uncommon. The case-record data on which these descriptions are based leave much to be desired, and findings of this sort require further careful assessment using structured or semi-structured assessment procedures, but they cannot be ignored. Inamdar *et al* (1979) noted the absence of motor agitation or retardation, delusions of guilt, and hopelessness in their sample of 30 depressed adolescents and, although these symptoms have been reported in adolescents with depression (Strober *et al*, 1981; Chambers *et al*, 1982; Kazdin & Petti, 1982; Friedman *et al*, 1983b), they may be rarer in childhood and early adolescence than in adulthood.

Difficult problems are encountered when attempting to deal with symptoms or types of behaviour that either do not occur in adulthood (such as school refusal—see Kolvin *et al*, 1984, for some informative data and discussion of depression and school refusal) or that are not usually regarded as being distinctively depressive, such as abdominal pains or headaches (Kazdin & Petti, 1982). Several authors have suggested that certain items of this sort are actually manifestations of depression in childhood and should be counted towards making the diagnosis rather than being regarded simply as associated phenomena. Ling *et al* (1970) and Weinberg *et al* (1973) included aggressive behaviour, worsening school performance, refusal to attend school, somatic complaints, and diminished socialization as diagnostic criteria. Pearce (1978), using case-note checklist data, found that depressed mood was significantly associated with morbid anxiety, irritability, refusal to attend school, phobias, alimentary disorders and abdominal pain, ruminations and obsessions, and altered perceptions, in addition to symptoms more commonly associated with depression. Birleson (1981) included ''wandering behaviour'' in his depression scale. If one attempts to include all of these possibilities, depression becomes just a catch-all diagnosis. This is as much of a mistake as the premature adoption of unmodified, non-developmental adult criteria. The truth is that we do not know much about the associations of depression in young people or whether age or developmental stage makes much difference to the phenomenology of these disorders, and the only way to remedy this situation is to take a middle path involving the measurement of the associations between a wide range of pathologies that might be associated with depression, while at the same time upholding the centrality of the triad of affective, cognitive, and behavioral manifestations that characterize the concept of depression in adulthood.

DEPRESSIVE PSYCHOSES AND BIPOLAR DISORDERS

Depressive psychoses have been well described even in prepubertal children (Chambers *et al*, 1982). However, several studies have documented the problem of distinguishing between schizophrenia and affective psychosis at this age (Haslam, 1978; Bowden & Sarabia, 1980; Joyce, 1984; Carlson & Strober, 1978; Carlson, 1985; Zeitlin, 1986). Nunn (1979) found some evidence that the onset of symptoms of subjects with mixed affective disorders occurred somewhat earlier than for those who had only had pure manic and depressive states. It would be interesting to know how many of the adolescents presenting with first episodes of affective disorder have mixed affective psychoses, since these conditions are often difficult to distinguish from schizophrenia if information about previous course is not available.

However, the confusion may not be all in one direction, since Zeitlin (1986) found that the diagnostic labels of schizophrenia and affective psychosis, as applied in adolescence, were often found to have been mistaken in the light of the later manifestations of the disorder. In this case, those who were thought to have been affectively ill were as likely to turn out to be schizophrenic as those who were said to be schizophrenic were to follow a typical manic-depressive course. In this area, careful longitudinal studies of the development and progress of psychotic disorders from their earliest manifestations into adulthood are urgently needed.

There is some debate over the status of mania in childhood. Cutting (1976) provides an interesting case report of a child with chronic mania and a radiological picture of cerebellar disease and includes a useful review of the small previous literature. In the adolescent population, mania is well recognized, though, as we have already discussed, it is often confused with schizophrenia. However, before puberty, classical mania or hypomania seem to be very rare (Anthony & Scott, 1960). Some workers have argued that it is more common than has been supposed (Weinberg & Brumback, 1976), but that the initial childhood presentation is often a confusing picture of episodically difficult, poorly controlled, hyperactive behaviour, which is likely to be interpreted as falling within the nosological ambit of conduct disorder or hyperactivity or attention-deficit disorder. Such children seem to be irritable and dysphoric rather than elated, and it may be that this is the result of a maturational change. Children do not show the usual adult euphoric response to amphetamine-like stimulants and it may be that they are incapable of manifesting manic euphoria (Puig-Antich, 1986). Given the association between conduct disorder and depression at the symptom and syndrome levels (see below), this idea is difficult to test, but careful longitudinal studies of children from families with a strong history of bipolar illness would provide valuable data.

In adolescence, the limited evidence suggests that depression and mania are equally common as the first episodes of bipolar disorders, but that mania predominates in the following episodes (Carlson & Strober, 1978). Depressed adolescents who later turned out to be bipolar were also found by the same group (Strober & Carlson, 1982) to be more likely to have family histories in three generations, hypomanic responses to tricyclics, and marked psychomotor retardation. There are also data suggesting that manic-depressive patients whose onsets of symptoms were during or before adolescence, rather than later, have more frequent episodes, are prone to rapid cycling, and are more likely to commit suicide (Olsen, 1961; Welner *et al*, 1979; Hassanyeh & Davison, 1980).

PHYSICAL AND MEDICAL PRESENTATIONS

Several studies have found high rates of depression in children and adolescents referred to medical assessment or treatment (see Table 1). Headaches (Ling *et al*, 1970) and chest pain (Kashani *et al*, 1982) unaccompanied by other neurological or chest disease seem to be highly associated with depression, as is chronic disability leading to hospital admission for orthopaedic procedures (Kashani *et al*, 1981). In an impressionistic paper, Vranjesevic *et al* (1972) describe high levels of depressive symptoms accompanying intracranial tumours, and consider that affective disturbances may be early manifestations of some of these lesions. Pfefferbaum-Levine *et al* (1983) have suggested that anti-depressants can have useful effects in raising the mood of children with a variety of types of cancer, although their work is far from adequately controlled.

BIOLOGICAL MANIFESTATIONS

In the early 1970s, Cytryn *et al* (1974) found evidence of abnormalities of catecholamine metabolism, using urinary excretion products as markers; but this line of enquiry does not seem to have been followed up. Cavallo *et al* (1987) found lower levels of melatonin secretion in a mixed group of depressed prepubertal and pubertal boys compared with normal control subjects, although there was no evidence of any alteration in the melatonin secretory rhythm. This is an interesting finding, because it may hold some promise as a trait marker of depression, albeit one that is capable of separating groups, but not individuals.

Much more interest has been shown in a variety of measures of hypothalamo-pituitary function. The greatest number of studies have been of cortisol hypersecretion and the dexamethasone suppression test (DST) (Puig-Antich *et al*, 1979b; De La Fuente & Rosenbaum, 1980; Crumley *et al*, 1982; Extein *et al*, 1982; Poznanski *et al*, 1982; Geller *et al*, 1983b; Hsu *et al*, 1983; Robbins *et al*, 1983; Targum & Capodanno, 1983; Ha, Kaplan & Foley, 1984; Klee & Garfinkel, 1984; Weller *et al*, 1984; Livingstone *et al*, 1984; Puig-Antich *et al*, 1984e; Burke *et al*, 1985; Doherty *et al*, 1986). In a review of the status of the DST in children, Leckman (1983) concluded that "the validity of the DST as a diagnostic test remains in doubt." The studies that have appeared since his review have done nothing to allay these doubts. While all find that DST abnormalities are present in only a subgroup of depressive patients, some studies indicate that the DST is quite highly specific for depression, while others find associations with a wide range of other conditions. Part of the problem clearly stems from a failure in most studies to follow the guidelines suggested by Carroll (1984), especially in respect of calibrating the DST at each laboratory to make the best discrimination between groups. The use of a pre-ordained cut-off score to determine non-suppression will result in poor discrimination by the DST, so that the uncertain position of the findings is hardly surprising. Given the present state of the evidence on the DST and depression in young people, it does not seem appropriate to adopt the DST as a diagnostic measure in this age group.

However, some other hypothalamo-pituitary regulatory abnormalities have been documented in the careful studies of Puig-Antich (1986), and Puig-Antich *et al* (1985a–e) found growth-hormone hyposecretion in response to insulin-tolerance tests in prepubertal endogenous major depressive patients. These findings parallel those observed in post-menopausal women, and preliminary evidence suggests that they disappear during puberty under the influence of high oestrogen levels. Thus it seems that "only during prepuberty and after menopause does GH response to ITT seem to reflect neuroregulatory mechanisms involved in depression." This group finds little in the way of abnormalities in the cortisol or prolactin responses to insulin-induced hypoglycaemia in either endogenous or nonendogenous depressive patients.

A number of studies of the sleep of depressed children and adolescents have appeared, again with conflicting results (Kane *et al*, 1977; Puig-Antich *et al*, 1982; Young *et al*, 1982; Lahmeyer *et al*, 1983; Puig-Antich *et al*, 1983; Hawkins *et al*, 1985; Puig-Antich, 1986). However, the best studies seem to suggest that the characteristic in-episode sleep abnormalities of adult endogenous depressives only emerge in late adolescence (Puig-Antich, 1986; Goetz *et al*, 1987). On the other hand, shortened REM latency may characterize children with depressive diatheses between episodes. The absence of striking polysomnographic findings during depressive episodes is not surprising when one considers the adult literature, in which age is found to be positively correlated with the probability of finding sleep disturbance during depressive episodes. There is a similar correlation between the frequency of occurrence of DST abnormalities and age, and these two phenomena probably reflect changes in neurotransmitter systems (Puig-Antich, 1986). Hawkins *et al* (1985) found a tendency towards the more frequent manifestation of hypersomnia in their young depressed patients (aged 17–25), and this finding deserves further exploration in still-younger subjects.

DEPRESSION AND CONDUCT DISORDER

Weinberg and Van den Dungen (1972) compared 35 depressive juvenile delinquents with 35 non-depressed adolescent delinquents and found that the former were more neurotic and introverted and possessed "more severely forbidding superego structures." Puig-Antich (1982) found that about a third of his sample of depressed children also had a conduct disorder. He also felt that the conduct disorder improved with antidepressant treatment, and that the conduct disorder was therefore secondary to the depression. Chiles *et al* (1980), using a semi-structured interview, found that 23% of 13–15-year-olds admitted to a correctional facility were depressed according to the RDC criteria. It seems, therefore, that mood disturbance is common in behaviourally disordered children, and the degree of mood disturbance may be related to the degree of behaviour disorder. For instance, Angold *et al* (1987, unpubl.) found a correlation of around 0.7 between parental reports of mood disturbance on the parent version of the Mood and Feelings Questionnaire and the Child Behaviour Checklist Externalizing factor score, which mainly measures behavioural disorder items. Findings such as this and Feinstein *et al's* (1984) work suggest that the mood disorder and the behaviour disorder may often not be separate conditions. The problem is that we have little evidence to suggest which should be regarded as primary when mixed conditions are found. The clinician will often consider which aspects of the mixed picture are most directly responsible for any psychosocial disability in answering this question. This is a sensible strategy and one that needs to be pursued more rigorously in the research literature.

SUICIDE AND PARASUICIDE

Suicidal and parasuicidal behaviour are also strongly associated with depression, or at least with marked misery in both childhood and adolescence (Robbins & Alessi, 1985). However, studies have been consistent in finding that a majority of children and adolescents who perform potentially self-harmful acts are not suffering from clear-cut depression (Shaffer & Fisher, 1981; Hawton, 1982; Shaffer, 1982, 1986; Brent *et al*, 1984; Taylor & Stansfeld, 1984a,b; McClure & Gould, 1984; Brooksbank, 1985). In clinical populations, there seems to be an association between the number of depressive symptoms shown by a child and that child's level of suicidal ideation or behaviour, but even here the link is by no means specific (Pfeffer *et al*, 1979, 1980, 1982, 1983, 1984; Carlson & Cantwell, 1982; Brent *et al*, 1986) and subgroups of suicidal children may exist, with only one group showing a strong link with depression (Pfeffer *et al*, 1983). It is also well known that suicide and parasuicide are very uncommon before puberty, and there is evidence that suicidal ideation is less common in prepubertal psychiatric clinic referred patients than in referred adolescents (Carlson & Cantwell, 1982). This fact underlines yet again the importance of considering developmental changes in the manifestations of depression (Shaffer, 1986).

OUTCOME OF CHILDHOOD AND ADOLESCENT DEPRESSIONS

The few studies that have attempted to assess the outcome of childhood depression have been uniform in finding a dismal prognosis, especially for those whose symptoms had already been present for a long time. Poznanski *et al* (1976) managed to follow up 10 of their original group of 14 depressed children and found that half of them still appeared to be depressed 6.5 years later. Pearce (1978) found that more than half of the children identified by an item checklist as suffering from a cluster of symptoms called "morbid depression" had had their disorder for more than a year, but then so had the nondepressed control group, and there was no difference between the two in terms of the overall duration of their symptoms.

The best study of this topic to date is that of Kovacs *et al* (1984a,b). The mean duration of major depression at the time of diagnosis was 32 weeks, while those with dysthymic disorder had already been suffering for 3 years. The median time to recovery after diagnosis for dysthmia was 3.5 years, although the recovery rate of MDD was much faster. However, within 5 years from diagnosis, 69% of the dysthymic patients had had an episode of major depression and 72% of the major depressive patients had had a second episode. The only groups to do well were those with adjustment disorder with depressive mood, who recovered relatively quickly and did not relapse, and the control group, of whom only 5% became depressed in the 5 years following their inception into the study. The interpretation of these dramatic results is, however, made less secure by the follow-up assessments not being performed blind to the initial assessments and diagnoses. But altogether, the evidence points to depression in this age-group being a potentially recurrent and disabling disorder. It may be objected that it is usually taught that 'neurotic' children have good outcomes. However, there is very little satisfactory evidence on this point, and it is quite possible that the outlook for depressed children is much worse than we have hitherto supposed.

TREATMENT

The published treatment studies have been exceedingly disappointing, being characterized by non-blind, non-placebo trials of tricyclic antidepressants (Lucas *et al*, 1965; Frommer, 1968, 1972; Ling *et al*, 1970; Kuhn & Kuhn, 1972; Polvan & Cebiroglu, 1972; Stack, 1972; Saraf *et al*, 1974; Ossofsky, 1974; Brumback *et al*, 1977; Rapoport, 1977; Puig-Antich *et al*, 1979a; Pallmeyer & Petti, 1979; De La Fuente & Rosenbaum, 1980; Petti *et al*, 1980; Puig-Antich, 1982; Weller *et al*, 1982; Geller *et al*, 1983a; Connors & Petti, 1983; Petti & Connors, 1983; Weller *et al*, 1983; Weller & Weller, 1984; Cytryn & McKnew, 1985). These studies have been interpreted as indicating that antidepressants are effective and do not cause unacceptable side-effects. Some workers have gone so far as to suggest that a therapeutic window exists for blood levels of antidepressant in children treated with imipramine (Puig-Antich *et al*, 1979a; Preskorn *et al*, 1982; Weller *et al*, 1982; Preskorn, 1984). However, the efficacy of these drugs has never been convincingly demonstrated in an adequate controlled, double-blind, placebo trial, and negative results have been reported from such studies (Kramer & Feiguine, 1981; Kashani, Shekim & Reid, 1984; Puig-Antich *et al*, 1987). Puig-Antich *et al* (1987) found evidence, from a sub-study examining the relationship between clinical response and blood levels of imipramine, that the failure of the active drug to improve clinical outcome (only 56% of those receiving the active drug [$n = 16$] were improved at the end of the 5-week study period, compared with 68% of those on placebo [$n = 22$]) was due to inadequate dosage, despite the mean daily dosage being 137 mg.

However, most clinicians have at least occasionally dealt with children who seemed to improve dramatically with antidepressant treatment, and it seems likely that there will turn out to be at least a subgroup of drug-responsive depressed children. At present, though, there is no strong evidence to support the routine administration of antidepressants to all those children whose symptoms warrant a DSM-III diagnosis of depression.

What evidence there is suggests that lithium is as effective in the treatment of bipolar disorders in young people as it is in other age-groups (Frommer, 1968; Annell, 1969a,b; Schou, 1972; De Long, 1978; Youngerman & Canino,

1978; Jefferson, 1982). No specific studies of lithium efficacy in relation to blood levels in childhood and adolescence are available, and so serum levels are recommended as for adults (Annell, 1969a,b; Shaffer, 1985). Likewise, side-effects parallel those known from adults. Effects on bone growth and growth-hormone regulation are theoretical possibilities (Birtch, 1980; Jefferson, 1982; Lal *et al*, 1978), but have not been observed as practical problems. Carbamazepine has been reported to have been effective in a couple of adolescents with lithium-resistant bipolar disorders (Hsu *et al*, 1983).

Sadly, other forms of treatment have hardly been assessed at all. Petti *et al* (1980) offer a case report of the evaluation and multimodality treatment of a depressed pre-pubertal girl and Weller *et al* (1984) provide a general discussion of possible therapeutic approaches. I am aware of no reasonable trial of any sort of psychotherapy, behavioural treatment, or family therapy specifically for childhood or adolescent depression.

CONCLUSIONS

Depression has been a major research area in child and adolescent psychiatry in the last few years, and much significant work has been done. Few now doubt the existence of prepubertal depression, and we know that the whole range of adult depressive symptoms may be expressed by children, certainly by the age of 6–8, and perhaps even younger (although the same cannot be said of the manic syndrome). The child is, much more than before, seen as the most important direct source of diagnostic information, as far as mood disorders are concerned, which is at least partly responsible for the increased rates being reported now, compared with 20 years ago. Some biological correlates have been found, and family and genetic factors are being progressively more strongly implicated in the aetiology of these disorders.

However, there has been a tendency to shy away from careful study of potential age and developmental-stage-associated changes in phenomenology, and a tendency to overvalue the DSM-III criteria as derived originally for adults. We also remain unsure where the borders of depression, as opposed to unhappiness or misery, should be drawn, with the result that tremendous differences in the reported rates of depression are found from different studies. What is more, it has still not been by any means unequivocally demonstrated that clearcut depressive disorders are by any means common, and, with the possible exception of adolescent bipolar disorders, none of the depressive syndromes is anywhere near fulfilling our criteria for disease status (Angold, 1988).

On the more positive side, the clinician faced with a miserable child can feel that the research evidence supports the taking of an 'adult-style' history (at least from the age of 7 or 8 up) from that child and using it as the central diagnostic tool. Parental reports provide supportive information and (in the case of younger children especially) more reliable information about the onset and timing of symptoms. Care should also be taken to investigate mood phenomena in conduct-disordered and hyperactive children, and depressive symptoms should be expected in children with anxiety disorders. If these are systematically pursued, then the reward can be a greater understanding of the child's world and a deepening of empathic contact between the child and the clinician. The clinician should also explore the specific links between particular areas of psychopathology and any psychosocial disability (such as school failure, or relationship problems) that the child may have. It seems sensible to label those disorders in which the mood change and its concomitants are making a major contribution to the disability 'depressive', while for those in which the mood change does not seem to be independently contributing, the term 'miserable' might be better.

The few available studies of outcome indicate that we should be very worried about children who have a good deal of adult-type depressive symptoms, because they may be at risk for continuing or relapsing affective illnesses. However, the studies present methodological problems and their results cannot be unequivocally accepted as yet. No therapeutic agent has been clearly shown to be effective, although a number of methodologically inadequate trials concur in suggesting that tricyclic antidepressants have a part to play in treatment, and lithium is effective in manic-depressive disorders.

Perhaps what is most exciting about the field is that we have the methodologies to examine many of these problems and supply answers to some of the questions (see Rutter, 1986b), especially in relation to diagnosis, outcome, and treatment. Aetiological studies should also be of particular interest to students of adult depression, since, in childhood, many of the factors that have been implicated in the causation of adult depressions are currently operative, so that their effects may be measured directly and even prospectively, rather than by recall many years later. Given the continuing interest in the field and the wide range of studies presently being conducted in a number of countries, many developments may be expected in the next 10 years, which may benefit many very unhappy children.

REFERENCES

Abraham, K. (1911) Notes on the psycho-analytical investigation and treatment of manic depressive insanity and allied conditions. In *Selected Papers on Psycho-Analysis* (ed. K. Abraham). London: Hogarth, 1927, New edition, London: Hogarth, 1949, New York: Basic Books, 1953.

—— (1949) The infantile prototype of melancholic depression. In *Selected Papers of Karl Abraham*. London: Hogarth Press.

American Psychiatric Association (1980) *Diagnostic and Statistical Manual of Mental Disorders* (3rd edn) (DSM-III). Washington DC: APA.

Angold, A. (1988) Childhood and adolescent depression: epidemiological and aetiological aspects. *British Journal of Psychiatry*, **152**, 601–617.

——, Weissman, M. M., John, K., Merikangas, K. R., Prusoff, B. A., Wickramaratne, P., Gammon, G. D. & Warner, V. (1987) Parent and child reports of depressive symptoms. *Journal of Child Psychology and Psychiatry*, **28**, 901–915.

Annell, A. J. (1969a) Lithium in the treatment of children and adolescents. *Acta Psychiatrica Scandinavica*, **Suppl. 207**, 19–30.

—— (1969b) Manic-depressive illness in children and effect of treatment with lithium carbonate. *Acta Paedopsychiatrica*, **36**, 292–301.

Anthony, J. (1967) Psychoneurotic disorders. In *Comprehensive Textbook of Psychiatry* (eds A. M. Freedman & M. S. Kaplan), pp. 1317–1406. Baltimore: Williams and Wilkins.

—— & Scott, P. (1960) Manic depressive psychosis in childhood. *Journal of Child Psychology and Psychiatry*, **1**, 53–72.

Berkson, J. (1946) Limitations of the application of fourfold table analysis to hospital data. *Biometrics*, **2**, 47–53.

Birleson, P. (1981) The validity of depressive disorder in childhood and the development of a self-rating scale. *Journal of Child Psychology and Psychiatry*, **22**, 73–88.

Birtch, N. J. (1980) Bone side-effects of lithium. In *Handbook of Lithium Therapy* (ed. F. N. Johnson), pp. 365–371. Lancaster, Pa.: MTP Press.

Bowden, C. & Sarabia, F. (1980) Diagnosing manic depressive illness in adolescents. *Comprehensive Psychiatry*, **21**, 263–269.

Bowlby, J. (1969) *Attachment and Loss: II. Loss: Sadness and Depression*. London: Hogarth Press.

Brent, D. A., Kalas, R., Edelbrock, E., Costello, A. J., Dulcan, M. K. & Conover, N. (1986) Psychopathology and its relationship to suicidal ideation in childhood and adolescence. *Journal of the American Academy of Child Psychiatry*, **25**, 666–673.

Brooksbank, D. J. (1985) Suicide and parasuicide in childhood and early adolescence. *British Journal of Psychiatry*, **146**, 459–463.

Brumback, R. A., Dietz-Schmidt, S. G. & Weinberg, W. A. (1977) Depression in children referred to an educational diagnostic center: diagnosis and treatment and analysis of criteria and literature review. *Diseases of the Nervous System*, **38**, 529–535.

Burke, P. M., Reicher, R. J., Smith, E., Dugaw, K., Mccauley, E. & Mitchell, J. (1985) Correlation between serum and salivary cortisol levels in depressed and non-depressed children and adolescents. *American Journal of Psychiatry*, **142**, 1065–1067.

Campbell, J. (1952) Manic-depressive psychoses in children. *Journal of Nervous and Mental Disease*, **116**, 424–439.

Cantwell, D. P. C. & Carlson, G. A. (eds) (1983) *Affective Disorders in Childhood and Adolescence: An update*. Lancaster, Pa.: MTP Press.

Carlson, G. A. (1985) Bipolar disorder in adolescence. *Psychiatric Annals*, **15**, 379–386.

—— & Cantwell, D. P. C. (1980) A survey of depressive symptoms, syndrome and disorder in a child psychiatric population. *Journal of Child Psychology and Psychiatry*, **21**, 19–25.

—— & —— (1982) Suicidal behaviour and depression in children and adolescents. *Journal of the American Academy of Child Psychiatry*, **21**, 361–368.

—— & Garber, J. (1986) Developmental issues in the classification of depression in children. In *Depression in Young Children: Developmental and Clinical Perspectives* (eds M. Rutter, C. E. Izard & P. B. Read), pp. 399–434. New York: Guilford Press.

—— & Strober, M. (1978) Manic depressive illness in early adolescence: a study of clinical and diagnostic characteristics in six cases. *Journal of the American Academy of Child Psychiatry*, **17**, 138–153.

Carroll, B. J. (1984) Dexamethasone suppression test. In *Handbook of Psychiatric Procedures* (eds R. C. W. Hall & T. P. Beresford) vol. 1. New York: Spectrum Publications.

Cavallo, A., Holt, K. G., Hejazi, M. S., Richard, G. E. R. & Meyer, W. J. (1987) Melatonin circadian rhythm in childhood depression. *Journal of the American Academy of Child and Adolescent Psychiatry*, **26**, 395–399.

Cebiroglu, R., Sumner, E. & Polvan, O. (1972) Etiology and pathogenesis of depression in Turkish children. In *Depressive States in Childhood and Adolescence* (ed. A. L. Annell), pp. 133–136. Stockhold: Almqvist and Wiksell.

Chambers, W. J., Puig-Antich, J., Tabrizi, M. A. & Davies, M. (1982) Psychotic symptoms in prepubertal major depressive disorder. *Archives of General Psychiatry*, **39**, 921–927.

Chiles, J. A., Miller, M. L. & Cox, G. B. (1980) Depression in an adolescent delinquent population. *Archives of General Psychiatry*, **37**, 1177–1184.

Connors, C. K. & Petti, T. A. (1983) Imipramine therapy of depressed children: methodologic considerations. *Psychopharmacology Bulletin*, **19**, 65–69.

Costello, E. J. (1986) Assessment and diagnosis of affective disorders in children. *Journal of Child Psychology and Psychiatry*, **27**, 565–574.

Crumley, F. E., Clevenger, J., Steinfink, D. & Oldham, D. (1982) Preliminary report on the dexamethazone suppression test for psychiatrically disturbed adolescents. *American Journal of Psychiatry*, **139**, 1062–1064.

Cutting, J. (1976) Chronic mania in childhood: case report of a possible association with a radiological picture of cerebellar disease. *Psychological Medicine*, **6**, 635–642.

Cytryn, L. & McKnew, D. H. (1972) Proposed classification of childhood depression. *American Journal of Psychiatry*, **129**, 149–155.

—— & —— (1985) Treatment issues in childhood depression. *Psychiatric Annals*, **15**, 401–403.

——, —— & Bunney, W. (1980) Diagnosis of depression in children. *American Journal of Psychiatry*, **137**, 22–25.

——, ——, Logue, M. & Desai, R. B. (1974) Biochemical correlates of affective disorders in children. *Archives of General Psychiatry*, **25**, 204–207.

Davidson, J., Turnbull, C., Strickland, R. & Belyea, M. (1984) Comparative diagnostic criteria for melancholia and endogenous depression. *Archives of General Psychiatry*, **41**, 506–511.

De La Fuente, J. R. & Rosenbaum, A. H. (1980) Neuroendocrine dysfunction and blood levels of tricyclic antidepressants. *American Journal of Psychiatry*, **137**, 1260–1261.

De Long, G. R. (1978) Lithium carbonate treatment of select behavior disorders in children suggesting manic-depressive illness. *Journal of Pediatrics,* **98,** 689–694.

Digdon, N. & Gotlib, I. H. (1985) Developmental considerations in the study of childhood depression. *Developmental Research,* **5,** 162–199.

Doherty, M. B., Madansky, D., Kraft, J., Carter-ake, L. L., Rosenthal, P. A. and Coughlin, B. F. (1986) Cortisol dynamics and test performance of the dexamethasone suppression test in 97 psychiatrically hospitalized children aged 3–16 years. *Journal of the American Academy of Child Psychiatry,* **25,** 400–408.

Edelbrock, C., Costello, A. J., Dulcan, M. K., Kalas, R. & Conover, N. C. (1985) Age differences in the reliability of the psychiatric interview of the child. *Child Development,* **56,** 265–275.

——, ——, ——, Conover, N. C. & Kalas, R. (1986) Parent-child agreement on child psychiatric symptoms assessed via structured interview. *Journal of Child Psychology and Psychiatry,* **27,** 181–190.

Eisenberg, L. (1986) When is a case a case? In *Depression in Young People: Developmental and Clinical Perspectives* (eds M. Rutter, C. E. Izard & P. B. Read) New York: Guilford Press.

Extein, I., Rosenberg, G., Pottash, A. L. C. & Gold, M. S. (1982) The dexamethasone test in depressed adolescents. *American Journal of Psychiatry,* **139,** 1617–1619.

Feighner, J. P., Robins, E., Guze, S. B., Woodruff, R. A., Winokur, G. & Munoz, R. (1972) Diagnostic criteria for use in psychiatric research. *Archives of General Psychiatry,* **26,** 57–63.

Feinstein, C., Blouin, A. G., Egan, J. & Connors, C. K. (1984) Depressive symptomatology in a child psychiatric outpatient population: correlations with diagnosis. *Comprehensive Psychiatry,* **25,** 379–391.

Fenichel, O. (1945) *The Psychoanalytic Study of the Personality.* New York: Norton.

Friedman, R. C., Clarkin, J. F., Corn, R., Aronoff, M. S., Hurt, S. W. & Murphy, M. C. (1982) DSM-III affective pathology in hospitalized adolescents. *Journal of Nervous and Mental Disease,* **170,** 511–521.

——, Hurt, S. W., Clarkin, J. F. & Corn, R. (1983a) Primary and secondary affective disorders in adolescents and young adults. *Acta Psychiatrica Scandinavica,* **67,** 226–235.

——, Hurt, S. W., Clarkin. J. F., Corn, R. & Aronoff, M. S. (1983b) Symptoms of depression among adolescents and young adults. *Journal of Affective Disorders,* **5,** 37–43.

Frommer, E. (1968) Depressive illness in childhood. *British Journal of Psychiatry,* **2,** 117–136.

—— (1972) Indications for antidepressant treatment with special reference to depressed preschool children. In *Depressive States in Childhood and Adolescence* (ed. A. N. Annell). Stockholm: Almqvist and Wiksell.

Gammon, G. D., John, K., Rothblum, E., Mullen, K., Tischler, G. & Weissman, M. M. (1983) Use of a structured diagnostic interview to identify bipolar disorder in adolescent inpatients: frequency and manifestations of the disorder. *American Journal of Psychiatry,* **140,** 543–547.

Geller, B., Perel, J. M., Knitter, E. F., Lycaki, H. & Farooki, Z. Q. (1983a) Nortriptyline in major depressive disorder in children: response, steady-state plasma levels, predictive kinetics and pharmacokinetics. *Psychopharmacology Bulletin,* **19,** 62–65.

——, Rogol, A. D. & Knitter, E. F. (1983b) Preliminary data on the dexamethazone suppression test in children with major depressive disorder. *American Journal of Psychiatry,* **140,** 620.

Gittelman-Klein, R. (1977) Definitional and methodological issues concerning depressive illness in children. In *Depression in Childhood: Diagnosis, Research and Conceptual Models* (eds J. G. Schulterbrandt & A. Raskin). New York: Raven Press.

Glaser, K. (1967) Masked depression in children and adolescents. *American Journal of Psychotherapy,* **21,** 565–574.

Goetz, R. R., Puig-Antich, J., Ryan, N., Rabinovich, H., Ambrosini, P. J., Nelson, B. & Krawkiec, V. (1987) Electroencephalographic sleep of adolescents with major depression and normal controls. *Archives of General Psychiatry,* **44,** 61–68.

Graham, P. (1974) Depression in prepubertal children. *Developmental Medicine and Child Neurology,* **16,** 340–349.

Ha, H., Kaplan, S. & Foley, C. (1984) The dexamethasone suppression test in adolescent psychiatric patients. *American Journal of Psychiatry,* **141,** 421–423.

Hardy, T. (1896) *Jude The Obscure.* Penguin edn 1972. Harmondsworth: Penguin Books.

Harms, E. (1952) Differential pattern of manic depressive disease in childhood. *The Nervous Child,* **9,** 326–356.

Haslam, A. T. (1978) A study of psychiatric illness in adolescence. *International Journal of Social Psychiatry,* **24,** 287–294.

Hassanyeh, F. & Davison, K. (1980) Bipolar affective psychosis with onset before age 16 years: report of 10 cases. *British Journal of Psychiatry,* **137,** 530–539.

Hawkins, D. R., Taub, J. M. & Van der Castle, R. L. (1985) Extended sleep (hypersomnia) in young depressed patients. *American Journal of Psychiatry,* **142,** 905–910.

Hawton, K. (1982) Attempted suicide in children. *Journal of Child Psychology and Psychiatry,* **23,** 497–503.

Herjanic, B. & Reich, W. (1982) Development of a structured psychiatric interview for children: agreement between child and parent on individual symptoms. *Journal of Abnormal Child Psychology,* **10,** 307–324.

Hsu, L. K. G., Molcan, K., Cashman, M. A., Lee, S., Lohr, J. & Hindmarsh, D. (1983) The dexamethasone suppression test in adolescent depression. *Journal of the American Academy of Child Psychiatry,* **22,** 470–473.

Hudgens, R. (1974) *Psychiatric Disorders in Adolescents.* Baltimore: Williams and Wilkins.

Inamdar, S. C., Siomopoulos, G., Osborne, M. & Bianchi, E. C. (1979) Phenomenology associated with depressed moods in adolescents. *American Journal of Psychiatry,* **136,** 150–159.

Jefferson, J. W. (1982) The use of lithium on the cognitive functions of normal subjects. *Journal of Clinical Psychiatry,* **43,** 174–177.

Joyce, P. R. (1984) Age of onset in bipolar affective disorder and misdiagnosis as schizophrenia. *Psychological Medicine,* **14,** 145–149.

Kane, J., Coble, P., Connors, C. K. & Kupfer, D. J. (1977) EEG sleep in a child with severe depression. *American Journal of Psychiatry,* **134,** 813–814.

Kashani, J. H., Lababidi, Z. & Jones, R. S. (1982) Depression in children and adolescents with cardiovascular symptomatology: the significance of chest pain. *Journal of the American Academy of Child Psychiatry,* **21,** 187–189.

——, Ray, J. S. & Carlson, G. A. (1984) Depression and depressive-like states in preschool-age children in a child development unit. *American Journal of Psychiatry,* **141,** 1397–1402.

——, Shekim, W. O. & Reid, J. C. (1984) Amitriptyline in children with major depressive disorder. A double-blind crossover pilot study. *Journal of the American Academy of Child Psychiatry,* **23,** 348–351.

——, Venzke, R. & Millar, E. A. (1981) Depression in children admitted to hospital for orthopaedic procedures. *British Journal of Psychiatry,* **138,** 21–25.

Kazdin, A. E., Esveldt-Dawson, K., Unis, A. S. & Rancurello, M. (1983a) Child and parent evaluations of depression and aggression in psychiatric inpatient children. *Journal of Abnormal Child Psychology,* **11,** 401–413.

——, French, N. H., Unis, A. S. & Esveldt-Dawson, K. (1983b) Assessment of childhood depression: correspondence of child and parent ratings. *Journal of the American Academy of Child Psychiatry,* **22,** 157–164.

——, Moser, J., Colbus, D. & Bell, R. (1985) Depressive symptoms among physically abused and psychiatrically disturbed children. *Journal of Abnormal Psychology,* **94,** 298–307.

—— & Petti, T. A. (1982) Self report and interview measures of childhood and adolescent depression. *Journal of Child Psychology and Psychiatry,* **23,** 437–457.

Kendell, R. E. (1976) The classification of depressions: a review of contemporary confusion. *British Journal of Psychiatry,* **129,** 15–28.

Klee, S. H. & Garfinkel, B. D. (1984) Identification of depression in children and adolescents: the role of the dexamethasone suppression test. *Journal of the American Academy of Child Psychiatry,* **23,** 410–415.

Klein, M. (1975) A contribution to the psychogenesis of manic-depressive states. *The Writings of Melanie Klein,* vol. 1, 262–239. London: Hogarth Press

Kolvin, I., Berney, T. P. & Bhate, S. R. (1984) Classification and diagnosis of depression in school phobia. *British Journal of Psychiatry,* **145,** 347–357.

Kovacs, M. (1986) A developmental perspective on methods and measures in the assessment of depressive disorders: the clinical interview. In *Depression in Young People: Issues and Perspectives* (eds M. L. Rutter, C. Izard & P. Read). New York: Guilford Press

—— & Beck, A. T. (1977) An empirical-clinical approach towards a definition of child depression. In *Depression in Childhood: Diagnosis, Research and Conceptual Models,* (eds J. G. Schulterbrandt & A. Raskin). New York: Raven Press.

——, Feinberg, T. L., Crouse-Novak, M. L., Paulauskas, S. L. & Finkelstein, R. (1984a) Depressive disorders in childhood. I: A longitudinal prospective study of characteristics and recovery. *Archives of General Psychiatry,* **41,** 229–237.

——, ——, ——, ——, Pollock, M. & Finkelstein, R. (1984b) Depressive disorders in children. II: A longitudinal study of the risk for a subsequent major depression. *Archives of General Psychiatry,* **41,** 643–649.

Kraepelin, E. (1921) *Manic, Depressive Insanity and Paranoia* (trans R. M. Barclay). Edinburgh: Livingstone.

Kramer, A. D. & Feiguine, B. A. (1981) Clinical effects of amitriptyline in adolescent depression: a pilot study. *Journal of the American Academy of Child Psychiatry,* **20,** 636–644.

Kuhn, V., & Kuhn R. (1972) Drug therapy for depression in children. In *Depressive States in Childhood and Adolescence* (ed. A. N. Annell). Stockholm: Almqvist and Wiksell.

Kuperman, S. & Stewart, M. A. (1979) The diagnosis of depression in childhood. *Journal of Affective Disorders,* **1,** 213–217.

Lachenmeyer, J. R. (1982) Special disorders of childhood: depression, school phobia and anorexia nervosa. In *Psychopathology in Childhood,* pp. 53–83. (eds J. R. Lachenmeyer & M. S. Gibbs).

Lahmeyer, H. W., Poznanski, E. O. & Bellur, S. N. (1983) EEG sleep in depressed adolescents. *American Journal of Psychiatry,* **140,** 1150–1153.

Lal, S., Nair, N. P. V. & Guyda, H. (1978) Effects of lithium on hypothalamic-pituitary dopaminergic functions. *Acta Psychiatrica Scandinavica,* **57,** 91–96.

Leckman, J. F. (1983) The dexamethasone suppression test. *Journal of the American Academy of Child Psychiatry,* **22,** 477–479.

Leon, G. R., Kendall, P. C. & Garber, J. (1980) Depression in children: parent, teacher and child perspectives. *Journal of Abnormal Child Psychology,* **8,** 221–235.

Lefkowitz, M. M. & Burton, N. (1978) Childhood depression: a critique of the concept. *Psychological Bulletin,* **45,** 716–726.

Ling, W., Oftedal, G. & Weinberg, N. (1970) Depressive illness in children presenting as severe headache. *American Journal of Diseases of Children,* **120,** 122–124.

Livingstone, R. E., Reis, C. J. & Ringdahl, I. C. (1984) Abnormal dexamethazone suppression test results in depressed and nondepressed children. *American Journal of Psychiatry,* **141,** 106–108.

Lobovits, D. A. & Handal, P. J. (1985) Childhood depression: prevalence using DSM-III criteria and validity of parent and child depression scales. *Journal of Paediatric Psychology,* **10,** 45–54.

Lucas, A. L., Lockett, H. J. & Grimm, F. (1965) Amitriptyline in childhood depression. *Diseases of the Nervous System,* **26,** 105–110.

Makita, K. (1973) The rarity of "depression" in childhood. *Acta Psychiatrica Scandinavica,* **40,** 37–44.

Malmquist, C. P. (1972) Depressive phenomena in children. In *Manual of Child Psychopathology* (ed. B. B. Wolman), New York: McGraw Hill.

McClure, G. & Gould, M. (1984) Recent trends in suicide among the young. *British Journal of Psychiatry,* **144,** 134–138.

McConville, B. J., Boag, L. C. & Purohit, A. (1973) Three types of childhood depression. *Canadian Psychiatric Association Journal,* **18,** 133–137.

Mokros, H. B., Poznanski, E., Grossman, J. A. & Freeman, L. N. (1987) A comparison of child and parent ratings of depression for normal and clinically referred children. *Journal of Child Psychology and Psychiatry,* **28,** 613–624.

Moretti, M. M., Fine, S., Haley, G. & Marriage, K. (1985) Childhood and adolescent depression: child-report versus parent-report information. *Journal of the American Academy of Child Psychiatry,* **24,** 298–302.

Murray, P. A. (1970) The clinical picture of depression in school children. *Irish Medical Journal,* **63,** 53–56.

Nunn, C. M. H. (1979) Mixed affective states and the natural history of manic-depressive psychosis. *British Journal of Psychiatry,* **134,** 153–160.

Olsen, T. (1961) Follow-up study of manic-depressive patients whose first attack occurred before the age of 19 years. *Acta Psychiatrica Scandinavica,* **Suppl. 162,** 45–51.

Orvaschel, H., Puig-Antich, J., Chambers, W. J. *et al* (1982) Retrospective assessment of prepubertal major depression with the Kiddie-SADS-E. *Journal of the American Academy of Child Psychiatry,* **4,** 392–397.

——, Weissman, M. M., Padian, N. & Lowe, T. (1981) Assessing psychopathology in children of psychiatrically disturbed parents: a pilot study. *Journal of the American Academy of Child Psychiatry,* **20,** 112–122.

Ossofsky, H. (1974) Endogenous depression in infancy and childhood. *Comprehensive Psychiatry,* **15,** 19–25.

Pallmeyer, T. P. & Petti, T. A. (1979) Effects of imipramine on aggression and dejection in depressed children. *American Journal of Psychiatry,* **136,** 1472–1473.

Pearce, J. (1977) Depressive disorder in childhood. *Journal of Child Psychology and Psychiatry,* **18,** 79–82.

—— (1978) The recognition of depressive disorder in children. *Journal of the Royal Society of Medicine,* **71,** 494–500.

Petti, T. A. (1978) Depression in hospitalized child psychiatry patients. *Journal of the American Academy of Child Psychiatry,* **17,** 49–59.

——, Bornstein, M., Delamater, A. & Connors, C. K. (1980) Evaluation and multimodality treatment of a depressed prepubertal girl. *Journal of the American Academy of Child Psychiatry,* **19,** 690–702.

—— & Connors, K. C. (1983) Changes in behavioural ratings of depressed children treated with imipramine. *Journal of the American Academy of Child Psychiatry,* **22,** 355–360.

Pfeffer, C. R., Conte, H. R., Plutchik, R. & Jerrett, I. (1979) Suicidal behavior in latency-age children: an empirical study. *Journal of the American Academy of Child Psychiatry,* **18,** 679–692.

——, ——, —— & —— (1980) Suicidal behavior in latency age children: an outpatient population. *Journal of the American Academy of Child Psychiatry,* **19,** 703–710.

——, Plutchik, R. & Mizruchi, M. S. (1983) Suicidal and assaultive behavior in children: classification, measurement and interrelations. *American Journal of Psychiatry,* **140,** 154–157.

——, Solomon, G., Plutchik, R., Mizruchi, M. S. & Weiner, A. (1982) Suicidal behaviour in latency-age psychiatric inpatients: a replication and cross validation. *Journal of the American Academy of Child Psychiatry,* **6,** 564–569.

——, Zuckerman, S., Plutchik, R. & Mizruchi, M. S. (1984) Suicidal behavior in normal school children: a comparison with child psychiatric inpatients. *Journal of the American Academy of Child Psychiatry,* **23,** 416–423.

Pfefferbaum-Levine, B., Kumor, K., Cangir, A., Choroszy, M. & Rosebery, E. A. (1983) Tricyclic antidepressants for children with cancer. *American Journal of Psychiatry,* **140,** 1074–1076.

Pinneau, S. R. (1955) Infantile disorders of hospitalism and anaclitic depression. *Psychological Bulletin,* **52,** 429–452.

Polvan, O. & Cebiroglu, R. (1972) Treatment with psychopharmacologic agents in children depression. In *Depressive States in Childhood and Adolescence* (ed. A. L. Annell). Stockholm: Almqvist and Wiksell, pp. 467–472.

Poznanski, E. O. (1982) The clinical phenomenology of childhood depression. *American Journal of Orthopsychiatry,* **52,** 308–313.

——, Carroll, B. J., Banegas, M. C., Cook, S. C. & Grossman, J. A. (1982) The dexamethasone test in prepubertal depressed children. *American Journal of Psychiatry,* **139,** 321–324.

——, Krahenbull, V. & Zrull, J. (1976) Childhood depression: a longitudinal perspective. *Journal of the American Academy of Child Psychiatry,* **15,** 491–501.

——, Mokros, H. B., Grossman, J. & Freeman, L. N. (1985) Diagnostic criteria in childhood depression. *American Journal of Psychiatry,* **142,** 1168–1173.

—— & Zrull, J. (1970) Childhood depression: clinical characteristics of overtly depressed children. *Archives of General Psychiatry,* **23,** 8–15.

Preskorn, S. H. (1984) Clinical usefulness of monitoring imipramine plasma levels in depressed children. In *Current Perspectives on Major Depressive Disorders in Children.* (eds B. Weller & R. A. Weller). Washington DC: American Psychiatric Press, 65–75.

——, Weller, E. B. & Weller, R. A. (1982) Depression in children: relationship between plasma imipramine levels and response. *Journal of Clinical Psychiatry,* **43,** 450–453.

Puig-Antich, J. (1982) Major depression and conduct disorder in prepuberty. *Journal of the American Academy of Child Psychiatry,* **21,** 118–128.

—— (1986) Psychobiological markers: effects of age and puberty. In *Depression in Young People: Issues and Perspectives* (eds M. Rutter, C. Izard & P. Read) New York: Guilford Press.

——, Blau, S., Marx, N., Greenhill, L. L. & Chambers, W. (1978) Prepubertal major depressive disorder: A pilot study. *Journal of the American Academy of Child Psychiatry,* **17,** 685–707.

—— & Chambers, W. (1978) Schedule for affective disorders and schizophrenia for school-age children (6–16 years). Second working draft. March 1978. Unpublished manuscript. University of Pittsburgh.

——, ——, Halpern, F. *et al.* (1979b) Cortisol hypersecretion in prepubertal depressive illness: a preliminary report, *Psychoneuroendocrinology,* **4,** 191–197.

—— & Gittelman, R. (1982) Depression in childhood and adolescence. In *Handbook of Affective Disorders* (ed. E. S. Paykel) London: Churchill Livingstone.

——, Goetz, R., Davies, M., Fein, M., Hanlon, C., Chambers, W. J., Tabrizi, M. A., Sacher, E. J. & Weitzman, E. D. (1984a) Growth hormone secretion in prepubertal children with major depression: II. Sleep related plasma concentrations during a depressive episode. *Archives of General Psychiatry,* **41,** 463–466.

——, ——, ——, Tabrizi, M. A., Novacenko, H., Hanlon, C., Sachar, E. J. & Weitzman, E. D. (1984b) Growth hormone secretion in prepubertal children with major depression: IV. Sleep related plasma concentrations in a drug-free, fully recovered clinical state. *Archives of General Psychiatry,* **41,** 479–483.

——, ——, Hanlon, C., Davies, M., Thompson, A., Chambers, W., Tabrizi, M. A. & Weitzman, E. D. (1982) Sleep architecture and REM sleep in prepubertal children with major depression. *Archives of General Psychiatry,* **39,** 932–939.

——, ——, ——, Tabrizi, M. A., Davies, M. & Weitzman, E. D. (1983) Sleep architecture and REM sleep measures in prepubertal major depressives: studies during recovery from a major depressive episode in a drug free state. *Archives of General Psychiatry,* **49,** 187–192.

——, Novacenko, H., Davies, M., Chambers, W. J., Tabrizi, M. A., Krawiec, V., Ambrosini, P. J. & Sacher, E. J. (1984c) Growth hormone secretion in prepubertal children with major depression: I. Final report on response to insulin-induced hypoglycemia during a depressive episode. *Archives of General Psychiatry,* **41,** 444–460.

——, ——, ——, Tabrizi, M. A., Ambrosini, P., Goetz, R., Bianca, J., Goetz, D. & Sachar, E. J. (1984d) Growth hormone secretion in prepubertal children with major depression: III. Response to insulin-induced hypoglycemia after recovery from a depessive episode and in a drug-free state. *Archives of General Psychiatry*, **41**, 471–475.

——, ——, Goetz, R., Corser, J., Davies, M. & Ryan, N. (1984e) Cortisol and prolactin responses to insulin-induced hypoglycemia in prepubertal major depressives during episode and after recovery. *Journal of the American Academy of Child Psychiatry*, **23**, 49–57.

——, Perel, J. M. & Lupatkin, W. (1979a) Plasma levels of imipramine (IMI) and clinical response in prepubertal major depressive disorder. *Journal of the American Academy of Child Psychiatry*, **18**, 616–627.

——, Perel, J. M., Lupatkin, W., Chambers, W. J., Tabrizi, M. A., King, J., Goetz, R., Davies, M. & Stiller, R. L. (1987) Imipramine in prepubertal major depressive disorders. *Archives of General Psychiatry*, **44**, 81–89.

Rapoport, J. L. (1977) Pediatric psychopharmacology and childhood depression. In *Depression in Childhood: Diagnosis, Treatment and Conceptual Models* (eds J. S. Schulterbrandt & A. Raskin). New York: Raven Press.

Reich, W., Herjanic, B., Welner, Z. & Gandhy, P. R. (1982) Development of a structured psychiatric interview for children: agreement on diagnosis comparing child and parent interviews. *Journal of Abnormal Child Psychology* **10**, 325–336.

Rie, H. E. (1966) Depression in childhood: a survey of some pertinent contributions. *Journal of the American Academy of Child Psychiatry*, **5**, 653–685.

Robbins, D. R. & Alessi, N. E. (1985) Depressive symptoms and suicidal behavior in adolescents. *American Journal of Psychiatry*, **142**, 588–592.

——, ——, Yanchyshyn, G. W. & Colfer, M. V. (1983) The dexamethasone suppression test in psychiatrically hospitalized adolescents. *Journal of the American Academy of Child Psychiatry*, **22**, 467–469.

Robertson, J. & Robertson, J. (1971) Young children in brief separation: a fresh look. *Psychoanalytic Study of the Child*, **26**, 264–315.

Rutter, M. (1980) Emotional development. In *Scientific Foundations of Developmental Psychiatry*. London: Heinemann Medical.

—— (1986a) The developmental psychopathology of depression: issues and perspectives. In *Depression in Young People: Developmental and Clinical Perspectives* (eds M. Rutter, C. E. Izard & P. B. Read). New York: Guilford Press.

—— (1986b) Depressive feelings, cognitions and disorders: a research postscript. In *Depression in Young People: Developmental and Clinical Perspectives* (eds M. Rutter, C. E. Izard & P. B. Read). New York: Guilford Press.

——, Graham, P., Chadwick, O. F. D. & Yule, W. (1976) Adolescent turmoil: fact or fiction? *Journal of Child Psychology and Psychiatry*, **17**, 35–56.

——, Izard, C. E. & Read, P. B. (eds) (1986) *Depression in Young People: Clinical and Developmental Perspectives*. New York: Guilford Press.

——, Shaffer, D. & Sturge, C. (1975) *A Guide to a Multi-Axial Classification Scheme for Psychiatric Disorders in Childhood and Adolescence*. London: Frowde & Co (Printers) Ltd.

——, Tizard, J. & Whitmore, K. (1970) *Education, Health and Behavior*. London: Longmans.

Sadler, W. S. (1952) Juvenile manic activity. *The Nervous Child*, **9**, 363–368.

Sandler, J. & Joffe, W. G. (1965) Notes on childhood depression. *International Journal of Psychoanalysis*, **46**, 88–96.

Saraf, K., Klein, D., Gittleman-Klein, R. & Grof, S. (1974) Imipramine and side effects in children. *Psychopharmacologia, 37,* 265–275.

Schou, M. (1972) Lithium in psychiatric therapy and prophylaxis. A review with special regard to its use in children. In *Depressive States in Childhood and Adolescence* (ed. A. N. Annell). Stockholm: Almqvist and Wiksell.

Shaffer, D. (1982) Diagnostic considerations in suicidal behaviour in children and adolescents. *Journal of the American Academy of Child Psychiatry, 21,* 414–416.

—— (1985) Depression, mania and suicidal acts. In *Child and Adolescent Psychiatry: Modern Approaches* (2nd edn) (eds. M. Rutter & L. Hersov). Oxford: Blackwell Scientific.

—— (1986) Developmental factors in child and adolescent suicide. In *Depression in Young People: Issues and Perspectives* (eds M. Rutter, C. Izard & P. Read). New York: Guilford Press.

—— & Fisher, P. (1981) The epidemiology of suicide in children and young adolescents. *Journal of the American Academy of Child Psychiatry, 20,* 45–65.

Shepherd, M., Oppenheim, A. N. & Mitchell, S. (1966) Childhood behaviour disorders and the child guidance clinic. An epidemiological study. *Journal of Child Psychology and Psychiatry, 7,* 39–52.

——, —— & —— (1971) *Childhood Behaviour and Mental Health.* New York: Grune and Stratton.

Spitz, R. A. (1946) Anaclitic depression. *Psychoanalystic Study of the Child, 2,* 313–342.

Spitzer, R. L., Endicott, J. & Robins, E. (1978) Research diagnostic criteria: rationale and reliability. *Archives of General Psychiatry, 35,* 773–782.

Stack, J. J. (1972) Chemotherapy in childhood depression. In *Depressive States in Childhood and Adolescence* (ed. A. L. Annell). Stockholm: Almqvist and Wiksell.

Strober, M. & Carlson, G. A. (1982) Bipolar illness in adolescents with major depression: clinical, genetic and psychopharmacologic predictors in a three-to-four-year prospective follow up investigation. *Archives of General Psychiatry, 39,* 549–555.

——, Green, J. & Carlson, G. (1981) Phenomenology and subtypes of major depressive disorder in adolescence. *Journal of Affective Disorders, 3,* 281–290.

Targum, S. D. & Capodanno, A. E. (1983) The dexamethasone suppression test in adolescent psychiatric inpatients. *American Journal of Psychiatry, 140,* 589–591.

Taylor, F. A. & Stansfeld, S. A. (1984a) Children who poison themselves: I. A clinical comparison with psychiatric controls. *British Journal of Psychiatry, 145,* 127–132.

Taylor, E. A. & Stansfeld, S. A. (1984b) Children who poison themselves: II. Prediction of attendance for treatment. *British Journal of Psychiatry, 145,* 132–135.

Toolan, J. (1962) Depression in children and adolescents. *American Journal of Orthopsychiatry, 32,* 404–414.

Vranjesevic, B., Radojicic, S. & Bumbasirevic, S. (1972) Depressive manifestations in children with intracranial tumors. In *Depressive States in Childhood and Adolescence* (ed. A. L. Annell). Stockholm: Almqvist and Wiksell.

Weinberg, J. & Van den Dungen, M. (1972) Depression and delinquency in adolescence: A psychodynamic study. In *Depressive States in Childhood and Adolescence* (ed. A. N. Annell). Stockholm: Almqvist and Wiksell.

Weinberg, W. A. & Brumback, R. A. (1976) Mania in childhood: case studies and literature review. *American Journal of Diseases of Children, 130,* 380–395.

——, Rutman, J., Sullivan, L., Penick, E. C. & Dietz, S. (1973) Depression in children referred to an educational diagnostic center: diagnosis and treatment. *Journal of Pediatrics*, **83**, 1065–1072.

Weissman, M. M., Orvaschel, H. & Padian, N. (1980) Children's symptom and social functioning self-report scales: comparison of mothers' and children's reports. *Journal of Nervous and Mental Disease*, **168**, 736–740.

Weller, R. A., Weller, E. B. & Herjanic, B. (1983) Adult psychiatric disorders in psychiatrically ill young adolescents. *American Journal of Psychiatry*, **22**, 52–58.

Weller, E. B., Weller, R. A., Fristad, M. A. & Preskorn, S. H. (1984) Dexamethasone suppression test in prepubertal depressed children. *American Journal of Psychiatry*, **141**, 290–291.

——, —— & Preskorn, S. (1982) Steady-state plasma imipramine levels in prepubertal depressed children. *American Journal of Psychiatry*, **139**, 506–508.

——, —— & Preskorn, S. (1983) Depression in children: effects of antidepressant therapy. *Journal of the Kansas Medical Society*, **84**, 117–119.

Weller, R. A. & Weller, E. B. (1984) The use of antidepressants in prepubertal depressed children. In *Current Perspectives on Major Depressive Disorders in Children* (eds E. B. Weller & R. A. Weller), pp. 65–75. Washington, DC: American Psychiatric Press.

Welner, A., Welner, Z. & Fishman, R. (1979) Psychiatric adolescent inpatients: eight to ten year follow-up. *Archives of General Psychiatry*, **36**, 698–700.

World Health Organization (1978) *Mental Disorders: Glossary and Guide to their Classification in Accordance with the Ninth Revision of the International Classification of Diseases* (ICD-9). Geneva: WHO.

Young, E., Knowles, J. B., Maclean, A. W., Boag, L. & McConville, B. J. (1982) The sleep of childhood depressives. Comparison with age-matched controls. *Biological Psychiatry*, **17**, 1163–1168.

Youngerman, J. & Canino, I. A. (1978) Lithium carbonate use in children and adolescents. *Archives of General Psychiatry*, **35**, 216–224.

Zeitlin, H. (1986) *The Natural History of Psychiatric Disorder in Children*, Institute of Psychiatry Maudsley Monograph No 29. London: Oxford University Press.

PART VI: DEPRESSION AND SUICIDE

23

Normal Children at Risk for Suicidal Behavior: A Two-Year Follow-up Study

Cynthia R. Pfeffer
Cornell University Medical College, New York, New York
New York Hospital
Robert Lipkins
New York Hospital
Robert Plutchik and Mark Mizruchi
Albert Einstein College of Medicine, Bronx, New York

Seventy-five preadolescents, mean age 12.1 ± 0.25 years, with no prior history of psychiatric care, and their mothers were extensively interviewed in this 2-year follow-up study. Among 67 children who reported on suicidal tendencies at follow-up, there were: 80.6% nonsuicidal, 17.9% with suicidal ideas, and 1.5% with suicidal threats. One hundred and one children studied initially included 88.1% nonsuicidal, 8.9% with suicidal ideas, 2.0% with suicidal threats, and 1.0% with mild suicidal attempts. Fifty percent reported suicidal ideas or acts initially and at follow-up. Of the children who were not initially suicidal, 15.3% were suicidal at follow-up. Suicidal tendencies at follow-up were associated with depression, death preoccupation, aggression, general psychopathology, and ego defenses of denial, reaction formation, and projection. Associations between suicidal tendencies and depression,

Reprinted with permission from the *Journal of the American Academy of Child and Adolescent Psychiatry,* 1988, Vol. 27, No. 1, 34–41. Copyright 1988 by the American Academy of Child and Adolescent Psychiatry.

This paper was presented at the 33rd Annual Meeting of the American Academy of Child Psychiatry, Los Angeles, California, October 1986.

This study was funded by a New York Hospital-Westchester Division Grant, the Herman Goldman Foundation, and National Institute of Mental Health Grant, No. 1ROMH37830–01.

Annual Progress in Child Psychiatry and Development

*death preoccupations, and general psychopathology were reported
also in the initial study. At follow-up, some factors not associated
with suicidal tendencies were: social status, age, sex, race/ethnic-
ity, impulse control, hopelessness, and parental depression. Implications of these findings are discussed.*

The present investigation, a continuation of our previous study (Pfeffer et
al., 1984) of schoolchildren with no prior history of psychiatric care, will
evaluate the prevalence of and psychosocial factors associated with suicidal
ideas and acts in the same schoolchildren 2 years after they were intially evaluated. More specifically, the present study will evaluate whether the same
variables, which were found to be associated with suicidal ideas and acts in
the initial study, will be associated with suicidal ideas and acts at the time of
follow-up. In addition, this study will determine whether the same children
exhibit suicidal ideas and acts both in the present study and at the initial time
of investigation 2 years previously.

There is relatively little information about prevalence rates of suicidal behavior in the general population of children and adolescents. Recent work
(Harkavy and Asnis, 1986; Josef et al., 1986) suggests that about 8% of adolescents in public school settings reported having attempted suicide within the
past year. In addition, preliminary data on the prevalence rates of depression
have been presented. Kandel and Davis (1982) reported that among 8,206 adolescents, aged 14 to 18 years, who were administered a self-report questionnaire, 19.7% reported feeling sad or depressed in the past year. Depressed
mood was more frequent among girls, and low levels of depressed mood correlated with high levels of attachment to parents and peers. Kashani et al.
(1983) investigated 955 9-year-olds in the Dunedin Multidisciplinary Child
Development Study with self-report measures and the K-SADS-E. They found
that there was a prevalence rate of 1.8% major depressive disorder and 2.5%
minor depressive disorder. There was no mention of suicidal behavior as a
factor evaluated in that study, however. Anderson et al. (1987) reported a prevalence of 1.8% of depression-dysthymia among 792 children, age 11 years,
from the Dunedin Multidisciplinary Child Development Study. These children
were evaluated with the Diagnostic Interview Schedule for Children. Kaplan et
al. (1984), using the Beck Depression Inventory self-report measure, found
that among 385 junior and senior high school students, 77.9% were not depressed, 13.5% were mildly depressed, 7.3% were moderately depressed, and
1.3% were seriously depressed. The younger adolescents were less depressed
than the older adolescents. This study noted that 23.8% of the adolescents
expressed suicidal ideation.

These studies, although they establish some index of prevalence rates within a given time period, have not followed the children over an extended period of time in order to identify the stability of suicidal behavior or depression. The present study will evaluate this issue.

METHOD

In our initial investigation, 101 schoolchildren, aged 6 to 12 years, were interviewed between December 1980 and June 1982 (Pfeffer et al., 1984). These schoolchildren were selected by stratified random sampling from a computerized roster of pupils in a large urban community. Stratification was on age, sex, and racial/ethnic distribution to match the comparable percentage of age, sex, and racial/ethnic distribution of a comparison group of 65 children who were previously studied in a voluntary hospital child psychiatry inpatient unit (Pfeffer et al., 1984). Of 1,565 children in the school roster, there were 71 boys and 30 girls chosen for our initial study. The mean age was 9.7 ± 1.2 years and the racial/ethnic distribution was 75.2% white and 24.8% black, Hispanic, or oriental. These children were predominantly from middle to low social status backgrounds. Any child who was in a special class for emotionally disturbed or neurologically handicapped was excluded from this study.

In the present 2-year follow-up study, 75 (74.3%) children who were originally studied gave informed consent to be reinterviewed. None of these children had a history of psychiatric treatment. Of the total sample of 75 children re-interviewed, data about the presence or absence of suicidal behavior were obtained for 67 children. Data about the presence or absence of suicidal behavior were not obtained for eight children, because the children refused to talk about suicidal behavior and the parents reported being unaware of whether or not such tendencies existed. Among the children not reevaluated at follow-up, 16 (15.8%) refused to participate and 10 (9.9%) children could not be located. These children, who were not re-interviewed, did not differ on distributions of age, sex, race/ethnicity, social status, religion, suicidal tendencies, and psychiatric diagnoses from the distributions of the same variables for the children who were re-interviewed.

Demographic features of the children at the initial (T_1) and at the 2-year follow-up (T_3) evaluations are presented in Table 1.

There were no significant differences in distributions of sex, race/ethnicity, social status, and religion between the children evaluated initially and at follow-up. Social status of the fathers, measured by the Hollingshead Two-Factor Classification (1958) was predominantly middle to low middle.

TABLE 1. *Demographic Features of Normal Children at Initial and at 2-Year Follow-up Evaluations*

	Initial (T₁)		Follow-up (T₃)	
	N	%	N	%
No. of children	101	100	75	100
Sex				
Boys	71	70.3	52	69.3
Girls	30	29.7	23	30.7
Race/ethnicity				
White	76	75.2	54	72.0
Other (black, Hispanic, Oriental)	25	24.8	21	28.0
Social status father	(N = 101)		(N = 72)	
I	7	7.1	1	1.4
II	4	4.1	4	5.6
III	19	19.4	16	22.2
IV	51	52.1	35	48.6
V	20	17.3	16	22.2
Religion				
Catholic	69	68.3	50	66.7
Protestant	18	17.8	13	17.3
Jewish	7	6.9	4	5.3
Other	7	6.9	8	10.7
Mean age (years)	9.7	±1.20	12.1	±0.25

Table 1. Demographic Features of Normal Children at Initial and at 2-Year Follow-up Evaluations

Each child and parent (usually the mother) was interviewed for up to 2 hours each by either a child psychiatrist or a child psychologist who was experienced in interviewing techniques, DSM-III criteria, and the use of the research instruments. To ensure that there was no bias in the follow-up interviews, the interviewers for this follow-up study were different from those who evaluated the children at the time of the initial assessment. In addition, they were not given information about the findings for the children in the initial study.

All interviews were conducted at the school the child attended. The interviews were semistructured to enable comprehensive gathering of data about the child's symptoms, behaviors, development, school performance, social functioning, and family history. All information obtained in the interviews was used to provide data required by the research instruments.

The battery of research instruments, called the Child Suicide Potential Scales, used in our initial and the present follow-up studies consisted of a Spectrum of Suicidal Behavior Scale, a Spectrum of Assaultive Behavior

Scale, a Precipitating Events Scale, Recent and Past General Psychopathology Scale, Child Concept of Death Scale, Family Background Scale, Ego Mechanism Scale, Ego Defense Scale, and Medical/Neurological History Questionnaire. For statistical analysis, a mean or total score could be determined for each scale. These scores were used in data analysis.

The Spectrum of Suicidal Behavior Scale defines and measures the severity of recent suicidal behaviors occurring in the 6-month period before evaluation. For purposes of statistical analysis, the Spectrum of Suicidal Behavior Scale is a 5-point scale ranging from nonsuicidal behavior (rated 1), suicidal ideas (rated 2), suicidal threats (rated 3), mild suicide attempts (rated 4), and serious suicide attempts (rated 5). Each child's score on the Spectrum of Suicidal Behavior Scale was determined by the highest degree of observed suicidal tendency. For example, those who had suicidal ideas and serious suicidal attempts were rated as making serious suicide attempts.

The presence of current DSM-III diagnoses at the time of follow-up were determined by the interviewer by applying DSM-III criteria to the clinical data (excluding the scores on the Child Suicide Potential Scales). The internal and interrater reliabilities and discriminative validity of the research instruments have been established previously and are high (Pfeffer et al., 1979, 1980, 1982, 1984). To provide a measure of the interrater reliability for the data collected in the present study, two clinicians simultaneously observed 15 child and parent interviews and separately recorded information on the research instruments. The ratings made by the two clinicians for the research instruments and current DSM-III diagnoses were intercorrelated. This was done separately for each scale and for the diagnoses. The product moment correlations representing interjudge reliability range from $r = 1.00$ to 0.60; these represent relatively high values.

In the present study, data were collected with the Child Suicide Potential Scales for three time periods. The initial period (T_1) was the time of the original assessments 2 years ago. The intervening time (T_2) was defined as the time between the initial assessment and 6 months before the follow-up evaluation. The follow-up time (T_3) involved the 6 months preceding and the time inclusive of the follow-up evaluation. Data for (T_2) were collected during the follow-up evaluation at (T_3).

In addition to these research instruments, each parent was asked to complete the Achenbach Child Behavior Checklist and Child Behavior Profile, which provided information about the child's present social competence in school, social, and activity spheres and about symptoms and behavior (Achenbach, 1978; Achenbach and Edelbrock, 1979). Each child was asked to complete the Children's Depression Inventory (Kovacs, 1980) and The Children's Hopelessness Scale (Kazdin et al., 1983). These self-report scales provide measures of the children's current perceptions of their own symptoms of depression and their sense of negative expectations.

Statistical Analysis

For statistical analysis, suicidal children were defined as those who showed evidence of suicidal thoughts or acts. The nonsuicidal children were those with no evidence of suicidal impulses. Continuous variables were analyzed with t tests or analysis of variance. Categorical variables were evaluated with chi-square tests.

RESULTS

Diagnosis

Prevalences of current DSM-III diagnoses for all the children studied at the initial (T_1) and at 2-year follow-up (T_3) evaluations are shown in Table 2.

With regard to the presence of a current psychiatric diagnosis, 57.3% of the children at follow-up (T_3), in contrast to 55.5% of the children at initial (T_1)

TABLE 2. *DSM-III Diagnoses of Normal Children at Initial (N = 101) and At Follow-up (N = 75) Evaluations*

Diagnosis	Initial (T_1)		Follow-up (T_3)	
	N	%	N	%
Axis I				
Overanxious disorder	28	27.7	20	26.7
Dysthymic disorder	14	13.9	17	22.7
Oppositional disorder	16	15.8	14	18.7
Adjustment disorder	3	3.0	8	10.7
Conduct disorder	6	5.9	6	8.0
Other disorders with physical symptoms	9	8.9	4	5.3
Attention deficit disorder	3	3.0	3	4.0
Major depressive disorder	0	0	1	1.3
Schizophrenia	1	1.0	0	0
Axis II				
Specific developmental disorder	15	14.9	12	16.0
Other personality disorder	5	5.0	3	4.0
Borderline personality disorder	0	0.0	2	2.7

Table 2. DSM-III Diagnoses of Normal Children at Initial (N = 101) and at Follow-up (N = 75) Evaluations

evaluation, were given a psychiatric diagnosis. There were a total of nine Axis I diagnoses and three Axis II diagnoses given at the time of follow-up (T_3), in contrast to eight Axis I diagnoses and two Axis II diagnoses given initially (T_1). If indicated, multiple diagnoses were used for each child.

The most prevalent Axis I diagnoses at the initial (T_1) and follow-up (T_3) evaluations were overanxious, dysthymic, and oppositional disorders. Specific developmental disorder was the most prevalent Axis II diagnosis at the time of both evaluations. The relation between follow-up diagnoses and suicidal behavior at follow-up was examined for those diagnoses that were given to at least five children. Using Fisher's exact test, there were no significant relations at the 0.05 level between a particular follow-up diagnosis and suicidal behavior at follow-up. Similarly, there were no associations between diagnoses and suicidal behavior assessed in the initial study (Pfeffer et al., 1984). When the children were grouped according to whether they were given any type of psychiatric diagnosis at the time of follow-up (T_3), however, significantly more suicidal children had a current DSM-III diagnosis than the nonsuicidal children ($\chi^2 = 4.62$, $df = 1$, $p < 0.03$).

Spectrum of Suicidal Behavior

Distributions on the Spectrum of Suicidal Behavior Scale for the children and their parents at the initial (T_1) and follow-up (T_3) evaluations are shown in Table 3.

At the 2-year follow-up, 17.9% of the children reported suicidal ideas and 1.5% indicated that they exhibited suicidal threats. No child attempted suicide: There was no difference between the boys and girls for the presence of suicidal ideas and/or threats. There was no difference in the severity of suicidal tendencies at the initial assessment (T_1) and the follow-up assessment (T_3) ($p < 0.06$).

| | Nonsuicidal | | Suicidal | | | | Suicide Attempts | | | | | |
| | | | Ideas | | Threats | | Mild | | Serious | | Suicide | |
	N	%	N	%	N	%	N	%	N	%	N	%
Children												
Initial evaluation (T_1)	89	88.1	9	8.9	2	2.0	1	1.0	0	0	0	0
Follow-up evaluation (T_3)	54	80.6	12	17.9	1	1.5	0	0	0	0	0	0
Parents												
Mother												
Initial evaluation (T_1)	75	74.3	21	20.8	5	5.0	0	0	0	0	0	0
Follow-up evaluation (T_3)	64	85.3	8	10.7	2	2.7	1	1.3	0	0	0	0
Father												
Initial evaluation (T_1)	95	94.1	5	5.0	1	1.0	0	0	0	0	0	0
Follow-up evaluation (T_3)	70	93.3	3	4.0	0	0	1	1.3	0	0	0	0

Table 3. Distributions on the Spectrum of Suicidal Behavior Scale for Children and Parents

Among the 13 children with suicidal tendencies, most (69.2%) were vague about having a plan for suicidal action. Among the methods considered were jumping from heights, stabbing, wrist cutting, and shooting.

Among the 149 parents, 10.1% expressed suicidal ideas and/or acts. There was no significant relation between the suicidal tendencies of the children and those of the mothers ($T = 0.08$, $df = 65$, $p < 0.94$). The data for the fathers should be considered tentative because most of the data about the fathers were obtained from the mothers.

Differences in Variables for Suicidal and Nonsuicidal Children at Follow-up

Table 4 shows significant differences between the 13 suicidal and the 54 nonsuicidal children for variables measured at 2-year follow-up for the time periods T_2 and T_3.

There were 35 variables analyzed for T_2 and T_3, and there were 11 significant differences between the suicidal and nonsuicidal children. The suicidal children had significantly higher scores on 10 of the 11 variables. Among these variables were depression at T_2 and T_3; death preoccupations at T_3; aggression at T_3; general psychopathology at T_2; and such ego defenses at T_3 as denial, reaction formation, and projection.

There were no significant differences between the suicidal and nonsuicidal children for a variety of factors measured at follow-up. Estimates at T_3 of IQ, reading/spelling/and arithmetic achievements, impulse control, hopelessness, and reality testing were not significantly different. Demographic features at T_3 such as social status, religion, race/ethnicity, age, and sex did not significantly

Variable (Range)[a]	Suicidal			Nonsuicidal			t	df	p
	N	X̄	S.D.	N	X̄	S.D.			
Depression (T₃) (0–13)	13	2.17	2.29	54	0.83	0.99	3.20	64.0	0.002
Death preoccupations (T₃) (0–10)	13	3.31	1.89	54	1.85	1.64	2.79	63.0	0.007
Child Depression Inventory score (T₃) (0–54)	13	10.08	6.76	52	4.92	3.88	2.64[b]	14.0	0.02
Depression (T₂) (0–18)	13	5.00	3.00	54	3.19	2.32	2.39	65.0	0.02
Denial (T₃) (1–3)	13	2.23	0.73	54	1.72	0.50	2.42[b]	14.9	0.03
Reaction formation (T₃) (1–3)	13	1.69	0.63	54	1.25	0.43	2.42[b]	14.9	0.03
Achenbach Aggressive Behavior (T₃) (55–100)	10	60.90	5.51	41	57.90	3.71	2.07	49.0	0.04
Mother's assaultive behavior (T₃) (1–6)	13	1.08	0.28	54	1.40	1.07	−2.00[b]	64.5	0.05
General psychopathology (T₂) (0–40)	13	10.54	5.50	54	7.59	4.53	2.02	65.0	0.05
Achenbach Sum of Behavior Problems (T₃) (30–100)	10	59.90	7.62	41	53.32	9.83	1.97	49.0	0.05
Projection (T₃) (1–3)	13	1.85	0.80	54	1.45	0.57	2.04	64.0	0.05

[a] Range of scores for each scale.
[b] Separate variance estimate.

Table 4. Significant Differences in Variables for Suicidal and Nonsuicidal Children Measured at Follow-up

differentiate the suicidal from the nonsuicidal children at follow-up. There were no differences for assaultive behavior at T_3. There were no differences for such family and environmental factors as environmental events at T_3, number of children in the family, ordinal position of the child in the family, parental separation, birth weight, pregnancy complications, history of parental problems such as chronic medical illness, depression, psychiatric hospitalization, alcohol/drug abuse, use of over-the-counter medication, and suicidal behavior of other relatives.

It should be noted that 33.3% of all of the children interviewed at follow-up experienced parental separation/divorce. Of the 75 children evaluated, 7.4% had at least one parent with symptoms of depression, 4.7% had at least one parent who abused alcohol and/or drugs, 6.7% had other relatives who attempted suicide, and 8.0% had relatives who committed suicide. The scores on all scales of the Achenbach Child Behavior Checklist and Profile at T_3 for the children as a group were within the normal range.

Stability of Variables

A comparison of initial (T_1) and follow-up (T_3) scores for the presence of suicidal tendencies and psychiatric diagnoses was made to evaluate the stability of these factors during the 2 years between the initial and follow-up period. For statistical analysis of these categorical factors, the children were grouped into four different groups depending upon whether each variable was present or absent at the initial and/or follow-up time (Table 5).

With regard to the stability of the presence of suicidal tendencies over the 2-year time, no suicidal tendencies were noted for 84.7% of the children at both the initial and follow-up assessment. Fifty percent of the children who initially reported suicidal tendencies also reported them at follow-up. In addition, 15.3% of the children reported suicidal tendencies at follow-up but not at the initial assessment.

With regard to the stability of DSM-III diagnoses during the 2-year time, there were significant differences among the four groups of children. Although 58.8% of the children did not have a psychiatric diagnosis at the initial assessment (T_1) and at follow-up (T_3), 41.2% who were without an initial diagnosis were diagnosed at follow-up. Of the children who were initially given a diagnosis, 70.7% were also given a diagnosis at follow-up. Of the children who initially had a diagnosis, 29.3% were not given a diagnosis at follow-up.

With regard to the stability of specific DSM-III diagnoses during the 2-year time of study, there were significant differences among the four groups of children for six diagnoses based on chi-square analysis. These diagnoses were overanxious disorder, other disorders with physical manifestations, oppositional, dysthymic, specific developmental, and other personality disorders. The

Variable	Presence of Variable Initially and at Follow-up[a]								χ^{2b}	P
	No[1] No[2]		No[1] Yes[2]		Yes[1] Yes[2]		Yes[1] No[2]			
	N	%	N	%	N	%	N	%		
Presence of suicidal ideas and/or acts (N = 67)	50	84.7	9	15.3	4	50.0	4	50.0	3.44	0.06
Having a DSM-III diagnosis (N = 75)	20	58.8	14	41.2	29	70.7	12	29.3	5.48	0.02
Axis I diagnoses										
Overanxious disorder (N = 75)	50	86.2	8	13.8	12	70.6	5	29.4	18.88	0.001
Oppositional disorder (N = 75)	55	88.7	7	11.3	7	53.8	6	46.2	10.17	0.001
Other disorder with physical manifestations (N = 75)	67	98.5	1	1.5	3	42.9	4	57.1	14.11	0.001
Dysthymic disorder (N = 75)	56	81.2	13	18.8	4	66.7	2	33.3	4.73	0.03
Conduct disorder (N = 75)	66	94.3	4	5.7	2	40.0	3	60.0	3.52	0.06
Attention deficit disorder (N = 75)	70	97.2	2	2.8	1	33.3	2	66.7	1.31	0.25
Adjustment disorder (N = 75)	64	88.9	8	11.1	0	0	0	0	0	1.00
Major depressive disorder (N = 75)	74	98.7	1	1.3	0	0	0	0	–	–
Eating disorder (N = 75)	74	98.7	1	1.3	0	0	0	0	–	–
Other disorders of childhood (N = 75)	73	97.3	2	2.7	0	0	0	0	–	–
Axis II diagnoses										
Specific developmental disorder (N = 75)	58	93.5	4	6.5	8	61.5	5	38.5	20.34	0.0001
Other personality disorder (N = 75)	69	98.6	1	1.4	2	40.0	3	60.0	9.43	0.002
Borderline personality disorder (N = 75)	73	97.3	2	2.7	0	0	0	0	–	–

[a] The superscript 1 refers to the initial data and superscript 2 refers to follow-up data. No[1] No[2], variable absent initially and at follow-up; No[1] Yes[2], variable present only at follow-up; Yes[1] Yes[2], variable present initially and at follow-up; Yes[1] No[2], variable present only initially.
[b] Yates corrected.

Table 5. Frequency of the Presence of Variables at Initial and Follow-up Times for Four Different Groups

most frequent diagnoses given initially and at follow-up were overanxious, dysthymic, or specific developmental disorder. For example, if a child was initially diagnosed with an overanxious disorder, 70.6% of these children were diagnosed as having overanxious disorders at follow-up.

For continuous variables such as general psychopathology, depression, and death preoccupations, the mean difference scores of each variable for the entire group of children at the initial (T_1) and follow-up (T_3) times are shown in Table 6.

Variable (Range)[a]	Score at T_1		Score at T_3		Mean Difference	S.D.	t	df	p
	Mean	S.D.	Mean	S.D.					
Depression (0–13)	1.85	1.82	1.11	1.39	0.74	1.91	3.35	73	0.0001
Death preoccupation (0–10)	3.09	2.11	2.15	1.78	0.94	2.16	3.51	64	0.001
General psychopathology (0–40)	3.47	3.25	2.70	2.30	0.77	3.23	2.05	73	0.04

[a] Range of scores of each variable.

Table 6. Mean Difference Scores of Variables at Initial (T_1) and Follow-up (T_3) Evaluations

There was a significant change in scores of general psychopathology, depression, and death preoccupations between the initial (T_1) and follow-up (T_3) evaluations. Mean scores for these variables were reported to be significantly lower at the time of follow-up.

Variables Associated with Change in Suicidal Status from Initial to Follow-Up Assessment

In order to determine which variables are associated with a change in suicidal status from the initial (T_1) to the follow-up (T_3) time, scores at T_1, T_2, and T_3 for selected variables were evaluated. The variables evaluated were: depression, general psychopathology, death preoccupations, mother's and father's suicidal behavior, and mother's and father's assaultive behavior. These variables were chosen because they were found to be associated with suicidal behavior of these children in our initial study (Pfeffer et al. 1984) or in this follow-up study (see Table 4). For statistical analysis, the children were classified into four groups depending on whether suicidal tendencies were present or absent at the initial (T_1) and/or follow-up (T_3) evaluations. There were too few children who were suicidal at both T_1 and at T_3 $(N = 4)$, and who were suicidal at T_1 but not at T_3 $(N = 4)$, to make statistical comparisons for these groups, however.

Scores of variables that were associated with a change in suicidal status from the initial (T_1) to follow-up (T_3) assessments are shown in Table 7. These are shown for the comparison of two groups of children: No[1] No[2] and No[1] Yes[2].

When children with no suicidal tendencies initially and at follow-up (No[1] No[2]) are compared with children with no initial suicidal tendencies but with suicidal tendencies at follow-up (No[1] Yes[2]), the children who were suicidal at the time of follow-up had higher mean scores on four variables. Assaultive behavior was the only variable measured at T_1 that was associated with a change in suicidal tendencies at follow-up.

Variable (Time Measured)	No[1] No[2] (N = 50)[a]		No[1] Yes[2] (N = 9)		*t*	*df*	*p*
	Mean	S.D.	Mean	S.D.			
Spectrum of assaultive behavior (T_1)	2.06	1.33	3.22	1.48	2.37	57	0.02
General psychopathology (T_2)	7.32	4.28	11.22	5.36	2.42	57	0.02
Depression (T_2)	3.08	2.18	5.00	3.04	2.28	57	0.03
Death preoccupations (T_3)	1.65	1.31	2.78	1.99	2.18	57	0.03

[a] The superscript 1 refers to initial data and superscript 2 refers to follow up data. No[1] No[2], no suicidal ideas or acts initially or at follow-up; No[1] Yes[2], suicidal ideas or acts only at follow-up.

Table 7. Variables Associated with Suicidal Tendencies in Two Groups at Follow-up

General psychopathology and depression measured at T_2, however, were associated with a change of suicidal tendencies at follow-up. Death preoccupation was the only variable measured at T_3 that was associated with a change in suicidal status.

DISCUSSION

We believe this to be the first reported follow-up study of suicidal behavior in a normal group of preadolescents. Approximately 74.2% of the original children participated in this follow-up study. This percentage is consistent with other follow-up studies of children with a similar time duration (Stanley and Barter, 1970). Furthermore, there were no differences in distributions of our selection variables of sex, race/ethnicity, religion, social status, suicidal tendencies, and diagnoses for those children studied initially and at follow-up. Thus, the children who were evaluated at this follow-up time can be considered representative of the entire sample of 101 children who were studied 2 years previously.

The results of this study indicate that factors associated with suicidal tendencies at the time of follow-up were similar to those found in our initial assessment of these children (Pfeffer et al. 1984). These factors included symptoms of depression, death preoccupations, and general psychopathology. Furthermore, no particular diagnosis was associated with suicidal tendencies initially or at follow-up. In addition, a wide variety of psychosocial variables were not associated with suicidal tendencies either initially or at follow-up. These factors included age, sex, social status, race/ethnicity, family size, IQ, academic achievement, impulse control, reality testing, parental separation/divorce, and parental medical or psychiatric symptoms that included suicidal tendencies, drug or alcohol abuse, or depression.

The Children's Depression Inventory and the Achenbach Child Behavior Checklist and Profile provided an additional check on the validity of the results determined by using the Child Suicide Potential Scales for depressive symptoms and general psychopathology. For example, the children identified as suicidal at the time of follow-up had significantly higher scores than the nonsuicidal children on the Children's Depression Inventory. This concurs with the findings that the suicidal children, compared with the nonsuicidal children, had higher scores for depressive symptoms measured by direct interviews using the Child Suicide Potential Scales. Suicidal children, in contrast to nonsuicidal children, scored higher on the sum score of the behavioral symptoms on the Achenbach Child Behavior Checklist and Profile. This score is a measure of general psychopathology. This finding agrees with the finding that the suicidal children, in contrast to the nonsuicidal children, had higher scores of general psychopathology measured on the Child Suicide Potential Scales. Furthermore, for the children as a group, the Achenbach Child Behavior Checklist and Profile scores were within the range of normality defined by this instrument. This suggests that, as a group, the children in this sample were functioning on a similar level to other normal children in the general population.

At the time of follow-up, 17.9% of the children reported suicidal ideas and 1.5% reported suicidal threats. In our initial assessment, 8.9% of the children had suicidal ideas and 3.0% had suicidal threats or mild attempts. This does not represent a significant change between the initial and follow-up assessments. These findings suggest that at a given time, a prevalence of suicidal ideas for normal preadolescents of between 8.9% and 17.9% can be expected at a given time. When individual children were evaluated over this 2-year study period, however, approximately 85% of the children had no suicidal tendencies initially or at follow-up, but approximately 15% of the children who were not suicidal initially were suicidal at follow-up. Furthermore, 50% who had suicidal tendencies at the initial assessment had suicidal tendencies at follow-up. This agrees with reports suggesting that a history of previous suicidal tendencies is associated with future suicidal ideas and/or acts (Eisenberg, 1984; Weissman, 1974).

This study yielded important information about the prevalences of psychiatric disorders and their stability over a 2-year time interval among these preadolescents with no history of psychiatric treatment. As a group, at the time of follow-up, 57.3% of the children were given a psychiatric diagnosis. This agrees with our previous observation that 55.5% of the children evaluated initially had a psychiatric disorder. In fact. 70.7% of the children who were given a DMS-III diagnosis initially were given a DSM-III diagnosis at follow-up evaluation. In addition, 41.2% of the children who did not initially have a psychiatric diagnosis had one at follow-up. These findings suggest that there is a high prevalence of predominantly mild psychiatric disorders among these schoolchildren and that such disorders are relatively stable over time.

Although these percentages appear high, there are no conclusive estimates of prevalence of psychopathology in the general population of children. Some estimates range from 11.8% in the United States (Gould et al., 1981; Offord, 1985) to 18% to 70% in New Zealand (Anderson et al., 1987; McGee et al., 1984). Variations in such estimates can be attributed to different research methodologies that were used in studies that estimate prevalence of child psychopathology. In fact, our sample of schoolchildren is not a representative epidemiological sample of the general population of that community because the children were chosen with a stratified random sampling method to match a previously studied group of child psychiatric inpatients for such demographic factors as age, sex, and racial/ethnic distributions (Pfeffer et al., 1984). Our study does highlight the fact that many psychiatric disorders are stable over this 2-year study period, however.

Specifically, the most prevalent DSM-III disorders noted initially and at the time of follow-up were overanxious, oppositional, dysthymic, and specific developmental disorders. The prevalence of 26.7% for overanxious disorder and 22.7% for dysthymic disorder at follow-up indicates that these nonpatient schoolchildren frequently suffer with symptoms of anxiety and depression. Furthermore, the diagnoses of overanxious, dysthymic, and specific developmental disorder were found to be stable over time. The results about the stability of dysthymic disorder in these preadolescents agrees with the findings from the longitudinal studies of Kovacs et al. (1984a,b), suggesting that preadolescent depressive disorders are chronic problems.

This study suggested that certain factors are associated with changes in suicidal tendencies during this 2-year follow-up time. The score at T_1 for assaultive behavior was a factor associated with an increase in suicidal tendency at follow-up. General psychopathology and depression at T_2 were associated with suicidal tendencies at follow-up. In addition, death preoccupations measured at the time of follow-up (T_3) were associated with suicidal ideas and acts at the time of follow-up. These findings suggest that changes in suicidal status are associated with risk indicators that have some predictive value over a 2-year period in preadolescents. The findings must be considered tentative, however, because of the small number of children evaluated in this way.

The main implications for prevention of suicidal behavior that can be derived from the results of this study are that children who warrant close follow-up and monitoring are those with a history of suicidal tendencies, depressive symptoms, past violent behavior, and recent preoccupations with death. Furthermore, the results of this study agree with the findings of Kaplan et al. (1984) of 23.8% of adolescents who report suicidal ideation. The percentages of the preadolescents in our study with suicidal ideas require some explanation.

One possible explanation for the percentage of suicidal thoughts found is that the criteria for identifying suicidal thoughts were too lenient in the present study. If having any fleeting thought of suicide was interpreted as defining a suicidal child, this may lead to an overdiagnosis of suicidal children. This is not likely in view of the actual comments made by the children. For example, an 8-year-old boy said "Sometimes when I'm really upset, I say I will shoot myself. When my brother gets on me, I feel like dying. Sometimes I wish my brother would die. Sometimes I say to my brother, I'm going to kill you. Sometimes I think of killing myself. I will take a pocketknife and stab myself." A 10-year-old boy said: "I think about dying a lot. I don't know how I would do it. I thought of hurting myself, cutting my wrist. I think about how it's going to be when I die. It keeps coming back.'' A 15-year-old girl said: ''When things get too hectic and I see no way out, I think of hurting myself. I was thinking, if I would kill myself, I would take pills. Sometimes I think I have to get out of the house or I will do something.''

Another explanation is that the interview permitted an in-depth discussion of any comments about suicide. This was not possible with survey methods in the few other recent studies. It should be kept in mind that the fact that these children had suicidal ideas did not necessarily mean that they had any suicidal plans or committed any suicidal acts. In fact, only 1.5% of the children reported any suicidal threats at the time of follow-up. Therefore, it appears that suicidal ideas may be approximately 10 times more prevalent than suicidal acts among these preadolescents, and that many factors must operate in order to influence a child to move from having a suicidal idea to carrying out a suicidal act. These risk factors are depression, death preoccupation, and general psychopathology.

REFERENCES

Achenbach, T. M. (1978), The child behavior profile I: boys aged 6–11. *J. Consult. Clin. Psychol.*, 46:478–488.

—— Edelbrock, C. S. (1979), The child behavior profile II: boys aged 12–16 and girls aged 6–11 and 12–16. *J. Consult. Clin. Psychol.*, 47:223–233.

Anderson, J. C., Williams, S., McGee, R. & Silva, P. A. (1987), DSM-III disorders in preadolescent children: prevalence of a large sample from the general population. *Arch. Gen. Psychiat.*, 44:69–76.

Eisenberg, L. (1984), The epidemiology of depression in children and adolescents. *Pediat. Ann.*, 13:47–54.

Gould, M. S., Wunsch-Hitzig, R. & Dohrenwend, B. (1981), Estimating the prevalence of childhood psychopathology: a critical review. *J. Am. Acad. Child Adolesc. Psychiatry*, 20:462–476.

Harkavey, J. M. & Asnis, G. M. (1986, May), *Adolescent suicidal behavior: preliminary study.* Paper presented at the New Research Program and Abstracts of the 139th Annual Meeting of the American Psychiatric Association, Washington, D.C.

Hollingshead, A. B. & Redlich, F. (1958), *Social Class and Mental Illness.* New York: Wiley.

Josef, N. C., Kinkel, R. J. & Bailey, C. W. (1986, May), *Suicide attempts by school-age adolescents.* New Research Program and Abstracts of the 139th Annual Meeting of the American Psychiatric Association, Washington, D.C.

Kandel, D. & Davis, M. (1982), Epidemiology of depressive mood in adolescents: an empirical study. *Arch. Gen. Psychiat.*, 39:1205–1212.

Kaplan, S. L., Hong, G. K. & Weinhold, C. (1984), Epidemiology of depressive symptomatology in adolescents. *J. Am. Acad. Child Adolesc. Psychiatry*, 23:91–98.

Kashani, J. H., McGee, R. O., Clarkson, S. E., et al. (1983), Depression in a sample of 9-year-old children: prevalence and associated characteristics. *Arch. Gen. Psychiat.*, 40:1217–1223.

Kazdin, A. E., French, N. H., Anio, A. S., Esveldt-Dawson, K. & Sherich, R. B. (1983), Hopelessness, depression, and suicidal intent among psychiatrically disturbed inpatient children. *J. Consult. Clin. Psychol.*, 51:504–510.

Kovacs, M. (1980), Rating scales to assess depression in school-aged children. *Acta Paedopsychiat.*, 46:305–315.

—— Feinberg, T. L., Crouse-Novak, M. A., Paulaushas, S. L. & Finkelstein, R. (1984a), Depressive disorders in childhood. *Arch. Gen. Psychiat.*, 41:229–237.

——, ——, ——, ——, (1984b), Depressive disorders in childhood. *Arch. Gen. Psychiat.*, 41:643–649.

McGee, R., Silva, P. A. & Williams, S. (1984), Behavior problems in a population of seven-year old children: prevalence, stability, and types of disorders—a research report. *J. Am. Acad. Child Adolesc. Psychiatry*, 25:251–259.

Offord, D. R. (1985), Child psychiatric disorders: prevalence and perspectives. *Psychiat. Clin. N. Amer.*, 8:637–652.

Pfeffer, C. R., Conte, H. R., Plutchik, R. & Jerrett, I. (1979), Suicidal behavior in latency age children: an empirical study. *J. Am. Acad. Child Adolesc. Psychiatry*, 18:679–692.

——, ——, ——, —— (1980), Suicidal behavior in latency age children: an empirical study of an outpatient population. *J. Am. Acad. Child Adolesc. Psychiatry*, 19:703–710.

—— Solomon, G., Plutchik, R., Mizruchi, M. S. & Weiner, A. (1982), Suicidal behavior in latency-age psychiatric inpatients: a replication and cross-validation. *J. Am. Acad. Child Adolesc. Psychiatry*, 21:564–569.

—— Zuckerman, S., Plutchik, R. & Mizruchi, M. S. (1984), Suicidal behavior in normal school children: a comparison with child psychiatric inpatients. *J. Am. Acad. Child Adolesc. Psychiatry*, 23:416–423.

Stanley, E. J. & Barter, J. T. (1970), Adolescent suicidal behavior. *Amer. J. Orthopsychiat.*, 40:87–96.

Weissman, M. M. (1974), The epidemiology of suicide attempts, 1960 to 1971. *Arch. Gen. Psychiat.*, 30:737–746.

24

Preventing Teenage Suicide:
A Critical Review

**David Shaffer, Ann Garland, Madelyn Gould,
Prudence Fisher, and Paul Trautman**
Columbia University, New York State Psychiatric Institute

This paper reviews the risk factors for suicide in teenagers to which prevention procedures could rationally be directed. A range of suicide preventive interventions, including hotline and crisis services, school based educational and screening procedures, effective treatment of suicide attempters, minimizing opportunities for suicide imitation, and controlling access to the methods most often used to commit suicide are described, and evidence for their efficacy is presented. Most suicides among teenagers occur in those with identifiable mental or character disorders, and increasing knowledge about risk factors may facilitate prediction in the future. The evidence for the efficacy of any existing intervention, however, is slender, and there is a clear need for more effective research into the management of high-risk groups.

Concern about teen suicide appears to have increased in recent years. This has been associated with a number of highly publicized outbreaks of suicide in teenagers and with evidence that, in contrast to the pattern found in other age groups, suicide among young (15- to 24-year-old) males has increased markedly since 1960. This concern has in turn led to the introduction of many school-based suicide prevention programs directed to unselected groups of high school students. In 1986 over 100 such programs existed in the United States, reaching approximately 180,000 students (Garland et al., submitted).

Reprinted with permission from the *Journal of the American Academy of Child and Adolescent Psychiatry,* 1988, Vol. 27 , No. 6, 675–687. Copyright 1988 by the American Academy of Child and Adolescent Psychiatry.

Prepared with the assistance of Grant R49 CCR202598-01 from the Centers for Disease Control and from Grants ROI MH 38198-04 and ROI MH416898-02, and Research Training Grant MH 16434, from N.I.M.H., and Faculty Scholar Award 84-0954-84 from the W.T. Grant Foundation.

Most of the programs appeared to operate on the assumption that, given sufficient stress, there is a universal potential for suicide and it is therefore appropriate to direct preventive interventions to unselected groups of young people.

The purpose of this paper is to review school-based and other suicide prevention strategies. Because the literature on suicide prevention in young people is limited, the review has been extended, where indicated, to include evaluations of preventive strategies directed mainly at adults. For the purposes of this review the term ''suicide'' covers any behavior that centers on a conscious or declared wish to bring about one's death. This comprises both suicides and suicide attempts; except after the event, there is no sure way of distinguishing between attempters who will go on to complete and those who will never make another suicide attempt.

In this paper, interventions that change attitudes of unaffected individuals that might predispose them toward suicide or that facilitate early identification and treatment of conditions known to increase the risk for suicide are grouped as *primary preventive measures.* Those that will reduce the potential for suicide among youngsters who have already made suicidal threats or attempts are considered *secondary and tertiary preventive measures.*

WHO IS AT RISK?

Adolescent suicide is uncommon; the rate in 1984 for all 15- to 19-year-olds was nine deaths per 100,000 population (Mortality Statistics Branch, Division of Vital Statistics, National Center for Health Statistics, 1986). This means that preventive efforts directed to the general population are likely to reach relatively few teenagers who will eventually commit suicide. For example, even if all of the school-based suicide prevention programs were completely successful (and the authors show below that this is questionable), they would prevent only 16 of the approximately 2,000 annual teen suicides. A more efficient strategy may be to target available resources to high-risk groups. Knowledge about these groups is reviewed below. This knowledge comes from death certificate data, prospective follow-up studies of groups thought to be at high risk, and retrospective enquiries about victims after their suicides (psychological autopsy studies).

Death Certificate Data

(Unless otherwise noted, data from death certificates are derived from the 1984 and preceding annual mortality surveys of the National Center for Health Statistics.)

Age. Very few children under age 12 commit suicide, although many threaten and some make suicide attempts. Suicide becomes increasingly common after puberty and its incidence increases in each of the teen years, reaching a peak in young people at age 23 (Shaffer and Fisher, 1981; see Fig. 1). It should be noted that the rate in adolescence, although higher than that in childhood, is less than that in adulthood. The highest rates of suicide are experienced by elderly men. This makes it unlikely that factors specific to adolescence are causally related to suicide.

Sex. In the United States nearly five times more teen boys commit suicide than girls. Data from a study currently in progress (Shaffer and Gould, 1987) indicate that sex differences are considerably less marked among Hispanics and somewhat less among blacks.

Ethnicity. In the United States suicide rates in whites are higher than in blacks at all ages, including the teens. The difference between black and white rates is greatest in the South and least in the north central states (Shaffer and Fisher, 1981). The incidence of suicide varies greatly among different native American groups (Shore, 1975). Some groups have rates more than 20-fold higher than the national average; others approximate that for the nation as a whole.

Geography. Youth suicide rates, uncorrected for ethnicity, are highest in western states and Alaska and lowest in the southern, north central, and northeastern states.

Suicide methods. In the United States adolescents of both sexes are most likely to commit suicide with a firearm. There is evidence (Brent et al., 1987) that substance abuse is more common among those suicide victims who use a

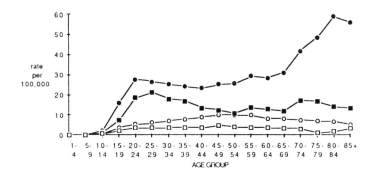

Figure 1. Suicide in different ages (1984). (●) white male; (○) white female; (Ü) nonwhite male; (□) nonwhite female.

firearm. The next most common method for boys is hanging, while for girls it is jumping from a height. Drug overdose, by far the most common method used in suicide attempts, accounts for few completed suicides in teenagers.

Secular trends. Over the past two decades suicide has become less common in the middle-aged and elderly but more common in the young. As Figure 2 shows, the increase is greatest (3-fold) among white males between ages 15 and 24, with the rate increasing nearly every year during this period. Black male rates have increased more slowly, and there has been no significant change in the suicide rate for either black or white females (National Center for Health Statistics, 1988). There is some suggestion (Brent, personal communication, 1987) that the increased rate in white male teenagers has occurred largely among those who committed suicide with discernible blood levels of drugs or alcohol.

Risk and imitation. Using death certificate data, Phillips and colleagues (Bollen and Phillips, 1981, 1982; Phillips, 1974, 1979, 1980, 1984; Phillips and Carstensen, 1986) and Wasserman (1984) demonstrated that prominent display of the news of a suicide in newspapers leads to a predictable increase in suicidal deaths—mainly among young people—during a 1- to 2-week period following the display. The relationship appears to be dose responsive, being most marked when there have been repeated showings of the program. Gould and Shaffer (1986), Holding (1974, 1975), Schmidtke and Hafner (1986), and Gould et al. (1988) have similarly shown that suicide completion and attempt rates increase after fictional television shows dealing with adoles-

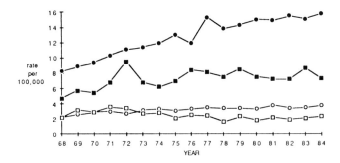

Figure 2. Adolescent suicide rates (15- to 19-year-olds) 1968 to 1984. (●) white male; (○) white female; (Ü) nonwhite male; (□) nonwhite female.

cent suicide. There are also documented examples of "copy-cat" suicides that have taken place within a few hours after a vulnerable teenager has seen a film, read a book, or seen a news story featuring suicide (Shaffer, 1974). The occurrence of suicide clusters is also thought to have an imitative basis (Gould and Davidson, 1988). Suicide clusters among 15- to 19-year-olds have been documented as occurring significantly more frequently than expected by chance alone. These findings may have implications for suicide prevention programs that show filmed vignettes of suicidal behavior or interviews with suicide attempters or survivors to a child or teen audience. There is yet no research about whether such imitative suicides are more or less or differently deviant from cases in which imitation is not a factor.

High-risk Follow-up Studies

High-risk follow-up studies provide reliable baseline information about suicide victims but this cannot be generalized for groups not included in the follow-up. Studies of this kind have been confined to psychiatric patients and suicide attempters. (Unless otherwise mentioned, all studies referred in this and the following sections deal primarily with adult attempters.)

Suicide and mental illness. Formerly hospitalized adult psychiatric patients have significantly higher suicide rates than nonpatients (Pokorny, 1964, 1983; Temoche et al. 1964). By contrast, a follow-up study of adults screened to exclude those with psychopathology showed that very few had committed suicide (Winokur and Tsuang, 1975).

Suicide attempts and later suicide. Although only a minority of teenage attempters go on to commit suicide, follow-up studies show that their suicide rate is considerably higher than that of the general population (see Table 1). Observed rates range from approximately 9% of a group of teen boys admitted to a psychiatric inpatient unit who had been depressed or who had made a suicide attempt (Motto, 1984; Otto, 1972) to less than 1% of boys who presented at an emergency room after an overdose but who were not admitted to a psychiatric hospital (Hawton and Goldacre, 1982). Similar proportions for girls range from 1% for former psychiatric inpatients to 0.1% for those who received no inpatient psychiatric care. In the 5- to 15-year follow-up described by Motto (1984), the symptoms of severe depression (psychomotor retardation, hopelessness, hypersomnia, etc.) best predicted later suicide. The prevalence of the predictors in noncompleters was high, so their specificity was limited. There are no studies relating suicidal death to earlier suicidal ideation; however, thinking about suicide is so common among high school students (Smith and Crawford, 1986) that it is unlikely that it serves as a very useful index of high risk.

Birth history. Salk et al. (1985), matching consecutive youth suicides to local birth records, noted an excess of obstetric complications among the suicides. This relationship could be mediated in a number of ways. Along with having complicated obstetric histories, the mothers of the potential suicides received less prenatal care and were more likely to have smoked and taken alcohol during pregnancy. The excess of suicide in their offspring could reflect such associated factors as the central nervous system consequences of birth complications, exposure to some teratogen during pregnancy, the heritability of psychopathology, or the effects of inappropriate parenting by deviant mothers.

Biological markers. In the past decade a number of biological correlates of suicide have been identified, all in adult studies (see Stanley and Mann, 1987, for a review). The most frequently replicated finding, first reported by Asberg et al. in 1976 in a study of depressed patients, is the presence of low concentrations of the serotonin metabolite 5-HIAA in the cerebrospinal fluid of suicide attempters and completers. Although CSF 5-HIAA derives from both brain and spinal cord, Stanley et al. (1985) have reported high correlations between brain and CSF 5-HIAA in autopsy studies. The relationship has been reported in suicidal individuals with a variety of primary diagnoses, specifically in depressed patients (Stanley and Mann, 1987), borderline and aggressive personality types (Brown et al., 1982), and violent prisoners who have attempted suicide (Linnoila et al., 1983).

These studies, although numerous, have in general involved small numbers and the specific behavioral correlates of the abnormal biochemistry have not been established, nor has the distribution of values in nonsuicidal populations been established. As a result, neither the sensitivity nor the specificity of this measure has been established. Asberg et al. (1986), however, determined that among 76 hospitalized adult suicide attempters followed over a one-year period, 21% of those whose CSF 5-HIAA was less than 90 μgms/ml went on to commit suicide during the follow-up period compared with only 2% of those with higher levels. Similar findings have been reported by Roy et al. (1986). The usefulness of CSF 5-HIAA as a predictor of suicide and therefore as an agent of prevention depends on whether or not serotonin indicators are stable over time (i.e., whether they are an index of a suicidal trait or rather of an abnormal state). Van Praag (1977), one of the early investigators in this field, found that low levels in depressed patients remained low in about half of the patients after their recovery. Traskman-Bendz et al. (1984), however, showed that some individuals had stable levels while others fluctuated. Asberg et al. (1987) reported on two patients whose levels of CSF5-HIAA continued to decline after their first attempt: both went on to commit suicide.

If declining or stable low levels predict a poor prognosis, then secondary or tertiary prevention could be served by routine CSF monitoring of patients who have made a suicide attempt, with special care being given to those with abnormally low levels. This is clearly an exciting field that may bring a new level of specificity to treatment and prevention.

Psychological Autopsies

A psychological autopsy is a retrospective enquiry about a deceased individual from a surviving informant or from contemporary records. This method, when based on consecutive reported suicides within a predefined geographical area, has potential for providing representative information that could not be obtained in any other way. Even though suicides may be systematically underreported, there is no evidence to suggest that under- or misreported suicides differ *systematically* from reported suicides (see Shaffer and Fisher, 1981 for a review of this subject). Information from psychological autopsies, however, will often be *incomplete,* being limited to whatever the informant has observed; an informant may understate such areas as undetected illegal activities and subjective mental states such as depression or anxiety. Missing information in naturalistic records may be truly absent or may have been present but not noted. Despite these limitations, the psychological autopsy is often the only method available to study the detailed characteristics of suicide victims.

Several uncontrolled psychological autopsy studies of child or adolescent suicide have been carried out (Jan-Tausch, 1964; Sanborn et al., 1974; Shaffer, 1974), but the only controlled studies reported so far (Brent et al., 1988; Shaffi, 1985) comprise small samples, and the study by Shaffi used acquaintance controls, which is likely to reduce case-control differences. The authors are currently undertaking a large population-based psychological autopsy study of completed suicides under age 20 that occurred over a 2-year period in the New York metropolitan region (N = 173), with both a randomly selected age-, ethnic-, and sex-matched normal control group and a matched comparison group of suicide attempters (Shaffer and Gould, 1987). Preliminary data from approximately two-thirds of this sample are referred to below.

Precipitants. The preliminary New York data (Shaffer and Gould, 1987) suggest that many teenagers commit suicide in the context of an acute disciplinary crisis or shortly after a rejection or humiliation (e.g., dispute with a girlfriend, an incident of being ridiculed or teased, or failing at some event), all with a brief stress-suicide interval. If these impressions are confirmed by a full analysis of the data, they would carry a negative implication for prevention because (a) these are common stresses not readily avoided and indeed they are often initiated by the type of psychopathology found in suicide victims, and (b) the short interval between stressor and suicide reduces the opportunity for preventive interventions.

Associated mental health problems. These have been found in the majority of suicides in representative psychological autopsy studies of adults (Barraclough et al., 1969; Dorpat and Ripley, 1960; Robins et al., 1959) and children (Shaffer, 1974). Only a very small proportion of suicides appear to be free of psychiatric symptoms prior to death. In the New York study (Shaffer and Gould, 1987), approximately half of all suicides had had previous contact with a mental health professional. The teenagers had suffered from a variety of psychiatric problems including depression, antisocial behavior, drug and alcohol abuse, and learning disorders: a subgroup with no behavior problems showed evidence of excessive anxiety, perfectionism, and distress at times of change and dislocation. Only a small proportion of teen suicides occurred among teenagers with manic-depressive or schizophrenic psychoses, although Brent et al. (1988) and Shaffi et al. (1985) found that bipolar symptoms were common in the suicide victims they studied.

Abnormal family history. In the New York study, a high proportion of the suicide completers had a first- or second-degree relative who had previously attempted or committed suicide (Shaffer and Gould, 1987). If this results from intra-familial imitation, a possible prevention strategy would be to stress the importance of minimizing exposure of vulnerable individuals to the example of suicidal behavior (e.g., emphasizing to the suicidal mother of a young child the potential risk of talking about her suicidal ideas in the presence of her children or, if exposure cannot be avoided, providing an intervention to vulnerable offspring or siblings). On the other hand, if the high familial incidence of suicide has a genetic basis, there is the hope that reliable predictive measures will be developed through biological markers.

A heuristic model that takes account of some of the observed correlates and the preventive implications of suicide in the young is shown in Figure 3. The model assumes that suicide does not occur randomly but only strikes certain individuals who are predisposed and that these individuals will only commit suicide if there are co-occurring triggering stresses and method opportunities. The individual predispositions include a major mood disorder and certain personality types. It can be assumed that very few individuals other than these will be at risk for suicide. Their suicide will often take place shortly after a stressful event induces some extreme emotion, most commonly fear or rage. Distorted affect may also follow from a depressed mood or intoxication with drugs or alcohol. Finally, the means of committing suicide will need to be at hand.

Preliminary findings from the New York study (Gould et al., in press) using the proportion of suicide completers and normal controls with a particular risk

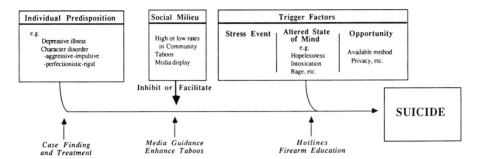

Figure 3. A model for suicide causation.

factor have been used, along with sex- and age-specific suicide rates from the general population (e.g., 15/100,000 for 15- to 19-year-old white boys), to estimate with Bayes' theorem (Fleiss, 1981) the probable incidence of suicide in various subgroups (see Table 2). The utility of these estimates lies primarily in their ranking rather than in any absolute number because estimates are based on univariate analyses only. A review of the small number of follow-up studies of teenagers who have been treated psychiatrically for suicide attempts or depression (see Table 1) shows suicide rates that are much higher than we would project from data on subjects in the New York study or from Goldacre and Hawton's (1985) study of attempters who for the most part received non-psychiatric treatment. The most plausible explanation for the difference is selection factors (i.e., that more severely disturbed patients are admitted for psychiatric treatment); however, one cannot rule out the possibility that hospital admission worsens the prognosis of attempters.

These data suggest that *the greatest preventive impact would come from effective intervention directed to teenage boys who have made a previous suicide attempt or who are depressed.* Attempters are potentially easy to identify because many are referred to emergency rooms for medical care after their

Study	N	Treatment	Length of Follow-up	Age Range	Suicide Rate %
Males					
Motto (1984)	122	I.P.	4–10 yr	10–19	9.0
Otto (1972)	321	I.P.	5 yr	10–20	11.3
Garfinkel et al. (1982)	124	I.P.	1–9 yr	8–19	5.0
Goldacre and Hawkins (1985)	641	O.P.	1–5 yr	12–20	0.7[a]
Females					
Otto (1972)	1,226	I.P.	5 yr	10–20	3.9
Garfinkel et al. (1982)	381	I.P.	1–9 yr	6–21	0.8
Goldacre and Hawkins (1985)	1,851	O.S.	1–5 yr	12–20	0.1[a]

[a] 16 to 20 years old.

Table 1. Suicide in Treated Suicide Attempters

Risk Factor	Normals[a] %	Suicides[b] %	Approximate Odds Ratio	Suicide Rate/ 100,000 Affected by Risk Factor
Males (general adolescent population)				14[c]
Prior attempt	1.2	21	22.5	270
Major depression	2	21	8.6	100
Substance abuse	7	37	7.1	70
Antisocial behavior	17	67	4.4	40
FH of suicide	17	41	3.0	35
Females (general adolescent population)				3.5[c]
Prior attempt	6	33	8.6	20
Major depression	2	50	49	80
Substance abuse	7	5	0.8	3
Antisocial behavior	12	30	3.2	8
FH of suicide	13	33	2.7	6

[a] Normal males: $N = 65$; normal females: $N = 20$.
[b] Male suicides: $N = 97$; female suicides: $N = 17$.
[c] N.C.H.S. Division of Mortality, unpublished data.

Table 2. Risk Factors for Suicide in Teenagers from a New York Adolescent Suicide Study

attempt (Kennedy et al., 1974). Furthermore, since they have already demonstrated suicidal behavior, there would be no concern about the introduction of suicidal preoccupations to individuals who may not be suicidal.

PRIMARY PREVENTION

Providing Psychiatric Services

Most individuals who commit suicide have evidence of a psychiatric disorder at the time of their death. Other factors being equal, the introduction of mental health services into a community should, by reducing the burden of mental illness, also reduce the suicide rate. This proposition was studied some time ago, although not specifically for children or teens. Walk (1967) examined suicide rates in the British county of Sussex and found no effect on suicide rates after the introduction of a community psychiatric service. Neilson and Videbech (1973) similarly found no effect on suicide rates after the introduction of a psychiatric service on the Danish island of Samso (with teenagers accounting for very few psychiatric cases). Neither study was controlled, so it is possible that the stable suicide rates observed were occurring at a time when rates elsewhere were increasing. More importantly, both studies were undertaken before the widespread use of antidepressants and lithium: therefore, they do not reflect the impact of current, effective therapies.

Restricting Access to Methods Used to Commit Suicide

Because youth suicide is often an impulsive act, it is reasonable to expect that limiting access to methods that are commonly used could reduce the teen suicide rate.

The so-called "British experience" is a frequently cited example of how reducing access to the means of suicide can significantly reduce the suicide rate. In 1957, the mean carbon monoxide content of domestic gas in Great Britain was 12%. Self-asphyxiation with domestic cooking gas accounted for over 40% of all British suicides (Hassall and Trethowan, 1972; Kreitman, 1976). By 1970, through the introduction of natural gas, the carbon monoxide content of domestic gas had been reduced to 2%. Over the same period British suicide rates from carbon monoxide asphyxiation declined steadily until by 1971 they accounted for fewer than 10% of all suicides, with the total suicide rate declining by 26%. Almost all of this decline can be attributed to the decrease in deaths from domestic gas asphyxiation. There was no compensatory increase in suicidal deaths by other methods, although during this period the incidence of attempts by overdose increased (Johns, 1977). It is implausible to suppose that individuals who would have committed suicide using domestic gas did not try another method when they felt suicidal. What may have happened was that the suicidal population, denied access to one universally available, nondeforming, nonviolent method, did not turn to other more violent (and more lethal) methods but rather chose another nonviolent method that also was readily available, namely self-poisoning. The impact of this may have been limited, however, because during that period, self-poisoning became progressively less dangerous, in part because of a decline in the use of highly toxic barbiturates and in part because of improved methods of resuscitation. Most significantly, however, British rates, in contrast to those in most other countries, remained at the new lower level (Farberow, 1985) for many years. The detoxification of domestic cooking gas also occurred in other European countries where it was not associated with a reduction in suicide rate. In these other countries, however, the base rate of self-asphyxiation from domestic gas was much lower than it had been in Great Britain.

The British example is not directly relevant to the United States where coal gas is not used for domestic purposes, although the introduction of automobile emission control systems has reduced the carbon monoxide content of automobile exhaust and this has coincided with a decline in suicide rates attributable to asphyxiation (Clark and Lester, 1987). Most suicides in the United States are committed with firearms, and it has been suggested (Boyd and Moscicki, 1986) that increased availability of firearms in U.S. households has been a reason for the recent increase in U.S. suicide rates. This reasoning is not entirely convincing because youth suicide rates have also increased in many European countries where changes in the availability of firearms do not parallel those in the United States. Furthermore, there seems to be a complicated association between sex, substance abuse (which in the New York Study is a common correlate among male suicides but not among females), and suicide by firearm (Brent et al., 1987), so that the increase in young male suicides through firearms may reflect the increasing number of substance abusers who commit suicide rather than being a direct effect of firearm availability. Given this relationship it would be sensible to deny ownership of firearms to individuals who share a household with a substance abusing or alcoholic member. Appropriate education programs could also be directed to parents of high-risk teenagers to discourage keeping firearms in the home except under the most secure conditions.

School-Based Programs

The growth in recent years of school-based programs seems to follow from public concern over serial suicides or clusters. Suicide clusters are often highly publicized and are frequently attributed by the public to specific stresses or faults in the community, such as the presence of a large number of recent migrants, an insensitive or "uncaring" school administration, or many working mothers with "latchkey" children. (These explanations are implausible because the putative stresses will nearly always have been present for some time, and if they did lead to the suicide outbreak, one might expect that the raised suicide rate would operate continuously rather than episodically). The authors have determined that in 1986 (Garland et al., submitted for publication) over 100 school-based programs were in operation in the United States, reaching approximately 180,000 teenagers. The description of school programs that follows is based on responses to a survey employed in that study and on an extensive review of manuals and other descriptive literature provided to describe individual programs. Most programs have the following goals:

1. *To heighten awareness of the problem.* This is sometimes done by showing taped vignettes of teenagers who have attempted suicide or by quoting disturbing statistics (e.g., that suicide is the second leading cause of death among teenagers).

2. *To promote case finding.* It is assumed that suicidal students are more likely to discuss suicidal feelings or intentions with other students than with responsible adults. Students are taught to recognize clinical features that may be warning signs of a presuicidal state and to pass these disclosures on to a responsible adult. Descriptions of warning signs usually comprise the symptoms of acute onset depression, along with what are held to be pathognomonic behaviors of suicidal intent, such as making a will, giving away valued possessions, or ambiguous references to the future. Disclosure of suicidal feelings is encouraged by presenting a model of suicide that is intended to be nonstigmatizing (i.e., that suicide is not a feature of mental illness but is a response to common adolescent stresses such as pressure to succeed, family upsets, res-

idential mobility, changing value systems, use of drugs and alcohol, etc.). Taped or filmed vignettes of youngsters who have made a previous attempt and who are glad that they survived are often shown. Pupils and staff may also be taught listening skills to promote trust and disclosure from potentially suicidal students.

3. *To provide staff and students with information about mental health resources,* specifically, how they operate and how they can be accessed.

4. A minority of programs set out *to improve teenagers' coping abilities* by training in stress management or coping strategies. Others aim to identify and support students who have drug or alcohol problems, failing grades, family problems, etc.

Some programs are directed solely at teachers with the expectation that they will apply the knowledge directly in their daily practice. In some programs teachers are required to pass on the information or techniques they have learned to their students. It is not uncommon for teachers to be called on to implement a program after a single training session from a mental health professional or from a training videotape.

Student programs are most often directed to students in the ninth grade or above, although sometimes younger students are involved. Programs may be given to small or large groups or both. Small groups focus on topics such as individual reactions to suicide; the difficulty a teacher, parent, or student may have in breaching confidentiality; and how best to communicate with teenagers. Larger meetings present information on the facts of teen suicide, resource information, and adolescent development and difficulties.

Course leaders are typically psychologists or social workers recruited from local mental health centers. A small number of programs use peer counselors, who may be known by such names as "natural helpers," "buddies," or "the care company." They are usually chosen by a panel of teachers and administrators are taught counseling techniques by a guidance counselor, sometimes earning class credits for their participation. One variation of peer counseling used previously suicidal students to address regular classmates in a special class.

Many programs distribute small, printed wallet cards or pamphlets with facts about suicide, warning signs, steps to take if one suspects that a friend or family member is suicidal, and telephone numbers of local hotlines and community groups.

Effectiveness of School Programs

At their most general level, didactic school-based suicide prevention programs can be criticized for following a *low risk strategy:* given the low base rate of teen suicide, very few of the adolescents receiving the programs are likely to attempt or commit suicide. Program leaders or designers, however, often counter this objection by indicating that, until individual students come forward and identify themselves, their high risk or low risk status remains unknown.

The only systematic controlled evaluation of school based programs (Shaffer et al., 1987) studied approximately 1000 students ranging in age from 13 to 18 who were exposed to one of three different programs in six different high schools. A similar number of students in five control schools who did not receive a program were also studied. Before exposure to a suicidal prevention program, most students held views and had knowledge that would generally be considered sound. They knew many of the warning signs, took the view that mental health professionals are helpful, and were aware that suicide threats should be taken seriously, that suicidal disclosures should be managed by consultation with responsible adults, and that suicidal preoccupations were best shared. The programs did not alter these views. The value of school-based screening programs was, however, demonstrated in the survey. Approximately 3% of the students identified themselves as being currently troubled or suicidal and wanting professional help.

Between 5 and 20% of the pupils in both experimental and control schools expressed views that would generally be regarded as inappropriate. They stated that under certain circumstances suicide was a reasonable solution to problems, and that they would not reveal the suicidal confidence of a friend or seek help from a mental health professional if they felt troubled. Unfortunately, the programs also had very little impact on these attitudes. These findings need to be interpreted with the caveats that (a) they record *attitudes* rather than behaviors, and there is no certainty that a given attitude will predict a related behavior in a time of crisis; (b) the absence of an effect may be a function of the very brief duration of exposure: none of the programs lasted more than 3 hours (although this was representative of the national pattern in which 76% of programs last 3 hours or less), and it may be that greater length of involvement is required to produce change. The three programs differed significantly in their techniques, and the program with the most experienced providers, using small group techniques to optimize engagement, was rated as significantly more interesting. None, however, was more effective than any other in changing attitudes.

Relatively few students believed either before or after exposure to a program that suicide was a feature of mental illness. In view of the evidence that suicide is a feature of mental illness, programs that choose to ignore the psychiatric correlates of suicide are either operating in ignorance or are misrepresenting the facts. They may also inadvertently enhance the chances of imitation, which the authors believe is especially likely if suicide is portrayed as an understandable, tragic, heroic, or romantic response to stresses emanating from uncaring adults or institutions. In the authors' view, suicide is less likely to be imitated if depicted as a deviant act by someone with a mental disturbance.

The findings thus do little to support the value of general educational programs. Most students do not need them, and those who do would probably be better served by an individualized approach to their clinical problems. This is not to say, however, that there is no place in the high school curriculum for more education about mental health and how to obtain help for emotional disorder.

SECONDARY AND TERTIARY INTERVENTIONS

In practice secondary and tertiary interventions overlap considerably with "treatment." A *secondary intervention* aims at preventing a presymptomatic condition, already established, from progressing to cause suffering or impairment. An example would be the successful treatment of a nonsuicidal depressive illness. A *tertiary intervention* would shorten the course of a condition that is already symptomatic, lessen the likelihood of its recurrence, and reduce its noxious consequences or complications. An example would be preventing a suicide ideator from attempting or completing suicide through crisis intervention on a suicide hotline.

Hotlines/Crisis Services

Rationale. A theory for suicide crisis intervention articulated by Shneidman and Farberow (1957) and Litman et al. (1965) can be summarized as follows. (1) Suicide is often associated with a critical stress event. (2) It is usually contemplated with psychological ambivalence; surviving attempters often report that the wish to die coexisted with wishes to be rescued and saved. (3) The wish to commit suicide as a solution to a problem arises in the context of mental disturbance. The suicidal individual has partial insight into the unsatisfactory nature of this solution (hence the ambivalence), and this can be identified and dealt with at the time of crisis by those with special training, reducing the impetus to commit suicide. If we accept the model of suicide presented in Figure 3, then crisis services have a potential for great efficiency because they operate at the final common pathway.

Description. Most crisis services are centered around a telephone service or "hotline." They are usually available outside usual office hours; obviate the need for a trip to a clinic or professional office; offer the caller in crisis an opportunity for immediate support; are anonymous, allowing callers to say shocking or embarrassing things that would be difficult in a face-to-face interview and giving those who are concerned with issues of control and power the freedom to hang up. Most meet Bridge et al.'s (1977) operational criteria by having (a) an identifiable individual in the community responsible for the service; (b) a 24-hour telephone or other emergency access; and (c) advertisement of their presence. Most centers are locally organized, an exception being the National Adolescent Runaway/Suicide Hotline. Many are staffed by volunteers who are supervised by social workers or other mental health professionals. Some hotlines, called "teenlines," are manned by teenagers (Simmons et al., 1986) who receive the same training as adult volunteers. Teenage volunteers, however, are likely to experience difficulty in dealing with sex calls, which are common, and their hours of availability are usually limited.

Some services target special groups such as college students and at least one has a telephone situated at a site on a bridge that has been used repeatedly for suicides (Glatt, 1987). Most give information about how to access appropriate services, although some, especially those that are part of a multi-service agency, carry out more active case management, making appointments with the appropriate clinical service and following up if the appointment is not kept. Relatively few offer direct therapy on the telephone and most will break confidentiality if they judge that it will avert a suicide. Many do not hesitate to call in police help, although most will ask a teenager's permission before contacting parents, others will do so without permission if the situation seems serious. An exception to many of these generalizations is the Samaritan organization, whose befriending process emphasizes acceptance, warmth, and confidentiality (Hirsch, 1981).

Effectiveness of Crisis Services and Hotlines

Only two evaluations of crisis services established specifically for young people have been found. Slem and Cotler (1973) systematically evaluated user satisfaction with a widely advertised teen hotline in suburban Detroit. The follow-up rate was low (58%), and the proportion of suicidal users was unspecified. The authors report that 68% of the responders had had a good experience. King (1977) determined client satisfaction in a survey of 3000 college freshmen. Most of the young women, but significantly fewer of the young men, had found the hotline helpful, although a third of the men and a fifth of the women reported that the advice given by the hotline had made their problem worse. A similar pattern was found among suicidal users, young men being significantly less likely to be satisfied with their experience than young women. Both sexes reported greater satisfaction when their call had been taken by an opposite-sexed operator.

A number of studies have addressed the very important question of whether the establishment of a suicide hotline reduces mortality from suicide. This research is correlational, lacking direct evidence about hotline usage and is thus subject to the "ecological fallacy." This problem was compounded in early studies (Lester, 1973; Litman and Farberow, 1969; Ringel, 1968; Weiner, 1969) that reported a reduction in suicide mortality in a community after the introduction of a hotline but that either used inappropriate controls or failed to account for demographic shifts that could have influenced the suicide rate (e.g., a decrease in the proportion of elderly men or of whites in a community, which can substantially lower the suicide rate). Bridge et al. (1977) took account of demographic shifts in a study of North Carolina hotlines and found no evidence that the introduction of a crisis center affected the suicide rate. An incidental finding of that study was that although the incidence of suicide was highest in communities with a high proportion of older, white, married persons, suicide centers were most often established in areas with younger, black, single people, groups who are certainly at high risk for other psychiatric conditions but who carry a relatively low rate of suicide. A British study (Bagley, 1968) that controlled for demographic shifts has been widely quoted as demonstrating the efficiency of suicide prevention centers (SPCs), but research using more elaborate matching techniques failed to replicate these findings (Barraclough et al., 1977; Jennings et al., 1978).

Most recently, Miller et al. (1984) examined age- and race-specific suicide rates in U.S. counties with and without, and before and after, the introduction of a suicide prevention center (SPC) and found the presence of a service to be associated with a small but significant reduction in the suicide rate (1.75/ 100,000) among young white women who are the most frequent SPC users. A more complete review of the efficacy of hotline services can be found in Shaffer et al., 1988.

The Limited Impact of Hotlines

There are several possible reasons for the limited impact of hotlines:

a. Low utilization rates in the suicide-prone population. Miller's 1984 findings suggest that hotlines might have more impact on the suicide rate if they could reach the groups at greatest risk. In the case of teenagers this would mean not only boys (for it seems that girls with their lower rates of suicide comprise the majority of hotline callers), but the age group as a whole. A small proportion of calls to general SPCs are made by teenagers (Litman et al., 1965), and in a study in Great Britain, teenage attempters were significantly less likely to know of the existence of hotlines than adult attempters (Greer and Anderson, 1979). It is likely that teenagers' knowledge about hotlines could be increased with appropriately targeted advertising. For example, 98% of community high school students recognized the name of a Detroit hotline after it had advertised its services among the high school population (Slem and Cotler, 1973) and a not insignificant 5.6% of these had made use of the service since its introduction 3 years previously, although most of these were girls.

   b. Inappropriate advice. Only a small proportion of callers comply with the advice they are given (Lester, 1970). This probably reflects both what advice they are given and how it is told. Slaiku et al. (1975) found that within a service with a uniform policy and training procedures, caller compliance varied with different telephone operators. The critical factors in responder variation have not been fully explored, but they seem to be unrelated to the conversational characteristics or whether the responder refers directly to suicide or uses some euphemism. Some responders provide poor quality information. In studies using simulated callers, Bleach and Claiborn (1974) and Apsler and Hodas (1975) found that some operators tended to give unvarying advice, using little judgment to obtain a "good fit" with the callers' problems. Other operators are dogmatic and hasty in their responses. Knowles (1979) and McCarthy and Berman (1979) found that untrained volunteers were commonly over-directive, offering advice prematurely on the basis of inadequate information. Also, experience seems to be no substitute for training; both are needed. Hirsch (1981) noted that untrained volunteers are less skilled than professionals in eliciting relevant past history and integrating caller information. Elkins and Cohen (1982) found that only volunteers who had received preliminary training improved their performance with experience. Training can improve the quality of information provided and also such qualities as empathy and warmth (Bleach and Claiborn, 1974; France, 1975; Genther, 1974; Kalafat et al., 1979).

   Compliance may also be a function of how much outreach the service provides. Sudak et al. (1977) reported exceptionally high compliance rates for a service in Cleveland where hotline operators routinely made clinic appointments for callers (instead of relying on the caller's own initiative) and undertook further follow-up if an appointment was not kept.

   It is probably a mistake to dismiss hotlines as well-intentioned but ineffective. Hotlines are widely available in the United States and provide help for a needy and otherwise underserved population. King's study (1977) showed that only 8% of callers were currently receiving other mental health services. There is abundant evidence that the suicide rate in hotline callers is many times that for the general population. In the survey of high school students referred to above (Shaffer et al., 1987), one of the few significant effects of attending a suicide prevention class was an increase in a declared willingness to use a hotline when experiencing emotional difficulties, there being no increase in willingness to use any other type of service.

Given the "fragility" of hotline systems, however, with their dependence on the vagaries of poorly trained operators, it is clearly important to develop a standardized, but clinically informed, screening procedure coupled with active case management procedures. It would also be desirable to broaden interest in hotlines, particularly among troubled boys, with appropriately directed advertising. Hotlines should be continuously and systematically assessed to determine the reasons for calling, the age and sex of callers (to determine whether a target group is being reached), and operator-specific rates of compliance, and to identify volunteers who might benefit from further training.

Treating Suicide Attempters

Although the literature is replete with suggestions for the appropriate treatment of teen suicide attempters (see Trautman and Shaffer, 1984 for a review), no satisfactory studies that have systematically evaluated such treatment (i.e., comparing outcome over a reasonable period of time with other treated or nontreated groups, using standard measures before the start of treatment and at follow-up, and random assignment to different treatment groups or the use of placebo or dummy interventions) have been found. Most of the studies referred to in this section have been done on predominantly adult attempters.

Compliance issues. Regardless of which treatment would help them most, the majority of suicide attempters who are treated in a medical emergency room for the medical effects of their attempt and who are then offered a psychiatric appointment will not keep this appointment. Is it reasonable to be complacent about this? Do teenagers not return because their crisis has passed? Is nonattendance associated with a good prognosis? The evidence suggests the reverse. In a small study of 27 adolescents, Litt et al. (1983) found that only 33% of first appointments were kept (similar to the proportion noted in several adult studies) and that failure to attend was more common in adolescents who had made a previous attempt, a factor known to be associated with attempt repetition and completion. Trautman et al. (1987), in a home visit study, compared teenagers who kept appointments with those who failed. Those who failed were more likely to have a parent with an untreated but significant psychiatric disturbance.

Experiences in the emergency room play some part in determining later compliance. In a study of nearly 300 emergency room cases (adults) managed by 15 different clinicians, Knesper (1982) found that while some clinicians were able to persuade most attempters to return for a further appointment, others persuaded very few. Specifically, clinicians who introduced the need for admission to a patient suddenly and without warning at the end of an examination had a very low rate of success in making referrals to an inpatient unit. Clinic procedures may also contribute to compliance rates. Kogan (1957) found that among adult attempters seen in an emergency room, only 37% kept an appointment when they were simply provided a name and telephone number; when an appointment was made for them in the emergency room, 82% kept it. Rogawski and Edmundson (1971), using a more stringent index of compliance (two appointments kept), found that only 30% of adult callers given a name and number kept their appointment, but 55% did so when an appointment was made for them.

Naturalistic treatment studies. Do patients who kept their appointment benefit from the treatment they receive? Naturalistic treatment studies rely on the natural variations in treatment experience that occur in a clinic. They typically compare the outcome of patients who attended for longer and shorter periods or who dropped out of treatment, or they compare the outcome of patients in a new program with those treated in a preexisting program. The results of these studies are difficult to interpret for a number of reasons. Nonattenders are a poor comparison group because they are likely to start off being more disturbed than attenders (see above). Differences between attenders and nonattenders might therefore reflect baseline differences and be unrelated to the effects of treatment. Studies that compare old and new programs may be misleading because the introduction of a new service may generate new referral sources, and with them a different type of patient. With these reservations in mind, there have been four studies that suggest that adult suicide attempters who receive psychiatric treatment have a better prognosis (with respect to repetition of suicide attempts) and one that suggests that treatment is ineffective.

Greer and Bagley (1971) contrasted adult suicide attempters discharged from a medical emergency room without a further appointment with those who had been given and who kept an appointment to attend a psychiatric clinic. The reattempt rate was significantly higher among those who had not been given an appointment, and those who attended only once did less well than those who attended more than once. The medical seriousness of the initial attempt did not predict reattempt. Kennedy (1972) found (after taking account of different rates of prior suicide attempts—usually a good predictor of further repetition) that suicide repetition rates were significantly lower among 142 attempters admitted for a short period to a suicide crisis unit than among six who had received outpatient care only and 56 who received no aftercare. Welu (1977) found higher attendance rates and fewer suicide repetitions during a brief 4-month follow-up period among 63 patients who were seen in a program with a strong outreach component than among 57 cases seen before the new program was introduced. Motto (1976) and Motto et al. (1981) offered after-care to 3005 predominantly adult hospitalized patients who had either made a previous suicide attempt or had been judged to be depressed during their admission. Of these, 862 declined, and the remainder were randomly assigned either to receive intermittent telephone contact at decreasing intervals over a 5-year period or to receive no further contact. During the first 2 years of follow-up, suicide was twice as common in the noncontacted group, but thereafter the rates converged. The contact rate in the experimental group was far from complete and diagnostic and other differences between compliers and noncompliers have not been described.

By contrast, no significant differences in suicide rates or social adjustments were found by Ettlinger (1975) in Denmark in a 6-year follow-up study of 670 consecutive adult patients attending a comprehensive treatment program, compared with 681 attempters seen before the service had been started. The program provided free access to mental health professionals, daytime hotline and walk-in clinics, home visits on request, close liaison with other hospitals, and proactive outreach for 1 year.

The optimal design for assessing the impact of a treatment is to assign similar types of cases randomly to different treatment conditions. This reduces the chance that a favorable outcome is due to some treatment-relevant referral bias, although randomization may fail if numbers are small.

The few experimental studies of this sort have not shown any significant treatment effect. Chowdhury et al. (1973) randomly assigned adult attempt repeaters to routine outpatient care or to an enhanced service that included emergency telephone access and walk-in facilities. Patients were visited at home when they failed to keep appointments. The groups did not differ from each other in reattempt rates nor on any measure of mental state at the end of a 6-month follow-up period, although the experimental group reported fewer social problems (difficulties with housing, employment, obtaining benefits, etc.) than the controls. One cannot conclude from this study that psychiatric care was not helpful because it was received by both groups, albeit in different amounts. Gibbons et al. (1978) and Gibbons (1980) randomly assigned 200 adult attempters each to a 3-month course of intensive, task-centered casework or to routine treatment (some cases being followed by a psychiatrist, others by a general practitioner). Cases judged to have high suicide intent were excluded from the random assignment. No differences in later adjustment were found between the two groups. Lieberman and Eckman (1981) randomly assigned a small group of adult attempters to either 32 hours of behavior therapy (social skills training, anxiety management, and contingency contracting) or to unlimited insight-oriented psychotherapy. No differences were found in the two groups with respect to repetition of suicide attempts, although the behavior therapy group had fewer symptoms, were less preoccupied with suicidal ideation, and made fewer threats.

Even if it is unreasonable to generalize from studies carried out with adults to adolescents, they are instructive for at least three reasons. First, they all treat attempted suicide as a single diagnostic entity, whereas there is good evidence that suicidal behavior is associated with several types of disorder and it is likely that patients with different types of disorder will have a different natural history and will respond differently to different interventions. Thus Chowdhury et al.'s (1973) study, quoted above, showed high suicide repetition rates in patients with a history of chronic personality disturbance, and according to Litman et al. (1965), this is the group of crisis service callers most likely to go on to commit suicide. Second, most use attempt repetition or death as an outcome measure. These are low frequency behaviors, which give the researcher little power even in a high-risk group. Third, there have been remarkably few psychopharmacological studies among suicide attempters (for a review, see Hirsch et al., 1982; Trautman and Shaffer, 1984). A small, controlled random assignment study with flupenthixol (a thiothixene) in a group of very high frequency attempt-repeaters resulted in a significant reduction in attempts but failed to take account of symptomatic or diagnostic differences in this heterogeneous population. There is clearly a great deal of scope in this area for well designed studies with a broader range of psychoactive drugs among diagnostically homogeneous groups.

POSTVENTION

Postvention refers to an intervention started after a suicide with family survivors or the school or community. The theoretical orientation or rationale for postvention activities is rarely described in the literature. Postvention could serve several preventive functions by (a) providing a structure for understanding the death, thus alleviating some of the guilt and isolation experienced by family survivors (Calhoun et al., 1982; Henley, 1984; Rogers et al., 1982); (b) minimizing the scapegoating that can affect parents, teachers, the school, or particular peers; and (c) reducing the likelihood of imitation either within the family or within the community or both.

The only evaluation research that we have noted in this area is an uncontrolled study by Rogers et al. (1982) of a volunteer-led survivors support group that lasted 2 months. At the start of the program most participants were reported to feel guilty, detached from the event, and abandoned. Many idealized the deceased. They scored high on the somatization, phobic, and obsessive-compulsive scales of the SCL–90 (Derogatis et al., 1973). At follow-up most of the participants felt that the program had been helpful and showed a decline in SCL–90 scores; however, as the study was uncontrolled, one does not know whether these would have occurred anyway.

A series of publications by Videka-Sherman was reported on the impact of a bereaved parent support group, the "Compassionate Friends" (Videka-Sherman, 1982a, 1982b; Videka-Sherman and Lieberman, 1985), which provides support to parents who have lost a child by any type of sudden death. The 2422 parents in the study were surveyed on two occasions, although the proportion made up of parents of suicides is not indicated. Comparisons were drawn between those who attended several meetings and those who either did not attend at all or who dropped out at an early stage. Only 28% of those surveyed responded at the time of the first survey and only 17% provided additional follow-up information. Responders were predominantly white and upper middle class. Depression scores declined equally in both groups, suggesting that attendance did not help with that aspect of adaptation. A relationship was noted between an early preoccupation with the memory of the child and persistent depression. Depression scores fell most in parents who immersed themselves in another activity or who had a "replacement" child. Persistent attendance at the group was not associated with either of these styles. Attendance did enhance altruistic activity; but this was not in itself associated with a higher-than-expected reduction in depression scores.

There are many questions outstanding with respect to postvention procedures in schools (e.g., is it a good or bad thing to hold large assemblies, to arrange small groups among close friends, to ignore or downplay the death, etc.). To date, there has been no systematic research in this area.

CONCLUSIONS

Predicting who will commit suicide has been dismissed as a futile enterprise in the general class of predicting rare events from common ones (Eisenberg, in press; Rosen, 1954; Temoche et al., 1964) with all of the problems of low specificity (high false positive rates) that are only acceptable if interventions are inexpensive or efficacious or both (far from the case in suicide). Although this argument certainly applies to low-risk interventions, it may not apply to focused high-risk interventions, especially if knowledge of specific risk factors improves. It is too soon to draw closure on suicide prevention.

REFERENCES

Apsler, R. & Hodas, M. (1975), Evaluating hotlines with simulated calls. *Crisis Intervention*, 6:14–21.

Asberg, M., Nordstrom, P. & Traskman-Bendz, L. (1986), Biological factors in suicide. In: *Suicide,* ed. A. Roy, Baltimore, MD: Williams and Wilkins.
——, ——, —— (1987), Cerebrospinal fluid studies in suicide. *Ann NY Acad. Sci.,* 487: 243–244.
——, Thorén, P., Träskman, L., Bertilsson, L. & Ringberger, V. (1976), Serotonin depression. *Science,* 191:478–480.
Bagley, C. (1968), The evaluation of a suicide prevention scheme by an ecological method. *Soc. Sci. Med.,* 2:1–14.
Barraclough, B. M., Bunch, J. & Nelson, B. et al. (1969), The diagnostic classification and psychiatric treatment of 100 suicides. *Proceedings of the Fifth International Conference for Suicide Prevention,* London.
——, Jennings, C. & Moss, J. R. (1977), Suicide prevention by the samaritans. *Lancet.*
Bleach, B. & Claiborn, W. L. (1974), Initial evaluation of hot-line telephone crisis centers. *Community Ment. Health J.,* 10:387–394.
Bollen, K. A. & Phillips, D. P. (1982), Imitative suicides. *American Sociological Review,* 47:802–809.
——, —— (1981), Suicidal motor vehicle fatalities in Detroit. *American Journal of Sociology,* 87: 404–412.
Boyd, J. H. & Moscicki, E. K. (1986), Firearms and youth suicide. *Am. J. Public Health,* 76:1240–1242.
Brent, D. A., Perper, J. A. & Allman, C. J. (1987), Alcohol, firearms and suicide among youth. *JAMA,* 257:3369–3372.
——, ——, Goldstein, C. E. et al. (in press), Risk factors for adolescent suicide. *Arch. Gen. Psychiatry,* 45:581–588.
Bridge, T. P., Potkin, S. G., Zung, W. W. et al. (1977), Suicide prevention centers. *Nerv. Men. Dis.* 164:18–24.
Brown, G. L., Ebert, M. H., Goyner, P. F. et al. (1982). Aggression, suicide, and serotonin. *Am. J. Psychiatry,* 139:741–746.
Calhoun, L. G., Selby, J. W. & Selby, L. E. (1982), The psychological aftermath of suicide. *Clinical Psychology Review,* 2:409–420.
Chowdhury, N., Hicks, R. C. & Kreitman, N. (1973), Evaluation of an after-care service for parasuicide (attempted suicide) patients. *Soc. Psychiatry,* 8:67–81.
Clarke, R. V. & Lester, D. (1987), Toxicity of car exhausts and opportunity for suicide. *J. Epidemiol. Community Health.* 41:114–120.
Derogatis, L. R., Lipman, R. S. & Covi, L. (1973), The SCL–90; an outpatient psychiatric rating scale. *Psychopharmacol. Bull.* 9:13–28.
Dorpat, T. L. & Ripley, H. S. (1960), A study of suicide in the Seattle area. *Compr. Psychiatry,* 1:349–359.
Eisenberg, L. (in press), Public policy: risk factor or remedy? In: *Risk Factors and the Prevention of Child Psychiatric Disorders.* ed. D. Shaffer, I. Phillips & N. Enzer. Washington, D.C.: ADAMHA.
Elkins, Jr., R. L. & Cohen, C. R. (1982), A comparison of the effects of prejob training and job experiences on nonprofessional telephone crisis counselors. *Suicide Life Threat. Behav.* 12:84–89.
Ettlinger, R. (1975), Evaluation of suicide prevention after attempted suicide. *Acta Psychiatr. Scand.* (Supp)260:5–135.
Farberow, N. R. (1985), Youth suicide. Report of the National Conference on Youth Suicide; Washington, D.C.: Youth Suicide National Center, pp 9–34.

Fleiss, J. L. (1981), *Statistical methods for rates and proportions*. 2nd Ed. New York: John Wiley.

France, K. (1975), Evaluation of lay volunteer crisis telephone workers. *Am J. Community Psychol.*, 3:197–220.

Genther, R. (1974), Evaluating the functioning of community based hotlines. *Professional Psychology,* 5:409–414.

Gibbons, J. S., Butler, J., Urwin, P. et al. (1978), Evaluation of a social work service for self-poisoning patients. *Br. J. Psychiatry,* 133:111–118.

—— (1980), Management of self-poisoning. In: *The Suicide Syndrome,* ed R. Farmer & S. Hirsch, London: Croon Helm.

Glatt, K. M. (1987), Helpline: suicide prevention at a suicide site. *Suicide Life Threat. Behav.,* 17:299–309.

Goldacre, M. & Hawton, K. (1985), Reception of self-poisoning and subsequent death in adolescents who take overdoses. *Br. J. Psychiatry,* 146:395–398.

Gould, M. S. & Davidson, L. (1988), Suicide contagion among adolescents. In: *Advances in Adolescent Mental Health, Volume III: Depression and Suicide,* ed. A. R. Stillman & R. A. Feldman. Greenwich, CT: JAI Press.

——, Shaffer, D. & Kleinman, M. (1988), The impact of suicide in television movies. *Suicide Life Threat. Behav.,* 18:

——, ——, Davies, M. (1988), Truncated pathways from childhood. In: *Straight and Devious Pathways to Adulthood,* ed. L. Robins & M. Rutter. Cambridge: Cambridge Univ. Press, (in press).

——, —— (1986), The impact of suicide in television movies. *N. Engl. J. Med.* 315:690–694.

Greer, S. & Anderson, M. (1979), Samaritan contact among 325 parasuicide patients. *Br. J. Psychiatry,* 135:263–268.

——, Bagley, C. (1971), Effect of psychiatric intervention in attempted suicide. *Br. Med. J.* 1:310–312.

Hassall, C. & Trethowan, W. H. (1972), Suicide in Birmingham. *Br. Med. J.* 1:717–718.

Hawton, K. & Goldacre, M. (1982), Hospital admissions for adverse effects of medicinal agents (mainly self-poisoning) among adolescents in the Oxford region. *Br. J. Psychiatry,* 141:106–170.

Henley, S. H. A. (1984), Bereavement following suicide. *Current Psychological Research & Reviews,* 3:53–61.

Hirsch, S. (1981), A critique of volunteer-staffed suicide prevention centres. *Can. J. Psychiatry,* 26:406–410.

Hirsch, S. R., Walsh, C. & Draper, R. (1982), Parasuicide. *J. Affective Disord.* 4:299–311.

Holding, T. A. (1974), The B. B. C. "Befriender" series and its effect. *Br. J. Psychiatry,* 124:470–472.

Holding, T. A. (1975), Suicide and "The Befrienders." *Br. Med. J.* 3:751–753.

Jan-Tausch, J., State of New Jersey Department of Education. Suicide of children 1960–63: New Jersey public school students. Trenton, N.J.: 1964.

Jennings, C., Barraclough, B. M. & Moss, J. R. (1978), Have the samaritans lowered the suicide rate? *Psychol. Med.* 8:413–422.

Johns, M. W. (1977), Self-poisoning with barbiturates in England and Wales during 1959–1974. *Br. Med. J.* 2:1128–1130.

Kalafat, J., Boroto, D. R. & France, K. (1979), Relationships among experience level and value orientation and the performance of paraprofessional telephone counselors. *Am. J. Community Psychol.* 5:167–179.

Kennedy, P. (1972), Efficacy of a regional poisoning treatment center in preventing further suicidal behavior. *Br. Med. J.* 4:255–257.

——, Kreitman, N. & Ovenstone, I. M. K. (1974), The prevalence of suicide and parasuicide (attempted suicide) in Edinburgh. *Br. J. Psychiatry*, 124:36–41.

King, G. D. (1977), An evaluation of the effectiveness of a telephone counselling center. *Am. J. Community Psychol.*, 5:75–83.

Knesper, D. J. (1982), A study of referral failures for potentially suicidal patients. *Hos. Community Psychiatry*. 33:49–52.

Knowles, D. (1979), On the tendency for volunteer helpers to give advice. *Journal of Counseling Psychology*, 26:352–354.

Kogan, L. S. (1957), The short-term case in a family agency. *Social Casework*, 38:296–302.

Kreitman, N. (1976), Age and parasuicide. *Psychol Med.*, 6:113–121.

——, Chowdhury, N. (1973), Distress behavior: a study of selected Samaritan clients and parasuicides (attempted suicide patients). *Br. J. Psychiatry*, 123:1–8/9–14.

Lester, D. (1973), Prevention of suicide. *J. A. M. A.*, 225:992.

—— (1970), Steps toward the evaluation of a suicide prevention center. *Crisis Intervention*, 2:42–45.

Lieberman, R. & Eckman, T. (1981), Behavior therapy vs. insight oriented therapy for repeated suicide attempters. *Arch. Gen. Psychiatry*, 38:1126–1130.

Linnoila, M., Virkkunen, M., Scheinin, M. et al. (1983), Low cerebrospinal fluid 5–hydroxyindoleacetic acid concentration differentiates impulsive from nonimpulsive violent behavior. *Life Sci.*, 33:2609–2614.

Litman, R. E., Farberow, N. L., Shneidman, E. S. et al. (1965), Suicide prevention telephone service. *J. A. M. A.*, 192:107–111.

——, —— (1969), Evaluating the effectiveness of suicide prevention. *Proceedings of the Fifth International Conference for Suicide Prevention*, London: 246–250.

Litt, I. F., Cuskey, W. R. & Rudd, S. (1983), Emergency room evaluation of the adolescent who attempts suicide. *J. Adolesc. Health Care*, 4:106–108.

McCarthy, B. W. & Berman, A. L. (1979), A student operated crisis center. *Personnel and Guidance*, 49:523–528.

Miller, H. L., Coombs, D. W., Leeper, J. D. et al. (1984), An analysis of the effects of suicide prevention facilities on suicide rates in the United States, *Am. J. Public Health*, 74:340–343.

Motto, J. A., Heilbron, D. C., Juster, R. P. et al. (1981), Communication as a suicide prevention program. *Depression et Suicide*, 148–154.

—— (1976), Suicide prevention for high-risk persons who refuse treatment. *Suicide Life Threat. Behav.*, 6:223–230.

—— (1984), Suicide in male adolescents. In: *Suicide in the Young*, eds. H. S. Segdak, A. B. Ford & N. B. Rushforth. Boston: John Wright PSG, pp. 227–244.

National Center for Health Statistics (1988), Department of Health and Human Services, Mortality Statistics Branch (published and unpublished data).

Neilson, J. & Videbech, T. (1973), Suicide frequency before and after introduction of community psychiatry in a Danish island. *Br. J. Psychiatry*, 123:35–39.

Otto, O. (1972), Suicidal acts by children and adolescents. *Acta Psychiatr. Scand. Supple.*, 233.

Phillips, D. P. (1980), Airplane accidents, murder and the mass media. *Social Forces,* 58:1001–1004.

—— (1974), The influence of suggestion on suicide. *American Sociological Review,* 39:340–354.

—— (1979), Suicide, motor vehicle fatalities, and the mass media. *American Journal of Sociology,* 84:1150–1174.

—— (1984), Teenage and adult temporal fluctuations in suicide and auto fatalities. In: *Suicide in the Young,* eds. H. S. Sudak, A. B. Ford & N. B. Rushforth. Boston, MA: John Wright PSG, pp. 69–80.

——, Carstenson, L. L. (1986), Clustering of teenage suicides after television news stories about suicide. *N. Engl. J. Med.,* 315:685–689.

Pokorny, A. D. (1983), Prediction of suicide in psychiatric patients. *Arch. Gen. Psychiatry,* 40:249–257.

—— (1964), Suicide rates in various psychiatric disorders. *J. Nerv., Ment. Dis.* 139:499–506.

Ringel, E. (1968), Suicide prevention in Vienna. In: *Suicidal Behaviors: Diagnosis and Management,* ed. H. L. P. Resnick. Boston: Little, Brown.

Robins, E., Gassner, S., Kayes, J. et al. (1959), The communication of suicide intent. *Am. J. Psychiatry,* 115:724–733.

Rogawski, A. B. & Edmundson, B. (1971), Factors affecting the outcome of psychiatric interagency referral. *Am. J. Psychiatry,* 127:925–934.

Rogers, J., Sheldon A., Barwick, C. et al. (1982), Help for families of suicide. Can. J. Psychiatry, 27:444–448.

Rosen, A. (1954), Detection of suicidal patients. *J. Consult. Psychol.,* 18:397–403.

Roy, A., Agren, H., Picker, D. et al. (1986), Reduced cerebrospinal fluid concentrations of homovanillic acid and homovanillic acid to 5–hydroxyindoleacetic acid ratios in depressed patients. *Am. J. Psychiatry,* 143:1539–1545.

Salk, L., Sturner, W., Reilly, B. et al. (1985), Relationship of maternal and perinatal conditions to eventual adolescent suicide. *Lancet* 1:624–627.

Sanborn, D. E., Sanborn, C. J. & Cimbolic, P. (1974), Two years of suicide. *Child Psychiatry Hum. Dev.,* 3:234–242.

Schmidtke, A. & Hafner, H. (1986), Die vermittlung von selbstmordmotivation und selbstmordhandlung durch fiktive modelle. *Nervenarz,* 57:502–510.

Shaffer, D., Garland, A., Underwood, M. & Whittle, B. (1987), *An evaluation of three youth suicide prevention programs in New Jersey.* Report prepared for the New Jersey State Department of Health and Human Services.

Shaffer, D., Garland, A. & Bacon, K. (in press), Prevention issues in youth suicide. In: *Risk Factors and the Prevention of Child Psychiatry Disorders,* eds. D. Shaffer, I. Phillips & N. Enzer. Washington, DC:P ADAMHA. In press.

—— (1974), Suicide in childhood and early adolescence. *J. Child Psychol. Psychiatry,* 15:275–291.

——, Fisher, P. (1981), The epidemiology of suicide in children and young adolescents. *This Journal,* 20:545–565.

——, Gould, M. (1987), Study of completed and attempted suicides in adolescents. Progress Report: National Institute of Mental Health.

Shaffi, M., Carrigan, S., Whittinghill, J. R. et al. (1985), Psychological autopsy of completed suicide in children and adolescents. *Am J. Psychiatry,* 142:1061–1064.

Shneidman, E. S. & Farberow, N. L. (1957), *Clues to suicide.* New York: Blakison.

Shore, J. H. (1975), American Indian suicide—fact and fantasy. *Psychiatry,* 38:86–91.

Simmons, J. T., Comstock, B. S. & Franklin, J. L. (1986), Prevention/intervention programs for suicidal adolescents. Prepared for: *The Prevention and Intervention Work Group of the Secretary of Health and Human Services' Task Force on Youth Suicide.* Oakland, CA.

Slaiku, K. A., Tulkin, S. R. & Speer, D. C. (1975), Process and outcome in the evaluation of telephone counseling referrals. *J. Consult. Clin. Psychol.,* 43:700–707.

Slem, C. M. & Cotler, S. (1973), Crisis phone services: evaluation of hotline program. *Am. J. Community Psychol.* 1:219–227.

Smith, K. & Crawford, S. (1986), Suicidal behavior among "normal" high school students. *Suicide Life Threat. Behav.,* 16:313–325.

Stanley, M., Traskman-Bendz, L. & Dorovini-Zis, K. (1985), Correlations between aminergic metabolites simultaneously obtained from human csf and brain. *Life Sci.,* 37:1279–1286.

——, Mann, J. J. (1987), Biological factors associated with suicide. In: *Annual Review of Psychiatry,* Vol. 7, eds. A. J. Frances & R. E. Hales. New York, N.Y.: American Psychiatry Press, Inc., pp. 334–352.

Sudak, H. S., Sawyer, J. B., Spring, G. K. et al. (1977), High referral success rates in a crisis center. *Hosp. Community Psychiatry,* 38:530–532.

Temoche, A., Pugh, T. F. & McMahon, B. (1964), Suicide rates among current and former mental institution patients. *J. Nerv. Ment. Dis.* 138:124–130.

Traskman-Bendz, L., Asberg, M., Bertilsson, L. et al. (1984), CSF monoamine metabolites of depressed patients during illness and after recovery. *Acta Psychiatr. Scand.,* 69:333–342.

Trautman, P. D., Lewin, M. A. & Krauskopf, M. A. (1987), Home visits with noncompliant adolescent suicide attempters. Presented at *The 34th Annual Meeting of the American Academy of Child & Adolescent Psychiatry,* Washington, D.C.; Vol. III.

——, Shaffer, D. (1984), Treatment of child and adolescent suicide attempters. In: *Suicide in the Young,* eds. H. S. Sudak, A. B. Ford and N. B. Rushforth. Boston, MA: John Wright PSG, pp. 307–323.

Van Praag, H. M. (1977), Significance of biochemical parameters in the diagnosis, treatment, and prevention of depressive disorders. *Biol. Psychiatry,* 12:101–131.

Videka-Sherman, L. (1982a), Coping with the death of a child. *Am. J. Orthopsychiatry,* 52:688–698.

—— (1982b), Effects of participation in a self-help group for bereaved parents. *Prevention in the Human Services,* 1:69–77.

——, Lieberman, M. A. (1985), The effects of self-help and psychotherapy intervention on child loss. *Am. J. Orthopsychiatry,* 55:70–82.

Walk, D. (1967), Suicide and community care. *Br. J. Psychiatry,* 113:1381–1391.

Wasserman, I. M. (1984), Imitation and suicide. *American Sociological Review,* 49:427–436.

Weiner, I. W. (1969), The effectiveness of a suicide prevention program. *Mental Hygiene,* 53:357–363.

Welu, T. C. (1977), A follow-up program for suicide attempters. *Suicide Life Threat. Behav.,* 7:17–30.

Winokur, G. & Ming, T. (1975), The Iowa 500. *Am. J. Psychiatry,* 132:650–651.

PART VI: DEPRESSION AND SUICIDE

25

Completed Suicide in Children and Adolescents

Harry M. Hoberman and Barry D. Garfinkel
University of Minnesota Medical School

Descriptive information on a large number of children and adolescents who had committed suicide was collected from medical examiners' records. A review of deaths of persons 19 and under from nonnatural causes identified 229 youth suicides. Characteristics of these youth were extracted from medical examiners' reports: no control groups were employed. Children and adolescents who committed suicide were most likely to be older males with a current psychiatric disorder, usually an affective disorder or alcohol or drug abuse. Suicides appeared to be impulsive and triggered by age-normative precipitants. Sex, age, and cohort differences are presented. Results are evaluated in light of previous research.

Despite the well-documented increases in the rate of completed suicide among adolescents (Center for Disease Control, 1986), accurate knowledge of the characteristics of youthful suicide completers is very limited. Moreover, even what little data are available suggest that the public as well as professionals possess erroneous conceptions of the nature of suicidal behavior. Such potential misconceptions have significant implications because they may determine the content and structure of intervention programs directed as suicidal youth. Consequently, there is a pressing need for systematic information designating the characteristics of children and adolescents who commit suicide.

Reprinted with permission from the *Journal of the American Academy of Child and Adolescent Psychiatry,* 1988, Vol. 27, No. 6, 689–695. Copyright 1988 by the American Academy of Child and Adolescent Psychiatry.

The authors wish to express their gratitude to Gary Peterson, M.D., J. D. and Michael McGee, M.D., Medical Examiners of Hennepin and Ramsey Counties, respectively. Their cooperation and support ensured the success of this endeavor. The authors are grateful to the Minnesota Medical Foundation and the Thorp Foundation for their generous support of this project.

Beyond Jan-Tausch's (1964) initial study of 41 child and adolescent suicides, only six studies have carefully attempted to delineate factors associated with self-inflicted death among younger persons in Western societies (Shaffer, 1974; Pettifor et al., 1983; Garfinkel and Golombek, 1983; Shaffii et al., 1985; and Thompson, 1987). Shaffer (1974) studied children fourteen years old and under who had committed suicide in England and Wales between 1962 and 1968 ($N = 31$). Pettifor et al. (1983) described differences between 40 adolescents seen at a mental health clinic in Alberta, who eventually committed suicide (between 1956 and 1979) and a matched group of nonsuicidal clinic outpatients. Garfinkel and Golombek (1983) examined coroners' and police reports and collected information on 1554 suicides by persons aged 10 to 24 in Ontario. Poteet (1987) studied medical examiners' reports for 87 suicides (ages 13 to 19) that occurred between 1970 and 1985 in Tennessee. Shaffi et al. (1985) have described the results of "psychological autopsies" conducted on 20 persons aged 19 and under. Finally, Thompson (1987) reported on 190 suicides by persons aged less than 20 in Manitoba from 1970 to 1982. Each of these studies has contributed significantly to our understanding of youth suicide, yet they all possess certain limitations. Several involve relatively small numbers of subjects and one study focuses on a potentially idiosyncratic group of patients (e.g., help-seeking persons). A number of the studies include persons whose suicide occurred a number of years ago (Garfinkel and Golombek, 1983; Pettifor et al., 1983; Poteet, 1987; Shaffer, 1974; Shaffi et al., 1985; Thompson, 1987) raising the question of potential cohort differences. Given the continuing increase in youth suicide rates over the past 30 to 40 years (Center for Disease Control, 1986), the characteristics of the youth who has recently taken his or her life may be quite different from those of one who committed suicide several decades ago. In brief, several methodological issues may comprise the application of the already limited knowledge available concerning child and adolescent suicides.

The present study provides a description of completed suicide among children and adolescents. As in the studies of Jan-Tausch (1964) and Shaffer (1974), the investigators examined medical examiners' records of a consecutive group of deceased children and adolescents. A detailed psychological autopsy (e.g., interviewing the decedent's family and friends) as described by Shaffi et al. (1985) was not conducted. Instead, a large number of youth suicide victims was studied over a number of years to examine differences between subgroups of those who died. In particular, this study attempted to characterize gender, age, and temporal differences in young suicides.

METHOD

Subjects consisted of deceased individuals 19 years and younger whose deaths occurred between January 1, 1975 and December 31, 1985. The deaths of those included in the study had been investigated by either the Hennepin Court medical examiner's office or the Ramsey County (Minnesota) medical examiner's office and were ruled to be the result of nonnatural causes: suicides, accidents, homicides, or undetermined. Hennepin and Ramsey counties contain the cities of Minneapolis and St. Paul, respectively. While they are predominately urban and suburban, they include rural areas as well. Each of the decedent's records was reviewed by one of three research assistants and information was obtained according to a structured format. The medical examiners' records contain a varied amount of information, depending upon the availability and cooperation of informants regarding the decedent at the time of death. Basic information found in the records of almost all decedents included demographic information concerning the decedent and information concerning the circumstances and means of death. Data concerning the psychosocial or behavioral aspects of the decedent were less consistently available.

All deaths not ruled as suicides were carefully reviewed. Ninety deaths that the medical examiners had determined to be accidental homicides, or undetermined were considered by the investigators to be suicides; these constituted 15% of the total group of youth suicides. Deaths were reclassified based upon criteria derived from previous studies of completed suicide among youth (e.g., Garfinkel and Golombek, 1983); characteristics of male gender, evidence of a depressive disorder, a stressor involving loss or conflict, and circumstances of the death were all applied in the decision making. All such reclassifications were based on unanimous agreement between the two investigators, who each rated the decedent separately. Later, two research assistants reviewed these records and coded the data into categories derived largely from those described in the Completed Suicide Informant Interview (Shaffer, 1985). This interview specifies a coding scheme for the classification of variables of interest regarding completed suicides (e.g., types of precipitants, relevant circumstances surrounding suicides). Thus, the coders noted whether the information in the medical examiner's record indicated, for example, if a relationship breakup occurred, if the decedent had made a previous remark regarding suicide, or if that decedent had numerous friends. A select number of cases (n = 30) were coded twice. Disagreements in coding were resolved through discussion. All recorded information was reviewed by both a clinical psychologist and a child psychiatrist.

In particular, information abstracted from the medical examiners' records was evaluated according to diagnostic criteria based upon Family History Research Diagnostic Criteria (Andreason et al., 1977). Additionally, ratings of blood alcohol based upon toxicology tests were available for selected decedents; other decedents were rated for the likelihood of being under the influence of alcohol or other illegal substances based on observers' reports or the presence of such substances at the scene of death.

Three comparisons were made within the larger group of suicides. First, male and female completers were compared. Second, comparisons were made upon the basis of age at the time of death. The groups were of persons 14 years old and under or of persons between the ages of 15 and 19 years, based upon the age divisions utilized by the Center for Disease Control. Lastly, in order to examine the possibility of temporal changes in the characteristics of youth suicide, comparisons were made between suicides occurring between 1975 and 1979 and those occurring between 1980 and 1985.

When differences between the various groups attained statistical significance, they are reported. Conversely, if no difference is noted, the groups obtained similar values on the variable in question. In general, percentages reported are absolute figures and reflect positive evidence for a particular variable. For most of the variables described, information was available for the entire sample. Because there is variability in the information contained in the records of the medical examiners, missing data might constitute either true or false negatives. In any case, these findings should be regarded as conservative estimates.

RESULTS

Demographics

Demographic features of the youthful suicides are presented in Table 1. Males predominated among youthful suicides (80%); the ratio of males to females was 4:1. Older adolescents (ages 15 to 19) constituted the overwhelming number of young suicides ($N = 208$); persons under 15 made up only 9% of the decedents ($N = 21$). Ninety-four percent of the suicides were Caucasian, 4% were black, and the remainder were members of other minority groups. Regarding occupation at the time of death 71% were students, 16% were laborers, 9% were otherwise employed, and 4% were unemployed. Only 2% were married; thus 98% were single. The great majority of the youthful suicides (79%) were living with their parents at the time of their deaths; the remainder lived with spouses, friends or roommates, with other relatives in an out-of-parental-home placement, or alone.

TABLE 1. *Age, Sex, and Cohort Differences for Suicides*

	N	%
Age (years)		
<14	21	9
15–19	208	91
Sex		
Male	184	80
Female	45	20
Cohort		
1975–1979	107	47
1980–1985	122	53

Table 1. Age, Sex, and Cohort Differences for Suicides

Male and female completers did not differ on the variables of age, race, or religion. Fewer female decedents were students and females were more likely to hold some type of clerical or sales position ($\chi^2 = 23.76$; $df = 6$; $p<0.0006$). Generally, there were no demographic differences between older and younger suicides. As might be expected, these groups tended to differ on the variable of occupation, with fewer of the older suicides being students; however, 18% of the 15- to 19-year-old group were employed as blue-collar laborers. No demographic variables differentiated between earlier and recent suicides.

Method of Death

The predominant means of suicide was firearms; 42% of the deaths resulted from such weapons. Hanging (17%), carbon monoxide poisoning (16%), ingestion (10%), and falls (7%) were the other leading causes of death. Only 1% of the suicides involved motor vehicle accidents. It should be noted that 38% of the fatal overdoses were from prescribed antidepressants, while 24% were from analgesics. The majority of antidepressant overdoses involved medicine prescribed for the decedent.

As can be seen in Table 2, females differed from males on their choices of method of suicide ($\chi^2 = 34.44$; $df = 7$; $p<0.0000$). While males were more than twice as likely to employ firearms or to hang themselves, females were much more likely to die by means of drug ingestion, carbon monoxide poisoning, falls, or suffocation. Males who committed suicide by drug overdose were more likely to ingest their own antidepressants, while females were more likely to take analgesics or other pharmacological agents.

Younger and older suicides differed in terms of their method of death ($\chi^2 = 25.53$; $df = 7$; $p<0.0006$) as can be seen in Table 3. Over half of the younger suicides (52%) hanged themselves; this was followed by firearms us-

	Males (N = 181) %	Females (N = 44) %
Firearms	47	21
Hanging	20	7
CO poisoning	14	25
Ingestion	6	27
Jumping	6	11
Suffocation	1	5
Other	6	14

Table 2. Gender Differences for Methods of Suicide of 225 Completers

	14 Years (N = 21) %	15–19 Years (N = 204) %
Firearms	24	44
Hanging	52	14
CO poisoning	5	17
Ingestion	14	10
Jumping	0	7
Other	5	8

Table 3. Age Differences in Method of Death of 225 Suicide Completers

age (24%). Older suicides, in contrast, were most likely to employ a gun as their means of death (44%) or carbon monoxide poisoning (17%).

Cohort differences were found for method of death (χ^2 = 22.32; df = 7; $p<0.002$). Deaths from firearms declined slightly, while suicides from hanging and carbon monoxide poisoning both doubled. Although not reaching statistical significance, the percentage of ingestion deaths from antidepressants increased sharply for recent suicides.

Circumstances of the Suicide

Slightly more than half (57%) of the suicides took place in the afternoon or evening. There was no seasonal difference in rates of suicides. The great majority of suicides occurred at the decedent's home (70%) with 22% taking place outdoors. In 30% of the cases, someone else was present at the time of the death; in another 29% of the cases, someone was likely to contact the decedent. Only 29% of the decedents took active precautions to avoid discovery. In 62% of the cases, the individual had made some remark about suicide before death; in most cases, such remarks were made on the day of death. Only 8% of the suicides showed evidence of definite preparation for death. In only 28% of the cases was there credible evidence of a plan to commit suicide and this typically appeared to be of brief duration. Approximately 50% of the youthful suicides left a note. On the day of the suicide, 45% of the suicides were rated as sad or despairing, while 21% and 18% were described as angry or calm, respectively. Twenty-eight percent of the decedents had consumed alcohol (unrelated to the cause of death) within 12 hours of their death; in another 17% of the cases there was evidence of probable alcohol consumption. In some cases, blood alcohol levels were as high as 0.30 meq/L.

No sex differences were found for time or location of death, the amount of precaution taken against being discovered, or the likelihood of being contacted at the time of the suicide. No differences were found for males and females regarding their mood prior to death or preparations for suicide. Males and females were equally likely to have consumed alcohol prior to the act of suicide. Females were nearly four times as likely to make a remark about suicide on the day of their death ($\chi^2 = 16.73$; $df = 7$; $p<0.02$). Additionally, more males were likely to write a suicide note before their death ($\chi^2 = 7.39$; $df = 2$; $p<0.02$).

Few age differences were found for circumstances of the suicide. Older suicides were equally likely to kill themselves during the morning as during later hours, while younger children never killed themselves early in the morning ($\chi^2 = 7.79$; $df = 3$; $p<0.05$). Older suicides were more likely to be described as either sad or despairing (49%), while younger suicides were more likely to be described as angry (40%) or nervous (40%) ($\chi^2 = 16.03$; $df = 6$; $p<0.01$). In addition, older suicides were more likely to have made a remark about suicide in the week before their death ($\chi^2 = 16.52$; $df = 6$; $p<0.01$).

No cohort differences were identified for the time or season of death, the degree of planning the suicide, leaving a suicide note, or the likelihood of being contacted at the time of the suicide. Recent suicides were more likely to take passive precautions against being discovered ($\chi^2 = 8.82$; $df = 2$; $p<0.01$) and were more likely to commit suicide at home ($\chi^2 = 10.74$; $df = 5$; $p<0.06$). For the variables regarding mood or alcohol consumption at the time of death or prior talk of suicide, no cohort differences emerged.

Psychiatric History

At the time of their death, 28% of the suicides were rated as suffering from a depressive disorder. Ten percent were characterized as alcohol abusers, while 12% were characterized as drug abusers. Conduct disorders were identified in 7% of the suicides. Two percent of the suicides were rated as schizophrenic and 2% were classified as having bipolar affective disorder. Overall, 50% of the decedents showed clear evidence (e.g., taking antidepressants, past chemical dependency treatment) of one or multiple psychiatric disorders. For the remainder of the subjects, no diagnosis was assigned either because the evidence did not support such a determination or because insufficient evidence was available.

The suicides were also evaluated for a past history of psychiatric disorders. Of the decedents, 16% showed evidence of a previous depressive disorder; past alcoholism or substance abuse characterized 9% and 11% of the suicides, respectively. Only 18% of the decedents were known to have made a prior suicide attempt.

While the results did not attain statistical significance, female decedents were more likely to have a current depressive disorder, while males were more likely to be characterized as alcohol abusers. Females were approximately twice as likely to have made a single previous suicide attempt ($\chi^2 = 12.08$; $df = 5$; $p<0.03$); they were also more likely to have made multiple previous suicide attempts ($\chi^2 = 15.84$; $df = 3$; $p<0.001$). Generally, these prior attempts were by drug ingestion or lacerations.

Although there were no significant differences between younger and older suicides regarding present psychiatric disorders, specific trends were evident. Younger suicides were much more likely to be described as having a conduct disorder; older suicides were more likely to be described as depressed or as abusing alcohol or other drugs.

There were no significant differences between earlier and recent studies regarding either present or past psychiatric history.

Precipitants

The occurrence of a variety of stressful situations in the three days preceding the suicide was rated for each decedent. Results are described in Table 4, with arguments being the most common precipitant. When they occurred, arguments were most likely to take place with a girlfriend or with either or

TABLE 4. *Precipitants to Suicide*

	%
Arguments	19
School problems	14
Disappointments	11
Police problems	10
Separation or threat of separation	8
Relationship breakup	5
Work problems	5

Note: $N = 229$.

Table 4. Precipitants to Suicide

both parents. Such arguments tended to occur within 12 hours of the suicide and concerned a variety of subjects; drug use, parenting issues, academic performance, and dating. School problems, disappointments, and problems with the police were common precipitants. Precipitants commonly occurred within the 24 hours preceding the suicide.

Generally, there were no sex differences in the types of precipitants to suicides. There were two precipitants that were unique to females: discovery of pregnancy ($\chi^2 = 4.87$; $df = -1$; $p<0.03$) and experience of recent assault ($\chi^2 = 8.44$; $df = 1$; $p<0.004$). Regarding arguments, female decedents were more likely to have argued with their mothers, while male decedents were more likely to have argued with their fathers ($\chi^2 = 24.83$; $df = 7$; $p<0.0008$). There were no differences, however, in the nature of the arguments that preceded the suicides.

The only precipitant that distinguished older from younger suicides was school problems ($\chi^2 = 5.49$; $df = 1$; $p<0.02$). A third of the younger suicides experienced this type of stressor before their death, which is twice the rate for older suicides. Younger children were much more likely to argue with their mother or father, while older children were equally likely to argue with a parent or with boy/girlfriend ($\chi^2 = 16.34$; $df = 7$; $p<0.02$).

More recent suicides were characterized by twice the rate of arguments prior to their suicides ($\chi^2 = 4.28$; $df = 1$; $p<0.04$) than earlier suicides. More of these arguments appeared to be with parents as opposed to a significant other, although this difference failed to reach statistical significance.

Psychosocial Characteristics

In terms of social adjustment, only 10% of the suicides were characterized as loners. Generally, suicide victims were seen as having friends and/or intimate relationships. Decedents were rated for personality characteristics as follows: 18% withdrawn; 10% lonely; 9% supersensitive; 7% angry; 5% impulsive; and 3% bizarre. Only 31% of the decedents were rated as being in good health. Chronic illnesses, physical disabilities, and a variety of illnesses and physical complaints were common. The majority of youthful suicides were described as poor students; additionally, in 76% of the cases, their academic performance had changed for the worse in the previous year.

Compared to males, females were more likely to be rated as having more friends and intimate relationships as well as being good students, although these differences did not attain statistical significance. In addition, no personality characteristic differentiated between male and female suicide completers.

Younger suicides were more likely to be described as impulsive ($\chi^2 = 12.12$; $df = 1$; $p<0.0005$) and tended to be described as angry. There

were no other psychosocial characteristics separating younger and older suicides. No cohort differences were found for personality characteristics, nature
of social relationships, or for change in academic performance. Such a difference was found for medical status (χ^2 = 15.23; df = 5; $p<0.009$); more
recent suicides were twice as likely to be described as being in good health,
but more likely to have had a physical disability.

DISCUSSION

The goal of the present study was to use information obtained from medical
examiners' records to characterize young people who had committed suicide
over a 10-year period. In addition, we were particularly interested in examining differences in suicide patterns based upon the characteristics of age and
gender of the decedent, as well as studying possible changes in suicide
over time.

Both Hawton (1986) and Shaffer and Fisher (1981) have argued that official
suicide statistics underestimate the true rate of suicide. In the present study,
that claim was substantiated; 15% of the deaths classified as suicides for this
study had not been so determined by the medical examiners' offices. There
was a tendency for older suicides to be judged more accurately. The difference
between the investigators and the medical examiners' judgment showed a cohort effect (χ^2 = 18.50; df = 1; $p<0.0000$). Fewer of the more recent suicides (5%) were misjudged relative to the earlier suicides (26%). This suggests
that current medical examiner practices, at least in metropolitan areas, have
become increasingly accurate in their determination of suicides.

Concerning demographic variables, the predominance of white, older adolescents among the suicide victims is similar to national epidemiological data
described by Shaffer and Fisher (1981) and by Poteet (1987). Shaffer (1974)
found no suicides before the age of 12. Suicides were extremely infrequent in
persons 14 and under, although three such deaths were noted in the current
study. Similarly, Thompson (1987) found only 16 suicides (7%) in persons
aged 14 and under. The rate among males of all ages was four times higher
than females; the male predominance tended to be most marked for middle
adolescents (4:1) and least among younger adolescents (2:1). The general population of adolescents in the two counties of the study is 89% white and 4%
black (Resnick et al., 1988); the rate of suicides among whites was somewhat
higher (94%) than would be predicted by population figures.

Firearms were the major method of death. This finding is in agreement with
the results of Garfinkel and Golombek (1983)—40%; Poteet (1987)—74% and
Thompson (1987)—56%. However, death from carbon monoxide poisoning
was twice the rate compared to the results of those studies, suggesting a pos-

sible regional or temporal idiosyncrasy. As in the studies by Garfinkel and Golombek (1983) and Thompson (1987), males were more likely to employ more violent methods (e.g., firearms). However, in Thompson's study and in a study by Holinger (1978), rates of overdoses were comparable for the genders. In the present study, more than four times the number of girls, relative to boys, were victims of self-poisoning. As in Shaffer's (1974) study of younger suicides, the youngest group in this study used hanging four times more frequently than the older group; CO poisoning was much more common for older suicides. That deaths from ingestions declined over time may suggest that this method allows greater opportunity for rescue or that emergency treatment is increasingly successful at preserving life. Given the high rate of depression among young suicides, the fact that antidepressant ingestion is becoming a significant cause of fatal self-poisoning (especially for male victims) indicates that great care must be employed in prescribing medication for depressed youths.

Circumstances of the suicides in this study correspond to findings of other researchers. As in Garfinkel and Golombek's (1983) study, most of the decedents committed suicide at home. Similarly, half of the suicides left a note; in Shaffer's (1974) study, 45% left notes, while in Poteet's (1987) and Thompson's (1987) reports, only 29% and 21%, respectively, did so. In studies of adult suicide, approximately one-third of the decedents left notes. Although Garfinkel and Golombek's (1983) study showed that only 5% of their sample had used intoxicants prior to their suicide, Poteet (1987) found that 45% of her subjects showed evidence of alcohol or drug use at the time of death; at least 45% of the suicides in the present study showed similar evidence. While Poteet (1987) found that one-third of her subjects showed signs of depression at the time of their deaths, nearly one-half of the subjects in this study were sad or despairing and another 20% were angry. Interestingly, younger suicides were much more likely to display anger before their suicide; Shaffer (1984) reported that 23% of his younger suicides left hostile suicide notes.

While Garfinkel and Golombek (1983) and Thompson (1987) reported an increase in youth suicide in the fall of the year, this study showed a consistent rate of death throughout the entire year. It was also striking that relatively few of the suicides in our study showed any evidence of preparation for their suicide; most suicides appeared to be a result of marked impulsivity. Similarly, Shaffer (in Holden, 1986) reported that in his most recent psychological autopsy study of adolescent suicides, there was no evidence of a lengthy "brooding" period before the suicides.

Garfinkel and Golombek (1983) identified significant psychiatric conditions in 25% of their sample (mostly depression), while Shaffer (1974) found that only 13% of his subjects did *not* show affective or antisocial symptoms. Poteet

(1987) indicated that 28% of the decedents in her study showed evidence of alcohol or substance abuse and 33% showed signs of depression or "mental problems." Shaffi et al. (1985) demonstrated high rates of several psychiatric disorders in his sample: 76% were depressed, 70% were alcohol or substance abusers, and another 70% had symptoms of antisocial behavior. Shaffer (in Holden, 1986) reported a preponderance of antisocial behavior and a limited occurrence of depression (20%) in his most recent study of adolescent suicides. Thompson (1987) found 33% had abused alcohol, while 17% were characterized by substance abuse. In the present study, half of the young suicides showed clear evidence of having a psychiatric disorder, mostly depressive disorders or alcohol or substance abuse. Most of these disorders appeared to be of a chronic nature, as opposed to more acute conditions. Affective disorders, in general, were more likely to characterize girls who committed suicide. Older adolescent suicides were also more likely to have affective disorders, while younger suicides were more likely to display antisocial behavior.

Additionally, a number of studies have demonstrated that neither parents (Leon et al., 1980; Weissman et al., 1980) nor teachers (Lefkowitz and Tesiny, 1980; Sacco and Graves, 1985) are generally accurate judges of depression in children or adolescents. Consequently, medical examiners' reports, which are based on parents, teachers, or employers as sources of information, are likely to underestimate the rate of affective disorders in younger persons. It is very likely that rates of affective as well as substance abuse disorders are underestimates of the true prevalence of these disorders among adolescent suicides. In the present study, the association between alcohol abuse and suicide seemed to increase, while the association between drug abuse and suicide decreased. This contrasts somewhat with the findings of Rich et al. (1986) that drug abuse diagnoses were strongly associated with suicides (70%) in persons under 30. The results of this and other studies of youth suicide indicate that younger suicides resemble older suicides concerning their degree and type of psychiatric disorder. In studies by Robins et al. (1959), Dorpat and Ripley (1960) and Barraclough et al. (1974) almost all adult suicides had experienced psychiatric episodes, predominantly affective disorders and alcohol abuse.

In the present study, evidence of previous suicide attempts were identified in less than 20% of the decedents. Thompson (1987) found evidence of previous attempts in 10% of his sample. These are somewhat lower figures than those found in other studies. Shaffer (1974) noted that 46% of his sample of younger suicides had previously discussed, threatened, or attempted suicide. Shaffi et al. (1985) reported that 40% of their sample had made a previous attempt, while 55% had made a suicide threat. Poteet (1987) found that 29% of her sample had displayed suicidal intent or made a suicide attempt. Generally, studies based upon medical examiners' records indicate lower rates of previous suicidal behavior, while those based upon more extensive "psychological autopsies" demonstrate higher rates. It is very likely that the present study underestimates rates of prior suicide attempts. In studies of older suicides, between 22% and 33% of the decedents were known to have made attempts (Robins et al., 1959; Dorpat and Ripley, 1960; Barraclough et al., 1974). The Thompson (1987) study and the present findings indicate females made twice the number of known prior attempts compared to males; while this may simply reflect the preponderance of females who attempt suicide, it might also suggest that males are more likely to commit suicide impulsively and without prior suicidal behavior. Pettifor et al. (1983) reported that suicidal ideation was the single variable that most discriminated between psychiatrically disturbed adolescents who did and did not eventually commit suicide.

Most of those studied in the present report were rated as having experienced a precipitant that appeared to be related to their suicide. Ninety percent of Shaffer's (1974) and 64% of Poteet's (1987) samples had experienced precipitants before their deaths. Most of the subjects in the present study had experienced arguments, problems with school, police, or work, or disappointing experiences such as relationship breakups or threats of separation. In Thompson's (1987) study, the rate for breakups was 26%, for family disputes 22%, and for legal problems 16%. Boys appeared much more likely to have experienced a discrete precipitant prior to their suicides, suggesting that girls may commit suicide more as a direct result of the course of their psychiatric disorders. Most girls were more likely to commit suicide after an assault, which agrees with Robbin's findings (in Holden, 1986) that being assaulted is strongly predictive of suicidal behavior.

These findings suggest a heterogeneity of personality characteristics that describe young persons who commit suicide. No single category defined more than 18% of the decedents. The most common descriptive categories were withdrawn, lonely, and super-sensitive. These results generally resemble those noted by Shaffer (1974) and Shaffi et al. (1985). In the former study, the two most common personality descriptors suggest a super-sensitive or withdrawn individual, while in the latter study, 70% of the youth were rated as having "inhibited personalities," defined by withdrawal and supersensitivity.

Because the source of the data base involved in this study is medical examiners' records, several methodological issues need to be considered. First, no control or comparisons groups are involved; thus, it is uncertain if the characteristics of the young suicide victims are uniquely related to suicide or are typical of any young person with a psychiatric disorder. More importantly, reliance on such records is likely to lead to an under-recognition of certain characteristics of young people who commit suicide. In particular, an archival study, like the present one, is likely to underestimate the frequency and type of psychiatric diagnoses (especially affective disorders, alcohol, and substance abuse), previous suicidal thoughts and attempts, and specific precipitants. Nonetheless, despite these potential methodological issues, the results of the present study are quite consistent with those of other studies of adolescent and young adult suicide. A number of conclusions appear to have a strong measure of support. In discussing these, it is important to emphasize that generalizations must be tempered with a sense that there is certainly heterogeneity in the characteristics of young suicides and that no single understanding of the nature of youthful suicide will suffice.

Suicide is primarily an act of white males and its frequency increases with age. As with adult suicide, psychiatric disorders appear to be the most significant precondition to youth suicide; most young persons who commit suicide are experiencing some episode of a psychiatric disorder. These disorders are generally of long duration or are chronic in nature. Conduct disorders appear to be strongly related to suicide in children and younger adolescents. More generally, affective disorders and alcohol and substance abuse demonstrate a particular relationship to suicide in the young as they do in older suicides. Moreover, the incidence of these types of disorders increases during the adolescent years. Each of these disorders is associated with a greater likelihood of suicidal ideation which in turn predisposes to suicide attempts. At the same time, most depressed or substance-abusing young people neither attempt nor complete suicide; even most attempters do not proceed to take their lives. Moreover, the incidence of depression is twice as great for females as for males, yet males predominate in completed suicide. Thus, it seems other characteristics must exist that differentiate those youth with psychiatric disorders who are at risk for suicide from those who are not. Shaffer (in Holden, 1986) has argued that boys may be at greater risk simply as a result of their comfort with, and their relative accessibility to, firearms. Males, as a group, may be more prone to impulsivity and emotional explosiveness. It is noteworthy that in this and in Shaffer's (1974) study, that the youngest suicides are more likely to be angry, aggressive, antisocial males.

The circumstances of young suicides also bear consideration. Precipitants appear to precede most suicides, yet these stressors generally appear to be the same type of life events that occur for most adolescents (Hoberman et al., 1986). Stressors, in and of themselves, do not likely pose a risk for the average adolescent. Instead, it appears to be their occurrence for particular individuals with pre-existing psychiatric conditions that creates a climate of risk. Some of the stressors may be a consequence of being depressed or abusing substances and may not be independently occurring traumatic events. Boys appear to be more affected by arguments in significant relationships and relationship break-ups. The greater degree of distress experienced by males after relationship breakups was demonstrated in a study of dating couples by Hill et al. (1976). Girls' suicides show an increasing association with assaults. Given the alarmingly high rate of sexual assaults experienced by adolescent females (e.g., Koss et al., 1987), this becomes an especially significant finding.

The seemingly impulsive, crisis nature of the actual suicides was impressive. Relatively few suicides showed evidence of advance planning or even precautions against being stopped or discovered at the time of the act. Additionally, the extent and degree of intoxication before death suggests a mental state of impaired judgment; it raises questions about the capacity for these young people to make rational judgments about their current life circumstances. It is also possible that intoxication may, in some cases, indicate an attempt at disinhibition in order to commit suicide.

Several studies have demonstrated that suicide prevention programs have not made a significant impact on the rate of suicides (Barraclough et al., 1978; Bridge et al., 1977; Miller et al., 1979). In recent years, a number of suicide prevention curricula have been developed specifically targeted at youth. Garfinkel (1986) has noted that many of these curricula focus to a great degree on the circumstances surrounding suicides and tend to deemphasize the relationship between psychopathology and suicide. It is apparent that a focus on precipitants, signs of premeditation, or planning is likely to be unproductive given the normative nature of the stresses experienced by young suicides and the apparently impulsive nature of the actual suicidal act. The likelihood of preventing particular suicides at the time of the act seems low. The emphasis in youth suicide prevention programs must be on the early identification and appropriate treatment of the episodes of psychopathology that underlie and precede most instances of suicide in young persons. Khuri and Akiskal (1983) have made a strong argument that energetic treatment and ongoing follow-up of patients with primary and secondary affective disorders will prove to be an effective method of preventing suicide. The authors believe this to be the approach most likely to slow or reduce suicide rates among youth. To contain the rising rates of adolescent suicide, programs are needed to train parents, teachers, and physicians to recognize depressive disorders and substance abuse in adolescents and make appropriate referrals. In the authors' experience, the most effective treatment for youth who are at elevated risk for suicide is a combination of multidimensional psychotherapy and appropriately administered medication. However, considerably more research is needed to better determine the most effective treatment for adolescents experiencing affective disorders or alcohol and substance abuse. Based upon the present findings, youth most at risk for completed suicide are males who have an affective disorder or alcohol or drug abuse and who have experienced an acute, proximal stressor that involves either a social loss or a blow to their self-esteem. Such information can begin to provide the foundation of realistic and effective strategies to reduce the rates of youth who tragically take their lives in an impulsive desire to manage the acute distress of their psychiatric disorders.

REFERENCES

Andreasen, N. C., Endicott, J., Spitzer, R. L. & Winokur, G. (1977), The family history method using diagnostic criteria. *Arch. Gen. Psychiatry,* 34:1229–1235.

Barraclough, B. M., Bunch, J., Nelson, B. & Sainsbury, P. (1974), A hundred cases of suicide. *Br J. Psychol.,* 125:355–373.

——, Jennings, C. & Moss, J. R. (1978), Suicide prevention by the Samaratian. *Lancet,* 2:868–870.

Berman, A. & Cohen-Sandler, R. (1982), Childhood and adolescent suicide research. *Crisis,* 3–5.

Bridge, T. P., Potkin, S. D., Sung, W. W. A. & Soldo, B. J. (1977), Suicide prevention centers. *J. Nerv. Ment. Dis.,* 164:18–24.

Center for Disease Control (November, 1986), Youth Suicide in the United States, 1970–1980 Department of Health and Human Services.

Dorpat, T. L. & Ripley, H. S. (1960), A study of suicide in the Seattle area. *Compr. Psychiatry,* 1:349–359.

Garfinkel, B. D. (1986). *School-based prevention programs.* Paper presented at the National Conference on Prevention and Interventions in Youth Suicide, Oakland, CA.

——, Golombek, H. (1983), Suicidal behavior in adolescents. In: *The Adolescent and Mood Disturbance,* ed. B. D. Garfinkel & H. Golombek. New York: International University Press, pp. 189–217.

Haim, A. (1974), *Adolescent Suicide.* New York: International University Press.

Hawton, K. (1986), Suicide in adolescents. In: *Suicide,* ed. A. Roy. Baltimore: Williams and Wilkins, pp. 135–150.

Hill, C., Rubin, Z. & Peplau, L. (1976), Breakups before marriage. *Journal of Social Issues,* 33:147–168.

Hoberman, H. M., Garfinkel, B. D., Parsons, J. H. & Walker, J. (1986, October), *Epidemiology of depression in a community sample of high school students.* Paper presented at the American Academy of Child Psychiatry, Los Angeles.

Holden, C. (1986), Youth suicide: new research focuses on a growing social problem. *Science,* 233:839–841.

Hollinger, P. C. (1978), Adolescent suicide: an epidemiological study of recent trends. *Am. J. Psychiatry,* 135:754–756.

Jan-Tausch, J. (1964), *Suicide in Children 1960–63.* Trenton, N.J.: New Jersey Public Schools, Department of Education.

Khuri, R. & Akiskal, H. S. (1983), Suicide prevention: the necessity of treating contributory psychiatric disorders. *Psychiatr. Clin. North Am.,* 6:193–207.

Koss, M. P., Gidycz, C. A. & Wisniewski, N. (1987), The scope of rape: incidence and prevalence of sexual aggression and victimization in a national sample of higher education students. *J. Consult. Clin. Psychol.,* 55:162–170.

Lefkowitz, M. M. & Tesiny, E. P. (1980), Assessment of childhood depression. *J. Consult. Clin. Psychol.,* 48:43–50.

Leon, G. R., Kendall, P. C. & Garber, J. (1980), Depression in children: parent, teacher, and child perspectives. *J. Abnorm. Child Psychol.,* 8:221–235.

Miller, H. L., Coombs, D. W., Mukherjee, D. & Barton, S. N. (1979), Suicide preventions services in America. *Ala. J. Med. Sci.,* 16:26–31.

Pettifor, J., Perry, D., Plowman, B. & Pitcher, S. (1983), Risk factors predicting childhood and adolescent suicides. *Journal of Child Care,* 1:17–49.

Petzel, S. V. & Cline, D. (1978), Adolescent suicide. *Adolesc. Psychiatry,* 6:239–266.

Poteet, D. J. (1987), Adolescent suicide: a review of 87 cases of completed suicide in Shelby County, Tennessee. *Am. J. Forensic Med. Pathol.,* 8:12–17.

Resnick, M. D., Blum, R. W., & Geer, L. (1988). *The Minnesota Adolescent Health Survey.* Adolescent Health Database Project, unpublished manuscript, University of Minnesota.

Rich, C. L., Young, D. & Fowler, R. C. (1986), San Diego suicide study I. Young vs. old subjects. *Arch. Gen. Psychiatry,* 43:577–582.

Robins, E., Murphy, G. E., Wilkinson, R. H., Gassner, S. Y. & Kayes, J. (1959), Some clinical considerations in the presentation of suicide based on a study of 134 successful suicides. *Am. J. Public Health,* 49:888–899.

Sacco, W. & Graves, D. (1985), Correspondence between teacher ratings of childhood depression and child self-ratings. *Journal of Clinical Child Psychology,* 4:353–355.

Shaffer, D. (1974), Suicide in childhood and early adolescence. *J. Child Psychol. Psychiatry,* 15:275–291.

—— (1985), *Completed suicide informant interview.* Unpublished manuscript, New York State Psychiatric Institute.

——, Fisher, P. (1981), The epidemiology of suicide in children and young adolescents. *J. Am. Acad. Child Adolesc. Psychiatry,* 20:545–565.

Shaffi, N., Carrigan, S., Whittinghill, J. R. & Derrick, A. (1985), Psychological autopsy of completed suicide in children and adolescents. *Am. J. Psychiatry,* 142:1061–1064.

Thompson, T. R. (1987), Childhood and adolescent suicide in Manitoba. *Can. J. Psychiatry,* 32:264–269.

Weissman, M., Orvaschel, H. & Padian, N. (1980). Children's symptoms and social functioning self-report scales. *J. Nerv. Ment. Dis.,* 168:736–740.

Part VII
OTHER CLINICAL ISSUES

Two papers in this section reflect the growing national concern with the impact of the AIDS epidemic. Although children and adolescents are being targeted for school-based AIDS education campaigns, and several states have already enacted statutes making AIDS education mandatory in public schools, many questions remain unanswered. The report by Brown and Fritz provides much needed baseline data concerning children's knowledge about and attitudes toward AIDS. They surveyed the entire seventh and tenth grade classes in two suburban school districts, who had not received any formal instruction in school about AIDS. A total of 908 students completed a 45-item questionnaire on knowledge, attitudes, and coping skills related to AIDS. Almost all adolescents, even 12-year-olds, know that AIDS is lethal, is transmitted sexually, is not transmitted by casual contact, and is found in "non-high-risk" groups. However, factual information regarding AIDS does not appear to influence attitudes and hypothetical behavior. Moreover, the least tolerant group of students demonstrated no clear distinguishing characteristics that would allow them to be readily identified and targeted for special education. The authors conclude that school-based programs that address AIDS-related knowledge and attitudes must be developed for all groups, but that further study is required to determine whether increased awareness and knowledge about the disease will also result in fear of intimacy, sexual anxieties, or, more desirably, avoidance of "risky" behaviors.

In their paper, "AIDS in Children and Adolescents," Belfer, Krener, and Miller predict that child psychiatry as a profession can expect an increased demand for services to AIDS patients. While work with AIDS patients will, of course, rest upon the broad-based experience and training of the child psychiatrist in the treatment of individuals and families and in consultation-liaison services, the unique characteristics of the epidemic pose special problems. The AIDS epidemic is having a broad impact upon the education of children, the psychological lives of both "at-risk" and "non-at-risk" children and youth, and on parent-child relationships. To assist practitioners as they cope with these new challenges, Belfer and his colleagues review the current state of knowledge with respect to the presentation of human immunodeficiency virus (HIV) infection in children and adolescents and consider the social and psychological issues involved in the development of appropriate clinical interventions.

The final paper in this section deals with a clinical issue of a very different sort: the pharamacological treatment of autism. The hypothesis that reduction of blood serotonin might be associated with clinical improvement in autism derives from the observation that blood serotonin is elevated in some 40% of autistic patients. The open treatment of 3 patients with fenfluramine, a diet drug known to lower blood serotonin, was sufficiently encouraging to lead to initiation of a multicenter study, under the auspices of the UCLA Neuropsychiatric Institute, to fully test the effects of fenfluramine on a large nationwide sample of autistic subjects. Although the results of the UCLA studies as well as other independent investigations have appeared in the professional literature, Verglas, Banks, and Guyer perform an important service in subjecting the various reports to critical review. The reviewed results indicate that fenfluramine has positive effects on the reduction of hyperactivity and stereotypic behaviors in 33% of subjects, the best responders being children with the highest baseline IQs. Cognitive performance did not show a similar improvement, and contrary to expectation, the best responders were seen among those children whose blood serotonin values were nearly normal. Mild negative side effects were observed in some children. The authors provide a thoughtful discussion of the implications of these research efforts, underscoring the need for future research to be conducted on sub-groupings of autistic children, defined both behaviorally and biochemically. Although fenfluramine does not offer a breakthrough in the treatment of autism, its usefulness as a pharmacologic probe in the study of neurotransmitter functions in autism may provide a basis for the development of distinct biochemical models for classification of the pervasive developmental disorders.

26

Children's Knowledge and Attitudes About AIDS

Larry K. Brown and Gregory K. Fritz

Rhode Island Hospital, Brown University Program in Medicine

Knowledge, attitudes, and coping skills were surveyed in 908 seventh and tenth grade students. The majority of students knew that AIDS was transmitted by sexual rather than casual contact. Correlations between knowledge and behavioral attitudes were minimal, so the impact of increasing knowledge about AIDS would seem unpredictable. A subgroup of least tolerant students (N = 57) could be distinguished from the other students only by differences in coping strategies.

AIDS has created a national health crisis, the control of which challenges every component of our society. Public concern about AIDS appears to be increasing rapidly, with the media reporting on this epidemic daily. Prevention has been advocated as the most realistic approach to controlling the illness (Institute of Medicine, 1986; U. S. DHHS, 1987). Children and adolescents are being targeted for school-based AIDS education campaigns, and several states already have statutes making AIDS education mandatory in public schools. The problem is urgent and the programs logical, but many questions central to the education effort are at present unanswered. The baseline levels of knowledge at different developmental stages are unknown. Does heightened AIDS awareness have side effects, such as increased prejudice or anxiety about sexuality and intimacy? Will risky behaviors be affected by increasing children's knowledge about AIDS?

An extensive literature search revealed only sparse data about AIDS-related knowledge and attitudes of children and adolescents. Three surveys of adoles-

Reprinted with permission from the *Journal of the American Academy of Child and Adolescent Psychiatry,* 1988, Vol. 27, No. 4, 504–508. Copyright 1988 by the American Academy of Child and Adolescent Psychiatry.

This work was funded in part by a grant from the American Foundation for AIDS Research.

cents done between 1984 and 1986 in Ohio, San Francisco, and Boston have been reported (DiClemente, et al., 1986; Price et al., 1985; Strunin and Hingson, 1987). Collectively, these studies suggest that adolescents are becoming increasingly knowledgeable. In 1985, only one-third surveyed knew that casual contact was not a route of AIDS transmission, compared with two-thirds of those surveyed in 1986. The number who knew that shaking hands was not a route of transmission rose from 75% in 1986 to 93% in 1987. In both of the most recent surveys, over 90% of teenagers knew that sexual intercourse was a route of transmission, with slightly less being sure about IV drug use as a route. Twenty-five percent of those surveyed in Boston in 1987 felt that children with AIDS should not be in school, despite "knowing" that casual contact would not lead to AIDS. The knowledge levels of elementary and middle school children are essentially unstudied.

The present study was undertaken to provide additional data concerning children's knowledge about AIDS. The authors were interested in exploring children's attitudes toward AIDS patients and homosexuals. By surveying the entire population of two different grades, it was hoped to examine any AIDS-related developmental differences and to use further statistical analysis to clarify the existing relationships between knowledge and attitudes. A specific evaluation of coping strategies seemed needed to properly understand children's response to this epidemic.

METHOD

The entire seventh and tenth grade classes in two suburban school districts in Rhode Island were surveyed. The students were 98% white and predominantly middle-class. Neither school district had given any formal instruction on AIDS, nor had any patients with AIDS been enrolled. In May 1987, 908 students (87% of total enrollment) completed a 45-item questionnaire on knowledge, attitudes, and coping skills related to AIDS. Confidential and anonymous, the questionnaire consisted of five demographic items, 12 knowledge questions, one item listing eight potential sources of AIDS information, 14 attitude statements, a 12-item coping scale, and an open-ended question soliciting emotional reactions to AIDS.

The attitude items were modeled in form after Harter's Self Perception Profile for Children (Harter, 1985). This form of assessment is understandable and provides a distribution of responses by asking students to first decide which of a pair of opposite statements best describes them and whether it is "really true for me" or "sort of true for me." Students could thus endorse a critical statement ("People with AIDS get what they deserve") or its opposite ("People with AIDS have gotten a bad deal'') and indicate the extent to which it applied to them.

The measure of coping skills used was the Kidcope, a preexisting scale with acceptable reliability and validity in other groups of children and adolescents (Spirito et al., 1987). In this measure students are given a hypothetical problem (''You learn that your friend has AIDS . . . '') and are then asked to rate ways they might cope with the problem. Possibilities range from denial and projection to problem-solving and intellectual mastery. The items of the scale are found in the Appendix.

RESULTS

The questionnaire was completed by 908 students (46% male), of which 434 were seventh graders and 474 were tenth graders.

Results of the 12 knowledge questions are presented in Table 1. The mean number of questions answered correctly was 9.01 (S.D. 1.32); 69% of stu-

Item	Correct Answer	% Correct $(N = 908)$[a]
AIDS is a disease caused by a bacteria.	F	42
All people with AIDS are gay.	F	96
AIDS is found only in men.	F	97
AIDS weakens the body's ability to fight infections.	T	95
There is no risk of getting AIDS giving blood.	T	34
One can get AIDS by touching or being near a person with AIDS.	F	91
AIDS is an inherited disorder.	F	73
You can get AIDS from sexual intercourse.	T	97
Somebody without symptoms could still be infected with the AIDS virus.	T	92
A positive blood test for AIDS means that the person will develop AIDS.	F	60
People with AIDS are likely to develop cancer.	T	29
At the present time, there is no known cure for AIDS.	T	97

[a] Mean no. correct, 9.01; S.D., 1.32.

Table 1. Seventh and Tenth Graders' Knowledge about AIDS

dents got 75% or more of the questions correct. Very highly known items (>95% correct) included: AIDS can be transmitted by sexual intercourse; it is not only found in men; not all people with AIDS are gay; and there is no cure for AIDS. Least known items (29 to 60% correct) included: AIDS patients are likely to develop cancer; donating blood is safe; and a positive HIV test does not mean that the person will get AIDS.

When rating sources of information about AIDS, 94% of students listed television as a source. Fifty-three percent rated television as the source that provided them with the most information, ranking it far ahead of other sources. Schools and family were listed as a source by half of the students. Health-care professionals were least likely to be acknowledged as a source (22%).

Attitudes related to AIDS are presented in Table 2. Avoiding any physical contact with AIDS patients was a concern of half of the students. A

Item	% "True for Me" (N = 813)
People related	
People with AIDS get what they deserve.	22
Students having the AIDS virus should be kept out of school.	38
It is best not to take a chance by touching someone with AIDS.	55
The AIDS problem is the fault of the homosexuals.	45
Behaviors	
They would have intercourse, even knowing about AIDS.	49
They would use IV drugs, even knowing about AIDS.	21
They would use condoms to avoid getting AIDS.	88
Reactions	
AIDS education in school is worthwhile.	90
Their parents know about AIDS and are more worried about teenage sex.	72
Descriptors	
They worry a lot about getting sick.	39
Their families talk about their problems.	68
There is a lot they can do to stay in good health.	91

Table 2. Attitudes Related to AIDS

substantial number of students attributed the cause of the AIDS epidemic to homosexuals. The percentages of students who would exercise caution in their sexual or drug-related behavior because of AIDS were substantial but lower than the percentages of students who knew the routes of AIDS transmission.

At least one-half of the students endorsed the following coping strategies in response to the hypothetical situation presented: cognitive restructuring ("try to see the good side"), problem solving, emotional expression, wishful thinking, and social support. Least likely to be highly rated (less than 20% endorsed) were blaming others and self-criticism.

Measures of students' fear of AIDS were included in several items. When asked to rank eight possible fears, AIDS was at the top of the list, as 75% of the students ranked it as one of their top three fears. Fifty-three percent of students said they would be "very" anxious, in response to the hypothetical question about a friend with AIDS; 72% indicated that their parents, knowing about AIDS, were now more worried about teenage sex.

Analysis by χ^2 revealed three significant differences between the sexes in expressed attitudes. Boys' attitudes were less tolerant of AIDS patients ($p<0.001$) and were more likely to attribute responsibility for AIDS to homosexuals ($p<0.0001$). Girls admitted to greater worry about general illness ($p<0.01$). There were no other significant differences between the sexes in other attitudes or in the total knowledge score.

These were some differences between the two grades. The total knowledge score of 10th graders (9.2) was significantly greater than the seventh graders (8.8), ($p<0.01$). Attitude differences between grades are in Table 3 analyzed by χ^2. Tenth graders indicated less tolerance than seventh graders as well as a greater likelihood to have intercourse and use condoms.

Attitude	7th Grade[a] % Agree	10th Grade[b] % Agree
AIDS patients "get what they deserve"	16	27**
Blame homosexuals for AIDS	40	50*
Would not touch AIDS patient	50	59*
Would have intercourse, despite knowing about AIDS	40	56***
Would use condoms	83	93***

[a] $N = 387$.
[b] $N = 426$.
* $p < 0.01$; ** $p < 0.001$; *** $p < 0.0001$.

Table 3. Age Differences in Attitudes

Two subsets of students were identified from their responses to the items tapping prejudicial attitudes. A "least tolerant" group (N = 57) agreed strongly (marking "really true for me") with the four "people-related" items that were critical of AIDS patients and homosexuals. Conversely, a "most tolerant" group (N = 71) agreed strongly with the opposite, noncritical statements. There were no differences between the two groups in knowledge about AIDS or in other expressed attitudes, with the exception that 97% of the most tolerant group said that AIDS education was worthwhile in school, as compared to 82% of the least tolerant group ($p<0.01$). Other attitudes (likelihood of having intercourse, using condoms, using IV drugs, worried about general illness, ability to influence one's own health, and families' tendency to discuss problems) were the same between groups. Analysis by χ^2 of the two groups' responses to the Kidcope revealed some statistically significant differences. Seventy-nine percent of least tolerant students were apt to rate the hypothetical situation (a friend with AIDS) as making them very anxious as compared with 32% of the most tolerant students ($p<0.001$). To deal with the hypothetical problem, the most tolerant students were much more likely than the least tolerant group to think of using cognitive restructuring or acceptance ($p<0.005$) and were far less likely to endorse blaming others ($p<0.001$).

Although computation of Pearson correlation coefficients between total knowledge score and attitudes did not result in any coefficient greater than 0.12, intolerant attitudes and anxiety were seen to relate to knowledge, to some degree. Table 4 indicates differences (by χ^2 analysis) between the most knowledgeable (total score >11), an average group (total score $=9$), and the least knowledgeable (total score <7). Students with more knowledge expressed less intolerance toward AIDS patients, worried less about general illness, and reported less anxiety to a friend's having AIDS. Other attitudes were the same between groups. Groups with more knowledge were also more likely to rate school as an important source of information about AIDS ($p<0.001$).

DISCUSSION

This study extends the findings of Strunin's (1987) telephone survey done in the Boston area with regard to student's baseline knowledge and reactions. Adolescents, even 12-year-olds, almost all know that AIDS is lethal, is transmitted sexually, is not transmitted by casual contact, and is found in "non-high-risk" groups. These are the facts most consistently seen in brief television reports on AIDS, and students in this study did rank television as their best source of information on AIDS. Students are far less likely to know other specifics of AIDS transmission or general medical facts about the illness. It is not surprising that students have nearly totally absorbed the basic mes-

	Low Know[a] % Agree	Average[b] % Agree	High Know[c] % Agree
Attitude			
Keep AIDS patients out of school	54	38	26**
Would not touch AIDS patient	66	51	48*
Worry a lot about illness	47	41	29*
Would get *very* anxious if friend had AIDS	67	50	49*
Source of most AIDS information			
Television	61	56	43*
School	5	11	23***

[a] $N = 96$.
[b] $N = 263$.
[c] $N = 102$.
* $p < 0.05$; ** $p < 0.01$; *** $p < 0.001$.

Table 4. Knowledge Differences: Attitudes and Sources

sages of the media. They report anxiety about AIDS for themselves and their parents, and 90% in this study favored AIDS education in schools. Difficult to quantify, but highly revealing, were the responses to the open-ended questions, "What upsets me the most about AIDS is. . . . " Students expressed great anxiety for themselves and their current or future relationships. As one 12-year-old girl poignantly wrote: "I've heard you can get AIDS from kissing, although I don't see how it could be true. This scares me because someday I'll be ready to be kissed." Another summarized her problem by writing, "You just don't know who to believe."

Although this exploration of attitudes with regard to AIDS is limited by the forced-choice nature and small numbers of attitude questions presented to the students, its findings suggest that a more extensive investigation of value judgments regarding AIDS is both warranted and necessary for appropriate education and intervention strategies.

Within this exploratory data, what kind of attitudes exist? Despite 91% of students knowing that you cannot get AIDS by touching someone, 55% indicated they would not "take a chance by touching someone with AIDS." About 4 of 10 students felt AIDS victims should not be in school and attributed responsibility to homosexuals for the AIDS problem. In the Strunin telephone survey (1987) a smaller number (25%) favored exclusion of AIDS victims from school. It is possible that adolescents felt inhibited about expressing intolerance on the phone survey but were more open using our anonymous questionnaire. It is likely that the personal contact of a phone interview is associated with greater pressure toward giving a socially desirable response (Lemon, 1973). The degree of intolerance suggested by this pilot study is of concern and indicates the need for further study of reactions to AIDS patients and homosexuals.

What coping strategies might students use to deal with AIDS? Perhaps indicative of the "newness" of AIDS and the fact that no one in our sample had had to deal with a friend getting AIDS is the finding that students rated highly a diverse group of coping strategies. Some highly ranked strategies, such as problem-solving or emotional support, would seem adaptive; while wishful thinking would seem less desirable. It may be that students responded with their generally preferred coping style, since they have had no direct experience with AIDS. Differences in coping strategies were the *only* variables that discriminated the "least tolerant" and the "most tolerant" students, pointing to the importance of including coping patterns in subsequent research and intervention programs.

If AIDS knowledge is correlated with attitudes, the relationship is neither clear nor strong. Pearson correlation coefficients did not show any meaningful correlation between the total knowledge score and any measured attitude in this study. Additionally, there were no differences in knowledge between the least tolerant and the most tolerant students. Tenth grade students were more knowledgeable than seventh graders, but this additional knowledge and their additional 3 years of maturity brought with it more, rather than less, intolerance. Although the two grades express the same degree of anxiety about AIDS, it may be that because issues of sexual intercourse and intimacy are increasingly relevant for older students, AIDS is of more concern to them. Thus, they may be more likely to scapegoat AIDS patients in an effort to cope with their uncertainties. There were not any age differences in the use of "blaming others" on the coping scale, however.

Will increasing knowledge lead to less intolerance and/or more responsible behavior? The present study cannot answer this important question, but it does provide for a more educated guess. Although no significant correlations between knowledge and attitudes were seen, the highly knowledgeable students did tend to be less intolerant, less anxious, and more in favor of AIDS education in school. It may be that this group was more "open" to a variety of experiences, thus likely to be tolerant of others' behaviors and also likely to have assimilated new information from the media. It might also be that these more knowledgeable students are also more intelligent or possess better reasoning skills with which to approach and cope with major social problems.

Other areas of health education have not found a large correlation between behavior, attitudes, and knowledge. In sex education, myths about sexuality have been seen to decrease with education (Kirby, 1980), but behavior is largely unrelated in knowledge (Chilman 1979; Pope et al., 1985). Students' attitudes toward the disabled can be modified, but correlations with knowledge about the disability are modest, at best (Karniski, 1978; Mabe et al., 1987).

To some, it may be surprising that these white, middle-class suburban adolescents knew as much as they did about AIDS and that they reacted to the disease so intensely. Further research, using a more extensive assessment of attitudes, is needed to corroborate these findings across socioeconomic groups and in other locales. How the attitudes of these students are related to those of their parents and teachers is unknown. As schools contemplate AIDS education at the elementary level, reports of knowledge and attitudes in even younger children become urgently needed.

Child psychiatrists can usefully aid schools that are attempting AIDS education. Adolescents are certainly ready to be taught. Even 12-year-olds already know something about AIDS and view the epidemic as relevant to their lives. Although the findings of this study suggest that factual information regarding AIDS does not influence attitudes and hypothetical behavior, the child psychiatrist's knowledge about expected age-appropriate anxieties (the seventh-grade girl who worries about kissing) and cognitive development (an adolescent's inability to think that something bad will happen to *him*) can help tailor curricula to be most effective and meaningful.

Existing prejudicial attitudes among adolescents make return of an AIDS patient to school difficult (Devine, 1986). The child psychiatrist can advocate for early, effective, and meaningful education and community involvement in these matters.

In this study, the least tolerant group of students demonstrated no clear distinguishing characteristics that would allow them to be readily identified and targeted for special education. Thus, programs that address AIDS-related knowledge and attitudes must be developed for all students rather than only a selected subgroup. It is hoped that this education will lead to a greater awareness of AIDS. Further study is needed to determine whether this increased awareness will also result in fear of intimacy, sexual anxieties, or avoidance of "risky" behaviors.

APPENDIX

1. I would think about something else, try to forget it, and/or go and do something like watch TV or play a game to get it off my mind.
2. I would stay away from people, keep my feelings to myself, and just handle the situation on my own.

3. I would try to see the good side of things and/or concentrate on something good that could come out of the situation.
4. I would realize that I brought the problem on myself and blame myself for causing it.
5. I would realize that someone else caused the problem and blame them for making me go through this.
6. I would think of ways to solve the problem, talk to others to get more facts and information about the problem, and/or try to actually solve the problem.
7. I would talk about how I was feeling; yell, scream, or hit something; try to calm myself by talking to myself, praying, taking a walk, or just trying to relax.
8. I would keep thinking and wishing this had never happened and/or that I could change what had happened.
9. I would turn to my family, friends, or other adults to help me feel better.
10. I would just accept the problem because I knew I couldn't do anything about it.

REFERENCES

Chilman, C. (1979), *Adolescent sexuality in a changing American society: social and psychological perspectives* (DHHS Publication No. NIH 79–1426). Washington, D.C.: U.S. Government Printing Office.

Devine, H. (1986), How and why we knowingly enrolled a student with AIDS. *The Executive Educator,* 8:20–21.

DiClemente, R., Zorn, J. & Temoshok, L. (1986), Adolescents and AIDS: a survey of knowledge, attitudes and beliefs about AIDS in San Francisco. *Am. J. Public Health,* 76:1443–1445.

Harter, S. (1982), The perceived competence scale for children. *Child Dev.,* 53:87–97.

Institute of Medicine, National Academy of Sciences, (1986), *Confronting AIDS: Directions for Public Health, Health Care, and Research.* Washington, D.C.: Author.

Karniski, M. (1978), The effect of increased knowledge of body systems and functions on attitudes toward the disabled. *Rehabilitation Counseling Bulletin,* 21:16–26.

Kirby, D. (1980), The effects of school sex education programs: a review of the literature. *J. Sch. Health,* 9:559–64.

Lemon, N. (1973), *Attitudes and Their Measurement.* New York: Wiley, pp. 57–60.

Mabe, P., Riley, W. & Treiber, F. (1987), Cancer knowledge and acceptance of children with cancer. *J. Sch. Health* 57:59–63.

Pope, A. J., Westerfield, C. & Walker, J. (1985), The effect of contraceptive knowledge source upon knowledge accuracy and contraceptive behavior. *Health Education,* 16:41–44.

Price, J., Desmond, S. & Kukolka, G. (1985), High school students' perceptions and misperceptions of AIDS. *J. Sch. Health,* 55:107–109.

Spirito, A., Stark, L. & Williams, C. (1987), *Coping in children and adolescents: development of a brief scale.* Manuscript submitted for publication.

Strunin, L. & Hingson, R. (1987), Acquired Immunodeficiency Syndrome and adolescents: knowledge, beliefs, attitudes and behaviors. *Pediatrics,* 79:825–828.

U. S. Department of Health and Human Services (1987), *Report of the Surgeon General's Workshop on Children with HIV infection and their families.* Washington, D.C.: U. S. Government Printing Office.

27

AIDS in Children and Adolescents

Myron L. Belfer
Harvard Medical School, Cambridge, Massachusetts
Penelope K. Krener
University of California Medical School, Davis
Frank Black Miller
Duke University Medical School, Durham, North Carolina

AIDS in children and adolescents is a significant medical illness with increasing impact on the psychological lives of infected and noninfected individuals. AIDS has impacted on the neuropsychological, psychological, and social functioning of children. The illness is imbedded in ongoing issues for the psychiatric care of children and adolescents. An understanding of the impact of AIDS for psychological development and the necessity of specialized support services for providers is discussed.

AIDS in children and adolescents is already known to be a medically devastating illness; however, its greatest potential influence is on the psychological development of youth. AIDS is currently a low-incidence, highly lethal disease found in certain specific, identifiable groups, but as a public health issue, the AIDS epidemic is having a broad impact upon the education of children, the psychological lives of "at risk" and non-"at risk" youth and upon parent-child relationships. The psychiatric impact of AIDS will be extensive and will outlast the search for a vaccine or cure; this provides a challenge to the clinician and researcher. This paper seeks to give a basic understanding of the presentation of human immunodeficiency virus (HIV) infection in children and adolescents, the magnitude of the problem in its several dimensions—social and psychological, and the issues in developing appropriate clinical intervention.

Reprinted with permission from the *Journal of the American Academy of Child and Adolescent Psychiatry,* 1988, Vol. 27, No. 2, 147–151. Copyright 1988 by the American Academy of Child and Adolescent Psychiatry.

As of November 30, 1987, 691 cases of AIDS in children younger than age 13 were diagnosed. In the age range 13 to 19, 195 cases were diagnosed. (Centers for Disease Control, 1987). More than 2,000 other children and adolescents had symptoms of AIDS but did not meet the CDC diagnostic criteria operative at that time (although they might meet newly broadened criteria). Particularly relevant to assessing the number of AIDS cases in children and adolescents is the limited knowledge of the full expression of the illness. Fifteen percent of cases are from transfusions. Two-thirds of cases are derived from mother-child transmission. Sixty-five percent of babies of infected mothers develop the disease.

When specifying patient status before the identification of the clinical syndromes of AIDS-related complex or AIDS, it is correct to refer to HIV infection, the etiologically significant infectious precursor. The full incubation period of AIDS is not known. The development of AIDS among those infected by HIV blood transfusions suggests a 15-year mean incubation and a high incidence of disease among carriers of the virus (Rees, 1987).

AIDS IN CHILDREN

A recent review of clinical, epidemiological, and public health aspects of AIDS in children generated a warning that a high level of suspicion by every provider is needed to ensure prompt diagnosis and reporting and to enable effective national monitoring (Rogers, 1985). The number of reported cases of AIDS is increasing because of better diagnosis and increased surveillance as well as greater occurrence. Numerous studies confirm that spread in pediatric populations occurs through known risk factors (Koenig et al., 1987).

The clinical presentation in children exhibits the full range of expression of the viral infection, manifesting both a lymphoablative pattern with encephalopathy and wasting, and a lymphoproliferative pattern with lymphoid interstitial pneumonia, cardiomyopathy, and recurrent infections (Oleske et al., 1983; Scott et al., 1984). Clinical patterns in pediatric patients have possibly different distributions, tumors being rarer and lymphoid interstitial pneunomitis more common. Morbidity is worse the younger the children are at the time the full infection establishes itself and is influenced by host factors such as nutrition and stress.

Neurological symptoms are as prominent in children as in adults (Epstein et al., 1987). Neurological findings in young children include developmental delay, loss of milestones, encephalopathy, seizures, microcephaly, and on CT scan, atrophy of the cortex (Snider et al., 1983). Myelopathy may be primary or secondary (Johnston and McArthur, 1987). Central nervous system complications include infections; tumors, both primary lymphomas and meningeal invasion by systemic lymphoma; vascular complications, deriving from bacterial thrombotic endocarditis or cerebral hemorrhage in a setting of thrombocytopenia; and nonspecific CNS problems evidenced as focal lesions of aseptic meningitis. The clinical picture, like that in adults, is one of eventual devastation of the nervous system by direct infection and opportunistic infections, preceded by moderate or severe subacute encephalitis with dementia or mild subacute encephalitis with no easily recognized neurological disorder (Jacobson and Seigelman, 1985; Shannon and Ammann, 1985).

Children infected with AIDS before or at birth are born to HIV-positive mothers. Many die within 2 to 4 years. Although more recently instituted aggressive therapies have extended the life span of these children, as a result of the illness and the treatments, they may survive in an institutionally dependent state. The lives of these children are frequently complicated by the death of one or more parents or the presence of such active parental illness that their parents are unable to care for them. In some instances, the same circumstances that have led the mother to become HIV-positive have undermined her child caregiving capacity. This further leaves the child "at risk" emotionally. The stigmatizing aspect of AIDS complicates the development of alternative care programs such as foster care or even institutional care. Recently, separate wards in hospitals have been opened to serve children unable to be served medically or socially in other surroundings.

AIDS IN ADOLESCENTS

The demographics of AIDS at this time suggest that adolescents most at risk for AIDS are probably not near the mean of the population curves of income, race, psychopathology, family stability, or drug use. It is known that AIDS is penetrating the heterosexual population first among low socioeconomic status groups, minorities, and persons in areas with anomie (lack of support of families) and disenfranchisement from educational and health care systems. Therefore, the adolescents more likely to be infected with HIV are those who are already handicapped by one or several other disadvantageous, physiological, psychological, or sociocultural conditions.

Consideration of the developmental aspects of the personality style of the adolescent and the tasks faced by the adolescent tends to highlight that this is the time when adolescents formalize behavioral decisions and practices with import for their adult lifestyles. This holds true for such normalizing life tasks as choice of occupation and the broad task of identity formation.

Subsumed under the task of identity formation may be included parameters with social and, therefore, moral dimensions such as sexual identity and orientation, choices about types and frequency of sexual activity, and use of recreational drugs. If the majority of adolescents, whether white or "minority," have been significantly sexually active by the time of high school graduation, the risk of AIDS, as the epidemic spreads within the general population, poses a task of enormous social importance for adolescents and those who care for them.

Known main routes of AIDS infection involve activities practiced by a high proportion of adolescents in certain groups. To develop psychological and educational strategies, child psychiatrists must understand the bases for the behaviors that add to an adolescent's being "at risk." Fifty percent of high school girls have had sexual intercourse, and 16% have had more than four partners. There are 1.2 million teen pregnancies in the United States annually, and one in seven teenagers has a sexually transmitted disease. In absolute numbers, the problem of adolescent pregnancy is greatest among disadvantaged black and Hispanic populations, but rates of teenage pregnancy are increasing fastest in white girls, aged 15 years or less.

There are not national statistics on IV drug abuse among adolescents distinct from the general population of drug users. Conservative estimates, however, suggest that more than 200,000 high school students have used heroin, and millions have used cocaine, stimulants, and other opiates—all of which can be used intravenously. Twenty-five percent of students drop out before graduating from high school, and these students likely have high rates of drug use (Quackenbush, 1987).

In a longitudinal study of drug abuse in a 15-year-old population of a cohort study, non-drug users and drug users were compared with reference to background data (Holmberg, 1985 a, b). Adolescents with chronic abuse differed most from the normal group. Prognostic factors for drug abuse were membership in a multi-problem family, child psychiatric care, contact with social welfare administration at an early age, truancy, placement in a special class, dropping out of school, and admitted high frequency drug use. Boys in this study had early contact with the juvenile justice system, and girls reported so-called nervous complaints. Over an 11-year follow-up, subjects who had more consumption of services for drug-related psychiatric and social care were more often on disability and assessed to be without income. As adults, more of the women had children before 20 years of age, and more of the men were exempted from military service.

Current statistics in the United States suggest that of individuals who have IV drug abuse with HIV/AIDS, 51% are female, 31% are sexual contacts of IV drug abusers, and 81% are black or Hispanic. Their mean age is 34 (range 15 to 39). Overall, 79% of IVDA are male, reflecting the drug-using population. Seventy-four percent reside in New York or New Jersey. Thirty percent of the IV drug abuse treatment center clients are women, who experience a 15%

fertility over an 18-month period (Rogers, 1985). Thus, the drug abusing and adolescent population overlap significantly, especially in poor, minority, inner-city populations.

CLINICAL INTERVENTIONS

Adolescent-focused

Given that IV drug abuse is one of the major transmission vectors of the HIV, and that the drug abuser is one of the most difficult to reach members of society, it would appear that child psychiatrists must make concerted and sustained efforts to reach such isolated populations. It is not enough simply to surrender to the now prevalent notion that once an individual becomes an IV drug abuser, she or he is unchangeable. The preventive approach mandates both more optimistic and useful consideration of such a problem. The logic is that one must find a point of purchase that permits access to this population and its problems.

The psychological impact of AIDS itself on the self-identity of being at risk cannot be underestimated in any subgroups (Forstein, 1984). Interventions must be adapted to specific subgroups. As suggested by Klein et al. (1987), programs designed to increase the sense of control over outcome might be most effective in more mature individuals, and appeals to peer group social norms may prove more successful in younger individuals. At-risk "antisocial youth" are notoriously resistant to didactic informational interventions, which although well-intended, still are perceived and experienced as condemnatory and judgmental. Many child psychiatrists are from racial and social backgrounds different from the poor inner city children at risk, differences which have been amplified by decades of education. Thus, without a reeducation into the at-risk culture, these psychiatrists may be unable to communicate effectively with the poor minority child. An alternative approach, which may produce quicker results, would be to supervise child psychiatrist extenders, i.e., peer counselors, more palatable to children already alienated from adults, particularly, authority figures such as health care professionals.

Therapists might serve as consultants to school systems or to health education programs, helping to educate peer counselors or "youth resource persons," who can present AIDS education in more accepted vehicles, such as youth-conducted rap or discussion groups. Once drug abusing adolescents have left school, they must be located and reached in novel ways, such as setting up similar education programs within runaway shelters, juvenile detention centers, and other likely places of contact.

Application of what child psychiatrists know about education of resistant students is necessary to equip vulnerable children and adolescents with needed information to protect themselves. A study of high school students' knowledge, beliefs, and sources of information, perceptions, and misperceptions concerning AIDS discovered that the students had very limited knowledge, although boys were more knowledgeable than girls. The majority were not personally worried about how little they knew or about contracting AIDS. The sources of students' information were TV, newspapers, magazines, and radio; schools were least often mentioned as a source of information (Price, 1986). When 1,326 San Francisco adolescents were surveyed to assess their knowledge, attitudes, and beliefs about AIDS, there was a marked variability in knowledge about informational items, particularly about the precautionary measures to be taken during sexual intercourse that may reduce the risk of infection (DiClemente et al., 1986). AIDS victims, even children, are described as modern pariahs (Scott, 1985), and it has been said that an educational blitz is needed to combat fear of this disease (Banning, 1985).

AIDS is stigmatizing, but it also has been identified as a special problem for adolescents for whom sexual identity is a present concern (Price et al., 1985). There are few studies of adolescent homosexuality beyond individual case reports of therapy. Remafedi (1987) anonymously interviewed 29 gay and bisexual male adolescents and learned that the majority had school problems related to sexuality, substance abuse, and/or emotional difficulties warranting mental health interventions. Half had had sexually transmitted diseases, had been runaways, or were in trouble with the law. A minority had been victims of sexual assaults or involved in prostitution. Those younger than age 18 had higher rates of psychiatric hospitalizations, substance abuse, high school dropout, and trouble with the law. In another review of medical problems of homosexual adolescents (Owen, 1985), health care providers were urged to take a complete and nonjudgmental medical history to explore the risk of four general groups of conditions in males: classical sexually transmitted disease, enterically transmitted diseases, trauma, and AIDS.

Knowledge about adolescent homosexuality is inadequate. In the age of AIDS, more than anecdotal or case knowledge about homosexual adolescents is needed. It is to be recognized that this is largely a secret population, in the process of developing a stigmatizing identity usually during early to middle adolescence. Even the size of this group in the nation's population is unknown at this point. Its response to the AIDS epidemic has not been adequately studied. Other than efforts based within various gay men's health projects, little energy is directed specifically to this population. Child psychiatric researchers need to focus survey efforts upon homosexual adolescents. Scientific and impartial study of this relatively unknown group of adolescents should further our understanding of how best to approach and help them in light of the on-coming AIDS epidemic.

Clinical observation of adolescents in psychiatric settings indicates that they are acutely aware of the danger of HIV infection and may fear it but that their anxiety is disorganizing, their defenses primitive, and their responses impul-sive (e.g., counterphobic sexual adventuring and magical hopes that a single negative antibody screening will ensure against future sexual transmission were observed in one frightened adolescent who had received many transfusions af-ter a gunshot wound). Another boy, exposed to risk through incestuous assault by a bisexual stepfather, fled from treatment after telling his therapist that he planned to have the antibody screening test. Generally, under stress of illness, adolescents will regress and become demanding, difficult, dependent, or de-pressed. Regression, cognitive backsliding, and acting out are characteristic of the age, and the evidence is that the threat of HIV infection propels the ado-lescent into a panic, which further excites these tendencies.

Health care providers, including child psychiatrists, might be able to assist in both alleviating patients' psychological distress and facilitating initial and continuing medical treatment of patients through psychological assessment and intervention. These interventions might affect positively the medical treatment of AIDS patients from a psychoneuroimmunological perspective (Coates, 1984).

In inpatient settings where such potentially disorganized and vulnerable ad-olescents will be found, child psychiatrists need to anticipate a likely future mandate of the Joint Commission on Accreditation of Hospitals to furnish sex and AIDS preventive education to each and every adolescent as is now re-quired for drug and alcohol abuse. Child psychiatrists can take the initiative to develop well-thought-out programs in order to help mobilize ego structures for every hospitalized adolescent and to advocate for such within their hospital practices. Issues such as informed consent of parents will be of no small im-port. Working through such issues within the controlled therapeutic milieu of family and inpatient work will provide sources of important experience for use in settings outside the hospital as our profession is called upon to move into responsible public health efforts.

Child-focused

AIDS in the young child population, whether present from birth or as the result of receiving contaminated blood products, presents many areas of concern to child psychiatrists. Among these are the following: clinical work with children with a chronic illness, intervention useful to sustain staff in clinical settings, development of psychologically appropriate strategies to educate children and adolescents, and support to ameliorate the impact of stigmatization.

With an increased medical armamentarium to deal with the biology of the illness, children are living longer in a debilitated, dependent state. The emotional stress, developmental distortions, losses, and grief yield a cumulative psychological burden requiring intervention. The role of the child psychiatrist, as a member of the team, is important in a number of ways.

Education about AIDS among children is controversial and requires knowledge about cognitive and psychological growth of children and adolescents. As it has become evident that infants may survive to school age, and that transfusion-related AIDS may emerge in later childhood, the problem of how to address AIDS education confronts the child psychiatrist. The American Academy of Pediatrics has developed a position on school attendance for children with AIDS syndrome (Rubenstein, 1986). Fear and prejudice obstruct equality of access to school services for the HIV-positive child. Child psychiatrists must assist schools in their communities to integrate these chronically ill and often stigmatized children into their classrooms both by school consultation to educators and by education of parents.

System-focused

What differentiates AIDS from other terminal illnesses is the diverse supportive needs of the family as well as the powerful social stigma that tragically depicts these victim families as pariahs. The degree to which a therapist is involved with AIDS families depends on the integrity of the family unit and availability of ancillary supports (Frierson, 1987). "The psychological stressors associated with AIDS are fear of contagion, revelation of lifestyle, notoriety, helplessness and grieving. Supportive therapy is essential for high risk persons who are concerned about AIDS" (Nichols, 1983). The disease tests a family's emotional stability by calling a host of feelings into play, from the guilt of giving AIDS to a child, to the shame of having the disease, to the anger of being a victim (Koocher and Berman, 1983).

Amchin and Polan (1986) pointed out that staff may feel unusually vulnerable to death and disease while both caring for these generally young, rapidly deteriorating patients and confronting their own anxieties and prejudices toward identified risk groups, particularly drug abusers and homosexuals. They further note that in the absence of scientific knowledge, more readily available now than at the outset of the epidemic, staff speculated about the dangers of treating such patients and were uncertain of treatment decisions. This resulted in a disruption of the therapeutic milieu. In response, a more medically-oriented model of treatment emerged and the AIDS patient was treated individually by his or her doctors. The shift to a medical model seemed to temporarily contain the overt expression of staff anxiety. With education and experience, there was a restitution of the therapeutic milieu model. The ability of patients to discuss AIDS openly paralleled the ability of staff to cope with their own fears about AIDS. A similar experience was noted in the care of an infant with AIDS in the hospital setting (Krener, 1987).

CONCLUSION

At the present time, AIDS is relatively restricted to child and adolescent populations that are not in the majority, such as homosexual youth, IV drug abusers, infants born to HIV-infected mothers, and hemophiliac youth who have been infected with the HIV through transfusions. However, the epidemic must be assumed to have the momentum to move outside of these groups through continued transmissions from infected youth via needle sharing and through sexual intercourse. Because the incubation period of the HIV is on the order of years, a significant portion of presently diagnosed adults were infected as adolescents. Therefore, it is imperative to realize that given time and continued operation of known risk-transmission vectors, AIDS will spread, especially among the adolescent population so prone to beginning now hazardous sexual activity at this developmental period.

Child psychiatry as a profession can expect to be asked to face the AIDS epidemic in its patient population in increasing numbers. The work with such patients and their families will draw upon the broad-based experience and training of the child psychiatrist practitioner who is accustomed to serving both the individual and family simultaneously. As medical practitioners, we are also experienced in work with the dying and will enlarge upon the tradition of consultation-liaison services in inpatient and outpatient services to these now terminally ill youth. Finally, our clinical services as consultants will be taxed to the utmost as we strive to meet the emotional needs of the clinical nursing staffs who will experience the drain of caring for ever increasing numbers of tragically and terminally ill children and adolescents.

Child psychiatrists will need to conceive of themselves as agents for promoting the public health as this epidemic marches through our populace, moving us from the setting of private, individual psychotherapy and from the confines and familiar protection of the hospital-based practice, out into the uncertain world of the competing and contradicting interests represented in our diverse population.

Our role must go beyond that of patient care. We must export our expertise derived from work with the developing ego of the child or adolescent. We must combat irrational use of the defenses we know through our clinical work, such as denial and projection, which impede the understanding of AIDS in children and adolescents. We must insist on rational knowledge and work to promote social awareness.

REFERENCES

Amchin, J. & Polan, J. H. (1986), A longitudinal account of staff adaption to AIDS patients on a psychiatric unit. *Hosp. Community Psychiatry,* 37:1235–1238.

Banning, J. (1985), Education blitz necessary to reduce fear of AIDS, *Canadian Nurse,* 81:10.

Centers for Disease Control (1987), Update: acquired immunodeficiency syndrome-United States. *Morbidity and Mortality Weekly Report.*

Coates T. J., Temoshok, L. & Mandel, J. (1984), Psychosocial research is essential to understanding and treating AIDS. *Am. Psychol.,* 38:1309–1314.

DiClemente, R. J., Zorn, J. & Temoshok, L. (1986), Adolescents and AIDS: a survey of knowledge, attitudes and beliefs about AIDS in San Francisco. *Am. J. Public Health,* 76:1443–1445.

Epstein, L. G., Goudsmit, L., Paul, D. A. et al. (1987), Expression of human immunodeficiency virus in cerebrospinal fluid of children with progressive encephalopathy. *Ann. Neurol.,* 21:397–401.

Forstein, M. (1984), The psychological impact of the acquired immunodeficiency syndrome. *Semin. Oncol.,* 11:77–82.

Frierson, R. L., Lippmann, S. B. & Johnson, J. (1987), AIDS: psychological stresses on the family. *Psychosomatics,* 28:65–68.

Holmberg, M. B. (1985a), Longitudinal studies of drug abuse in a fifteen year old population. 2. Antecedents and consequences. *Acta Psychiatr. Scand.,* 71:80–91.

—— (1985b), Longitudinal studies of drug abuse in a fifteen year old population. 5. prognostic factors. *Acta Psychiatr. Scand.,* 71:207–210.

Jacobson, H. G. & Seigelman, S. S. (1985), Intracranial lesions in the acquired immunodeficiency syndrome, *JAMA,* 253:393–396.

Johnston, R. T. & McArthur, J. C. (1987), Myelopathies and retroviral infections. *Ann. Neurol.,* 21:113–115.

Klein, D. E., Sullivan, G., Wolcott, D. L., Landsverk, J., Namir, S. & Fawzy, F. (1987), Changes in AIDS risk behaviors among homosexual male physicians and university students. *Am. J. Psychiatry,* 144:742–747.

Koenig, R. E., Pitlaluga, J., Bogart, M. et al. (1987), Prevalence of antibodies to the human immunodeficiency virus in Dominicans and Haitians in the Dominican Republic. *JAMA,* 257:631–634.

Koocher, G. P. & Berman, S. J. (1983), Life threatening and terminal illness in childhood. In: *Developmental Behavioral Pediatrics,* ed. M. D. Levine, W. B. Carey, A. C. Crocker & R. T. Gross. Philadelphia: W. B. Saunders, pp. 488–520.

Krener, P. G. (1987), Impact on the diagnosis of AIDS on hospital care on an infant. *Clin. Pediatr. (Phila.),* 26:30–34.

Nichols, S. E. (1983), Psychiatric aspects of AIDS. *Psychosomatics,* 24:1083–1089.

Oleske, J., Minnefor, A., Cooper, R., Jr., et al. (1983), Immune deficiency syndrome in children. *JAMA,* 249:2345–2355.

Owen, W. F., Jr. (1985), Medical problems of the homosexual adolescent. *J. Adolesc. Health Care,* 6:278–285.

Price, J. H. (1986), AIDS, the schools, and policy issues. *J. Sch. Health,* 56:137–140.
Price, J. H., Desmond, S. & Kukulka, G. (1985), High school students' perceptions and misperceptions of AIDS. *J. Sch. Health,* 55:107–109.
Quackenbush, M. (1987), *Educating youth about AIDS.* Focus, University of California San Francisco, AIDS Health Project, vol. 2, pp. 1–2.
Rees, M. (1987), The sombre view of AIDS. *Nature,* 326:343–345.
Remafedi, G. (1987), Adolescent homosexuality: psychosocial and medical implications. *Pediatrics,* 79:331–337.
Rogers, M. F. (1985), AIDS in children: a review of the clinical, epidemiological and public health aspects. *Pediatr. Infect. Dis.,* 4:3–11.
Rubenstein, A. (1986), Schooling for children with acquired immune deficiency syndrome. *J. Pediatr.* 109:301.
Scott, D. (1985), AIDS victims: modern pariah. *Postgrad. Med.,* 5:21–24.
Scott, G. B., Buck, B. E., Leterman, J. G., Bloom, F. L., & Parks, W. P. (1984), Acquired immunodeficiency syndrome in infants. *N. Engl. J. Med.,* 310:76–82.
Shannon, K. M. & Ammann, A. J. (1985), Acquired immune deficiency syndrome in children. *J. Pediatr.* 106:332–342.
Snider, W. D., Simpson, D. M., Nielsen, S., Gold, J. W. M., Metroka, C. E. & Posner, J. B. (1983), Neurological complications of acquired immune deficiency syndrome. Analysis of 50 patients. *Ann. Neurol.* 14:403–418.

28

Clinical Effects of Fenfluramine on Children with Autism: A Review of the Research

Gabrielle du Verglas
Autism Training Center, College of Education, Marshall University
Steven R. Banks
Special Education, College of Education, Marshall University
Kenneth E. Guyer
Biochemistry, School of Medicine, Marshall University

A review of research studies published to date on the effects of fenfluramine on children with autism is presented. The current status of the fenfluramine research on children with autism is assessed. The review analyzed the methodological aspects of the research, the toxicity of fenfluramine, and the relationship between fenfluramine, neurotransmitter activity, cognitive ability, and subsequent behavioral change. The review of published data indicated that fenfluramine had positive effects on the reduction of hyperactivity and stereotypic behaviors in 33% of the subjects. The best responders were children with the highest baseline IQs. The conclusions address the need for appropriate subgrouping of autistic syndromes, which may lead to identification of responders to pharmacological treatments. The need for further study of the possible long-term adverse side effects of fenfluramine is noted. Further experimental research on the effects of fenfluramine on children with autism is endorsed.

Reprinted with permission from the *Journal of Autism and Developmental Disorders*, 1988, Vol. 18, No. 2, 297–308. Copyright 1988 by the American Psychiatric Association.

INTRODUCTION

The syndrome of infantile autism is classified as a pervasive developmental disorder with the onset of symptoms prior to 30 months after birth (DSM–III; American Psychiatric Association, 1980). The diverse nature of autism has led researchers to examine a variety of genetic, perinatal, and biochemical causes for this disorder (Coleman & Gillberg, 1985).

One of the accepted biochemical findings has been the elevated blood serotonin levels in approximately 40% of autistic patients (Ritvo et al., 1984). Thus, the possibility that elevated serotonin levels may be associated with the symptomatology of autism was investigated. A number of researchers attempted various pharmaceutical treatments to reduce blood serotonin levels and the symptoms that were possibly associated with serotonin elevation. Recently, a multicenter study consisting of 24 separate research centers throughout North America has examined the effects of fenfluramine in reducing the blood serotonin levels in an effort to alleviate the symptoms of autism. Though individual centers published their results and Ritvo et al. (1986) summarized the results on 81 subjects, no comprehensive review of all the fenfluramine research has been published.

This review analyzes the results of the published fenfluramine studies and offers possible avenues for further study. We have examined the methodology of the studies, the toxicity of fenfluramine, and the effects of fenfluramine on biochemical, cognitive, and behavioral indices.

REVIEW OF THE RESEARCH

Fenfluramine is an anorexigenic amine which has been used to treat obesity in adult humans (Shoulson & Chase, 1975). Fenfluramine is similar in structure to the amphetamines, though its behavioral manifestations are much more variable (Campbell, Deutsch, Perry, Wolsky, & Palij, 1986). The Food and Drug Administration (FDA) has approved it only for the treatment of obesity in adults. Its initial use in the treatment of three autistic patients produced dramatic increases in IQ scores and a significant reduction in symptomatology (Geller, Ritvo, Freeman, & Yuwiler, 1982).

These initial positive results encouraged the UCLA Neuropsychiatric Institute investigators to propose a multicenter study to fully test the effects of fenfluramine on a large, nationwide sample of autistic subjects. The research design was either a double-blind placebo crossover procedure or a double-blind placebo controlled procedure. The subject selection criteria were uniform for all centers and involved both DSM–III diagnosis (confirmed by Ritvo from existing records) and a medication-free period of 2 months prior to participation in the study. Other standardized procedures included blood serotonin assays; parental daily log of the child's behavior; intelligence test scores at specified intervals; and adaptive behavior scales. The multicenter study consisted of 24 separate centers with data collected on 190 subjects. To date, results from 9 centers have been summarized by Ritvo et al. (1986). Of the 24 centers, 5 have separately published their results.

Table 1 presents the five separately published reports from the multicenter study of fenfluramine that was initiated by the UCLA Neuropsychiatric Institute.

Ritvo et al. (1986) summarized the initial results from nine centers. This report included data on 81 subjects and contained data reported previously by separate center publications. Among the major findings of the study was the relationship between fenfluramine and serotonin. Blood serotonin levels fell an average of 57% while the subjects were on fenfluramine. During a subsequent placebo phase, blood serotonin values rebounded to slightly above baseline levels. The principal investigators from the nine centers were asked to list subjects who showed strong clinical improvements, subjects who showed no improvements, and subjects who did not justify placement in either of the first two categories. On the basis of this ranking, the principal investigators classified 27 of the 81 subjects in the strong-responder category, 12 subjects in the no-improvement category, and 42 subjects in the no-classification category. The no-classification group was termed moderate responders by Ritvo et al. (1986).

In addition to these subjective ratings, the clinical observation rating scales indicated that there was a significant reduction in motor disturbances while the subjects were under the fenfluramine treatment. The other significant findings

	Ho (Vancouver)	Stubbs[a] (Portland)	Klykylo (Cincinnati)	August[a] (Galveston)	Ritvo (Los Angles)
Subjects	7	8	10	9.	14
Male	7	4	N/A	8	11
Female	0	4	N/A	1	3
Age range (years)	3–16	3–13	N/A	5–13	2.5–18
Baseline IQ	33–107	15–55	N/A	27–88	N/A
Tests used	Wechsler; Leiter; ITPA; PPVT	Cattell; Stanford-Binet; Ritvo-Freedman; Alpern-Boll	Stanford-Binet; Wechsler Merrill-Palmer; Alpern-Boll	Stanford-Binet; Wechsler; Conner's; Merrill-Palmer	Stanford-Binet; Wechsler; Merrill-Palmer; Ritvo-Freeman
Side effects	Weight loss	Irritability; mood swings; appetite loss	Lethargy; weight loss	Weight loss; lethargy	Irritability; lethargy
Results	High IQ subjects showed some improvement	Significant decreases in abnormal motor behavior were found. Some positive improvements were noted in other areas in high IQ subjects.	Significant behavior improvements in 2 subjects. No overall significant trends in the total sample.	Significant decreases were found in hyperactivity, distractibility, and in abnormal motor behavior.	Significant increases in IQ levels in 7 IQ subjects; Significant improvements in total sample in motor behavior and in social skills.

[a]Double-blind placebo control design.

Table 1. Fenfluramine Multicenter Studies

from the multicenter study were in the relationship between blood serotonin levels and IQ. There was a significant inverse correlation between baseline serotonin values and performance IQ. Baseline serotonin values also showed a significant inverse relationship with good clinical response.

Some of the reported adverse side effects were irritability, lethargy, and slight weight loss. All the side effects were reported as mild and nearly all side effects subsided after the first month of drug administration.

In summary, the results of the multicenter study indicated that some behavioral improvements did occur, especially in motor behavior and attention span. However, cognitive performance did not show a similar improvement. The initial pilot study results (Geller et al., 1982), indicating that fenfluramine produced dramatic increases in IQ, were not substantiated. Their original hypotheses, that the most dramatic improvements would occur in patients with the highest baseline levels of serotonin, was not confirmed. Overall, the best clinical responses were with those subjects who had the highest baseline IQs and the lowest baseline blood serotonin levels.

In addition to these multicenter studies, an independent study by Deutsch et al. (1984) reported significant improvements in their subjects' clinical ratings after treatment with fenfluramine. Campbell et al. (1986) also completed an independent study on the effects of fenfluramine on children with autism. Their study used 10 subjects with a mean average of 4.15 years. The protocols involved an initial baseline period followed by 8 weeks of treatment with fenfluramine. Using the Children's Psychiatric Rating Scale, this study found that 5 of the 14 items showed a significant reduction in symptoms under fenfluramine treatment. The items indicating significant reduction were fidgetiness; hyperactivity; withdrawal; negative, uncooperative behavior; and stereotypies. In contrast to other studies the most significant improvements were seen in children with low IQs. Another difference between this study and previous studies was in the flexible dosage levels employed by the researchers. Campbell et al. (1986) began fenfluramine administration at 10 mg/day with increases in dose levels occurring gradually at previously established intervals. Dosage was regulated individually with increments ceasing when positive effects were observed. Dosage was reduced when adverse side effects occurred. Optimum levels for the 10 subjects ranged from 1.1 mg/kg to 1.8 mg/kg.

Though nearly all studies of fenfluramine on children with autism indicated that some of the most notable effects were with hyperactivity and attention disorders, this result was not confirmed in a study of children who had only attention deficit disorders (Donnelly, Rapoport, & Ismond 1986). Ten male children participated in a 10-week double-blind placebo-controlled design study. The results did not indicate any significant improvement with the fenfluramine therapy. Therefore, the authors concluded that serotonergic activity was not mediating the activity of stimulant drugs in children with attention deficit disorders.

Piggott, Gdowski, Villaneuva, Fischoff, and Frohman (1986) reported on the side effects of eight subjects in their portion of the multicenter study. Four of eight autistic children developed side effects while receiving fenfluramine at a dosage of 1.5 mg/kg. The side effects included lethargy, decreased appetite, and irritability. Side effects were reversed in three subjects when the dosage was decreased. A fourth child severely regressed at a dosage of 1.5 mg/kg. He was dropped from the study and his adverse side effects ceased 4 to 5 days after cessation of medication. Development of a gastric ulcer in one child was noted, but Piggott et al. (1986) stated that it was questionable whether the ulcer was caused by fenfluramine.

Realmuto et al. (1986) also completed a multicenter report on the adverse side effects of fenfluramine of children with autism. This study examined 14 subjects in a double-blind placebo crossover design. Using a structured parental diary as their measurement method, Realmuto et al. found a number of significant side effects. Significant increases in food refusal, moodiness, listlessness, and agitation were found. Realmuto et al. also reported four case studies from other multicenter studies. These case studies indicated the need for careful monitoring of children with autism who are administered fenfluramine.

A number of questions have been raised concerning the neurotoxicity and efficacy of fenfluramine, especially long-term effects on serotonergic neurons (Gualtieri, 1986; Harvey & McMaster, 1975; Schuster, Lewis, & Seiden, 1986). Findings have indicated some possible toxicity in certain general regions of the brain (Clineschmidt, Zacchei, & Tataro, 1978) or specifically in the hippocampus (Schuster et al., 1986).

In the 1970s a series of articles reported that fenfluramine caused neurotoxicity in the midbrain of rats (Harvey & McMaster, 1975, 1977 Harvey, McMaster, & Fuller, 1977). These findings led the FDA to request that the Armed Forces Institute of Pathology (AFIP) review the data supplied by Harvey et al. and to analyze other relevant data on the neurotoxicity of fenfluramine. The findings by the AFIP indicated that there was a methodological error in Harvey's research that invalidated his interpretation of the data. The AFIP concluded that no neurotoxicity was apparent with the use of fenfluramine. These results were reported at the June 13, 1978 meeting of the Peripheral and Central Nervous System Drugs Advisory Committee. Subsequently, similar findings concerning Harvey's research were reported by Powers et al. (1979).

Previous reviews of the neurotoxicity of fenfluramine (Gualtieri, 1986; Schuster et al., 1986) did not indicate that the FDA had reviewed the neurotoxicity question and found no apparent neurotoxicity with proper administration of fenfluramine.

DISCUSSION

There are three major issues that need to be addressed in analyzing the present result of the fenfluramine research: (a) the question of methodological problems in the multicenter study. Such problems may compromise the validity of the multicenter study and may suggest different procedures in future research; (b) the question of possible adverse side effects in the fenfluramine therapy because of the relative toxicity of amphetamine derivatives; (c) the relationship between fenfluramine, neurotransmitter changes produced by fenfluramine, and subsequent positive behavioral outcomes.

Methodology

One of the methodological problems with the multicenter study is reflected in the loss of control over measurement and data collection procedures that were produced by a number of different research sites. Different IQ measures were used at the various centers and may have contributed to the wide variations seen in IQ performance among the different sites. The same problem also occurred with the different motor and behavior rating scales used at the research centers. With both the cognitive and behavioral measures the problem of equating different test values makes interpretation of the combined multicenter report difficult. The different means and standard deviations used with some of the measures required statistical transformations of the data that were not evident in the Ritvo et al. (1986) multicenter publication. A third difficulty with the study was the ranking system used by the principal investigators. The use of a subjective ranking by the principal investigators was not a part of the original research protocols. Besides this questionable practice of using a measure that was not in the protocols, the problems of subjectivity and possible experimenter bias may be indicated.

Another methodological problem with the multicenter study is in the relationship between intelligence and overall functioning in children with autism. Research studies examining the intellectual functioning of autistic children have demonstrated repeatedly the importance of IQ as a predictor in the child's general development and prognosis (Rutter & Schopler, 1978). Studies utilizing autistic subjects should select subjects matched on IQ in order to avoid the confounding effects of IQ with other variables (Rutter & Schopler,

1978). If the multicenter study had controlled for IQ, their final results might have been different.

In addition to these problems with the different measurements, variations in research designs pose additional problems. Of the multicenter studies that have been published, three of the five studies used the double-blind placebo cross-over design. August, Raz, and Baird (1985) and Stubbs, Budden, Jackson, Terdal, and Ritvo (1986) used a placebo controlled design. Campbell et al. (1986) also used a placebo controlled design. Since the two different designs were not equivalent, the results obtained from these designs may not be comparable. In addition to the differences in designs, the problems with the placebo control design include threats to the internal validity of the design in the areas of experimenter bias and order effect bias. However, it should be noted that in the separate multicenter publications the double-blind placebo control studies produced 5 strong responders from a sample 18 subjects (August et al., 1985; Stubbs et al., 1986). In the double-blind placebo crossover design studies there were 9 strong responders out of a total of 25 subjects (Ho, Lockkitch, Eaves, & Jacobson, 1986; Klyklo, Feldis, O'Grady, Ross, & Halloran, 1985; Ritvo et al., 1984). From these results it does not appear that design differences produced significant differences in the results.

Toxicity

The issue of adverse side effects with fenfluramine therapy remains to be fully examined. Though no actual toxicity has yet been associated with the appropriate administration of fenfluramine in human subjects, the absence of such findings does not rule out this possibility. In the multicenter study mild negative side effects were observed in some children. However, the claims made that fenfluramine produces permanent damage to serotonergic neurons has not been supported by currently available data. Subjects' serotonin levels were reported to rebound to above baseline levels after the cessation of the treatment phase. This type of rebound would be unlikely if extensive damage had occurred to serotonergic pathways.

The concern expressed by Gualtieri (1986) that fenfluramine research has produced unwarranted prescriptions by physicians is justified. Parents of children with autism must understand that the efficacy of fenfluramine has not yet been established. It has been approved by the FDA for the treatment of children with autism. Thus, it is advisable that fenfluramine research be continued only under carefully monitored experimental conditions. If such research is not continued, important questions with regard to the long term safety and effective use of fenfluramine will not be adequately addressed.

Biochemistry

Another important aspect of this review was to assess the relationship between fenfluramine, neurotransmitter activity, cognitive ability, and subsequent behavioral change. Even though it is generally acknowledged that autism is a cluster of different disorders with separate etiologies (Coleman & Gillberg, 1985), one subgroup appears to have had a positive response to fenfluramine. Future study of this subgroup will be facilitated through the development of a biochemical model analogous to the one used for the dopamine hypothesis used in the treatment of schizophrenia (Meltzer & Stahl, 1976).

In most studies presently published, the blood levels of serotonin have had a definitive response to fenfluramine. It also appears that fenfluramine had a positive effect on certain behavioral indices, particularly stereotyped movements and attention deficits. The improvements in the motor and attention areas appear to be the main reason why the principal investigators rated 33% of the subjects in the multicenter study as having improved.

One of the serendipitous findings in the multicenter study has been the paradoxical relationship between baseline blood serotonin levels and response to fenfluramine. With the exception of the Campbell et al. (1986) study the medication has had its most dramatic results with those subjects whose IQ scores have been the highest, but whose serotonin levels have been closest to normal values. Thus, in looking at the biochemical model of autism, the relationship between fenfluramine and serotonin appears somewhat equivocal. It appears that if high levels of serotonin are directly related to the behavioral deficits of autism, the effects of fenfluramine would be most dramatic in those subjects who had the highest initial blood levels of serotonin. However, these subjects, whose serotonin values were nearly normal and who had the highest IQs, showed the best response to fenfluramine.

There are a number of possible explanations for the equivocal relationship between fenfluramine, serotonin, and the behavioral changes associated with autism. One possibility is that blood serotonin levels are an inaccurate index of CNS levels of serotonin functioning. The relationship between the peripheral measures of serotonin and CNS indicator of serotonin are still being debated (Boullin, Coleman, & O'Brien, 1971; Cohen, Caparulo, Shaywitz, & Bowers, 1977; Hanley, Stahl, & Freedman, 1977). In a study with monkeys, Raleigh et al. (1986) reported a parallel effect on whole blood serotonin and cerebral spinal fluid 5–HIAA (a metabolite of serotonin) during treatment with fenfluramine as well as after cessation of treatment. Future studies of fenfluramine need to address the relationship between blood serotonin and CNS levels of serotonin or its metabolites.

If the blood serotonin levels are a relatively accurate measure of CNS functioning, a second possibility is that fenfluramine is having a pronounced effect on other neurotransmitters in addition to serotonin. Fenfluramine would then be having its major effect on other neurotransmitters, perhaps norepinephrine or dopamine, with a secondary or even spurious effect on serotonin. A similar viewpoint has been expressed by August et al. (1984). They noted that drugs such as the amphetamines, which have served as agonists for dopamine, tended to produce a negative impact on autistic subjects. In contrast, haloperidol, which serves as an antagonist for dopamine, has been shown to produce some symptomatic improvements in some autistic subjects.

A third possible explanation is that there is an interaction between the neurotransmitters or their metabolites when the subjects are receiving the fenfluramine medication. This type of interaction could occur in a variety of ways. It could be an interaction between the major transmitters, due to the possible effects of fenfluramine on different pathways. It is also possible that fenfluramine acts on the metabolites of dopamine or serotonin within these pathways in some yet unspecified way.

Future Research

Future biochemical models of autism need to address the possibility that one subgroup of children with autism has both abnormal serotonin levels and a deficit in the normal functioning of the dopaminergic system. This possibility has also been noted by Sandyk and Gillman (1986). Such an approach does offer some avenues for further research. Certainly, it points to the need in future fenfluramine research for biochemical assays of catecholamine levels in addition to accurate serotonin measures. A further examination of the total process of catecholamine synthesis and degradation in autistic subjects is also needed.

One problem with previous biochemical models of autism has been the global classification of the disorder. When the different studies of the biochemical aspects of autism are examined, there does appear to be a distinct need for separate diagnostic subclassifications. In the present area of fenfluramine research the most obvious differentiation is between the autistic syndrome with retardation and the autistic syndrome without retardation. In the multicenter study the differences between the high IQ autistic group and low IQ autistic appear to warrant treating these two groups as responding differently to the fenfluramine medication. In addition to IQ as a subgroup marker, there may be a need to classify subgroups on the basis of Fragile-X syndrome, familial incidence of autism, electroretinograms, and diagnosed neurological dysfunctions (Coleman & Gillberg, 1985).

Another possible consideration for future study is that the IQ levels are an approximate marker for the degree of neurologic insult sustained by the autistic individual. The greater the degree of insult, as indicated by a low IQ, the less the chance for any recovery. Therefore, the low IQ group may have too much overall impairment to show any significant signs of improvement.

Future research studies should focus on the relationship between dosage levels and positive behavioral outcomes. All the multicenter studies used a standard dosage of 1.5 mg/per body kg. However, the study by Campbell et al. (1986) varied the dosage levels of fenfluramine in order to enhance the response of each subject to the medication. They found wide individual differences in the optimal response to the medication. Thus, the relationship between optimal dosage levels, reduced serotonin levels, and positive behavioral outcomes needs further investigation. Extreme caution should be used in such a study as the parameters for safe and effective dosage levels have not yet been established.

Future studies should utilize only the double-blind placebo crossover design to avoid any possible threats to the validity of the study. Most important, future studies need to match or covary on the basis of IQ scores (Rutter & Schopler, 1978).

In summary the reviewed results indicate that fenfluramine administration appears to be most effective with the subgroup of autistic children who have the highest IQ levels, the lowest serotonin values, and who exhibit hyperactivity with motor stereotypies. Though fenfluramine does not offer a breakthrough in the treatment of autistic syndromes, it has produced a positive line of research. Subsequent research in this area should further confirm the initial indications of which subgroup of children with autism will be most responsive to fenfluramine. Additional research should also examine the questions of neurotransmitter change under fenfluramine administration and the dose-dependent parameters that would be most effective with the medication. Resolving such questions may enable future researchers to produce a specific biochemical model for certain syndromes of autism and eventually an appropriate treatment regimen for these syndromes.

REFERENCES

American Psychiatric Association. (1980) *Diagnostic and statistical manual of mental disorders* (3rd ed.). Washington DC: Author.

August, G. J., Raz, N., & Baird, T. D. (1985). Effects of fenfluramine on behavioral, cognitive, and affective disturbances in autistic children. *Journal of Autism and Developmental Disorders, 15*, 97–106.

August, G. J., Raz, N., Papanicolaou, A. C., Baird, T. D., Hirsh, S. L., & Hsu, L. L. (1984). Fenfluramine treatment in infantile autism. Neurochemical, electrophysiological, and behavioral effects. *Journal of Nervous and Mental Disease, 172,* 604–612.

Boullin, D. J., Coleman, M., O'Brien, R. A. (1971). Laboratory predictions of infantile autism based on 5–hydroxytryptamine efflux from blood platelets and their correlation with the Rimland E–2 score. *Journal of Autism and Childhood Schizophrenia, 1,* 63–71.

Campbell, M., Deutsch, S. I., Perry, R., Wolsky, B. B., & Palij, M. (1986). Short-term efficacy and safety of fenfluramine in hospitalized preschool-age autistic children: an open study. *Psychopharmacology Bulletin, 22,* 141–147.

Clineschmidt, B. V., Zacchei, A. G., Tataro, J. A. (1978). Fenfluramine and brain serotonin. *Annals of the New York Academy of Sciences, 305,* 222–241.

Cohen, D. J., Caparulo, B. K., Shaytwitz, B. A., & Bowers, M. B. (1977). Dopamine and serotonin metabolism in neuropsychiatrically disturbed children. *Archives of General Psychiatry, 34,* 545–550.

Coleman, M., & Gillberg, C. (1985). *The biology of the autistic syndromes.* New York: Prager Press.

Deutsch, S. I., Campbell, M., Green, W. H., Small, A. M., Perry, R., & Wolsky, B. B. (1984). Efficacy and safety of fenfluramine in hospital preschool-age autistic children: A pilot study. *Proceedings of American Academy of Child Psychiatry.*

Donnelly, M., Rapoport, J. L., & Ismond, D. R. (1986). Fenfluramine treatment of childhood attention deficit disorder with hyperactivity: A preliminary report. *Psychopharmacology Bulletin, 22,* 152–154.

Geller, E., Ritvo, E. R., Freeman, B. J., & Yuwiler, A. (1982). Preliminary observations on the effect of fenfluramine on blood serotonin and symptoms in three autistic boys. *New England Journal of Medicine, 307,* 165–169.

Gualtieri, C. T. (1986). Fenfluramine and autism: Careful reappraisal is in order. *Journal of Pediatrics, 108,* 417–419.

Hanley, H. G., Stahl, S. M., & Freedman, D. X. (1977). Hyperserotonemia and amine metabolites in autistic and retarded children. *Archives of General Psychiatry, 34,* 521–531.

Harvey, J. A., & McMaster, S. E. (1975). Fenfluramine: Evidence for a neurotoxic action on midbrain and a long-term depletion of serotonin. *Psychopharmacology Communications, 1,* 217–228.

Harvey, J. A., & McMaster, S. E. (1977). Fenfluramine: cumulative neurotoxicity after chronic treatment with low dosages in the rat. *Communications in Psychopharmacology, 1,* 3–17.

Harvey, J. A., McMaster, S. E., & Fuller, R. A. (1977). Comparison between the neurotoxic and serotonin-depleting effects of various halogenated derivatives of amphetamine in the rat. *Journal of Pharmacology and Experimental Therapeutics, 202,* 581–589.

Ho, H. H., Lockitch, G., Eaves, L., & Jacobson, B. (1986). Blood serotonin concentrations and fenfluramine therapy in autistic children. *Pediatric Pharmacology and Therapeutics, 108,* 465–469.

Klykylo, W. M., Feldis, D., O'Grady, D., Ross, D. L., & Halloran, C. (1985). Clinical effects of fenfluramine in ten autistic subjects. *Journal of Autism and Developmental Disorders, 15,* 417–423.

Meltzer, H. Y., & Stahl, S. M. (1976). The dopamine hypothesis of schizophrenia: A review. *Schizophrenia Bulletin, 2,* 19–76.

Piggott, L. R., Gdowski, C. L., Villanueva, D., Fischoff, J., & Frohman, C. F. (1986). Side effects of fenfluramine in autistic children. *Journal of the American Academy of Child Psychiatry, 25,* 287–289.

Powers, J. M., Mann, G. T., Jones, R., Ward, J. W., Elsea, J. R., & Smith, H. M. (1979). A reassessment of the significance of dark neurons in serotonergic cell groups. *Neuropharmacology, 18,* 383–389.

Raleigh, M. J., Brammer, G. L., Ritvo, E. R., Geller, E., McGuire, M. T., & Yuwiler, A. (1986). Effects of chronic fenfluramine on blood serotonin, cerebrospinal fluid metabolites, and behavior in monkeys. *Psychopharmacology, 90,* 503–508.

Realmuto, G. M., Jensen, J., Klykylo, W., Piggott, L., Stubbs, G., Yuwiler, A., Geller, E., Freeman, B. J., & Ritvo, E. (1986). Untoward effects of fenfluramine in autistic children. *Journal of Clinical Psychopharmacology, 6,* 350–355.

Ritvo, E. R., Freeman, B. J., Yuwiler, A., Geller, E., Yokata, A., Schroth, P., & Novak, P. (1984). Study of fenfluramine in outpatients with the syndrome of autism. *Journal of Pediatrics, 105,* 823–828.

Ritvo, E. R., Freeman, B. J., Yuwiler, A., Geller, E., Schroth, P., Yokota, A., Mason-Brothers, A., August, G. J., Klykylo, W., Leventhal, B., Lewis, K., Piggott, L., Realmuto, G., Stubbs, E. G., & Umansky, R. (1986). Fenfluramine treatment of autism: UCLA-collaborative study of 81 patients at nine medical centers. *Psychopharmacology Bulletin, 22,* 133–140.

Rutter, M., & Schopler, E. (1978). *Autism: A reappraisal of concepts and treatment.* New York: Plenum Press.

Sandyk, R., & Gillman, M. A. (1986). Infantile autism: A dysfunction of the opioids? *Medical Hypotheses, 19,* 41–45.

Shoulson, I., & Chase, T. N. (1975). Fenfluramine in man: Hypophagia associated with diminished serotonin turnover. *Clinical Pharmacology Therapy, 17,* 616.

Schuster, C. R., Lewis, M., & Seiden, S. S. (1986). Fenfluramine: neurotoxicity. *Psychopharmacology Bulletin, 22,* 148–151.

Stahl, S. M. (1977). The human platelet. *Archives of General Psychiatry, 34,* 509–516.

Stubbs, E., Budden, S., Jackson, R., Terdal, L., & Ritvo, E. (1986). Effects of fenfluramine on eight outpatients with the syndrome of autism. *Developmental Medicine and Child Neurology, 28,* 229–235.

Part VIII
ADOLESCENT ISSUES

Although the three papers in this section are reports of studies of adolescents, the relevance of the findings extends far beyond the teenage years. While the identification of conditions that place children and adolescents exposed to them at risk of maldevelopment has long been in the forefront of investigative efforts, the complementary study of protective factors has been much less systematically pursued. Beardslee and Podorefsky address this issue in their study, "Resilient Adolescents Whose Parents Have Serious Affective and Other Psychiatric Disorders." The investigation reports on a group of 18 young men and women between the ages of 13 and 19 years, whose parents had major affective disorders, often in combination with other psychiatric disorders, who were selected from a larger sample on the basis of their good behavioral functioning at the time of initial assessment. When re-examined two and a half years later, 15 of the 18 were still functioning well. Protective factors included considerable self-understanding, which included accurate cognitive appraisal of the stress to be dealt with and a realistic assessment of what might constitute effective action; a deep commitment to relationships; and the ability to think and act separately from their parents. Many had assumed considerable responsibility for the care of their ill parents. The findings are of importance in underscoring the fact that while exposure to "risk" factors increases the likelihood of maldevelopment, undesirable outcome is not inevitable. Furthermore, the findings suggest directions for the clinician working with the offspring of individuals with serious affective illnesses, by highlighting the importance of enhancing separateness from the parents' illness system, facilitating the development of strong intimate relationships and self-understanding.

The paper by Flament and her colleagues describes an epidemiological study of obsessive-compulsive disorder in adolescence. A county-wide population of high school students was studied using a two-stage procedure. In the first stage, a survey questionnaire that included the 20-item survey form of the Leyton Obsessional Inventory-Child Version, as well as measures of eating, depressions, and anxiety symptoms, was administered to students in each of eight high schools. In the second stage, clinicians conducted semistructured interviews of students selected on the basis of the survey responses. The minimum estimates obtained for the prevalence rates of OCD in the general adolescent population were 0.35% for current prevalence rate and 0.40% for lifetime prevalence. The minimum prevalence rate for compulsive personality disorder was about 0.3%. An additional 0.27% of the population surveyed in stage 1 were found to have what the authors characterized as sub-clinical OCD. Although the relationship between ''sub-clinical OCD'' and ''true OCD'' is unclear at the present time, and awaits follow-up study for clarification, the estimates of OCD among adolescents was considerably higher than anticipated. The pattern of obsessions and compulsions in these epidemiologically derived OCD cases, of whom only 20% had ever received treatment, was similar to that seen in a clinical series of obsessive compulsive patients. Cleaning rituals were most frequently found, with checking and straightening compulsions also common. The most frequent obsessions were fear of dirt or contamination and thoughts of harm coming to self and/or family members. Clinically referred cases tended not to be more severe, but rather to have somewhat more observant caretakers than those who were uncovered in the course of this epidemiologic survey. Among those survey cases who had consulted psychiatrists, help was most often sought for anxiety or depression, and obsessive-compulsive symptomology was rarely disclosed. Clinicians need to be aware of the secrecy that many obsessive-compulsive patients have about their conditions, if the recently recognized effective treatments are to be made available to individuals with this chronic and frequently disabling disorder.

The Supreme Court is currently considering the constitutionality of the death penalty for juveniles. Thus, Dorothy Lewis et al.'s review of ''Neuropsychiatric, Psychoeducational, and Family Characteristics of 14 Juveniles Condemned to Death in the United States'' is both timely and persuasive. Following methods developed in the course of many years of work with violent juvenile offenders, Lewis and her colleagues evaluated approximately 40% of the juvenile death row population. Juveniles condemned to death in the United States are multiply handicapped, tending to have sustained injuries to the CNS and to have suffered since early childhood from a multiplicity of psychotic symptoms and cognitive impairments. In addition, histories of physical and sexual abuse were common. A thoughtful and incisive discussion makes an important contribution to forensic psychiatry, as Lewis explores the reasons why these vulnerabilities routinely fail to be uncovered before sentencing, when they might be considered as factors mitigating against the imposition of the death penalty.

PART VIII: ADOLESCENT ISSUES

29

Resilient Adolescents Whose Parents Have Serious Affective and Other Psychiatric Disorders: Importance of Self-Understanding and Relationships

William R. Beardslee and Donna Podorefsky
The Children's Hospital, Boston, Massachusetts

Eighteen young men and women whose parents had major affective disorders, often in combination with other serious psychiatric disorders, were selected from a larger sample on the basis of their good behavioral functioning as adolescents at initial assessment. When they were reassessed an average of 2½ years later, 15 of the 18 were still functioning well. Considerable self-understanding, a deep commitment to relationships, and the ability to think and act separately from their parents characterized these young people. Many of them were taking care of their ill parents. The implications of these findings for preventive and clinical intervention are discussed.

Although extensive empirical research has documented serious psychopathology in the children of parents with affective illness,[1-6] no studies have

Reprinted with permission from the *American Journal of Psychiatry,* 1988, Vol. 145, No. 1, 63–69. Copyright 1988 by the *American Psychiatric Association.*

Supported by the William T. Grant Foundation, NIMH grant MH-34780 in conjunction with the Boston center of the National Institute of Mental Health-Clinical Research Branch Collaborative Study on the Psychobiology of Depression (grant MH-25475), the Harris Trust through Harvard University, the Overseas Shipholding Group, the George P. Harrington Trust, and a Faculty Scholar Award of the William T. Grant Foundation to Dr. Beardslee.

The authors thank Robert Selman, Leon Eisenberg, and Chester Pierce for comments on drafts of the manuscript.

appeared on youngsters in this risk group who are adapting well. Such study forms a necessary complement to the description of psychopathology.[7] The best predictors of later functioning are often indices of adaptation rather than psychopathology.[8,9] Moreover, knowledge about what is protective—what characterizes young people at risk who are functioning well—should provide a basis for the development of both clinical intervention and prevention programs for youngsters whose parents have affective disorders.

There has been considerable interest in studying the adaptation of children and adolescents in various other high-risk situations, resulting in longitudinal studies of youngsters at risk because of diminished economic resources, minority status, or other factors,[8,10,11] epidemiological studies,[11] studies of response to particular stressful circumstances such as medical illness,[12] and studies of the children of schizophrenic parents,[13] including some studies of successful adaptation.[14] Several findings from these studies guided the design of our investigation. Researchers have agreed that the description of the subjects' current behavioral functioning is the essential first step in describing adaptation and resiliency.[7] This approach has the advantage of being reliable and objective, since ratings are made on actual behavior or reported behavior rather than inferred processes. Second, relationships have been found to be protective in a wide variety of risk situations.[10,15–17] Because parental affective illness seriously impairs relationships within the family,[18–20] the possible protective effects of relationships are relevant to the study of resilient offspring of parents with affective disorders. Finally, investigators have recognized the importance of other protective factors in resilient youngsters. These include constitutional factors, for example, certain temperamental characteristics.[21] Also important are ways of responding, thinking, and acting, for example, certain coping styles,[12,22] positive self-esteem, and a sense of being in control.[23]

Within this broad domain, previous work of the first author[24–26] demonstrated that self-understanding was an essential component of resilient individuals who dealt successfully with various stressful situations; thus, it was a focus of the current study. Self-understanding is of interest because it is potentially amenable to intervention. The reflections of young people who have seriously affectively ill parents give a clear sense of exactly what experiences are troublesome and difficult for them. Also, given the lack of standardized and validated measures of resiliency, investigation of a subject's own perceptions of what enabled him or her to function effectively provides important information for understanding the psychological processes involved in such adaptive behavior.

METHOD

A group of resilient adolescents was selected by objective criteria from a larger sample of child and adolescent subjects who had been part of a previous study of the impact of parental affective illness. This small group was reinterviewed 1½–3 years after the initial interview to assess the stability of their adaptive functioning, to characterize their adaptive behavior, and to allow them to describe their experiences with ill parents and their understanding of themselves. It was hypothesized that young people who were adapting well to parental affective illness had developed and would manifest considerable self-understanding.

Sample Selection in the Larger Study

Inclusion in the larger study required that the families be Caucasian and English speaking, that they have children 6–19 years old who lived with their mothers, and that there be data available on both biological parents.

Subjects were drawn from three main sampling groups: parent subjects recruited from a large study of the course and outcome of serious affective illness,[27] subjects recruited through a door-to-door survey of neighborhoods in which families with clinically identified affective illness lived, and a random sample of subjects from a prepaid health plan. We used this sampling design in order to assess whether the impact of affective illness identified by community survey or random sampling was similar to that for parent subjects being treated in clinical centers. This proved to be the case. Previous analyses[6] had shown that combining these sampling groups into a single pool of subjects was in general a reasonable approach.

Initial Interview Assessments

A standard structured research interview, the Schedule of Affective Disorders and Schizophrenia (SADS),[28] scored according to the Research Diagnostic Criteria (RDC),[29] was used to characterize parental lifetime psychopathology.[1,6] Lifetime psychopathology in the children was assessed according to *DSM-III* criteria by a consensus rating on standardized interviews with the youngsters (Diagnostic Interview for Children and Adolescents)[30,31] and with the mothers about their youngsters on the parent version of the same diagnostic interview. The adaptive functioning of the youngsters was assessed by means of the Garmezy Child Interview[32] and, from the mother's perspective about the child, by means of the Rochester Adaptive Behavior Inventory.[33,34]

Parents were interviewed separately from their offspring by an interviewer blind to any knowledge of the findings on the children. Only biological parents were assessed because the overall study design called for the exploration of family patterns of inheritance. All mothers were interviewed; both biological parents were interviewed whenever possible, and when this was not possible, information on the fathers was obtained from the mothers. This occurred in the majority of the cases.

Each subject was assigned an overall rating of adaptive functioning (6 and summary scale for the Rochester Adaptive Behavior Inventory [L. Wynne, personal communication]) for the 3 months before interview on the basis of all information collected from the child and from the parent about the child. Ratings were made on a 9-point scale (1 = above-average functioning, 9 = seriously disturbed). The overall rating of adaptive functioning was based primarily on specific ratings of discrete areas of behavioral functioning, i.e., school performance, work performance, involvement in other activities, and relationships with mother, father, siblings, and friends. In meetings between the interviewers and a senior psychiatrist, consensus ratings for diagnoses and adaptive functioning were made from the reports of the parents and children according to specified criteria for resolving discrepancies between the accounts.

The main findings of the larger study—much higher rates of general psychopathology and of major depression as well as lower overall adaptive functioning in the youngsters at risk than in those not at risk—have been previously described,[1,2] as has the relative weight of various parental risk factors in relation to youngsters' outcomes.[6]

Selection of Sample of Resilient Young People

Subjects with good overall ratings of behavioral functioning (adaptive function scores of 1–3) at initial assessment and without major current psychiatric disorder were considered for the follow-up study if they met the following inclusion criteria: 1) they were at least 12 years old at the time of initial assessment, 2) they were at least 6 years of age at the time of some parental affective illness, 3) they were living with the ill parent at the time of parental illness, and 4) there was a history of serious parental affective illness. These criteria were used to ensure that the subjects had experienced the parental affective illness when they were old enough to remember it and that they themselves were old enough to reflect about their experiences. Clinical review of the cases was also conducted to ensure that the youngsters had been exposed to serious disorder and had been functioning well at initial assessment. From a large number of families with serious affective disorders who had children over age 12, 19 families providing 23 subjects met all the requirements. Three potential subjects were excluded from the follow-up study because they would have been markedly older than the rest of the sample at follow-up. All the remaining subjects were recontacted at 18 (90%) from 14 families agreed to be reexamined. Informed consent was obtained from all subjects in the study.

Subsequent Interview

Two separate domains, behavioral functioning and self-understanding, were examined at reinterview. The major areas of previously studied behavioral adaptive functioning during the 3 months before interview were systematically reassessed by a shortened version of the initial research interview with the youngsters themselves. The major important diagnoses identified in the adolescents in the previous study—affective disorder, substance abuse, and conduct disorder—were reassessed with a shortened version of the Diagnostic Interview for Children and Adolescents[30,31] for the interval since first assessment.

On the basis of previous work,[24-26] we developed an interview that addressed systematic questions to the subjects about their awareness, experience, and understanding of their parents' illness. They were directly asked what they believed had enabled them to deal with the illness, what aspects were most difficult for them, and what advice they would give to others. Most of the subjects were seen in their own homes for several hours, and in all cases they were interviewed by the same research associate (D.P.) who had interviewed them initially.

The interviews were summarized by the interviewer, and these summaries were reviewed separately by the interviewer and by the senior researcher (W.R.B.) to determine the main content areas. Behavioral functioning was summarized for each individual by using the scales developed in the initial study (overall adaptive functioning and specific 5-point scales, ranging from 1 = outstanding to 5 = poor, that measured relationships with peers, friends, mother, and father and functioning in school, at work, and in other activities). Three components of self-understanding were identified and examined in the 18 summaries: awareness of the parent's illness, specific response to parental illness, and capacity to observe and reflect on the experience of parental illness and other matters.

FINDINGS

The mean age of the parents at initial assessment was 43 years (range = 34–53 years). The most common lifetime RDC diagnosis was major depressive disorder (12 cases), followed by alcoholism (10 cases) and intermittent depression (eight cases). Seventeen of the 28 parents had experienced affective illness, sometimes in combination with nonaffective disorder; four had never been ill; and seven had experienced nonaffective illness only. The presence of only nonaffective diagnoses for some parents is explained by the fact that some individuals with affective illness had spouses with a nonaffective illness. Most of the illnesses were chronic; for example, the mean duration of a child's lifetime exposure to parental affective disorder was 4.5 years (range = 8 weeks to 15 years, median exposure = 4.4 years). In 10 of the 14 families, both parents were ill. The rate of divorce or separation was 64% (nine of 14 families).

The young men and women ranged in age from 13 years to 19 years and 10 months at the time of the first assessment. They were reassessed an average of 30 months after the first assessment, when they ranged in age from 14 years and 6 months to 22 years and 8 months; the mean age was 19. There were eight young men and 10 young women.

No history of serious medical problems in this group was elicited at either assessment. The overall IQ of the subjects was well above average; the lowest full-scale IQ was 92 and the highest was 137, with a mean of 113.5. There were no instances of diagnosable learning disorders in this group. At initial assessment, four youngsters had met criteria for a *DSM–III* disorder at some time during their lives.

Quantitative Findings: Follow-up Assessment

Fifteen of the 18 individuals had overall adaptive functioning scores that represented good functioning (between 1 and 3 on the 9-point scale) at both assessments, whereas three individuals had scores above 3 at the time of the second assessment. Examination of the component ratings that contributed to the overall score showed consistently high scores for the 15 with good ratings.

In terms of *DSM–III* diagnoses in the interval between the first and second assessments, no subjects had developed conduct or substance abuse disorders, but three subjects had had depressive disorders; two of them were episodes of major depression and one was a dysthymic disorder. One of these occurred in a young woman who had had a previous episode of depression.

Of the 18 young men and women, 16 described themselves as valuing close, confiding relationships and emphasized that these relationships were a central part of their lives. These relationships were with a wide variety of individuals (11 subjects were extremely close to their mothers, four to their fathers, 11 to siblings, and 13 to friends).

Thirteen subjects were attending school. Most of these were extensively and deeply involved in their academic pursuits, and several were attending or planned to attend prestigious colleges. In addition to academic work, they reported deep involvement in and commitment to their jobs. Of the seven in college, all had part-time and summer jobs, and of the six in high school, three had part-time jobs. Of the remaining five, four had at least one full-time job and three held two jobs. They manifested the ability to persist in their work; all but one had good work and academic histories. The one young person with a poor school and work history had such a history only for the recent past.

Furthermore, all but two of the 18 subjects reported having intensive and varied activities outside of work and school and took pleasure in these outside activities. Several were deeply involved in athletics, particularly those who were still in school.

Description of the Experience of Parental Affective Illness

All of the young men and women were deeply aware of their parents' illness. They described their experience of parental illness in terms of changes in parental behavior or outlook. Observable changes in parents included irritability, sadness, lack of energy, and for some, excessive drinking. Many of the respondents reported the loneliness and isolation of their parents' lives. Several commented that their parents tried not to show their distress and attempted to keep their depression to themselves.

The young people's accounts focused on the disruption of their own lives that was associated with or was a consequence of parental illness, rather than on the identification of the parents' behavior as the sequelae of depression. This disruption included economic hardship and change of house or apartment, as well as lack of parental awareness and involvement.

The young people described in detail major life events associated with their parents' illness and often related the parental illness to the presence of painful life events. Especially important were parental divorce, deaths in the family, and for a few, serious medical illnesses of the parents.

The young people described their experiences as full of disillusionment, confusion, and feelings of helplessness. Many described the loss of a role model or an idealized loved one. An important theme in their accounts was the sick parent's unavailability to perform usual tasks, as well as their own considerable initial anger and frustration about not knowing what was going on. Nine individuals specifically mentioned turning to an identified other person during episodes of severe parental illness in order to make sense of the experience or to derive comfort.

More generally, relationships were crucial for many of these young people in allowing them to separate from their parents, whether this was during an acute illness episode of the parent or not. Two subjects reported turning to an adult outside the family in this process, and two turned to a sibling perceived as a best friend. Four individuals felt the need to flee the family and found that close friends provided a refuge and base away from the family despair so that they were able to continue their own lives.

Eleven young men and women assumed a caretaking role either within the family or outside it. This included taking charge of all the family functions, managing finances and living situations, caring for younger children, and calling attention to the parent's illness, which in some cases led to assistance and recovery. They served as peacemakers, supported younger siblings, and cheered up depressed mothers. Two other young women, although they were not involved in a major caretaking role within their families, were pursuing careers in the helping professions. Three others were the siblings of those who were caretakers and thus might not be expected to assume that role.

Understanding of the Parents' Illness and Subjects' Relation to It

Understanding of themselves and their parents' illness was evident in many ways in the 15 individuals who were coping well. First, they were able to reflect on changes over time in themselves and in their parents' behavior. They were able to talk about their concerns when they first became aware of their parents' illness and about the ways in which they came to see both themselves and their parents' situation differently over time.

Second, they were able to distinguish clearly between themselves (and their own experiences) and their parents' illness. Thus, they were able to talk about their parents' difficulties and, in many cases, be saddened by them and empathic and yet not be overwhelmed. For example, they did not expect that their own life experiences in the future would be the same as those of their parents. Third, they were clearly able to think and to act separately from their parents' illness system. Finally, before the interview, they had reflected on their relationships and their experiences with their parents. They had somehow made peace with or come to an understanding of the experience, and this was important to them; the interview tapped into this ongoing process of understanding.

In all cases, the young people who functioned well had noticed that there was something wrong with their parents and had concluded that they were not the cause of their parents' illness. They claimed that the realization that they were not the cause was crucial to understanding what was happening and to their capacity to deal with the experience of having a sick parent. This understanding of what was happening in the life of the parent and that they were not to blame was markedly absent in the three young people who were not functioning well at the second assessment. These three had not separated from their parents; they felt left out and angry or saw themselves as the ill parent's lifeline. The parents of these three subjects had not discussed their depression with them. Two of these young people had themselves experienced depression in the interval since the first assessment.

DISCUSSION

Behaviorally defined good adaptation was relatively stable in these individuals, since 15 of the 18 subjects had high ratings at the two assessment times. This was the first study, to our knowledge, to examine the stability of the adaptive functioning of resilient young people in this risk group, and the finding of such stability points to the value of a behaviorally rated adaptive function measure in identifying resilient individuals. Furthermore, it is the first study to report the considerable extent of such young people's awareness of their parents' affective illness and their reflections on their experiences.

The young men and women who adapted well were doers and problem solvers. Their accounts reflected a deep pride and sense of efficaciousness in their actions. This is the opposite of the helplessness and hopelessness so often described as accompanying depression.[35] Several subjects commented that it was this problem-solving, action orientation—a rejection of extraneous thoughts—which enabled them to function so well.

Taken together, these accounts reflect the association of good adaptive functioning with self-understanding. This was not a prospective study and so self-understanding cannot yet be described as a protective factor for the individuals in the sample. With that qualification, however, the accounts of these individuals allow for a definition of the components of self-understanding in those who were functioning well.

1. Accurate cognitive appraisal of the stress to be dealt with. The importance of adequate cognitive appraisal has been emphasized by a number of researchers in stress and coping,[12,36] primarily in response to medical illness or immediate situational stresses. In the present study cognitive appraisal involved an awareness of various aspects of parental illness over a period of time and changes in the awareness as the parent's illness changed.

2. Realistic assessment of one's capacity to act and realistic expectations of the consequences of the action. These young men and women were able to delineate what they were and were not responsible for in relation to their parents' illness system. As an example, many of them had wished to save or change their parents and had tried to do so, but over time they had come to

accept the fact that they could not cure their parents, although they could in certain important ways contribute to their well-being. Moreover, their assessments were accurate in the sense that they did not see themselves as responsible for the illness. Self-reflection was an important part of this process.

3. Actions that reflect understanding or are congruent with it. These individuals described themselves as separate from their parents' illness system and not responsible for it. They acted without depending on their parents, seeking independent relationships and functioning independently at work and in school.

The use of objective criteria to define the sample and the recruitment of 90% of the available subjects who met the criteria increase the generalizability of the findings, since these subjects were representative of resilient young people in the various sampling groups we studied. The use of the in-depth life history method in combination with structured assessments of psychopathology and behavioral functioning allowed a fuller and more detailed understanding of the subjects' experiences with their sick parents than either method alone would have provided. An important life dimension for many of them was the caretaking role that they assumed in relation to the parent who was ill. Interestingly, although they were separate and able to function independently, they remained very involved with their ill parents. For example, all of those who attended college did so in the metropolitan area in which their families lived rather than going to other cities. All remained connected to at least one parent.

These subjects were selected because they had had a period of good functioning in the 3 months before the first interview. They were selected without reference to prognosis or history of past difficulties, and the time interval between the two assessments was relatively short. They are now entering the age that is at highest risk for the onset of affective disorders and are at risk in the future because of both genetic factors and their psychosocial exposure to chronic impairments in parental functioning.[37]

These youngsters faced and were affected by multiple serious stresses, not simply episodes of pure affective illness in a parent. These included divorce or separation in the majority of cases, illness of both parents in the majority of cases, and nonaffective psychiatric disorders, especially alcoholism, in the parents. Given the nature of the sample, it is likely that these multiple stresses in combination are encountered by the majority of youngsters growing up in homes where there are serious parental affective disorders.

The ratings and descriptions of the processes of self-understanding were made by the two investigators in the project and were based on clear definitions of the concepts for specific content areas in the interview. Such an approach was necessary because of the large amount of interview material involving reflections at different points in time. In the future, specific quantitative ratings of dimensions of self-understanding applicable to clinical and research endeavors need to be developed.

A prospective study of the development of self-understanding, the various stages in its unfolding, and its role as a protective factor against future difficulties would provide different and needed information. Clearly, self-understanding of these young people evolved over time. They were at a point in their development (late adolescence and early adulthood) when an appropriate developmental task is separating from parents, and this requires self-reflection. It is likely that both the role and the nature of self-understanding are different at other points in development.

This was not a study of the etiology of the young people's resiliency. Clearly they had certain constitutional factors, such as above-average intelligence, lack of serious medical illness, and lack of neurodevelopmental disabilities, that contributed to their adaptation and may well have contributed to their capacity to understand themselves. Furthermore, they clearly manifested a variety of important psychological qualities and ego strengths, including courage, motivation, and a strong sense of personal integrity. The method of inquiry and focus on self-understanding provides a useful way of obtaining information about and characterizing these dimensions, yet they are clearly distinct from self-understanding.

Both the role of self-understanding and the role of caretaking in other samples of subjects in this risk situation and in other risk situations, especially parental alcoholism, deserve much fuller study.

These individuals were deeply aware of and deeply affected by their parents' illness. The actual stresses that they faced varied, for example, psychiatric illness in the mother or the father, divorce, and physical disease in a parent. Clinicians working with youngsters who have parents with serious affective illnesses should carefully inquire about the presence and meaning of individual experiences as they try to help these young people make sense of what has occurred. In this study, what bothered the subjects was often associated with, but different from, the parent's affective illness itself and was different for different subjects.

Depression and other affective illness in parents are public health problems of major proportions. Fully 20% of women and 8%–12% of men will experience an episode of major depressive disorder during their lifetimes.[38] The number of youngsters growing up in families exposed to these conditions is considerable; thus, there is a need for preventive strategies.[39] One preventive approach that grows naturally from our work is to develop strategies for all youngsters in this risk situation for enhancing separateness from the parent's illness system, strong intimate relationships, and self-understanding which characterized the resilient young men and women in this study.

REFERENCES

1. Beardslee WR, Klerman GL, Keller MB, et al: But are they cases? Validity of *DSM-III* major depression in children identified in a family study. Am J Psychiatry 1985; 142:687–691
2. Beardslee WR, Keller MB, Klerman GL: Children of parents with affective disorders. Int J Family Psychiatry 1986; 6:283–299
3. Weissman MM, Prusoff BA, Gammon GD, et al: Psychopathology in the children (ages 6–18) of depressed and normal parents. J Am Acad Child Psychiatry 1984; 23:78–84
4. Welner Z, Welner A, McCrary MD, et al: Psychopathology in children of inpatients with depression: a controlled study. J Nerv Ment Dis 1977; 164:408–413
5. McKnew DH, Cytryn L, Efron AM, et al: Offspring of patients with affective disorders. Br J Psychiatry 1979; 134:148–152
6. Keller MB, Beardslee WR, Dorer DJ, et al: Impact of severity and chronicity of parental affective illness on adaptive functioning and psychopathology in children. Arch Gen Psychiatry 1986; 43:930–937
7. Beardslee WR: Need for the study of adaptation in the children of parents with affective disorder, in Depression in *Young People: Developmental and Clinical Perspectives*. Edited by Rutter M, Izard CE, Read PB. New York, Guilford Press, 1986
8. Vaillant GE, Vaillant CO: Natural history of male psychological health, X: work as a predictor of positive mental health. Am J Psychiatry 1981; 138:1433–1440
9. Kohlberg L, LaCrosse J, Ricks D: The predictability of adult mental health from childhood behavior, in *Manual of Child Psychopathology*. Edited by Wolman BB. New York, McGraw-Hill, 1972.
10. Rutter M: Protective factors in children's response to stress and disadvantage, in *Primary Prevention of Psychopathology, vol III: Social Competence in Children*. Edited by Rolf R, Kent MD. Hanover, NH, University Press of New England, 1979
11. Werner EE, Smith RS: *Vulnerable But Invincible: A Longitudinal Study of Resilient Children and Youth*. New York, McGraw-Hill, 1982
12. Cohen F, Lazarus RS: Coping and adaptation in health and illness, in *Handbook of Health, Health Care, and the Health Professions*. Edited by Mecham R. New York, Free Press, 1983
13. Watt NF, Anthony J, Wynne LC, et al (eds): *Children at Risk for Schizophrenia: A Longitudinal Perspective*. New York, Cambridge University Press, 1984
14. Kauffman C, Grunebaum H, Cohler B, et al: Superkids: competent children of psychotic mothers. Am J Psychiatry 1979; 136:1398–1402
15. Eisenberg L: A friend, not an apple, a day will help keep the doctor away. Am J Med 1979; 66:551–553
16. Rutter M: Meyerian psychobiology, personality development, and the role of life experiences. Am J Psychiatry 1986; 143:1077–1087
17. Lieberman MA: The effects of social supports on response to stress, in *Handbook of Stress: Theoretical and Clinical Aspects*. Edited by Goldberger L, Breznitz S. New York, Free Press, 1982
18. Rounsaville BJ, Weissman MM, Prusoff BA, et al: Process of psychotherapy among depressed women with marital disputes. Am J Orthopsychiatry 1979; 49:505–510

19. Weissman MM, Paykel ES, Klerman GL: The depressed woman as mother. Soc Psychiatry 1972; 7:98–108
20. Billings AG, Cronkite RC, Moos RH: Social-environmental factors in unipolar depression: comparisons of depressed patients and nondepressed controls. J Abnorm Psychol 1983; 92:119–133
21. Porter R, Collins GM (eds): Temperamental Differences in Infants and Young children: Ciba Foundation Symposium 89. London, Pitman, 1982
22. Rutter M: Stress, coping and development: some issues and some questions. J Child Psychol Psychiatry 1981; 22:323–356
23. Garmezy N: Stressors of childhood, in *Stress, Coping and Development in Children.* Edited by Garmezy N, Rutter M. New York, McGraw-Hill, 1983
24. Beardslee WR: *The Way Out Must Lead In: Life Histories in the Civil Rights Movement.* Westport, Conn, Lawrence Hill, 1983
25. Beardslee WR: Commitment and endurance: a study of civil rights workers who stayed. Am J Orthopsychiatry 1983; 53:34–42
26. Beardslee WR: Self understanding and coping with cancer, in *The Damocles Syndrome: Psychosocial Consequences of Surviving Childhood Cancer.* Edited by Koocher GP, O'Malley JE. New York, McGraw-Hill, 1981
27. Katz MM, Klerman GL: Introduction: overview of the clinical studies program. Am J Psychiatry 1979; 136:49–51
28. Spitzer RL, Endicott J: Schedule for Affective Disorders and Schizophrenia (SADS), 3rd ed. New York, New York State Psychiatric Institute, Biometrics Research, 1977
29. Spitzer RL, Endicott J, Robins E: Research Diagnostic Criteria (RDC), for a Selected Group of Functional Disorders, 3rd ed. New York, New York State Psychiatric Institute, Biometrics Research, 1977
30. Herjanic B, Reich W: Development of a structured psychiatric interview for children, part 1: agreement between child and parent on individual symptoms. J Abnorm Child Psychol 1982; 10:307–324
31. Reich W, Herjanic B, Welner Z, et al: Development of a structured psychiatric interview for children, part 2: agreement on diagnosis comparing child and parent interviews. J Abnorm Child Psychol 1982; 10:325–336
32. Finkleman D, Garmezy N: Child interview used in Project Competence studies, in Technical Reports: Project Competence. Minneapolis, University of Minnesota, 1979
33. Jones F: The Rochester Adaptive Behavior Inventory: a parallel series of instruments for assessing social competence during early and middle childhood and adolescence, in *The Origins and Course of Psychopathology.* Edited by Strauss J, Babisian H, Roff M. New York, Plenum, 1977
34. Garmezy N: Rochester Adaptive Behavior Inventory, modified for use in Project Competence, in Technical Reports: Project Competence. Minneapolis, University of Minnesota, 1979
35. Seligman MEP, Peterson C: A learned helplessness perspective on childhood depression: theory and research, in Depression in *Young People: Developmental and Clinical Perspectives.* Edited by Rutter M, Izard CE, Read PB. New York, Guilford Press, 1986
36. Lazarus RS, Rolkman S: *Stress, Appraisal, and Coping.* New York, Springer, 1984

37. Beardslee WR: Familial influences in childhood depression. Pediatr Ann 1984; 13:32–36
38. Weissman MM, Myers JK: Affective disorders in a US urban community. Arch Gen Psychiatry 1978; 35:1304–1311
39. Philips I: Opportunities for prevention in the practice of psychiatry. Am J Psychiatry 1983; 140:389–395

30

Obsessive-Compulsive Disorder in Adolescence: An Epidemiological Study

Martine F. Flament, Judith L. Rapoport
Carol Zaremba Berg, and Walter Sceery
National Institute of Mental Health, Bethesda, Maryland
Agnes Whitaker, Mark Davies,
Kevin Kalikow, and David Shaffer
Columbia University, College of Physicians and Surgeons,
New York, New York
New York State Psychiatric Institute

In the second part of a two-stage epidemiologic study of obsessive-compulsive symptoms in nonreferred adolescents, clinicians interviewed high school students selected from screening measures administered in the first stage. Of the 356 students interviewed, 93 scored above clinically derived thresholds on the 20-item Leyton Obsessional Inventory-Child Version, 188 scored below the clinical threshold but positively on at least one other screen for psychopathology, and 75 scored negatively on all screens. The Leyton inventory had a sensitivity of 75%, a specificity of 84%, and a predictive value of 18% as a screen for obsessive-compulsive disorder (OCD). The OCD cases identified had characteristics similar

Reprinted with permission from the *Journal of the American Academy of Child and Adolescent Psychiatry,* 1988, Vol. 27, No. 6, 764–771. Copyright 1988 by the American Academy of Child and Adolescent Psychiatry.

This research was supported by BRSG (NYS Psychiatric Institute) and NIMH Grant # 1–RO3–MH40527–01 (Eating Disorders in Adolescents: An Epidemiological Study) awarded to Dr. Whitaker, and NIMH Grant # ST32 MH16434 (Research Training in Child Psychiatry) and NIMH Clinical Research Center Grant # 30906–07.

We gratefully acknowledge the students, school teachers, and administrators who made this study possible. The authors would like to thank John Bartko, Ph.D., for his statistical advice and Eleanor Brown and Susan Braiman, C. S. W., for their assistance.

to those of clinical cases, except for the nonpredominance of males. There was a high frequency of associated disorders, but only four of the 18 cases had been under professional care. OCD is much more common during adolescence than has been previously thought; it is both underdiagnosed and undertreated.

Obsessive-compulsive disorder (OCD) has fascinated clinicians for hundreds of years, but because of the high proportion of cases with childhood onset, the disorder holds particular interest for child psychiatrists. The early clinical descriptions of Freud (1955, 1958) and Janet (1903) mention children 11 and 5 years of age with classical presentation of the disorder. Systematic studies have affirmed that from one-third (Black, 1974) to one-half (Pitres and Regis, 1902) of adult cases have had their onset by age 15. Moreover, unlike depression and schizophrenia, the disorder in childhood appears in a form virtually identical to that seen in adults.

Recent research has refocused attention on this disorder. Adult epidemiologic, pharmacological and clinical descriptive studies, studies of related disorders, and a large prospective study of children with severe primary OCD ongoing at the National Institute of Mental Health (NIMH) suggest that the disorder is more common than previously thought and reaffirms intriguing neurological links. Questions that apply equally to adult and child patients with OCD concern the continuity of OCD with normal development and with personality disorder, the nature of the association between OCD and other disorders, etiology (with focus on neurobiological components), and long-term prognosis. This last issue is particularly important in the light of the newer treatments.

The clinical literature describing childhood obsessive-compulsive disorder is meager. Previous studies on the prevalence of OCD during childhood were mainly retrospective chart reviews in child psychiatric populations. Berman (1942) found six cases of obsessive-compulsive neurosis among more than 3,000 pediatric cases admitted to Bellevue Hospital or the Bradley Home in a 5-year period, a prevalence of 0.2%. A retrospective chart examination of 405 children seen at UCLA Neuropsychiatric Institute yielded five cases that met diagnostic criteria for obsessive-compulsive neurosis, representing 1.2% of the child psychiatric cases (Judd, 1965). More recently in the same center, only 17 cases were found in a retrospective examination of more than 8,000 inpatient and outpatient clinical records, a prevalence of 0.2% of child psychiatric cases (Hollingsworth et al., 1980). To date, the only study investigating the prevalence of OCD in an unselected pediatric population is the survey of over 2,000 10- and 11-year-olds on the Isle of Wight in England (Rutter et al., 1970). While no "pure" cases of OCD were described, a total of seven children were seen with "mixed obsessional/anxiety disorders," a prevalence of up to 0.3%, depending on how these cases were classified.

In the United States, the recent Epidemiologic Catchment Area (ECA) surveys of large community samples (Regier et al., 1984) have estimated prevalence rates of OCD in adulthood. In each of the five sites of the study, the lifetime prevalence rate for OCD was unexpectedly high: 1.2 to 2.3% of the general adult population (Karno et al., in press), about twice as much as for schizophrenia or panic disorder (Robins et al., 1984). These figures, however, are based on lay diagnostic interviews. In the Baltimore site (Anthony et al., 1985), the 1-month prevalence rate for OCD was 1.3% when the lay interviews alone were used and 0.3% after reexamination by psychiatrists.

In the NIMH study of children and adolescents with OCD (Flament and Rapoport, 1984), the large number of children referred from the Baltimore and Washington area alone was more than would have been expected given previous prevalence estimates. These clinically referred cases of children had characteristics similar to adults with the exceptions that depression is relatively rare, males outnumber females 2:1, and the disorder appears for the most part discontinuous from trait (i.e., the disorder seems to often arise de novo in a child with otherwise unremarkable development).

The present report is based on the second part of a two-stage epidemiologic study of obsessionality in a county-wide high school population, the first such study of childhood/adolescent obsessive-compulsive disorder. This part of the study addressed several questions:

1. How efficiently does the 20-item Leyton identify cases of obsessive compulsive disorder in a nonreferred adolescent population?
2. What is the prevalence of OCD in a nonreferred adolescent population?
3. Are the characteristics of a community-derived sample similar to those of referred cases, particularly with regard to clinical picture, sociodemographic variables, and associated psychopathology?

METHOD

This study was part of a broader two-stage epidemiological investigation of eating, depressive, and anxiety symptoms in high school students (Whitaker et al., in press).

The target population consisted of the entire 9th through 12th grade enrollment (5,596 students) in a semirural, middle-class, predominately white county. In the first stage, a survey questionnaire that included the 20-item survey form of the Leyton Obsessional Inventory-Child Version as well as measures of eating, depressions, and anxiety symptoms was administered to students in each of the eight high schools in the county in October 1984. In the second stage, clinicians conducted semistructured interviews of students selected on the basis of scores on the LOI-CV and other measures in the first stage.

A companion paper (Berg et al., 1988) describes the study population, completion rates, and norms for survey form of the LOI-CV.

Stage I Summarized

The target population consisted of the entire 9th through 12th grade enrollment (5,596 students) in a single semirural county. In the first stage, the 20-item survey form of the Leyton Obsessional Inventory-Child Version (Berg et al., 1986), as part of a large questionnaire containing other measures of psychopathology, was administered to students in each of the eight high schools in the county during one week in October 1984. The Leyton survey form asks for the presence or absence of a number of obsessive preoccupations and behaviors as well as, for each positive response, a rating of interference in personal functioning (range 0 to 3, no interference to interferes a lot). Valid questionnaires were returned by 5,108 of the 5,596 students. An additional 557 students did not respond to 50% or more yes items on the 20-item Leyton; thus, the total number of students who completed the 20-item Leyton was 4,551 (81.3%) (Berg et al., 1988).

Sampling Procedure

The sample for the second stage of the study was a stratified random sample selected from the 5,108 respondents to the survey questionnaire. For seven of the schools, six characteristics were used to cross-classify the entire population into the strata. These characteristics comprised the school that the student attended and scores on five screens (the screen for obsessive-compulsive disorder, and screens for depressive disorder, bulimia, anorexia nervosa, and panic disorder). In the eighth school (a general public high school), two additional screens, one for shyness and the other for Type A-B behavior were included in the stratification. The sampling fraction within each stratum varied considerably. The entire stratum was sampled for the very high levels of screening scales for OCD, major depression, bulimia, and anorexia nervosa. Students who were negative on all screening scales were sampled at a rate of approximately 2%. A total of 468 students were included in the sample. Of these, 356 or 76.1% participated in the second stage interviews. For these 356 clinical interviews, individual weights were assigned that reflect the sampling design and the participation rates. These rates yield unbiased estimates for the population parameters.

Cutoff scores for the obsessive sample were chosen to be in the range suggestive of psychopathology and to yield a sub-sample of the population of appropriate size for clinical examination: 15 or more for the *Yes Score,* 20 or more for the *Interference Score.* The Interference Score, in the authors' experience, had been the best indicator of psychopathology, but also of interest was the possibility of selecting "healthy" or even "supernormal" individuals with noninterfering, ego-syntonic obsessional features. Therefore, two distinct groups of subjects were defined as "positive" on the obsessive-compulsive screen. The first group, called *High Yes/Low Interference* (shortened to *High Yes*), consisted of all subjects with a Yes Score of 15 or more and an Interference Score of 10 or less. The second group, termed here *High Interference,* included all the subjects scoring 25 or more for interference regardless of the Yes Score. It should be noted that subjects with a high Yes Score (≥ 15) but an Interference Score between 10 and 25 are considered "negative" on the obsessive-compulsive screen. These individuals were included in other strata and might have been chosen for interview at stage 2.

Table 1 shows that 35 subjects (1%) of the population surveyed were selected from stage 1 into the High Yes category, and 81 (2%) into the High Interference category. Therefore, the total number of students with positive obsessive-compulsive screen was 116, 2% of the population. Of the 116, 49 scored positive only on the obsessive-compulsive screen, but 67 also scored positive on one or more of the other screens.

Also selected for stage 2 clinical examination were the subjects positive in stage 1 on one or more of the other screens, e.g., the depression screen, the eating disorders screen, and/or the panic disorder screen. The screens and sam-

	Evaluation			
	Subjects Selected		Subjects Interviewed	
Screening Status	N	% of Population	N	% of Subjects Selected
High yes/low interference	35	0.7	26	74.3
High interference	81	1.6	67	82.7
Either "positive" obsessive-compulsive screen	116	2.3	93	80.2
Other positive screens control group	253	5.0	188	74.3
Negative screens control group	99	1.9	75	75.8
Total	468	9.2	356	76.1

Table 1. Evaluation

pling process for these subjects is described elsewhere (Whitaker et al., in press). For the present report, they provide a large *Other Positive Screens* comparison group of 253 subjects, 5% of the population. Finally, 99 students (2%) were randomly selected from subjects with negative scores on all stage 1 screens as a *Negative Screens* comparison group.

Interview Instrument and Administration

Obsessive-compulsive pathology in the interview stage was assessed with the OCD section of the Diagnostic Interview for Children and Adolescents (DICA) (Herjanic and Campbell, 1977), the Addendum for Compulsive Personality Disorder from the Interview Schedule for Children (Kovacs, unpublished data) and a few additional questions regarding checking habits, tics, and extracurricular activities. The other parts of the interview were the Eating Symptoms Interview (Whitaker et al., in press); the Columbia Clinical Interview (Shaffer et al., in preparation); the Adolescent Panic Attack Interview (Kalikow, unpublished); demographic and socio-familial items, questions on psychosocial stressors, and mental status examination from the DICA; and a brief medical history. In addition, the students completed the Achenbach Behavior Checklist (Achenbach and Edelbrock, 1979), and, in two schools, the Beck Depression Inventory (Beck et al., 1961). Finally, the clinician rated the child on the Children's Global Assessment Scale (GAS) (Shaffer et al., 1983), which assesses the child's most impaired level of general functioning during the past month on a continuum from 0 to 100.

The interviews were conducted between January and August 1985 by a team of 13 clinicians who were blind to each subject's screening status. The interviewers included five child psychiatrists, two child psychiatry fellows, three psychologists, two social workers, and one registered nurse, all with experience in adolescent psychiatry. The interviews were conducted in the schools, or occasionally at home upon parent's request, and were about 75 minutes in duration.

Completion Rate

As shown in Table 1, interviews could be completed for 83% of the subjects in the High Interference group and 74% in the High Yes group, an overall completion rate of 80%. Eighty-four of the students (90%) were interviewed in their schools of attendance, and nine (10%) during home visits. Not interviewed were 16 subjects who refused to participate, two who had moved away and could not be located, and five who could not be identified by name from stage 1. Completion rate for the Other Positive Screens group was 74%, and for the Negative Screens control group, 76%.

Diagnostic Classification

Based on the interviews, all cases were written up with brief clinical vignettes, and provisional multiaxial *DSM–III* diagnoses were given by the interviewer.

The interviews allowed for current as well as lifetime diagnosis of OCD. For obsessive-compulsive personality disorder, we used the *DSM–III* criteria of constant (lifelong) patterns or rigidity, stubbornness, indecisiveness, preoccupation with details, etc. We were not prepared for the high frequency of a phenomenon we labeled "subclinical OCD," since it defied *DSM–III* classification. In numerous instances (see Table 2), we noted one or two obsessive-compulsive symptoms that had a definite date of onset but did not appear developmentally continuous or accountable by situation or personality, and was seen as abnormal or undesirable. These subjects did not meet full criteria for OCD (or another disorder). For example, a 16-year-old girl had a 1-year history of washing the walls of her room for 3 hours every week. She did not exhibit enough interference from this habit to be significant, but the behavior had begun rather suddenly and was regarded as undesirable by the girl and her family. Other instances were mild but senseless straightening or cleaning rituals, infrequent by egodystonic obsessive thoughts, etc. Finally, for some cases, clear obsessive-compulsive symptoms appeared to be part of the clinical picture of a *DSM–III* disorder other than OCD, and this was also reported separately.

The range of diagnoses therefore available to the interviewers comprised current or past OCD; compulsive personality disorder, "subclinical OCD" (current); other (lifetime) *DSM–III* disorders with obsessive-compulsive features; other (lifetime) *DSM–III* disorders; and no diagnosis. Except when mutually exclusive, multiple diagnoses were permitted.

Current Clinical Diagnosis	Screening Status				
	High Interference[a] (N = 67)	High Yes[a] (N = 26)	Other Positive Screens Controls (N = 188)	Negative Screens Controls (N = 75)	Total Interviewed (N = 356)
OCD	12	2	4[b]	0	18
Compulsive personality disorder	4	2	4[c]	1	11
"Subclinical OCD"	7	2	4	1	14
Other psychiatric disorders with obsessive-compulsive features	9	2	5	0	16
Other psychiatric disorders (no obsessive-compulsive symptoms)	12	2	46	9	69
No diagnosis	23	16	125	64	228

[a] Refer to the Yes score and Interference score on the Leyton Obsessional Inventory–Child Version.
[b] Two had onset of OCD since initial survey; one had: Yes = 20, Interference missing; one had Yes = 15, Interference = 17.
[c] Yes and Interference missing.

Table 2. Clinical Diagnoses Given to Subjects in the Four Groups Derived from Screening Questionnaire in a Population of 5108 High School Students

Diagnostic Agreement

One of the authors (M. F.) received both the protocol and the summary vignettes from 81 cases interviewed by the other clinicians, blind to their diagnoses. The interrater overall agreement for the six diagnostic categories described above was expressed using the kappa statistic (Cohen, 1960). The kappa value was 0.85 ($p < 0.0001$). Diagnostic disagreements were resolved by consensus.

Statistical Analysis

Comparisons between different groups of students were obtained by chi square test statistics, Yates corrected where appropriate, for discrete characteristics and by analysis of variance for measures that were assumed to be approximately Gaussian in distribution. Prevalence rates were calculated using both raw and weighted data to reflect the sampling design.

RESULTS

The Screening Instrument

How efficient was the screening instrument, the 20-item Leyton, for identifying OCD cases? As can be seen in Table 2, 14 of the 18 current OCD cases diagnosed in stage 2 were positive on the obsessive-compulsive screen in stage 1 (12 had an Interference Score ≥ 25, two more had a Yes Score ≥ 15). The remaining four cases came from the Other Positive Screens control group. Two of these were recent cases that had developed after the initial survey, while the other two had a high Yes Score (with Interference Score either missing or in the medium range). None of the subjects in the Negative Screens control group had a diagnosis of OCD. The obsessive-compulsive screen also picked up most but not all of the cases of compulsive personality as well as a number of subjects having intriguing obsessive-compulsive symptoms without the full picture of the disorder.

On the other hand, of the 67 subjects selected for their high Interference score, 21 had a psychiatric disorder other than OCD (with or without associated obsessive-compulsive features), and 23 had no diagnosis at all.

Thus, the screening procedure yielded very few false negative cases but a large number of false positives. To look at the screen's properties, the two cases with onset of OCD postdating the survey were excluded. Using a cutoff score of 25 or more for Interference (the High Interference group), the sensitivity of the instrument for OCD is 75%, its specificity 84%, and its positive predictive value 18%. Using a selection criterion of 15 or more on the Yes score (High Interference and High Yes groups combined), the sensitivity increases to 88%, the specificity is 77% and the positive predictive value, 15%. The 20-item Leyton was not designed to identify compulsive personality disorder, but the broader selection criterion (Yes score ≥ 15) gives the instrument a sensitivity for obsessive compulsive personality disorder of 64%.

Prevalence Rates

A total of 18 current cases of OCD were found among the 356 adolescents interviewed in stage 2, that is 0.35% of the population surveyed in stage 1. An additional two subjects had histories of past episodes of OCD. From these data, a minimum figure of 0.35% is estimated for the point-prevalence rate of OCD in the adolescent population and a minimum figure of 0.40% for its lifetime prevalence rate. If the sample is weighted to reflect the sampling design, then the prevalences are 1 (± 0.5)% and 1.9 (± 0.7)%, for current and lifetime, respectively.

The 11 cases of compulsive personality disorder identified in the current study suggest a minimum prevalence rate for this disorder in the general adolescent population of about 0.3%.

Clinical Characteristics and Correlates

The main clinical characteristics of the OCD cases (lifetime and current combined) identified are presented in Table 3. It should be noted that a total of 20 cases are described, as two cases with past but not current OCD were diagnosed from other positive groups. Eleven were males and nine were females. The mean age of the cases was 16.2 years (range, 14 to 18 years), compared with a mean age of 15.6 years in the whole population. Age of onset varied from 7 to 18 years (mean age at onset, 12.8 years). Onset was most often gradual, but sudden in some cases; in general, no precipitating events were acknowledged by the subjects. One boy had an early episode of obsessions between the ages of 8 and 9, then relapsed at age 16. Although duration of the disorder had been from 6 months to 7 years, only four subjects had ever been under brief psychiatric care, three for associated depression or anxiety (they had been in psychotherapy for a few months). One severely ill girl had received medication; she was hospitalized following her interview.

Only one boy (5% of the cases) had isolated obsessions without rituals (intrusive thoughts of having a ski accident). All other subjects had compulsive rituals, usually related to obsessive thoughts of fear of contamination (35%) or fear of hurting self and/or familiar persons (30%); one boy had "neutral" obsessive thoughts. The most common rituals were washing and cleaning rituals (85% of the cases), compulsive checking (40%), and straightening (35%). Three subjects (15%) had to repeat their actions and three had to do things "just right." One girl avoided touching certain objects, one boy had obses-

Age	Sex	Main Symptoms		Duration of Disorder (by Age)	Other Symptoms/ Disorders	Treatment	GAS[a]	LOI-CV[b] Scores		Other Positive Screens[c]
		Obsessions	Compulsions					Yes	Interference	
16	M	Thoughts of traps	Checking	13-current	Overanxious disorder		70	17	51	Depression, panic
18	M	Thoughts of ski accident	No	8–9 and 16-current	None		90	16	3	
15	M	Fear of contamination	Washing	13-current	ADD-residual type, history of one panic attack		70	18	40	
14	M		Cleaning, checking things, "just right"	12-current	ADD-residual type, compulsive personality disorder			16	36	Depression
14	M		Cleaning, checking	9-current	None		81	15	17	Eating
14	M	Fear of contamination	Washing, straightening	7-current	None		72	14	27	
17	M		Washing, cleaning, straigtening, slowness	15-current	Compulsive personality disorder		68	14	37	
17	M		Cleaning, checking, straightening	14-current	Past separation anxiety disorder (age 3–12)		81	15	27	
16	F	Fear of contamination	Handwashing, avoiding touching, checking, straightening, re-reading	15-current	None		65	20		Eating, depression
17	F		Washing, cleaning	13-current	Two past episodes of adjustment disorder with depressed mood		75	16	27	
17	F	Thoughts of hurting self or others	Handwashing, checking	13-current	Phobia of strangers, history of one panic attack	Psychotherapy for 4 months	61	9	25	
18	M	Thoughts of getting hurt, fear of contamination	Things "just right," cleaning	15-current	Simple phobias (ladders, tarantulas)		75	16	31	
16	F		Handwashing, re-doing papers	13-current	Overanxious disorder, bulimia		50	14	30	Eating, depression
16	M	Fear of hurting others	Closing/opening drawers, straightening, checking	7-current	Dysthymic disorder, history of one panic attack	Psychotherapy last 2 months	80	15	0	Panic
16	F		Handwashing	15-current	Bulimia, major depression		60	19	38	Eating, depression, panic
16	M	Thoughts of hurting others	Handwashing, checking	14-current	Major depression, overanxious disorder, compulsive personality disorder		57	15	28	Eating, depression

Table 3 continues

Table 3. Clinical Characteristics of Lifetime and Current OCD Cases Identified in the Epidemiological Study of a High School Student Population (N = 5108)

TABLE 3—*Continued*

Age	Sex	Main Symptoms		Duration of Disorder (by Age)	Other Symptoms/ Disorders	Treatment	GAS[a]	LOI-CV[b] Scores		Other Positive Screens[c]
		Obsessions	Compulsions					Yes	Interference	
18	F	Thoughts of hurting children	Handwashing, cleaning, straightening	18[d]-current	Atypical eating disorder, major depression		50	8	6	Eating
16	F	Fear of contamination	Handwashing, cleaning, straightening things "just right"	16[d]-current		Imipramine, lithium	50			Depression
18	F	Fear of contamination	Handwashing	10-11 Not current	Bulimia, major depression	Psychotherapy last 3 months	60	13	16	Eating, depression
15	F	Fear of contamination	Handwashing	13-13 Not current	Episodes of generalized anxiety, atypical eating disorder, subclinical panic attacks		70	12	23	Eating, depression, panic

[a] GAS indicates the Children's Global Assessment Scale.
[b] LOI-CV indicates the Leyton Obsessional Inventory–Child Version.
[c] From initial survey questionnaire.
[d] Symptoms developed after the survey.

Table 3. (*Continued*)

sional slowness. Most subjects (70%) had multiple obsessions/compulsions.

As can be seen in Table 3, 15 of the 20 adolescents with a lifetime history of OCD (75%) had one or more other lifetime psychiatric diagnoses, and 10 of them (50%) had at least one other current diagnosis. Associated disorders were most frequently major depression (five cases), dysthymia (one case), bulimia (three cases), and overanxious disorder (four cases); two subjects had a phobic disorder and four had histories of isolated or subclinical panic attacks. No case had Tourette's or other tic disorder. Three boys with OCD (17% of the cases) also met criteria for compulsive personality disorder. Except for the three cases with associated OCD, most of the subjects with compulsive personality showed no evidence of other psychopathology, three had symptoms of an eating disorder, two had phobias, and one had dysthymia.

The adolescents with OCD or obsessive-compulsive personality disorder did not differ from the population as a whole in terms of family constellation or socioeconomic status, race, religious affiliation, grade point average, or current physical health. Subjects with obsessive-compulsive *symptoms,* (but not those with compulsive personality disorder) were more likely to report having "poor" or "very poor" emotional health ($p < 0.001$).

DISCUSSION

This is the first epidemiologic study of obsessive-compulsive disorder in adolescents. A county-wide population of high school students has been studied using a two-stage procedure. The minimum estimates obtained for the prevalence rates of OCD in the general adolescent population, 0.35% for current prevalence rate and 0.40% for lifetime prevalence, were much greater than expected but are probably still minimal figures. The weighted prevalence figures, in keeping with the NIMH Epidemiologic Catchment Area figures, of 1% and 1.9% take into account the stratified sampling for this second stage and give greater weight to positive cases in lower risk groups. They also support the authors' clinical experience that the disorder is common and usually not seen and/or recognized by health care professionals. There are several reasons why the authors believe the true rates to be even higher. First, the sample was school-based and the most severely disturbed adolescents would not be attending school. Secondly, the 557 cases not completing the survey questionnaire would, based on clinical experience, be likely to contain a higher than chance proportion of subjects with obsessive-compulsive symptomatology (difficulty making choices, secretiveness, difficulty completing the task on time, etc.). Another factor that might have affected the estimate of the lifetime prevalence rate of OCD is the screening procedure. The 20-item Leyton screens for current symptomatology; the past cases of the disorder could only be diagnosed through clinical interview. The two cases with past episodes of OCD came from the Other Positive Screens comparison group; it is possible that a few more cases existed among the subjects not interviewed.

On the other hand, there were no true "false negative" cases of OCD in the control groups, using as a screening instrument for OCD the 20-item Leyton. In the authors' clinical experience, almost 50% of referred OCD patients have a few, albeit severe, symptoms, thus generating a relatively low Yes Score on which the Interference Score is based. The same did not seem to be true in the current epidemiologic sample. The 20-item Leyton appeared to serve its screening purpose, selecting a heterogeneous group of subjects among which the true positive cases could be identified by subsequent clinical interview.

The methodological weaknesses in the current study included: (1) The survey did not include institutionalized adolescents or high school dropouts. (2) The time-lag between screening and clinical interview, although kept to a minimum (3 to 10 months), allowed psychopathological changes for some subjects. (3) Survey respondents with 'Low' and 'High' Interference Scores were included but not sampled at a high rate. (4) Time limitations prevented open clinical interview, and so diagnosis relied entirely on a structured interview section of the DICA.

The study has relative strengths. First, the good screening properties of the 20-item Leyton, whose high sensitivity and lower specificity were compatible with the two-stage screening/clinical interviews method used. The low-positive predictive value is a property shared by all screens for rare disorder (Williams et al., 1982). Second, the interrater diagnostic agreement for the subjects interviewed was acceptable (kappa = 0.85). The interviewers were all trained clinicians, all interviews were reviewed by child psychiatrists, the interview instrument contained detailed questions on all diagnostic criteria of OCD and for obsessive-compulsive personality disorder, and the final diagnoses were not algorithmically derived but based upon clinical judgment. The diagnostic category that was introduced, "subclinical OCD," although not satisfying for nosological purposes, might have contributed to a better interrater reliability for the "true" cases: in epidemiologic studies, the extremes are more easily defined than are cases near diagnostic threshold.

The sizeable "subclinical OCD" subgroup is particularly intriguing. The adolescents in this group did not meet *DSM–III* criteria for compulsive personality disorder nor did they for the most part show tendencies in this direction. Their symptoms seemed discrete and they adapted their lives around them, but the usual history of abrupt onset (the subject could often name the month it started even if this had occurred a year or two before the interview) and some acknowledgment that the behavior was different from that of peers, some attempt to hide the behavior, etc., suggested a mild or early form of the disorder. Interestingly, these individuals come close to the ICD-9 diagnosis of Anankastic Personality in which discrete and unwelcome thoughts or impulses occur but are below threshold for obsessional neurosis. An ongoing, long-term follow-up of these "subclinical OCD" cases will elucidate their relationship to "true" OCD. At present, however, the relationship in childhood between OCD, compulsive-personality disorder, and what the authors call "subclinical OCD" remains unclear. Follow-up of diagnosed cases of OCD, also underway, will also help validate the initial diagnosis as well as assess the prognosis of this untreated community sample.

The minimal point-prevalence figure of OCD obtained in this study, 0.35% of an unselected adolescent population, is quite similar to the 0.3% 1-month-prevalence rate found among adult residents in the Baltimore site of the ECA survey (Anthony et al., 1985). Comparison across studies, however, it is not possible because thresholds for diagnostic sensitivity may differ considerably. Furthermore, the long-term prognosis of adolescent OCD is not known. Rasmussen and Tsuang (1986), however, find two peaks of maximal incidence for the disorder, one at 12 to 14, the second at 20 to 22 years of age. If, as has been suggested, half of adolescent cases remit (Warren, 1960) then the rates for adolescents and adults may be comparable. Although most clinical reports of childhood OCD find that males outnumber females 2 to 1 (Despert, 1955; Flament and Rapoport, 1984; Hollingsworth et al., 1980), the current study found the equal representation seen in adult clinical (Black, 1974; Rasmussen and Tsuang, 1984) as well as epidemiological (Robins et al., 1984) series. It is possible that the overrepresentation of boys in child-clinical samples is due to greater severity of the disorder in young males, as boys have more severe symptoms than girls, and an earlier age of onset (Flament et al., 1985). The present community-based sample, as expected, contained several subjects who were less severely ill than our clinic sample.

The survey population was relatively homogeneous demographically being mostly white, rural, and middle class. As in the ECA study (Robins et al., 1984), OCD subjects did not differ from others for race or any socioeconomic variable recorded. Family size and ordinal position did not distinguish OCD cases, although an overrepresentation of firstborn or only children in OCD has been described (Kaylon and Borge, 1967; Snowden, 1979). The only significant medical event reported by OCD subjects in the current study was past history of head injury. This is interesting in the light of several reports of increased frequency of birth trauma (Capstick and Seldrup, 1977) or neurological dysfunction (Baxter et al., 1987; Jenike, 1974) in OCD patients.

The pattern of obsessions and compulsions in these epidemiologically derived OCD cases was quite similar to that seen in clinical series of obsessive-compulsive patients. As in the NIMH pediatric sample (Flament and Rapoport, 1984), cleaning rituals were most frequently found with checking and straightening compulsions also common. The most frequent obsessions were fear of dirt or contamination and thoughts of harm coming to self and/or familiar figures. Obsessions without rituals were rare while multiple obsessions/compulsions was the rule. The existence of similar presentations in OCD across ages and across cultures (Aktar et al., 1975; Insel, 1984; Lo, 1967; Rachman and Hodgson, 1980; Rasmussen and Tsuang, 1986) is particularly striking in this disorder. The clinically referred cases tended, not surprisingly, to be more severe and, seemingly, to have somewhat more observant caretakers.

The most striking dissimilarity between child and adult OCD patients is the relative infrequency of compulsive personality, which is reported in more than 50% of adult OCD patients (Rasmussen and Tsuang, 1986; Rosenberg, 1967) but which was seen in only three boys (17%) of the OCD cases. For the other subjects, the obsessive-compulsive symptoms appeared discontinuous from earlier developments.

Conversely, in the current study, 14 subjects were diagnosed as having compulsive personality disorder, a minimum prevalence rate of 0.35% of the general adolescent population, and only three of these had concurrent OCD. Except for those three, these cases were functioning quite well; few had symptoms of eating disorders, phobia, or dysthymia.

In adult OCD patients, the most commonly associated psychiatric disorder is depression, occurring before, concurrently, or after the onset of OCD in 71% of 149 cases in a St. Louis study (Welner et al., 1976). In our epidemiological adolescent sample, major depressive disorder affected five (25%) of the OCD cases, and anxiety disorders were seen commonly (a pattern found also in the NIMH clinical sample of referred OCD adolescents). Three adolescent girls had both obsessive-compulsive disorder and bulimia, an association reported elsewhere in adults (Weiss and Ebert, 1983; Solyom et al., 1983). Although several authors have reported a high frequency of obsessive-compulsive traits or symptoms in Tourette's disorder patients (Grad et al., 1987; Pauls et al., 1986), the reverse does not seem to be true in this nonreferred sample.

Finally, only four (20%) of the 20 lifetime cases of OCD identified in our study had ever sought treatment, although most rated themselves as having poor emotional health. Three of the four treated cases had sought help for depression or anxiety and had not ever disclosed their obsessive-compulsive preoccupations to their therapist. This confirms the secrecy that many obsessive-compulsive patients have about their condition, undoubtedly contributing to the underdiagnosis of the disorder. Social disablement (inability to carry out accustomed work or social duties) may occur years after onset and the first psychiatric contact is usually sought still later: on average 7.5 years after onset (Pollitt, 1957).

The present study has major implications for mental health practice. The unexpected high frequency of cases found in the current epidemiologic study, the chronic nature of the untreated disorder, and recent recognition of effective treatment (Flament et al., 1985; Wolff and Rapoport, 1988) calls for greater sensitivity to this diagnosis.

REFERENCES

Achenbach, T. & Edelbrock, C. (1979), The Child Behavior Profile. *J. Consult. Clin. Psychol.*, 47:223.

Aktar, S., Wig, N. N. & Varma, V. K. (1975), A phenomenologic analysis of symptoms in obsessive-compulsive neurosis. *Br. J. Psychiatry*, 127:342–348.

Anthony, J. C., Folstein, M., Romanoski, A. J. et al. (1985), Comparison of the lay diagnostic interview and a standardized psychiatric diagnosis. *Arch. Gen. Psychiatry*, 42:667–675.

Baxter, L. R., Phelps, M. E., Mazziotta, J. C., Guze, B. H., Schwartz, J. M. & Selin, C. E. (1987), Local cerebral glucose metabolic rates in obsessive-compulsive disorder. *Arch. Gen. Psychiatry*, 44:211–218.

Beck, A. T., Ward, C. H., Mendelson, M., Mock, J. E. & Erbaugh, J. K. (1961), An interview for measuring depression. *Arch. Gen. Psychiatry*, 4:561–571.

Berg, C. Z., Rapoport, J. L. & Flament, M. (1986), The Leyton Obsessional Inventory-Child Version. *J. Am. Acad. Child Adolesc. Psychiatry*, 25:84–91.

—— Whittaker, A., Davies, M., Flament, M. F. & Rapoport, J. L. (1988), The survey form of the Leyton Obsessional Inventory-Child Version. *J. Am. Acad. Child Adolesc. Psychiatry*, 27:759–763.

Berman, L. (1942), The obsessive-compulsive neurosis in children. *J. Nerv. Ment. Dis.*, 85:26–39.

Black, A. (1974), The natural history of obsessional neurosis. In: *Obsessional States*, ed. P. H. Hock & J. Zubin. London: Methuen and Co. Ltd., pp. 19–54.

Capstick, N. & Seldrup, J. (1977), Obsessional states: a study in the relationship between abnormalities occurring at the time of birth and the subsequent development of obsessional symptoms. *Acta. Psychiatr. Scand.*, 56:427–431.

Cohen, J. (1960), A coefficient of agreement for nominal scales. *Educational and Psychological Measurement*, 20:37–46.

Despert, L. (1955), Differential diagnosis between obsessive-compulsive neurosis and schizophrenia in children. In: *Psychopathology of Childhood*, ed. P. H. Hoch & Zubin. New York: Grune and Stratton.

Flament, M. & Rapoport, J. L. (1984), Childhood obsessive compulsive disorder. In: *New Findings in Obsessive Compulsive Disorder*, ed. T. R. Insel. Washington, D.C.: American Psychiatric Press, Inc., pp. 23–43.

—— Rapoport, J. L., Berg, C. J. et al. (1985), Clomipramine treatment of childhood obsessive compulsive disorder. *Arch. Gen. Psychiatry*, 42:977–983.

Freud, S. (1955), Obsessions and phobias. In: *Collected Papers I*, ed. J. Strachey. London: Hogarth Press, pp. 128–137.

—— (1958), The predisposition to obsessional neurosis. In: *The Standard Edition of the Collected Works on Sigmund Freud, Vol. 12*, ed. J. Strahey, London: Hogarth Press, pp. 311–326.

Grad, L., Pelcovitz, D., Olsen, M., Matthews, M. & Grad, G. (1987), Obsessive-compulsive symptomatology in children with Tourette's disorder. *J. Am. Acad. Child Adolesc. Psychiatry*, 26:69–73.

Hollingsworth, C. E., Tanguay, P. E., Grossman, L. & Pabst, P. (1980), Long-term outcome of obsessive-compulsive disorder in childhood. *J. Am. Acad. Child Adolesc. Psychiatry*, 19:134–144.

Herjanic, B. & Campbell, W. (1977), Differentiating psychiatrically disturbed children on the basis of a structured psychiatric interview. *J. Abnorm. Child Psychol.*, 5:127–135.

Insel, T. R., (1984), *New Findings in Obsessive-Compulsive Disorder*. Washington, D.C.: American Psychiatric Press.

Janet, P. (1903), Les Obsessions et la Psychasthenie, *Vol. I*, Paris: Felix Alcan.

Jenike, M. A. (1984), Obsessive-compulsive disorder: a question of a neurological lesion. *Compr. Psychiatry*, 25:298–304.

Judd, L. L. (1965), Obsessive compulsive neurosis in children. *Arch. Gen. Psychiatry*, 12:136–143.

Karno, M., Golding, J., Sorenson, S. & Burnham, M. (in press), The epidemiology of obsessive compulsive disorder in five U.S. communities. *Arch. Gen. Psychiatry*.

Kaylon, L. & Borge, G. F. (1967), Birth order and obsessive compulsive character. *Arch. Gen. Psychiatry*, 17:751–754.

Lo, W. H. (1967), A follow-up study of obsessional neurotics in Hong-Kong Chinese. *Br. J. Psychiatry* 113:823–832.

Pauls, D., Leckman, J., Towbin, K., Zahner, G. & Cohen, D. (1986), Tourette's syndrome and obsessive compulsive disorder. *Arch. Gen. Psychiatry*, 43:1180–1182.

Pitres, A. & Regis, E. (1902), *Les Obsessions et Les Impulsions*. Paris: Doin.

Pollitt, J. (1957), Natural history of obsessional states. A study of 150 cases. *Br. Med. J.*, 1:194–198.

Rachman, S. J. & Hodgson, R. J. (1980), *Obsessions and Compulsions*. Englewood Cliffs, N.J.: Prentice-Hall.

Rasmussen, S. A. & Tsuang, M. T. (1984), The epidemiology of obsessive compulsive disorder, *J. Clin. Psychiatry,* 45:450–457.

——, —— (1986), Clinical characteristics and family history in *DSM–III* obsessive compulsive disorder. *Am. J. Psychiatry,* 143:317–322.

Regier, D. A., Myers, J. K., Kramer, M. et al. (1984), The NIMH epidemiologic catchment area program. *Arch Gen. Psychiatry,* 41:934–941.

Robins, L. N., Helzer, J. E., Weissman, M. M. et al. (1984), Lifetime prevalence of specific psychiatric disorders in three sites. *Arch. Gen. Psychiatry,* 41:949–958.

Rosenberg, C. M. (1967), Familial aspects of obsessional neurosis. *Br. J. Psychiatry,* 113:405–413.

Rutter, M., Tizard, J. & Whitmore, K. (1970), *Education, Health and Behavior.* London: Longmans.

Shaffer, D., Gould, M. S., Brasic, J. et al. (1983), The Children's global assessment scale. *Arch. Gen. Psychiatry,* 40:1228–1231.

Snowdon, S. (1979), Family size and birth order in obsessional neurosis. *Acta Psychiatr. Scand.,* 60:121–128.

Solyom, L., Freeman, R. J., Thomas C. D. & Miles, J. E. (1983), The comparative psycholpathology of anorexia nervosa. *International Journal of Eating Disorders,* 3:3–14.

Warren, W. (1960). Some relationships between the psychiatry of children and adults. *Journal of Mental Science,* 106:815–826.

Weiss, S. R. & Ebert, M. H. (1983). Psychological and behavorial characteristics of normal-weight bulimics and normal weight controls. *Psychosom. Med.,* 45:293–303.

Welner, A., Reich, T. & Robins, E. (1976), Obsessive-compulsive neurosis. I. Inpatient record study. *Compr. Psychiatry,* 17:527–539.

Whitaker, A., Davies, M., Shaffer, et al. (in press), The struggle to be thin: a survey of anorectic and bulimic symptoms in a nonreferred adolescent population. *Psychol. Med.*

Williams, P., Hand, D. & Tarnopolsky, A. (1982). The problem of screening for uncommon disorders—a comment on the Eating Attitudes Test. *Psychol. Med.,* 12:431–434.

Wolff, R. & Rapoport, J. (1988), Behavioral treatment of childhood anxiety disorders. *Behav. Modif.,* 12:252–266.

31

Neuropsychiatric, Psychoeducational, and Family Characteristics of 14 Juveniles Condemned to Death in the United States

Dorothy Otnow Lewis, Jonathan H. Pincus, Barbara Bard, Ellis Richardson, Leslie S. Prichep, Marilyn Feldman and Catherine Yeager

New York University School of Medicine
Georgetown University School of Medicine, Washington, DC
Department of Special Education, Central Connecticut State University, New Britain

Of the 37 juveniles currently condemned to death in the United States, all of the 14 incarcerated in four states received comprehensive psychiatric, neurological, neuropsychological, and educational evaluations. Nine had major neurological impairment, seven suffered psychotic disorders antedating incarceration, seven evidenced significant organic dysfunction on neuropsychological testing, and only two had full-scale IQ scores above 90. Twelve had been brutally physically abused, and five had been sodomized by relatives. For a variety of reasons the subjects' vulnerabilities were not recognized at the time of trial or sentencing, when they could have been used for purposes of migitation.

The purpose of this paper is twofold: to describe the biopsychosocial characteristics of 14 juveniles sentenced to death in the United States and to ex-

Reprinted with permission from the *American Journal of Psychiatry*, 1988, Vol. 145, No. 5, 584–589. Copyright 1988 by the American Psychiatric Association.

Presented at the annual meeting of the American Academy of Child and Adolescent Psychiatry, Washington, D.C., Oct. 21–25, 1987.

Supported by the law firm of Shearman and Sterling as part of their pro bono program.

plore the implications of these findings for imposition of the death penalty on juveniles.

The execution of juveniles in America dates back to the seventeenth century when, in 1642, a child was executed for the crime of bestiality.[1] Since then, 272 juveniles have been executed in the United States.[2] This figure includes the execution in 1985–1986 of three boys who were condemned as juveniles but who were not executed until after they reached their majority. During our study (1986–1987), the number of juveniles awaiting execution rose from 33 to 37.

U.S. law permitting the execution of juveniles is based on English common law.[3,4] Blackstone, in his *Commentaries on the Laws of England*,[5] commented, "If it appear to the court and jury that he was *doli capax*, and could discern between good and evil, he may be convicted and suffer death."

Although U.S. law regarding the responsibility of children has rested heavily on the commentaries of English jurists such as Blackstone, modifications based on case law have occurred.[6] For example, in the case of *State v. Aaron*,[7] in which an 11-year-old slave was accused of murdering a younger child, the 11-year-old's conviction and sentence of death were overturned by the Supreme Court of New Jersey. The presumption of innocence had not been refuted by "strong and irrefutable evidence that he had sufficient discernment to distinguish good from evil."

The outcome was quite different in the case of *Godfrey v. State*,[8] in which a slave of approximately 11 years of age hacked a 4-year-old to death. Covered with blood, the accused child blamed the act on imaginary Indians. The child was sentenced to death, and in spite of clear evidence of infantile reasoning, he was executed.

We seem to have inherited a paradoxical set of traditions. We have a juvenile justice system that recognizes the emotional and intellectual immaturity of juveniles and holds them less culpable than adults; at the same time, in the case of certain kinds of serious offenses, juveniles are tried in the criminal justice system and their punishment for these offenses, including execution, is meted out as though juveniles were as responsible as adults.

Little or nothing is currently known about the mental condition and cognitive capacities of juveniles sentenced to death. Given the dearth of information regarding the biopsychosocial status of condemned juveniles, we welcomed the opportunity to conduct comprehensive assessments of approximately 40% of the 37 juveniles who are currently awaiting execution in the United States.

METHOD

Our subjects were 14 boys who were sentenced to death for a capital offense committed before they reached age 18. The subjects comprised all the juve-

Annual Progress in Child Psychiatry and Development

niles sentenced to death in four states with statutes that permit the execution of minors. The subjects were chosen because of their youth and not because of any known psychopathology. They therefore can be presumed to be representative of the juvenile death row population in general. Their ages at the time of their offenses ranged from 15 years 10 months to 17 years 10 months, (mean, 16 years 6 months). Their ages at the time of their evaluation ranged from 17 years 10 months to 29 years, 2 months (mean, 22 years 3 months). There were six black subjects, seven white subjects, and one Hispanic subject. Informed consent was obtained from subjects and their attorneys.

The diagnostic evaluation consisted of psychiatric, neurological, psychological, neuropsychological, educational, and EEG examinations. The psychiatric examination consisted of a semistructured interview based on an expanded version of the Bellevue Adolescent Interview Schedule. This schedule, consisting of 160 questions, was devised because no existing diagnostic instrument for children or adults dealt adequately with topics such as medical history, history of neuropsychiatric symptoms (e.g., psychomotor symptoms), characteristics of temper, or history of physical abuse. A trial of this instrument before its use in this study revealed that data obtained were appreciably more comprehensive than those elicited after a routine 2-week evaluation on an inpatient teaching service on adolescents.

Detailed neurological histories were obtained by the psychiatrist and the neurologist. Whenever histories of CNS insults were elicited, attempts were made to corroborate the histories through physical examination (e.g., scars, neurological signs), record reviews, and specialized tests (e.g., EEG). Standard neurological examinations were performed on 12 of the 14 subjects (in two cases, scheduling precluded a neurological examination). The neurologist also performed a mental status examination. Paranoid ideation was evaluated by both clinicians because of its importance in previous studies[9] and because of the subjectivity inherent in the assessment of this particular symptom. In only one case did their ratings differ, and in that case, the subject was coded as not having paranoid symptoms.

Certain other information was obtained independently by both the psychiatrist and the neurologist. Both tried to ascertain whether a child had been the victim of abuse or had been witness to extreme family violence. A subject was considered to have been physically abused if he had been punched; beaten with a stick, board, pipe, or belt buckle; or beaten other than on the buttocks with a belt or a switch. A subject was not considered to have been physically abused if he had been struck only with an open hand or beaten only on the buttocks with the leather part of a belt. A subject was considered to have been sexually abused if older persons had fondled his genitals or penetrated his anus or if he had been forced to perform sexual acts on an older person of either sex.

A neurometric quantitative EEG was performed on all subjects. For the purpose of this phase of the study, 2 minutes of artifact-free quantitative EEG data were analyzed visually in order to determine the existence of sharp waves and/or actual seizure activity. Neuropsychological testing consisted of the WAIS, Revised,[10] Bender-Gestalt test,[11] Rorschach Test,[12] House-Tree-Person Test,[13] and the Halstead-Reitan Battery of Neuropsychological Tests.[14] Educational testing included the Woodcock-Johnson Psycho-Educational Battery,[15] the Mini-Screen subtest from the Test of Adolescent Language (E. Prather, unpublished), the Story subtest from the Test of Written Language,[16] and a speech screening test.

Findings were made available to individual attorneys if requested.

FINDINGS

Table 1 presents evidence of CNS trauma. As can be seen, eight subjects had had injuries that were severe enough to result in hospitalization, and/or indentation of the cranium (subjects 1, 2, 4, 7, 8, 12, 13, 14). For example, one subject was hit by a truck at age 4 years, was comatose for days, and was hospitalized for 11 months; another was hit by a car at age 6 years and hospitalized for 6 months.

Table 2 illustrates the neurological and EEG findings. In nine cases serious neurological abnormalities were documented, including evidence of focal brain injury (subjects 1 and 13), major neurological abnormalities such as abnormal head circumference or a positive Babinski sign (subjects 5, 10, 12), a history

Subject	Nature of Trauma	Objective Evidence
1	Automobile accident at age 12 (loss of consciousness); repeated blows to the head by father in infancy	Deep indentation of cranium behind right ear
2	Hit by truck at age 4—fractured skull, coma	11-month hospitalization
3	Fall from tree at age 11 (loss of consciousness)	Multiple scars on head
4	Shot in right temple at age 16	Indentation in right temporal area; many scars on face
5	Blow to head at age 8—amnesia for 2 weeks	No documentation
6	Fell from roof at age 10 (loss of consciousness); motorcycle accident at age 15	Multiple scars on head
7	Car accident at age 10 (loss of consciousness); hit in head with board during early childhood	Indentation of forehead
8	Fell from bunk bed at age 7; serious bicycle accident in later childhood	Indentation of cranium in center of forehead; multiple facial scars
9	Motorcycle accident in adolescence	No documentation
10	Fell from bed onto face in infancy; car accident with head injury; fell down flight of stairs in early childhood	Deviated septum from first accident; scars on chin and upper lip
11	Car accident in early childhood (possible loss of consciousness); motorcycle accident at age 17	No documentation
12	Hit by car at age 6 (loss of consciousness); fell from roof onto chin in later childhood	6-month hospitalization for first accident; scar in occipital area
13	Fell from tree at age 7; ran into car while riding bicycle at age 13	Prominent bump on right side of forehead; scar behind left ear
14	Severe bicycle accident at age 12 (loss of consciousness)—broke nose and was told he "cracked skull"	Surgery to repair nose; multiple facial scars

Table 1. Head Injuries of 14 Juveniles Condemned to Death

Subject	Subjective Symptoms	Objective Evidence
1	Lapses of fully conscious awareness; frequent, severe headaches	Suggestion of focal damage (e.g., extinguished left visual field); EEG: increased slow waves in right temporal and bilateral parieto-occipital regions, possible sharp waves; evidence of diffuse cerebral dysfunction
2	Dizzy spells, falling, confusion; multiple psychomotor symptoms	Neurologist suspects seizures; EEG attempted but data not obtained
3	Bizarre, violent behavior with memory impairment; multiple psychomotor symptoms	Neurological exam not performed; EEG: sharp waves in left temporal region
4	Lapses of awareness; migraine headaches	Normal findings on neurological exam; EEG: bilateral temporal sharp waves
5	Severe headaches	Babinski sign on right side; EEG attempted but data not obtained
6	History of grand mal seizures; multiple psychomotor symptoms	Mild left-sided weakness; bilateral unsustained clonus; EEG attempted but data not obtained
7	Multiple psychomotor symptoms	Hyperactive deep tendon reflexes; EEG: severe abnormalities in left temporal and right frontal regions
8	Occasional dizziness and lapses of awareness	Neurological exam not performed; EEG: sharp waves throughout record, especially in left temporal area
9	Episodes of dizziness	Saccadic eye movements, otherwise normal findings on neurological exam; EEG: possible sharp waves
10	Hypergraphia, micropsia; possible lapses of awareness	Unsustained bilateral ankle clonus, multiple "soft" signs; EEG: equivocal sharp waves in temporal and central regions
11	Lapses of awareness; dizzy spells; multiple psychomotor symptoms	Multiple soft signs; EEG: equivocal sharp waves in right parietal and posterior temporal regions
12	Severe headaches; impaired memory of behavior	Macrocephaly; EEG attempted but data not obtained
13	Lapses of awareness; impaired memory of behavior; frequent déjà vu	Left ankle clonus; poor rapid alternating movements on left side; "evidence of right hemisphere dysfunction"; EEG: diffusely abnormal
14	Lapses of awareness; multiple psychomotor symptoms	Normal findings on neurological exam; EEG: possible sharp activity

Table 2. Signs and Symptoms of Neurological Dysfunction in 14 Juveniles Condemned to Death

of grand mal seizures (subject 6), and symptoms or EEG findings strongly suggestive of a previously undiagnosed seizure disorder (subjects 2, 7, 8).

Table 3 illustrates the severe psychopathology characteristic of the 14 juveniles. As can be seen, seven of the subjects were psychotic at the time of their evaluations or had been so diagnosed in earlier childhood (subjects 1, 2, 3, 6, 9, 12, 14). An additional four subjects had histories consistent with diagnoses

Subject	Recent Psychiatric Signs and Symptoms	Childhood Indicators of Psychopathology
1	Paranoid ideation; command hallucinations; rambling, illogical speech	Severe emotional and behavioral problems since kindergarten; required special classes
2	Grandiosity, racing thoughts, insomnia; episodically paranoid; suicide attempts	Psychiatrically hospitalized age 15, diagnosed as having "organic psychosis"
3	Auditory hallucinations; paranoid ideation	None
4	Questionable paranoid ideation	None
5	Severely depressed and suicidal during interview; episodes of racing thoughts and insomnia	Recurrent depressions since childhood; suicide attempt at age 11
6	Auditory and visual hallucinations during interview; paranoid ideation	Visual and auditory hallucinations beginning at age 9
7	Auditory hallucinations; manic episodes and depressive episodes	Psychiatric symptoms requiring evaluation at age 8
8	Paranoid ideation	None
9	Paranoid ideation; auditory hallucinations	None
10	Suggestion of bipolar mood disorder, insomnia, racing thoughts, hypergraphia, hyperactivity	Psychiatric treatment at age 12 for compulsive sexually deviant behaviors
11	Paranoid misperceptions; one episode of auditory hallucinations; depressive and euphoric periods	Depressive symptoms since early childhood
12	Illogical; delusional; paranoid; inappropriate smiling (paranoid schizophrenic)	Multiple psychiatric evaluations and treatments since age 6
13	Questionable paranoid ideation	Drug abuse since age 8; alcohol abuse since age 10
14	Visual and auditory hallucinations; bizarre behavior (e.g., drinking blood, sticking tacks in head)	Auditory hallucinations since age 6

Table 3. Psychiatric Characteristics of 14 Juveniles Condemned to Death

of severe mood disorders (subjects 5, 7, 10, 11). The three remaining subjects experienced periodic paranoid ideation, at which times they often assaulted their perceived enemies. Seven of the subjects suffered from psychiatric disturbances that were first manifested in early or middle childhood.

Table 4 presents data from selected subtests of the psychoeducational test batteries. This table illustrates that only two subjects had IQ scores above 90. Of particular importance was the finding that 10 subjects scored significantly below grade level on the concept formation subtest, and nine subjects made more than 50 errors on the categories subtest. Both subtests are indicators of impaired abstract reasoning. The reading comprehension subtest scores of the Woodcock-Johnson Psycho-Educational Battery indicated that only three juveniles were reading at grade level. In fact, three subjects did not learn to read until their incarceration on death row.

As shown in Table 5, 12 of the subjects had been brutally, physically abused and five had been sodomized by older male relatives. Therefore, not only did older family members fail to protect these adolescents, but they also often used the subjects to vent their rages and to satisfy their sexual appetites. Alcoholism, drug abuse, psychiatric treatment, and psychiatric hospitalization were prevalent in the histories of the parents.

DISCUSSION

Our data, based on evaluations of approximately 40% of the juvenile death row population, indicate that juveniles condemned to death in the United

	WAIS-R IQ			Halstead-Reitan Battery			Woodcock-Johnson Battery		
Subject	Verbal	Performance	Full-Scale	Categories (errors)[a]	Tactile Performance (minutes)[b]	Impairment Index[c]	Reading Comprehension (grade equivalent)	Calculation (grade equivalent)	Concept Formation Score
1	67	63	64	113	37.0	1.0	2.3	3.0	1.0[d]
2	85	84	85	57	9.4	0.4	7.6	3.3	5.8[d]
3	76	82	77	57	10.8	0.7	6.6	7.5	1.0[d]
4	75	76	74	96	23.3	0.7	5.8	7.5	2.2[d]
5	88	88	86	90	9.5	0.6	12.9	5.0	12.8
6	80	87	82	93	27.3	0.9	10.6	6.6	8.6
7	84	71	77	93	25.0	0.7	5.6	5.0	4.6[d]
8	75	85	77	66	18.6	0.7	8.6	5.3	3.0[d]
9	84	85	83	38	21.6	0.7	8.6	8.0	5.8[d]
10	112	99	106	15	8.4	0.1	12.9	12.9	7.1[d]
11	68	91	81	23	12.7	0.4	1.1	6.6	3.6[d]
12	71	77'	73	91	15.6	0.5	2.0	2.6	1.0[d]
13	86	94	88	11	6.4	0.0	9.5	6.2	10.8
14	115	125	121	19	8.9	0.0	12.9	12.9	19.9

[a]More than 50 errors indicates significant brain dysfunction.
[b]More than 15 minutes indicates significant brain dysfunction.
[c]An overall index of 0.7 or greater indicates brain damage.
[d]Subject functions significantly below his appropriate grade level.

Table 4. Neuropsychiatric and Psychoeducational Scores of 14 Juveniles Condemned to Death

Subject	Physical Abuse	Sexual Abuse	Family Violence and Psychiatric Illness
1	Beaten by father, mother, step-father; blows to head	None	Violence between parents; father alcoholic; mother alcoholic and drug abuser
2	Hit in head with hammer by stepfather	Sodomized by stepfather and grand-father throughout childhood	Violence between parents; mother psychiatri-cally hospitalized
3	Placed in children's shelter in early childhood	None	Violence between parents; mother medicated for "nerves"
4	Whipped all over body by step-father; mother broke plate over subject's head	None	Violence between parents
5	Punched by father; beaten on legs and buttocks by mother	None	Violence between parents
6	Seated on hot burner by stepfa-ther (scars on buttocks)	Sodomized by stepfather and his friends; possible sexual abuse by mother and brother	Father beat mother during pregnancy; mother had several "nervous breakdowns"
7	Punched and hit in head with board by father (broke teeth)	None	Violence between parents; mother had multi-ple hospitalizations and seizures
8	Beaten by father with bullwhips and boards	None	Violence between parents; father possibly alcoholic
9	Beaten by stepfather all over body with cords	None	Siblings beat up stepfather for his mistreat-ment of subject
10	None	None	None
11	Beaten by mother, father, grandmother	Sodomized by uncle and male cousin from age 5 to 11; sexually abused by older female cousin at age 4	Violence between parents; father alcoholic and psychotic; both parents take medica-tion for "nerves"
12	Beaten by father and mother, sometimes in the face	None	Father alcoholic; mother depressed and alco-holic
13	Beaten and stomped by older brother; whipped by mother; kicked in head by relative	Sodomized by older cousin in early childhood; sexual assault attempted by male relative	Extreme violence with weapons by several family members
14	Beaten from infancy by father, mother, and grandfather	Sodomized by family member and family friend in childhood	Stepfather extraordinarily violent (e.g., pre-ferred "hunting men" to animals); mother medicated for "nerves"

Table 5. Physical and Sexual Abuse, Family Violence, and Family Psychiatric Illness of 14 Juveniles Condemned to Death

States are multiply handicapped. They tend to have suffered serious CNS in-juries, to have suffered since early childhood from a multiplicity of psychotic symptoms, and to have been physically and sexually abused.

Theoretically, all of the vulnerabilities described—neurological impairment, psychiatric illness, cognitive deficits, and parental abusiveness—were poten-tially mitigating factors that, coupled with youthfulness, would have argued against the imposition of a death sentence. Unfortunately, these cognitively handicapped juveniles had little if any recognition of the existence of these vulnerabilities, much less of their relevance to issues of mitigation. In fact, they almost uniformly tried to hide evidence of cognitive deficits and psy-chotic symptoms. They frequently told examiners, "I'm not crazy" or "I'm not a retard." It required comprehensive, specialized evaluations to obtain ac-curate clinical information.

Similarly, these juveniles were ashamed of their parent's brutality toward them and tried to conceal or minimize it. Only painstaking, lengthy inter-views, inquiring in detail about injuries, the origin of visible scars, and the existence of "scars I can't see" revealed the extent to which they had been victimized. Suffice it to say that a history of sexual abuse was even more difficult to elicit. Thus, these juveniles systematically concealed factors in their lives that were most likely to mitigate a death sentence.

Unfortunately, the parents, who should have assisted in their children's defenses, were inadequate to this task by virtue of their own psychopathology. They also had vested interests in concealing their own abusiveness, misconduct that would have constituted mitigating circumstances. In fact, we have found that in several adult and juvenile capital cases, family members have requested that histories of abuse be minimized, have cooperated with the prosecution, have testified against their own family members, or have urged the judge to impose a death sentence.

Conceivably, the juveniles' lawyers might have been relied upon to unearth and make use of the kinds of clinical data described in this paper. Such was not the case. The time and expertise required to document the necessary clinical information were not available. Furthermore, the attorneys' alliances were often divided between the juveniles and their families. In fact, on several occasions, attorneys who chose to make use of our evaluations requested that we conceal or minimize parental physical and sexual abuse to spare the family any embarrassment.

Thus, some of the very factors that led to the juveniles' aggression in the first place also contributed to an inadequate defense during the sentencing phase of their trials. Brain damage, paranoid ideation, physical abuse, and sexual abuse, all relevant to issues of mitigation, were either overlooked or deliberately concealed. Of note, in only five cases were any pretrial evaluations performed at all. These tended to be perfunctory and provided inadequate and inaccurate information regarding the adolescents' neuropsychiatric and cognitive functioning.

Adolescence is well recognized to be a time of physiological and psychological change and stress. Normal adolescents are distinguished from adults by their intensity of feeling, immature judgment, and impulsiveness. Our data indicate that, above and beyond these maturational stresses, homicidal adolescents sentenced to death have had to cope with brain dysfunction, cognitive limitations, severe psychopathology, and violent, abusive households.

At this time the clinical and legal services necessary to try to uncover these vulnerabilities are routinely unavailable to this population of juveniles. Moreover, even when such services are made available, the very family members on whom these juveniles must rely to assist in their defenses often collude with each other, the juvenile, and the attorney to minimize or conceal entirely the violence and abusiveness experienced in the home. Thus juveniles accused of a capital offense are uniquely vulnerable; they lack the maturity or insight to recognize the importance of psychiatric or neurological symptoms to their defense, and they are dependent on family for assistance in a way that adult offenders are not. Our data shed light on some of the special difficulties encountered when adolescents are treated as though they were as responsible as adults and are condemned to death.

REFERENCES

1. Seligson T: Are they too young to die? Parade Magazine, Oct 19, 1986, pp 4–7
2. National Coalition against the death penalty: A call to abolish the death penalty for juvenile offenders. Washington, DC, NCADP, 1987
3. Platt AM: *The Child Savers: The Invention of Delinquency.* Chicago, University of Chicago Press, 1969
4. Knell BEF: Capital punishment: its administration in relation to juvenile offenders in the nineteenth century and its possible administration in the eighteenth. Br J Delinquency 1965; 5:198–207
5. Blackstone W: *Commentaries on the Laws of England.* Oxford, England, Clarendon Press, 1796
6. State v Doherty, 2 Tenn 79 (1806)
7. State v Aaron, 4 NJ L 263 (1818)
8. Godfrey v State, 31 Ala 323 (1858)
9. Lewis DO, Shanok SS, Pincus JH, et al: Violent juvenile delinquents: psychiatric, neurological, psychological, and abuse factors. J Am Acad Child Psychiatry 1979; 18:307–319
10. Wechsler D: The Wechsler Intelligence Scale for Children, Revised. Middleburg Heights, Ohio, Psychological Corp, 1974
11. Bender L: The Bender Visual Motor Gestalt Test. New York, American Orthopsychiatric Association, 1946
12. Rorschach H: Rorschach Test. Bern, Switzerland, Hans Huber Publishers, 1945
13. Hammer EF: *The House-Tree-Person Clinical Research Manual.* Beverly Hills, Calif, Western Psychological Services, 1955
14. Halstead WC, Reitan RM: *The Halstead-Reitan Battery.* Tucson, University of Arizona, 1979
15. Woodcock RW, Johnson MB: Woodcock-Johnson Psycho-Educational Battery. Hingham, Mass, Teaching Resources Corp, 1977
16. Hammil DD, Larson SC: Test of Written Language. Austin, Tex, Pro-Ed, 1978, 1983

Part IX

SPECIAL ISSUES

This section includes two reviews of considerable interest to those concerned with the emotional well-being of children. Stella Chess provides an account of the past 50 years of child and adolescent psychiatry from the vantage point of one who has been an active practitioner and researcher for a considerable portion of that time period. Dr. Chess characterizes the development of child and adolescent psychiatry in dialectic terms. Fifty years ago, empirical knowledge of either the normal or pathologic behavioral development of children was limited, psychological disorders were considered to be biologically determined, and prospects for treatment were bleak. This period was followed by a period of antithesis—during which the environmental factors, as shaped by the interplay of psychodynamic defense mechanisms during the first few years of life, were considered primary influences on behavioral development. The current period, encompassing the past 20 years, has been one of synthesis, characterized by increasing integration between biological and environmental effects on developmental course. Theories of both normal and deviant child development have come to be based on the recognition of how much the biological mediates environmental stimuli and demands in shaping the child's behavior from birth onward. Of importance in facilitating this growing synthesis has been the explosion of information, deriving from methodologically sophisticated studies (see paper by Meltzhoff in this volume) regarding the competence of even very young infants to engage in active social communication and imitation of adults. The recognition of individual differences in temperamental organization and their influences on psychological development have enhanced our understanding of varieties of normal behavioral organization, as well as more deviant developmental patterns. Continuities and discontinuities in development (see paper by Clarke and Clarke in this volume) are better understood, leading to an increased appreciation for the capacity of the human mind for adaptation, integration, and mastery with regard to new and stressful events (see paper by Beardslee and Podorefsky in this volume). For the future, Dr. Chess urges increased cooperation between clinicians and researchers, and encourages both the clinical and experimental investigator not to abdicate to statisticians responsibility for the design of research and the interpretation of results. Most importantly, she cautions us all against seeking and expecting to find simple solutions to the complex problems posed by disturbed children and adolescents.

A member of the original Head Start planning committee, Edward Zigler has been a longtime student of intervention programs for young children. In this paper he, together with Nancy Hall, brings his expertise to bear on a consideration of the effect of day care on children. This overview, prepared for pediatricians, is useful for all those who are in a position of helping the parents of young children to evaluate arrangements for child care. The review considers the types of substitute care available in the United States today, studies the demographics of the various types of care, and summarizes a representative sample of the literature on the effects of alternative care on children's development. The authors point out that there are no easy answers that will be right for every family. Decisions about employment, child care, and family priorities are intensely personal and must be made by every family on an individual basis. The task of experts in child health and development is not to make decisions for families or to mandate a particular child care arrangement. Rather, the professional is a source of information for families and a source of support and understanding in the face of problems. The information base provided by this review will assist professionals in helping parents find quality day care for their children.

PART IX: SPECIAL ISSUES

32

Child and Adolescent Psychiatry Come of Age: A Fifty-Year Perspective

Stella Chess
New York University Medical Center

The author surveys some of the major developments in child and adolescent psychiatry over the past 50 years. Her account emphasizes those issues that have impressed her personally in the period when this specialty has grown dramatically and has now come of age. Increasing knowledge has challenged a number of previously accepted ideas and practices, has provided new insights in many areas, and, at the same time, has posed new challenges for both the clinician and researcher.

CHILD AND ADOLESCENT PSYCHIATRY IN THEIR INFANCY

Fifty years ago, child and adolescent psychiatry were truly in their infancy periods as scientific disciplines. Only a limited body of empirical knowledge of the normal and pathological behavior of children and adolescents had been gathered. The mechanistic biological view, which had dominated concepts of the child's development in previous decades, still retained many adherents, with diagnostic labels such as "constitutional inferior" and "constitutional psychopath," and an emphasis on the hereditary basis of psychopathology. Also, if psychological disorders were biologically determined and hereditary, then the prospects for treatment were indeed gloomy. The IQ score was reified as an absolute measure of "intelligence" with a fixed hereditary basis. It was only 10 years previously that the U.S. Supreme Court had upheld the Virginia sterilization law in the case of a young mother with an allegedly feeble-

Reprinted with permission from the *Journal of the American Academy of Child and Adolescent Psychiatry,* 1988, Vol. 27, No. 1, 1–7. Copyright 1988 by the American Academy of Child and Adolescent Psychiatry.

minded child in which the mother, and her mother, both had subnormal scores on the Stanford-Binet IQ test, with the chilling statement that "Three generations of imbeciles are enough." No thought was given that three generations of low IQ scores might be the result of an impoverished education and might not necessarily prove a genetically transmitted mental retardation.

By 1937, this pessimistic constitutional-hereditary view was being increasingly challenged and discredited. Freud and Pavlov had demonstrated how much of behavior that had been labeled as preformed and predetermined actually arose out of the child's life experiences. Psychodynamic-psychoanalytic ideas based on Freud's work took hold in child psychiatry, whereas behaviorism, based on Pavlov's studies of conditioning, in the main became an important influence among clinical and experimental psychologists.

Although both psychoanalysis and behaviorism made crucial contributions to child psychiatry, each emphasized primarily the significance of the life experiences of the first few years of life. For psychoanalysis, middle childhood became a latency period in which substantial psychological changes did not occur. Adolescence, by contrast, was viewed as a period of turmoil brought on by the revival of unresolved conflicts of early childhood that could no longer be repressed because of the adolescent's dramatic physical and emotional changes. This presumed turmoil and unstable psychological equilibrium led most psychiatrists to conclude that the adolescent was an unfavorable subject for any effective psychotherapy. If child psychiatry was in its infancy, adolescent psychiatry was as yet unborn.

The mechanical biological view was strongly adult-oriented in its formulations. With this concept, the newborn infant was considered a homunculus, an adult in miniature, who already possessed all the physical and psychological attributes that would characterize him or her as an adult. Child psychoanalysis correctly rejected this view but then developed its own adult-oriented version of the infant's mind. Superficial resemblances between the newborn and adult's behavior led to labels such as "infantile omnipotence" and "infantile narcissism." Paradoxically, such complex cognitive traits were attributed to a neonate who, in that era, was considered incapable of even the simplest sensory and perceptual abilities. The 3-year-old girl was similarly endowed with elaborate ideas of penis envy, and the boy of the same age with even more complicated emotional and cognitive concepts, subsumed under the theory of the Oedipus Complex.

Beyond these unidimensional and adult-oriented imperfections, child psychiatry suffered from an isolation from other more advanced scientific disciplines to which it should have been closely linked: developmental and social psychology, pediatrics, and the neurosciences. This isolation was detrimental to all concerned. The child psychiatrists could have benefited enormously from the knowledge and scientific standards of these other fields and at the same time could have contributed to them the unique findings that were beginning to emerge from their work with disturbed children. It is only in recent years that this gap has begun to be bridged, with immeasurable benefit to both theory and practice in child psychiatry.

A few pioneering child psychiatrists, such as Bender, Kanner, Levy, and Allen, challenged the unidimensional views that labeled the child's behavior as either nature or nurture and, instead, pointed to the need for a theoretical direction that could encompass both biology and environment in an interactional unity. They also warned against speculations and formulations that did not have a solid foundation in factual empirical data. But it took many years before the mainstream of child psychiatrists began to heed these early "cries in the wilderness."

THE ERA OF PURE ENVIRONMENTALISM

By the 1940s, the constitutional-hereditary view of the infant as a homunculus had been thoroughly discredited. As so often happens, however, the pendulum swung to the opposite extreme, and the neonate now became a tabula rasa, a blank slate on which the environment would inscribe its influence until the adult personality was etched to completion. It was the first few years of life that were considered crucial in this process. Given this premise, it was no surprise that child psychiatrists began to place the blame for a child's disturbed behavior on the parents, especially, the mother. This thesis was buttressed by the reports and formulations of a number of influential figures. Perhaps most important was the study done by Bowlby (1951) for the World Health Organization on the mental health of homeless children. He concluded that "mother love in infancy and childhood is as important for mental health as are vitamins and proteins for physical health." Although he has modified some of his early formulations, in a more recent volume (1969) Bowlby reaffirmed his conviction that the loss of the mother figure in early life is capable of "generating responses and processes that are of the greatest interest to psychopathology."

Concepts such as the "schizophrenogenic mother" became so widely accepted that they were used without attribution (see Jackson, 1960). This "double bind" theory put forward by the anthropologist, Gregory Bateson, and his colleagues, and such concepts as the "hostile rejecting mother," began to dominate child psychiatrists' thinking and practice. Circular reasoning was rampant. If the mother appeared psychologically healthy and devoted to her child, who was suffering from some psychological disorder, this only meant that her conscious attitudes were reaction formations against unconscious hostility and rejection of the child.

This mal de mere ideology (Chess, 1964) caused untold guilt and anxiety to innumerable mothers. There were, of course, unstable, rejecting, and even child-abusing mothers who were basically responsible for their children's ills. But these were a minority. Most mothers whose children had behavior problems or serious illness, such as autism or schizophrenia, were committed to their children's welfare. In addition to their confusion and distress over their difficulties in care-giving, the mothers were made to feel responsible for their child's disorder by mental health professionals. The pressure on the mothers in those days was vividly described in 1954 by Hilda Bruch, one of the few prominent psychiatrists who viewed this development with alarm: "An unrelieved picture of model parental behavior, a contrived image of artificial perfection of happiness, is held up before parents who try valiantly to reach the ever receding ideal of 'good parenthood' like dogs after a mechanical rabbit. . . . The new teaching implies that parents are all-responsible and must assume the role of preventive Fate for their children." I certainly shared Bruch's concerns and could not as a clinician make the linear one-to-one correlation between parental attitudes and practices and the child's psychological development. Although our skepticism was confirmed by reviews of the research literature (Orlansky, 1949), the "blame-the-mother" ideology, with its simple, uncomplicated explanation for all kinds of complex clinical problems in children, continued unchallenged.

Psychoanalysis played a progressive role in those early days by substituting a dynamic viewpoint and a focus on the child's early life experiences for the static, pessimistic, constitutional formulations that paid little if any attention to the individual child's real life. It offered a comprehensive theoretical system of the developmental process and promised therapeutic relief through the special techniques it had formulated. However, it also contributed strongly to the blame-the-mother ideology and ignored the biological in favor of a purely psychogenic approach. (Psychoanalysis is often considered to be a biological theory because of its basic concept of inborn instinctual drive states. In practice, however, the vicissitudes of these instinctual drives and their effect on the child's development were presumed to be shaped by psychological influences and psychodynamic defense mechanisms). As Detre (1987) recently commented, "One by-product of our nearly exclusive reliance on psychosocial explanatory theories was that we rid ourselves of problems that did not fit our newly found identity. We abandoned the epileptics, the demented, the developmentally disabled and the retarded, and asked the police to take care of the alcoholics, the substance abusers, and the delinquents."

In the 1950s and 1960s, the domination of child, adolescent, and adult psychiatry by psychoanalytic theory was overwhelming. I remember many meetings of the American Academy of Child Psychiatry in those years in which papers were presented with titles purporting to refer to child psychiatry as a whole but which consisted of a purely psychoanalytic viewpoint. I was usually the sole discussant to protest that a psychoanalytic paper was relevant but should not be equated with child psychiatry as a whole. The speakers would agree politely with me, but this did not change their attitudes. Eisenberg (1986) reported a similar experience at the 1962 American Psychiatric Association Conference on Psychiatric Education. He expressed his concern with the preoccupation in teaching intensive individual psychotherapy, in spite of the lack of evidence that long-term psychoanalytic psychotherapy was superior to brief psychotherapy. After these remarks, he described "a veritable stampede of Department Chairmen to the floor microphones. . . . Just about every eminent figure present rose to defend the primacy of psychoanalysis as the 'basic science' of psychiatry; not one supported my critique in the public forum."

Change did occur, however. By the 1976 APA Conference, " 'deemphasis on a psychoanalytic orientation' was listed as first among the shifts in professional training goals that had occurred over the previous decade" (Eisenberg, 1986). What was responsible for this dramatic change in emphasis? A number of factors were responsible. Specialists in our field have been increasingly formulating specific investigative hypotheses capable of critical testing through the identification of appropriate samples and populations for study, with adequate control groups and with methods that are replicable, reliable, and statistically analyzable. Developmental psychologists and psychiatrists have placed more emphasis on the study of children in naturalistic life situations rather than relying primarily on laboratory experiments that could be carefully controlled but might bear little relevance to the child in real life (McCall, 1977). A number of prospective longitudinal studies, including our own New York Longitudinal Study (Chess, 1979), have followed cohorts of children from infancy onward, with findings that have refuted previous speculations based on the dubious accuracy of retrospective memories of biased samples of adults undergoing psychiatric treatment. New techniques of observing and testing neonates and young children, starting with the pioneering studies of the visual capacities of very young infants by Fantz and Nevis (1967), and the neurobehavioral responses of the neonate by Brazelton (1973) have radically revised our concepts of the psychological competences of the newborn infant. On the theoretical side, the previous categorical opposition of the biological and the environmental—the traditional nature-nuture controversy—was resolved by the geneticists and biologists in terms of the concept of the unity of these opposites. "A defensible generalization is what a species' genetic constitution contributes in some manner to the development of *all* behavior in *all* organisms, as does milieu, developmental context, or environment" (Schneirla, 1957, p. 79). The geneticist Dobzhansky (1966) spelled this concept out further for human beings. "What is biologically inherited are not body parts or even traits, but the ways in which the body reacts to the environment. . . . Our genes enable us to learn and to deliberate. What we learn comes not from the genes but from the associations, direct and indirect, with other men."

From the 1950s, there has also been a mounting wave of modifications and new influences on traditional psychoanalytic theory. Many factors have been responsible for this development. Most noteworthy has been the emphasis on sociocultural factors by many investigators, especially the classic volume, *Childhood and Society* (Erikson, 1950), and the acceptance of autonomous ego functions as a legitimate focus of psychoanalytic theory and practice (Hartman, 1950; Loewenstein, 1950).

All of these developments have led to an explosion of new knowledge and new ideas in child and adolescent psychiatry, a revision or rejection of a number of formerly upheld theoretical and practical concepts, and the development of new approaches to prevention and treatment. We also know more clearly what we do *not* know, what new questions have to be asked, and what research is necessary to answer them. Our new knowledge and ideas have also begun to influence concepts and practice in adult psychiatry, just as the new findings and expanding horizons of adult psychiatry have been affecting our field. I will summarize those developments that I believe are most significant and that have contributed to the coming of age for child and adolescent psychiatry.

INTEGRATION OF THE BIOLOGICAL
AND THE ENVIRONMENTAL

Perhaps the most dramatic change in the past 20 years in our concepts of normal and deviant child development has been the recognition of how much the biological mediates environmental stimuli and demands in shaping the child's behavior from birth onward. The infant is not a tabula rasa, but his or her biological characteristics play an active role at all times in affecting the psychological influences of the family and the extrafamilial environment.

Temperament and Its Functional Significance

Our own studies (Ciba Foundation, 1982; Chess and Thomas, 1984; Thomas and Chess, 1977) of temperamental individuality and its significance for the child's development, initiated in 1956, were perhaps the first systematic application in child psychiatry of Dobzhansky's (1966) formulation that "what is biologically inherited. . . . the ways in which the body reacts to the environment." (After a few years Dr. Herbert Birch joined our study and made a number of basic conceptual and methodological contributions to its development until his untimely death in 1973.) A number of previous investigators, including Freud, Gesell, Escalona, and Fries, observed that specific individual behavioral differences in very young infants might be intrinsic to the child and significant for his or her psychological development. Pavlov had made a similar formulation from his vantage-point as a neurophysicologist with his description of different types of nervous systems, with differences in patterns of excitation and inhibition in the formation of conditioned reflexes. However, none of these investigators made a systematic, comprehensive study of these differences and then traced the sequential development of a sufficiently large cohort of infants into later childhood and adolescence to determine whether and how these differences influenced the child's psychological development. This task we accomplished with the New York Longitudinal Study. These individual differences in behavior we have called temperament (a term already in the psychological literature), comprising the style or *how* of behavior, as contrasted to motivations *or* the why of behavior, and abilities or the *what* of behavior. Our own findings, which have been confirmed by studies in a number of other research centers in this country and abroad, have shown that the child's temperamental traits significantly influence the effects of the attitudes and practices of care-givers, mental health professionals, pediatricians, educators, and nurses. Also, the same set of child care practices will affect children of different temperaments in different ways.

Some workers have proposed modifications of our scheme of temperamental characteristics and have suggested various hypotheses regarding their biological basis. However, a consensus exists that temperament is a significant variable in shaping a child's development, that it has a biological origin, which may be both genetic and constitutional, and that it is not immutable to modification or change by the environment. It is important to emphasize that, contrary to the views of a few investigators, temperament is *not* equivalent or isometric with personality. Temperament plays its part in influencing development, as do many other variables, and the child's evolving personality is shaped by the interaction among these many variables at all age-stage levels of development.

The Infant as a Competent Human Being

In the past, as a prominent developmental psychologist has stated, "it was thought that in the early weeks of life a baby's senses were not yet capable of taking in any information from the outside world, so that to all intents and purposes he was deaf and blind. Unable to move much either, he seemed a picture of psychological incompetence, of confusion and disorganization. Only the regularity of his experience, provided principally by his parent, was thought to bring order to the baby's mind. Until this was achieved, all he could do was feed and sleep" (Schaffer, 1977).

This view has been radically revised by the research of the past 20 years. It is now quite clear that the newborn is capable of recognizing visual patterns, can localize the direction from which the sound comes, has a wide range of behavioral integrative processes, begins to learn actively, and can engage in active social communication and imitation of adults (Field and Fox, 1985; Kagan, 1984; Lipsitt, 1986). As a leading researcher in infant development, Daniel Stern (1977), has stated, "The infant comes into the world bringing formidable capabilities to established human relatedness. Immediately he is a partner in shaping his first and foremost relationship."

The biological endowment of the human newborn thus makes her an independent human being from the beginning. She needs to be nurtured and cared for, of course, but she is capable of responding to these care-giving necessities in her own independent, responsive, and actively communicating fashion. This new view of the newborn, based on the solid research of the past few decades, makes obsolete such formulations as "normal autism," "mother-infant symbiosis," and "hatching" of the infant as a separate individual at 3 or 4 months. Beyond this, the detailed information on the infant's behavioral capabilities and sequences of development have caused a number of psychoanalysts to question the basic assumptions of traditional psychoanalytic theory, based as they were largely on the retrospective memories of psychologically disturbed adults undergoing psychoanalytic treatment. Thus, Stern (1985), a psychoanalyst as well as one of our most sophisticated professional "baby watchers," concludes that "Many basic psychoanalytic conceptions about drives, their allegiance to id or ego, (or even such a notion as allegiance), and their developmental sequencing all need to be reconceptualized when confronted with the infant as observed."

Brain Dysfunction and the Environment

We have learned how much the child's biological endowment (some would call it the biological preprogramming of the brain) mediates and shapes the effect of environmental influences, but the opposite is also true. Brain dysfunction—whether caused by a convulsive disorder, brain trauma, toxic chemical effects as in phenylketonuria, a genetic chromosomal fault as in Turner's syndrome, the damage resulting from intrauterine infection with the Rubella virus or any other type of brain pathology—has deviant behavioral consequences that can be diverse and crippling. In the past, such behavior was considered to be the direct consequence of the brain dysfunction and irremediable except for a few medications such as the anticonvulsant drugs.

As a medical student I learned from an instructor in surgery that "around the lesion there is a person"—a rare insight in those days from a medical specialist. Simultaneously, I discovered that Lauretta Bender was applying this principle to all of the children with brain dysfunction under her care. She wrote little on this subject but constantly reminded us that the afflicted child's behavior could not be explained solely by the brain lesion but was also determined in a give-and-take relationship with environmental factors. The reaction of parents, sibs, peers, and adults to the child's deviant behavior could affect profoundly the child's functioning and self-image. For example, a brain-damaged child with perseverative speech and behavior could meet with patient understanding and encouragement or with impatient scolding over his repetitive questions. In the first instance, the child could develop confidence in his ability to communicate with others and gain much needed self-confidence in the process. If treated with impatience, however, he would all too likely feel inept, frustrated, and socially isolated.

I also learned to identify the handicapped child's strengths, and teach her and her caretakers to give maximal attention to exploiting and maximizing these assets. These propositions appear elementary these days, but 50 years ago there were only a few psychiatrists who held any optimistic view of the possibilities of the treatment of the brain-damaged child. This optimism depended on the recognition of the integration of the biological and the environmental in the child's behavioral functioning.

SIGNIFICANCE OF EARLY LIFE EXPERIENCE

The ascendency of the environmentalist view in the 1930s and subsequent decades brought with it a number of formulations, too numerous to detail here (see Thomas and Chess, 1980, Ch. VIII), which emphasized the decisive role of the child's early life experiences for his or her later development. These concepts were very tempting both theoretically and practically. A simple linear model of development was sufficient, and different outcomes in later life could be traced back directly to causative factors in early life. On the practical side, treatment of the disturbed child and adult could be structured from the beginning so as to uncover and change the pathogenic influences carried over from early life.

As indicated earlier in this paper, this emphasis on the child's early life inevitably put the blame on the mother as the most important care giver in those years for the host of behavior problems and even some serious mental illnesses that some children developed. Even many mothers whose children were doing very well were bedevilled by the fear that they might be transmitting some pathogenic attitude to their child unconsciously.

Fortunately, the research studies of the past quarter century tell a different story. Significant data have come from the major long-term longitudinal studies, including our own. With an impressive unanimity, these studies have reported the unpredictability of later functioning from early life experience and behavior (Chess, 1979). Careful reviews of the literature by Clarke and Clarke (1976), Rutter (1972), and Sameroff (1975) have all come to the same conclusion. There are so many factors that influence an individual's life at all stages of development, and so many unpredictable maturational changes that emerge, that any formulation concentrating primarily on the first few years of life is bound to be inadequate. The human mind is remarkable for its capacity for adaptation, integration and mastery with regard to new and stressful events. A good start in infancy is important physically and mentally, but what happens in middle childhood, adolescence, and adult life is also important. As I have stated in another context, "As we grow from childhood to maturity, all of us have to shed many childhood illusions. As the field of developmental studies has matured, we now have to give up the illusion that once we know the young child's psychological history, subsequent personality and functioning are *ipso facto* predictable. On the other hand, we now have a much more optimistic vision of human development. The emotionally traumatized child is not doomed, the parents' early mistakes are not irrevocable, and our preventative and therapeutic intervention can make a difference at all age-periods" (1979).

NEW APPROACHES TO THE DEVELOPMENTAL PROCESS

The concept of development as a linear one-to-one unidimensional progression from early infancy onward has been discredited by the weight of the research data, as indicated above. Related models of invariant psychological developmental schemes, including those derived from the monumental pioneering work of Piaget, have also received critical evaluations from a number of sources for their inadequate attention to sociocultural factors, the narrowness and rigidity of their formulations, their methodological problems, and the questions raised as to their universitality by the empirical data provided by an increasing number of studies (see Thomas and Chess, 1980, pp. 128–131). Development is characterized by both change and continuity, and one cannot occur without the other. Development proceeds from the simpler to the more complex, and sequential stages can often be identified in this process. Such sequential stages, however, are the categorization of group trends for specific populations with specific sociocultural backgrounds. Individual variability between and within groups is significant and widespread.

With the abandonment of unidimensional theories of development, a consensus has developed among developmental psychiatrists and psychologists that a multifactorial approach is necessary that takes into account the interaction of biological, psychological, and sociocultural influences at all age-stage levels of functioning. This new emphasis is reflected in the DSM-III, which is developmentally oriented and provides a phenomenologically based multiaxial system of diagnosis that has summarized much of our available knowledge with respect to clinical characteristics, natural history, associated factors, complications, predisposing factors, prevalence, and familial patterns.

A multifactional approach that takes into account the many interacting variables that can influence personality development poses complex challenges to the research worker and the clinician. As Rutter stated, the multifactorial interactionist view indicates that "It is difficult to make valid, broad, sweeping generalizations about human behavior. Attention must be paid to the specificities of person-situation interactions. . . . it may be suggested that it is preferable to take an ideographic approach which explicitly focuses on the individuality of human beings—not just in the degree to which they show particular traits or even in terms of the traits which are relevant to them, but more generally in terms of the idiosyncrasies which make each person uniquely different from all others" (1980, p. 5).

Rutter's formulation highlights a fundamental issue in child and adolescent, as well as adult, psychiatric research. The growth of a scientific base for developmental psychiatry requires the conceptualization of general principles that can be applied to separate individuals and their life experiences. Yet, how do we proceed to gain these generalizations if we have to take an approach "which explicitly focuses on the individuality of human beings. . . . in terms of the idiosyncrasies which make each person uniquely different from all others"?

This dilemma is evident in the research efforts to identify high risk factors that predispose to behavior problem development. Werner and Smith (1982), in their large-scale longitudinal study of the children of Kauai, Hawaii, point up this issue most emphatically. "In this cohort of 698, 204 children developed severe behavior or learning problems *at some time* during the first two decades of their lives. . . . Yet there were others, also *vulnerable*—exposed to poverty, biological risks, and family instability, and reared by parents with little education or serious mental health problems—who remained *invincible* and developed into competent and autonomous young adults who 'worked well, played well, loved well and expected well.'" Gordon (1987) used the apt phrase "defiers of negative prediction" to designate such children, and we have found a number of dramatic illustrations of such cases in our own longitudinal studies.

A basic challenge to our field is identifying the many variables that can affect personality development and the risk of behavior disorder development

(Marmor [1983] identifies at least 13 such important variables) as well as their mutual influence on each other over time. Addressing this issue involves the concept of "goodness of fit." If the demands, expectations, and opportunities of the environment are consonant with the temperament, abilities, and motivations of the child, there is a "goodness of fit," and positive psychological development is likely. If the environment, however, makes demands that are excessive or otherwise inappropriate for the child's characteristics, there is "poorness of fit," with unfavorable consequences for the child's development. We have found this concept empirically useful in analyzing the life-course of our longitudinal study subjects and in the formulation of therapeutic strategies. A number of other investigators have begun to use similar formulations (Chess and Thomas, 1984).

Goodness or poorness of fit cannot be rated in the abstract but only within the social context in which the individual is functioning. Also, in an individual, a particular characteristic and a particular environmental demand may be the prime interactional determinants in the development of a behavior disorder, whereas in another case, the significant pathogenic factors may be different. Similarly, the crucial elements making for a "goodness of fit" and a healthy developmental course may vary from one child to another.

Application of this "goodness of fit" model requires clinical judgment when applied to an individual case. The overall concept itself, although it appears to be heuristically valuable, is still in its earliest stages of formulation and application.

THE STATISTICAL APPROACH

When confronted with the mass of data and variables in long-term developmental studies, many psychiatrists and psychologists have turned to the statistician and the computer.

There is no question but that the increasing use of statistical methods has been a powerful tool for the enhancement of the scientific level of our research activities. Quantitative ratings can be subjected to various types of statistical analysis capable of identifying significant correlations when these are not apparent by clinical inspection. Conversely, a statistical evaluation may indicate that a relationship between two or more variables that appear impressively high on tabulation is, in some instances, likely to be the result of chance alone. The demand for reliable quantitative ratings has also forced us to sharpen and objectify our diagnostic criteria.

The statistical methods and the computer should be the servant and not the master of the researcher, however. Also, it does not follow that the use of a more complex and mathematically sophisticated method will necessarily provide more decisive answers to our clinical problems. These statements may appear to be truisms. Unfortunately, there are too many studies that report elaborate reliability ratings of questionnaire data that are then subjected to complex computer analyses and the results reported with little if any thought given to their relevance of "real children growing up in real families and in real neighborhoods" (McCall, 1977, p. 334).

Too many researchers are also easily satisfied with the finding of a statistically significant correlation. A correlation of 0.50 is impressive in a behavioral study, but it actually only accounts for 25% of the variance. In other words, 75% of the significant factors in the study have not been identified. To be satisfied with the finding of the statistical correlation alone would be to ignore the richness of findings that could emerge from a simultaneous clinical qualitative study of the data. After all, the basic contributions of Kraepelin, Bleuler, Freud, Kanner, and Piaget, to mention a few, were based on careful clinical studies and creative, systematic generalizations from the data they had accumulated. These pioneers in no way were restricted by their inability to use statistical strategies such as correlation coefficients, factor analysis, or structural equations.

The clinical or experimental investigator cannot abdicate his or her responsibilities to the computer. As one statistician has emphasized, "It is the researcher who decides what data to collect and how, what analytic techniques to use, how to enter the data into the analysis, how to interpret the results, who is right or wrong" (Kraemer, 1981).

NO COOKBOOK RECIPES

What we have learned over the past 50 years has given us new concepts of normal and deviant development, has sharpened our diagnostic and therapeutic skills, and has opened up many avenues of intervention for high-risk children. It is clear, however, that the search for simple formulas that can be applied like cookbook recipes to all children and adolescents is, indeed, a search for "fool's gold." Children are different, parents and families are different, and communities are different. The interplay of these factors will influence the course of psychological development and ensure that the flowering of true individuality can take many forms. The newborn's capacity to learn, the plasticity of developmental pathways, the individual differences in temperament, the active role played by the child in interaction with the environment from the moment of birth onward, the enormous variability in the cultural influences brought to bear on the developmental process, the subtleties and complexities of the relationships among language, thought, and emotion—all promote a diversity of healthy or abnormal psychological functioning from one individual to another.

No one-sided approach can hope to do justice to the needs of troubled children. As Eisenberg (1986) has warned, the advances in our biological knowledge and techniques raise the danger that we will substitute a mindless psychiatry for the brainless psychiatry of the past. Advances in psychopharmacology give us an increasing armamentarium of useful medications for many psychiatric disorders. But hyperactive children or depressed adolescents need more than a drug prescription. They also need help in overcoming the consequential psychological damage to their self-esteem and their problems in social functioning. The realization that effective treatment of a child with a psychiatric disorder may require the simultaneous treatment or counseling of the family does not mean that a sick child always means a sick family. And, the combination of medication and psychotherapy, or individual and family therapy, cannot be blueprinted ahead of time with the idea that they can be applied in precisely the same way with all cases.

Furthermore, we have learned that our traditional role as advocates for the troubled children carries many responsibilities. These responsibilities do not stop in our professional offices but take us into the schools, courts, day-care centers, and the many governmental and voluntary agencies that are concerned with disturbed or abused children and their families.

THE CLINICIAN AND THE RESEARCHER

As a final comment, it is disturbing to see how often the clinician and researcher still view themselves as antagonists. The clinician may resent the researcher's prestige and academic status, and the researcher may belittle the value of the clinician's reliance on his or her empirical clinical experience.

In reality, the clinician and researcher must relate to each other in a deeply cooperative and collegial fashion if our field is to continue advancing. Researchers provide clinicians with new data approaches, which the clinicians can apply to their patients and to the development of new programs of early intervention for high risk children and families. Clinicians provide the researchers with new ideas and problems gleaned from their practices to be tested by the researcher. Clinicians also feed back to researchers their practical experience with the usefulness of new preventative or therapeutic strategies that have been suggested by new investigations.

This reciprocal, positive relationship of clinician and researcher is, of course, not unique to child and adolescent psychiatry but is true in all clinical medicine. It ensures the continued scientific advance of our field. It also guarantees that we will not become abstract in our theorizing and not try to fit the child rigidly into one or another conceptual Procrustean bed. Rather, the clinician and the researcher, assisted when necessary by the statistician, ideally will continue to expand our knowledge and strengthen our ability to help each disturbed child or adolescent in terms of his or her own individuality and life situation.

REFERENCES

Bowlby, J. (1951), *Maternal Care and Mental Health.* Geneva: World Health Organization.

—— (1969), *Attachment.* Vol. I. *Attachment and Loss.* New York: Basic Books.

Brazelton, T. B. (1973), Neonatal behavioral scale. *Clin. Dev. Med,* No. 50.

Bruch, H. (1954), Parent education or the illusion of omnipotence. *Am. J. Orthopsychiatry,* 24:723–732.

Chess, S. (1964), Mal de mère. *Am. J. Orthopsychiatry,* 34:613–614.

—— (1979), Developmental theory revisited: findings of a longitudinal study. *Can. J. Psychiatry,* 24:101–112.

—— (1986), *Temperament in Clinical Practice.* New York: Guilford Press.

—— Thomas, A. (1984), *Origins and Evolution of Behavior Disorders.* New York: Brunner/Mazel.

Ciba Foundation Symposium 89 (1982), *Temperament Differences in Infants and Young Children.* London: Pitman.

Clarke, A. M. & Clarke, A. D. B. (1976), *Early Experience: Myth and Evidence.* London: Open Books.

Detre, T. (1987), The future of psychiatry. *Am. J. Psychiatry,* 144:621–625.

Dobzhansky, T. (1966), A geneticist's view of human equality. *The Pharos,* 29:12–16.

Eisenberg, L. (1986), Mindlessness and brainlessness in psychiatry. *Br. J. Psychiatry,* 148:497–508.

Erikson, E. H. (1950), *Childhood and Society.* New York: Norton.

Fantz, R. L. & Nevis, S. (1967), Pattern preferences and perceptual-cognitive development in early infancy. *Merrill-Palmer Q.,* 13:77–108.

Field, T. M. & Fox, N. A. ed. (1985), The roots of social and cognitive development: models of man's original nature. In: *Social Perception in Infants.* Norwood, N.J.: Ablex Publishing.

Hartman, H. (1950), Comments on the psychoanalytic theory of the ego. *Psychoanal. Study Child,* V:74–96.

Jackson, D. D. ed. (1960), *Etiology of Schizophrenia.* New York: Basic Books.

Kagan, J. (1984), *The Nature of the Child.* New York: Basic Books.

Kraemer, H. C. (1981), Coping strategies in psychiatric clinical research. *J. Consult. Clin. Psychol.,* 49:309–319.

Lipsitt, L. P. (1986), Learning in infancy: cognitive development in babies. *J. Pediatr.,* 109:172–182.

Loewenstein, R. (1950), Conflict and autonomous ego development during the phallic phase. *Psychoanal. Study Child,* V: 47–52.

Marmor, J. (1983), Systems thinking in psychiatry: some theoretical and clinical implications. *Am. J. Psychiatry,* 146:833–838.

McCall, R. B. (1977), Challenges to a science of developmental psychology. *Child Dev.*, 48:333–344.

Orlansky, H. (1949), Infant care and personality. *Psychol. Bull.*, 46:1–48.

Rutter, M. (1972), *Maternal Deprivation Reassessed.* Middlesex: Penguin Books.

—— (1980), Introduction. In: *Scientific Foundations of Developmental Psychiatry,* ed. M. Rutter. London: Heinemann, pp. 1–7.

Sameroff, A. J. (1975), Early influences on development: fact or fancy? *Merrill-Palmer Q.*, 20:275–301.

Schaffer, R. (1977), *Mothering.* Cambridge, Mass.: Harvard University Press.

Schneirla, T. C. (1957), the concept of development in comparative psychology. In: *The Concept of Development,* ed. D. B. Harris. Minneapolis: University of Minnesota Press.

Stern, D. (1977), *The First Relationship.* Cambridge, Mass.: Harvard University Press.

—— (1985), *The Interpersonal World of the Infant.* New York: Basic Books.

Thomas, A. & Chess, S. (1980), *The Dynamics of Psychological Development.* New York: Brunner/Mazel.

—— —— (1977), *Temperament and Development.* New York: Brunner/Mazel.

Werner, E. E. & Smith, R. S. (1982), *Vulnerable but Invincible.* New York: McGraw-Hill.

33

Day Care and Its Effect on Children: An Overview for Pediatric Health Professionals

Edward Zigler and Nancy W. Hall

Yale University, New Haven, Connecticut

There is a quiet revolution going on, today, in the composition and dynamics of the American family. The demographics in our society are changing; as a result, parents are facing a host of new dilemmas about how best to enhance the healthy development of their children. Perhaps the most controversial areas are those that concern mothers working out of the home, and the issues and consequences of supplemental child care.

There are no easy answers that will be right for every family. Decisions about employment, child care, and family priorities are intensely personal, and must be made by every family on an individual basis; an almost impossible juggling of schedules has come to typify many American families. Parents must weigh the costs and benefits of different arrangements and decide on the basis of personal and economic need what is right for their family. Our task, as experts in child health and development, is not to make this decision or to mandate a particular child care arrangement. Instead, we must supply parents with the information they need to make such decisions, and provide support and understanding in the face of problems. Many parents will ask their children's pediatrician about day care and work, but too many others will assume that this issue does not fall under the purview of pediatrics. Instead, they will turn to family members and friends for advice, or will make these important decisions in isolation. We feel that it is vitally important that pediatricians become involved in the day care debate, that they become knowledgeable

Reprinted with permission from *Developmental and Behavioral Pediatrics*, 1988, Vol. 9, No. 1, 38–46. Copyright 1988 by Williams & Wilkins Co.

about the research in this area, and that they let parents know that they are available to discuss concerns regarding day care in an informative and support-ive way.

In this paper, we will present an overview of what we know about day care in America today. We will examine the types of substitute care available, and look at who tends to use what type of care arrangement. Next, we will review a representative sample of the literature on the effects of day care on children's development, and discuss some policy options that might improve supplemen-tal child care in America. Finally, we will summarize points that pediatricians may find especially helpful when dealing with parents' concerns in this area, and make some practical suggestions for them to pass on to parents.

THE DEMOGRAPHICS OF DAY CARE

Where Are the Mothers?

Of all the demographic changes in America today, perhaps the most striking is the increasing number of mothers of young children entering the out-of-home work force. At present, 62% of the women in this country with children at home are employed outside of the home.[1] This figure has increased 10-fold since the end of World War II[2] and has not yet reached a peak. Current esti-mates are that by 1990, 75% of American mothers will be in the out-of-home work force.[3] Within this rapidly rising group, analysis by age of the youngest child reveals differential trends that are even more remarkable. The fastest-growing subgroup of working mothers is that with children under 1 year old. In 1977, 44% of mothers of children under 3 years and 34% of those with infants under 1 year old were employed. By 1982, those figures had increased by 15% and 22%, respectively.[4–6]

Before we describe the child care arrangements made by these families, we want to put to rest once and for all the notion that there is something frivolous or self-indulgent about mothers joining the out-of-home work force. American mothers work for the same reasons that American fathers work: personal choice and economic necessity. The very structure of the American family is changing. Although the divorce rate in this country has begun to level off, it has done so at an alarming level: between one-third and one-half of the mar-riages that take place this year will end in divorce. Births to single women are also on the rise. One child out of four today lives in a single-parent household, usually headed by the mother. Among our nation's black families, this ratio is higher than 2 out of 4. Many of these women do not have a choice; working outside the home is essential. A 1983 *New York Times* poll revealed that 71% of working mothers surveyed about their reasons for employment responded that they worked to help support their families.[1] A recently released Congressional report corroborates this finding, and praises the working mothers of America for their willingness to, in words of Congressman David Obey from Wisconsin, assume a role that "carries with it both the anguish of worrying about children left in others' care and the fatigue and frustration of working longer hours, usually at lower pay than (that) given working men."[7] The Congressional report indicates that, although the median family income in America fell 3.1% between 1973 and 1984, if mothers had not joined the work force to support their families, the drop in median income would instead have been 9.5%. It is clear that such a drastic decline in family income would have had immediate, concrete, and devastating effects on children and families. Other research[8] has indicated that work outside the home is as important for women as it is for men in other respects as well. The workplace can provide an important source of support networks, and work force participation can provide stimulation, and a sense of accomplishment and self-worth.

Many women do not wish to work outside the home, and do not do so. For others, it is a personal or economic necessity. It is important for pediatricians to recognize the range of feelings that parents may have about work outside the home. We know that it is common for mothers to have conflicting ideas and feelings about how to balance work and child care.[9-11] Even a mother who wants to work outside the home and who can afford child care that enables her to do so may feel guilty and defensive when asked about her child care arrangements. The sensitive pediatrician will recognize these ambivalent feelings and be supportive of the needs of the mother and the family, regardless of the nature of the decision.

Pediatricians should be acquainted with the new facts of American family life. The family is changing, and social supports for the family must change as well. It may be helpful to bear in mind that the distinction between "working mothers" and "full-time" mothers is inappropriate. All mothers work, and women who are apart from their children for a portion of each day to go to work outside the home do not cease to be mothers during this period.

WHERE ARE THE CHILDREN?

There is an enormous range of day care settings in America, but most fall into one of three types: home care, center care, and family day care. Even though these differ greatly from each other, we have found that parents' decisions about what day care arrangement to use rest largely on two factors: cost and distance from home. Many other variables ought to be considered, however, and in this section we will characterize the day care opportunities now available in America.

In-Home Care

According to the most recent U.S. Bureau of Census figures for day care use,[12] 26% of the children of working parents are in home care, in which one person, a relative or nonrelative, comes to children's homes to care for them, or in which one child is taken to the caregiver's home to receive individual care. By far, the smallest portion of this group, about 6%,[9] is cared for by regular sitters, nannies, or housekeepers. The remainder are cared for by grandparents, fathers, or other relatives, or by the mother herself, taking turns with someone else. The advantages of home care are obvious. Children are in a familiar environment and parents need not spend time in transit (unless, of course, the sitter must be brought to the child). If the parent is very fortunate, the caregiver may also do a little housework or cooking, freeing parents to spend more time with the child. There are reasons this arrangement is uncommon, however.[9,11] First, it is far more costly. To have one person caring for one child, or one family's children, is expensive. Second, such arrangements are often difficult to make. Qualified, congenial people are difficult to find, and parents are unlikely to be able to offer much in the way of employment benefits. Many are uncomfortable about advertising widely for such a person, preferring to find someone through friends. In addition, a good nanny or sitter may be difficult to keep. The informality of such arrangements and the lack of benefits do not lend great security to this situation. Many of these caregivers are students, or recent immigrants who may or may not speak the family's language.[9] Although excellent caregivers exist, there is little stability in such a system; changes in school schedule or work status may suddenly leave parents with no caregiver. There is also no backup if the sitter is ill or has to be absent for some other reason, again with little possibility of advance warning. In such a case, parents must struggle to make alternative arrangements, or must themselves miss work to care for their children.

Day Care Centers

Approximately 18% of American children in non-maternal care attend day care centers. Although centers serve a relatively small proportion of children, this type of arrangement tends to be the most highly visible. The centers fall into two subcategories: for-profit centers, including large chains like Kinder-Care, and not-for-profit centers, such as those run by churches, community centers, and employers. Little is known to date about how quality of day care differs between for-profit and non-profit child care centers, although Dr. Lynn Kagan at Yale University's Bush Center in Child Development and Social Policy is currently completing a nationwide comparison of non-profit and for-profit centers. Center care tends to be less expensive than in-home care because resources are distributed among a larger group of children, with more parents contributing directly. Centers are more likely than private sitters to offer a sliding scale of fees, or discounts for parents who enroll more than one child. Centers are also more likely to be well-equipped with attractive toys and other materials. Centers are reliable on a daily basis. Unlike the nanny or grandparent, the center is unlikely to cancel care due to vacations or illness.

One drawback, however, is that because centers cater to the needs of many children, the individual needs of a particular child could be overlooked. Many children may do fine in such a setting, but the child who needs a great deal of individual attention may not receive sufficient amounts, and the child who is easily stimulated by relatively large numbers of people may be overwhelmed. Neither can most centers cater to the individual time demands of parents. The relative lack of flexibility in hours means that parents must work around the center's schedule. Children must be dropped off and picked up as the center dictates. For some parents, this means frequently being late to work, or having no leeway for overtime or trips to the dry cleaners or grocery.

Another potential problem associated with centers is the problem of arranging for care when children fall ill. The Swedish government has responded to this phenomenon by instituting leaves that can be taken by a parent when a child is ill. Mothers and fathers make equal use of such days. In America and Canada, some facilities are being created to care for ill children, or for children whose care arrangements unexpectedly break down. Some of these care centers room all sick children together. Others segregate by symptom: sneezes and sniffles in this room, intestinal disturbances in that. The practicality, cost, and wisdom of such arrangements remains to be seen. In the meantime, the need for reliable, safe arrangements for the ill children of working parents must be recognized.

Family Day Care

By far the largest group of children in substitute care in America can be found in family day care. Although such care is conducted in private homes, it differs from in-home care in that a number of children, typically four to six, come from different families to be cared for under one roof. Fifty-six percent of all children receiving supplemental care are in family day care.[12] Over two-thirds of these children are between 3 and 5 years old.[13] In spite of the large numbers of children enrolled in such care, it is the least researched. The vast majority of family day care homes are unlicensed and unregulated.[14,15] Because of the lack of regulation of such facilities, we know little about the quality of family care, in general. As a group, they can be characterized only by their heterogeneity. A study conducted by the National Council of Jewish Women[16] examined day care facilities of this type and revealed that only 10% provide "superior" care; half provide only custodial care, meeting basic physical needs but going no further, and 11% provide care that was rated "poor." The superior settings were warm, homelike, loving places with an appropriate number of children, interesting and safe things to do, and affectionate and stable caregivers. Poor quality settings were characterized by some or all of the following: overcrowded, dirty, unstimulating and/or dangerous, with day care providers who are more interested in increasing cash flow than enhancing development. Some settings are so bad that they constitute neglectful or abusive environments. Most fall somewhere in between these two extremes. Half of the day care facilities surveyed in this study provided adequate care, but no better, seeing only to the basic needs of their charges.

Family day care's ready availability and affordability contributes to its popularity. Compared with centers, it is generally conveniently located and more flexible about dropoff and pickup times. Many family day care providers do not mind taking in a child with a cold or other minor illness. Family day care, because of its homelike setting, smaller numbers of children, and greater flexibility, is by far the most widely used by parents of infants. Although there are a number of good quality centers for infants and toddlers, they are often far too costly for most families (they now run $120–$140 per week in urban centers). Again, however, because of the lack of regulation and licensing, the possibility of finding some very bad family day care settings is quite high.

It is essential to keep this heterogeneity in mind when speaking with parents about all types of day care. It is the right and responsibility of parents—and their support network, of which the pediatrician should be a part—to investigate care settings carefully, and to choose the best available. Later in this article, we will outline some simple guidelines for parents to follow when evaluating care settings.

AGE-SPECIFIC ISSUES

Most of what is written about day care does not differentiate between day care for children of different ages. We feel strongly, however, that it is important to take a developmental perspective on day care, as on other child-related issues. The impact and outcomes of day care for the 3-month-old babies and their families will be very different from those for the preschooler, and these, in turn, will be different from the effects of day care on the school-age child. We believe it is most useful to distinguish among three groups of children: from birth to about 2½ years, preschoolers up to age five, and school age children. Quality care is always essential, but for the infant and school-age groups, there are specific issues of which we should be aware, and concerning which we must work together to educate parents and day care providers.

Infant Day Care

Much of what we hear about day care in the popular press concerns infant day care. In some places, infants as young as six and even 3 weeks of age are placed in substitute care so that their mothers can return to work. As yet, little research has been conducted on day care's effects on children of this age. We do know, however, that some crucial developmental landmarks occur at this time.[17] During infancy, particularly soon after birth, parents and children begin to get to know one another. The work of Stern[18,19] and others[2] demonstrates the need for parents to spend time with their infants to learn about their individual temperaments, and give the children and parents an opportunity to get into "synch" with one another's rhythms. Family systems theory contributes the idea that the period after the birth of a new baby is a time for redefinition of family roles and a time for each family member to adjust to the changes the new addition occasions.[20,22] Others[2,9] have documented the guilt and impaired sense of self-esteem that can arise when parents who would prefer to stay home have no choice but to put their infants into day care in order to maintain their jobs. We believe that parents who desire to spend the early months of their child's life at home should have the opportunity to do so. These parents would benefit from the implementation, at the federal level, of a paid infant care leave similar to that already in place in so many other nations.[23] This would allow them to take the time to get to know each other.

The crucial task of infants during this period is the formation of secure attachments to their primary caregiver. While we acknowledge that infants do form multiple attachments, and that significant others play important roles in infant development, we know that infants require continuity of care in the form of one primary caregiver whom they can learn to love and trust.[24,25] Only after such an attachment has been securely formed can the infant feel that there is a safe base from which to explore the world. This is the beginning of independence, and a strong basis for the establishment of other relationships. Whatever the nature of the child care arrangements during this period, they must be characterized by good quality, affection, and continuity.

School-Age Children

Even though they get the least attention in both the academic journals and the popular media, school-age children comprise the largest group of day care users. Two-thirds of child care needs in this nation are for children over six.[26]

This largely unmet need has contributed to the growing number of "latchkey children"—those who fend for themselves after school and during vacations. The latchkey phenomenon is one of the newest manifestations of changing American demographics. As with infant day care, theoretical stances in this area vary, and more research is needed to determine the effects of being a latchkey child. Some research[27,28] has failed to demonstrate any ill effects. At least one worker has gone on record as believing that self-care has positive features contributing to independence in children.[29] We do not agree. Recent research in this area[30,31] has demonstrated that latchkey children are more fearful and anxious than their adult-care peers. Teachers in one study, asked to rate their pupils on several factors without knowing their after-school status, rated latchkey boys (but not girls) as less likeable than adult-care boys. Others have indicated positive correlations between self-care and juvenile delinquency[32] and have linked safety hazards with unattended children. For instance, one out of six fires in the state of New Jersey each year is started by an unsupervised child.[33] Involvement in a fire is but one of the many safety risks for latchkey children, of whom over 6,000 are injured every year.[34] Perhaps most telling was the recent testimony before Congress of a number of latchkey children who told their own stories.[13] They spoke of being afraid, of not knowing what to do during emergencies, even of being sexually abused.

Parents must be educated to understand the necessity of adequate supervision for children of all ages. Parents in many communities have begun to set up nonacademic after-school programs for older day-care recipients, making use of school facilities that would otherwise remain empty at such times.[13] School-age children may go to these programs after school and on holidays to play, read, do homework, or rest, all in a safe and familiar environment, and under the supervision of trained child care workers. Detailed models are being developed for the general establishment of such programs.[35] Because they make use of existing facilities designed for children in locations convenient and familiar to parents, such programs have proven to be a cost-effective solution to the latchkey problem. The Child Development Associate, a child development specialist certified on the basis of training and experience in child care, rather than merely on the basis of formal education, is the ideal worker for such programs.[36] Some of these programs are subsidized wholly by the local school system, and these are available to all parents, free of charge or at a nominal cost. However, others are paid for by the parents, and are thus usually available only to the upper- and middle-class families who can afford them.

We urge pediatricians and parents to investigate such models and work with local educational authorities to implement accessible after-school programs in every community. For all age groups, our greatest concern is the quality of care the child receives. Bad quality care is bad for children of all ages. Parents, teachers, and day care providers must cooperate to provide an environment for them which is developmentally appropriate, safe, and stimulating.

THE EFFECTS OF DAY CARE
ON CHILD DEVELOPMENT

A great deal of research exists on the effects of day care on child development. Workers in this area have taken a range of positions on the issue of day care effects. At one end of this spectrum is the view held by Clarke-Stewart and her colleagues,[37,38] who not only believe that day care has no appreciable ill effects on children, but who feel that it may be beneficial. Clarke-Stewart believes day care children to be better off than exclusively mother-reared children, and describes them as more socially mature, independent, and knowledgeable about the world. At the opposite end of this spectrum is Burton White's view.[39] He states that day care is bad for children, and counsels women to stay at home until their children are at least 3 years old. This advice seems well-intentioned but unrealistic. As we have demonstrated, the vast majority of employed mothers in America are in the out-of-home workforce because they must be. Telling them that they must stay at home or risk damaging their children is not a constructive solution to the child care crisis.

In between these two extremes are a range of views: Fraiberg[40] tends to agree with White that children are harmed by day care; Ainsworth[41] feels that mother-child attachment formation may be compromised by early day care. Brazelton,[2] too, is concerned, and urges parents to stay home with the child whenever possible. Others take a middle-ground position. Rutter[42] is cautious but not overly concerned about the effects of good quality, well-staffed day care. Caldwell[43] and Kagan[44] are sanguine about the effects of day care, though it should be noted that most of their research was conducted in very high quality day care. Scarr[11] also feels that the effects of day care of reasonable quality are essentially benign. What, then, is the "truth" about day care? We believe that the most realistic picture is complex, and includes few absolutes. Research has shown us that the effect of day care depends upon a number of interrelated factors, characteristics of both the child and the care setting. When interpreting the results of research on day care, we must keep this in mind.

To date, there have been a number of important and comprehensive reviews of the literature on the effects of day care.[11,38,42,45–48] Because these are readily available and widely cited, we will review only the major findings. Most of this research has focused on the effects of day care on infants and toddlers. Unless otherwise noted, the work we describe here concerns this group.

Effects of Infant and Toddler Day Care on Attachment

Much of the research on the effects of day care has focused on the quality of children's attachment to their mother. Many parents fear that their child will direct their attachment to the day care provider rather than to the parents, but research has indicated this concern is unnecessary.[38,42,46-47]

A great deal of research, however, has indicated that day care participation may affect the *nature* of attachment to the mother. Early research in this area failed to demonstrate any connection between day care and the insecurely attached infant-mother relationships.[49] Later research has indicated that mothers whose young children were in out-of-home care prior to the age of one were more likely to exhibit insecure attachments to their mothers than were their home-care peers.[50] Follow-up studies of these children have shown insecure attachment status. This group was related to increased oppositionality and decreased compliance with mother's directions when the children were assessed again at 24 months.

Interaction Effects of Stress and Day Care

Gamble and Zigler[47] have proposed that an "additive model" (p. 29) be used when looking at the socioemotional effects of infant day care. This model emphasizes the importance of environmental stressors in the day care child's life in determining the effect of out-of-home care. Within this model, quality of attachment, maternal stress, the family's financial status, absence of one or both parents, stability in the child's home, and other factors, such as the child's temperament, must be considered, along with the type and quality of the child's day care setting. As Gamble and Zigler[47] note, "The risk for damage increases if the child who experiences poor infant day care also comes from a highly stressed home environment or one without a father. . . ." (p. 29).[50,53-55] In fact, the likelihood of insecure attachments in the Vaughn et al.[50] study mentioned above was greater for early day care children from non-intact families and families with higher levels of maternal stress.

Social Relations and Day Care

Research conducted on the social relations of day care children versus those reared exclusively at home by parents has yielded mixed findings, but, in general, the consensus is that group care for infants and toddlers does have some deleterious effect on both peer interactions and adult-child interactions.[45,47] Again, whereas some have demonstrated that positive social effects may accrue from participation in high quality day care,[37] others have found that early group care leads to aggression and peer, rather than adult, orientation.[47,56]

Gender Effects

Many researchers have indicated that gender also interacts with environmental features, including type of care, to produce differential outcomes. Day-care boys, but not girls, have often been found to be more aggressive than their parent-care peers.[53,56–57] This effect was often found several years *after* the child's day care experience.[58–59] This finding is an important indication that the effects of day care may be long-lasting, and, even more important, that day care may have "sleeper effects."

In summary, we feel that caution is in order when interpreting research findings on the effects of day care on child development. We find it striking that so much of the early research found no effect or positive effects, whereas more recent research has begun to discover negative consequences from some day care. This trend is well-illustrated by looking at Belsky's two excellent reviews of day care research. In an early review,[46] he expressed little concern about the effects of infant day care. In his most recent review of this body of literature,[45] he takes a more concerned view. He notes that a number of studies have demonstrated negative outcomes from day care, that long-term outcomes and sleeper effects remain to be examined, and that many facets of the child's environment that interact with day care have not yet been adequately studied. Thus, Belsky's conclusions are similar to those adopted by Gamble and Zigler.[47]

We are further inclined to caution regarding the effects of day care by the caveats of such a major worker as Rutter.[42] Although he concludes that the effects of infant day care are essentially benign, he qualifies his position with a lengthy postscript on the necessity of good quality care. An essential element of this quality, in Rutter's eyes, is the provision of appropriate staff:child ratios. Rutter's caveat concerning quality becomes important in view of the evidence[15] that only three states have infant day care licensing requirements that meet Rutter's staff:child ratio standards.

In conclusion, it seems clear to us that day care does affect child development and behavior. The magnitude of such effects depends to a great extent on the child's whole ecosystem, the nature of the care, and the child's home environment, personal characteristics, family, and community.[60]

Some standards, we believe, are essential for day care to be a constructive experience for the child. It must be of high quality. This is the case for children of all ages, in all types of day care. We can only be sanguine about the effects of supplemental child care for children over 2½ or 3 years old; too little is known about the dynamics of care for infants and young toddlers. A comprehensive approach must be taken, which takes into consideration such elements as the level of stress at home, maternal attitudes about working, the degree of support received by working parents from the community and significant individuals in their lives, and finally, the child's personal characteristics.

With such factors in mind, we would hope that future research on the effects of day care on child development will focus on four areas: (1) broad outcomes of day care participation, beyond the results of artificially contrived separation-reunion studies, (2) the effects of mediocre and poor quality day care, (3) differential effects of day care on children of different ages, genders, and temperaments, and with different levels of environmental stress, and (4) the long-term effects of day care.

SOCIAL POLICY CONSIDERATIONS FOR CHILDREN AND FAMILIES

Day Care Standards

What do we mean by "good quality" day care? Several comprehensive studies have been conducted on the effects of day care characteristics on child development.[61] In this section, we will review these efforts to establish criteria for quality in child care, and look at some of the steps that have been taken to regulate quality in day care.

We are nearing the end of the 18th year of the struggle to implement day care standards at the federal level.[62,63] In 1968, when the first effort to review day care was made public, and again in 1977, when the National Day Care Study was published, staff:child ratios became a matter of concern.[61] These findings linked enhanced development of children in out-of-home care with certain staff:child ratios. Development was assessed with regard to teacher behaviors, child social behaviors, teacher-child interaction, verbal development, and scores on preschool intelligence measures. Children performed better on all measures, and teachers were more child-oriented, when the ratio of teachers to children was high, 1:6, for example, rather than 1:12. The Federal Interagency Day Care Regulations, or FIDCR,[64,15] proposed a set of guidelines mandating staff:child ratios, although the FIDCR proposals represent *minimal* rather than optimal standards. The FIDCR would set staff:child ratios for infant day care at no lower than 1:3, and the ratio for toddlers at 1:4. For family day care, the ratio would be 1:5, with no more than two of these children under 2 years old. Unfortunately, the FIDCR proposals were withdrawn in 1980, and the federal role in setting standards for day care remains ambiguous.

The recently enacted Model Child Care Standards Act, Public Law 98-473,[65,66] contains no firm regulations about staff:child ratio, but leaves the setting of such a ratio to the discretion of individual states. At present, 16% of the states have no mandated ratio for children under two. As stated earlier, only three states meet the withdrawn FIDCR standards.[15]

The authors of the National Day Care Study felt group size to be still more important than staff:child ratios. The summary of findings concludes:

> In smaller groups, as contrasted to larger ones, lead teachers engage in more social interactions with children and less observation of children; children show more cooperation, verbal initiative, and reflective/innovative behavior; children show less hostility and conflict and are less frequently observed to wander aimlessly or to be uninvolved in tasks or activities; and children make greater gains on the Preschool Inventory and Peabody Picture Vocabulary Test[61] (p. 77).

The FIDCR proposes a group size of six for infant day care and 12 for toddler care.[64] Only 38% of states have set any limits for group size; these range from six to 20 for infants and from six to 35 for toddlers.[15]

Caregiver qualifications are also addressed in these documents. The National Day Care survey[61] stressed that caregivers with training and/or education in topics relevant to the care and development of young children provide better care. Specialized training in development was found to be of more value than even an advanced degree in general education. The FIDCR, too, proposed specialized training for child care providers, and specified that directors and caregivers should have qualifications relevant to their responsibilities.[64] Still, more than half of the states permit individuals with no training in child care or development to direct day care centers, and only eight states require caregivers to have any training in child care.[15] Public Law 98–473 focuses its attention on "training in the prevention, detection, and reporting of suspected child abuse"[66] (p. 51), but does not specify what such training might be, nor does it require other, more developmentally oriented forms of training.

Standards for program content and curricula were also delineated by the withdrawn 1980 FIDCR, but again, few states have complied voluntarily with these standards. Only 42% of the states mandate developmentally appropriate programs. In the remaining programs, 58% of states' program specifications include only such items as having refrigeration available for food and water.[15] For family day care homes, only 10 states meet the FIDCR program requirement that programs include appropriate developmental activities.

Many important issues are not addressed by any of these model federal day care standards. Minimum age for entry to group care is left to the discretion of states. No specific guidelines for staff training are provided. It is not difficult to see that enforced standards for child care are desperately needed. Because of the laxity of the present regulations, and the lack of federal responsibility with regard to regulation, child care in the United States continues to be extremely heterogeneous. Even though there is a consensus on what constitutes good quality child care, ambivalence remains concerning who should take responsibility for seeing that such standards are put into place. With the absence of federal standards, the responsibility for maintaining quality in day care rests at this time with the individual states. Here, too, however, there is great variation. Although a few states have adequate regulations, others are lax or nonexistent. In one state, for instance, a high-school dropout with no training or experience in child care could legally be solely responsible for the care of eight infants. We feel it is important for pediatricians and others who work with families to be familiar with the standards for their state. These are listed on a state-by-state basis for both center care and family day care in Young and Zigler.[15]

Infant Care Leaves

Earlier, we spoke of the desirability of giving parents and infants the opportunity to become comfortable with one another. Such a period enhances parents' confidence in their ability to care for their new baby. This is particularly important for first-time parents. It is also important to allow mothers to recuperate physically from pregnancy and childbirth, and to adjust to mothering before their return to work outside the home.[67] More than two-thirds of the nations of the world have implemented policies of paid parental infant care leave, which allows parents to stay home with the new baby or newly adopted child for weeks or months, with a guarantee that their jobs will be waiting when they return.

During 1984 and 1985, the Yale University Bush Center in Child Development and Social Policy sponsored an intensive research effort into the possibility of implementing such a policy in the United States. Chaired by Edward Zigler, the Advisory Committee on Infant Care Leaves consisted of a panel of experts from the fields of child development, pediatrics, government, law, and business, including T. Berry Brazelton, Urie Bronfenbrenner, Bettye Caldwell, Jerome Kagan, Sheila Kammerman, Sally Provence, and Julius Richmond. One of the most striking features of the committee is that, although its members held a wide range of views about early day care, all agreed on the necessity of a policy of paid infant care leave in this nation. The committee's summary statement[23] includes recommendations for paid infant care leaves, available to either parent, for a minimum of 6 months. Job benefits would continue for the entire period, with partial income replacement available for the first 3 months. Job protection would be available for the entire 6 months. The committee further recommended that all families have access to good quality, affordable child care, and that the federal and state governments work together with employers and parents to implement such policies. (Detailed research findings and recommendations for implementing such a policy are available from the Committee.) It is time for us to recognize that mothers of young children and women entering their childbearing years make up a significant part of the American work force. We must deal with this situation in a way that will prove optimal for parents and children.

CONCLUSIONS

Much remains to be learned about the effects of day care on children of all ages. However, this cannot be an excuse for inaction on the part of those concerned with the welfare of children and families. The pediatric health professional has two crucial roles to play in the enhancement of supplemental child care. The first is that of the social activist. Begin by becoming aware. Find out what the day care standards are for your state. Listen to parents, community leaders, and local media sources to find out what types of care are available in your area, and at what cost. Use the lobbying power of the American Academy of Pediatrics and the American Medical Association to push for day care standards, paid infant care leaves, and cost defrayal of these efforts. Lend your expertise in child health and development to legislators at the federal, state, and local levels, and let them know that these efforts are of vital importance to children and families.

Second, become a central part of a working parents support system. Parents will often turn to their pediatrician for expert advice on day care. Let them know that this is appropriate by being informed and supportive. As pediatricians, child development specialists, and psychologists, it is our job to educate and help parents to make the best choices for their children.

Day care information and referral services exist at several levels in many communities. Some employers and churches provide such information, as do some child welfare and other government offices. The National Association for the Education of Young Children in Washington, D.C., publishes a checklist for parents to use in evaluating day care settings. We suggest that you obtain some of these checklists from the NAEYC, and make them available. Scarr[11] features a similar checklist in her book.

Other points to keep in mind when working with parents include:

- Whether or not a mother works outside of the home is a personal decision and must be made on the basis of what is best for parents and children in each family.
- It is the parents' right and responsibility to provide the best care they can afford for their child. Help parents to find information and referral services that will enable them to investigate all of their day care options. The family day care home down the block may be convenient, but it may not be optimal. Reinforce parents' efforts to find and use the best quality care they can.
- Until day care standards are uniformly enacted by federal and state governments, it will be up to the parents to see that their children are in a good quality setting. Again, it is their right and responsibility to investigate day care settings *before* enrolling their children. Parents should not hesitate to go in and observe. They should talk to the day care provider, and, if it is a center, to the director. Parents should feel free to enquire about group size, staff:child ratios, and caregiving training. They should use the NAEYC checklist, or Scarr's suggestions, as guidelines.

Working out of the home and making appropriate child care decisions are important issues that should be approached with sensitivity. Most parents will welcome the opportunity to talk to a supportive and well-informed pediatrician about these decisions. They will also welcome concrete advice about choosing the most appropriate setting for their child. Above all, remember, and help parents to remember that, in selecting a day care option, they are not just buying a service. They are choosing an *environment* in which their children will spend a large part of their early lives and which will therefore be an important determinant of their development. It is our job to help them to be informed and thoughtful in their choice.

REFERENCES

1. Joint Economic Committee of the U.S. Congress. Working mothers are preserving family living standards. A staff study prepared for the use of the Joint Economic Committee, Congress of the United States, May 9, 1986
2. Brazelton TB: Issues for working parents. Am J Orthopsychiatry 56:14–25, 1986

3. Zigler E: Child care: Beginning a national initiative. Testimony before the House Select Committee on Children, Youth and Families, April 4, 1984, Washington, DC

4. Hayghe H: Working mothers reach record numbers in 1984. Monthly Labor Rev 31–34, December 1984

5. Klein RP: Caregiving arrangements by employed women with children under 1 year of age. Dev Psychol 21:403–406, 1985

6. O'Connell M, Rogers CC: Child care arrangements for working mothers. Current Population Reports, Series P–23, No. 129. Washington, DC, U.S. Government Printing Office, 1983

7. Joint Economic Committee of the U.S. Congress. Press release: Obey releases report on working mothers. May 10, 1986

8. Repetti RL: *The social environment at work and psychological well-being.* Unpublished doctoral dissertation. New Haven, CT, Yale University, 1985

9. Fallows D: *A mother's work.* Boston, MA, Houghton Mifflin Company, 1985

10. Maynard F: *The child care crisis.* Markham, Ontario, Viking, 1985

11. Scarr S: *Mother care/other care.* New York, Basic Books, 1984

12. U.S. Department of Commerce Bureau of Census, Current Population Reports. Series P–23, No. 129, June. Washington, DC, Author, 1982

13. Select Committee on Children, Youth and Families. Families and child care: Improving the options. Washington, DC, U.S. Government Printing Office, 39–146–0, September 1984

14. Ruopp R, Travers J: Janus faces day care: Perspectives on quality and cost, in Zigler E, Gordon E (eds): *Day care: Scientific and social policy issues.* Boston, MA, Auburn House Publishers, 1982, pp 72–101

15. Young KT, Zigler E: Infant and toddler day care: Regulations and policy implications. Am J Orthopsychiatry 56:43–55, 1986

16. Keyserling M: Windows on Day Care. New York, National Council of Jewish Women, 1972

17. Emde R, Gaensbauer T, Harmon R: *Emotional expression in infancy: A biobehavioral study.* New York, International Universities Press, 1976

18. Stern D: Mother and infant at play: The dyadic interaction involving facial, vocal and gaze behavior, in Lewis M, Rosenblum L (eds): *The effect of the infant on the caregiver.* New York, John Wiley, 1974

19. Stern D: *The interpersonal world of the infant: A view from psychoanalysis and developmental psychology.* New York, Basic Books, 1985

20. Belsky J: Experimenting with the family in the newborn period. Child Dev 56:407–414, 1985

21. Goldberg WA, Easterbrooks MA: Role of marital quality in toddler development. Dev Psychol 20:504–514, 1984

22. Minuchin P: Families and individual development: Provocations from the field of family therapy. Child Dev 56: 289–302, 1985

23. Advisory Committee on Infant Care Leave. Statement and Recommendations. New Haven, CT, Yale Bush Center in Child Development and Social Policy, 1985

24. Bretherton I: Attachment theory: Retrospect and prospect. Monogr Child Dev 50:3–35, 1985

25. Parke R: *Fathers.* Cambridge, MA, Harvard University Press, 1981

26. Zigler E, Muenchow S: Infectious diseases in day care: Parallels between psychologically and physically healthy care. Rev Infect Dis 8:514–520

27. Leishman K: When kids are home alone: How mothers make sure they're safe. Working Mothers 3:21–25, 1980
28. Rodman H, Pratto D: How children take care of themselves: Preliminary statement on magazine survey. Report submitted to the Ford Foundation, 1980
29. Langway L, Abramson P, Foote: The latchkey children. Newsweek, February 16, 1981, pp 96–97
30. Ginter MA: *An exploratory study of the "latchkey child": Children who care for themselves.* Unpublished predissertation project. New Haven, CT, Yale University, 1981
31. Long TJ, Long L: Latchkey children. National Institute of Education. Contract No. 400–76–0008, 1982
32. Garbarino J: "Latchkey children": How much of a problem? Educ Digest February, pp 14–16, 1981
33. U.S. News and World Report. September 14, 1981
34. Accident Facts. Chicago, IL, National Safety Council, 1981
35. School Age Child Care Project. School-age child care, in Zigler E, Gordon E (eds): *Day care: Scientific and social policy issues.* Boston, MA, Auburn House, 1982, pp 457–475
36. Zigler E, Kagan SL, Muenchow S: Preventive interventions in the schools, in Reynolds CR, Gutkin TB (eds): *The handbook of school psychology.* New York, John Wiley, 1982, pp 774–795
37. Clarke-Stewart A: *Day Care.* Cambridge, MA, Harvard University Press, 1982
38. Clarke-Stewart A, Fein G: *Day care in context.* New York, John Wiley, 1973
39. White B: *The first three years of life.* Englewood Cliffs, NJ, Prentice-Hall, 1975
40. Fraiberg S: Every Child's Birthright: In *Defense of mothering.* New York, Basic Books, 1977
41. Ainsworth MD, Bell SM: Attachment, exploration and separation: Illustrated by the behavior of one-year-olds in a strange situation. Child Dev 41:49–67, 1970
42. Rutter M: Social-emotional consequences of day care for preschool children, in Zigler E, Gordon E (eds): *Day care: Scientific and social policy issues.* Boston, MA, Auburn House, 1982, pp 3–32
43. Caldwell BM, Wright CM, Honig AS, Tannenbaum BS: Infant day care and attachment. Am J Orthopsychiatry 40:397–412, 1970
44. Kagan J, Kearsley R, Zelazo P: Infancy: Its place in human development. Cambridge, MA, Harvard University Press, 1980
45. Belsky J: Infant day care: A cause for concern? Zero to Three 6:1–7, 1986
46. Belsky J, Steinberg L: The effects of day care: A critical review. Child Dev 49:924–949, 1978
47. Gamble T, Zigler E: Effects of infant day care: Another look at the evidence. Am J Orthopsychiatry 56:26–42, 1986
48. Riccuiti H: Effects of infant day care experience on behavior and development: Research and implications for social policy. Prepared for the Office of the Assistant Secretary for Planning and Evaluation, Department of Health, Education and Welfare, Washington, DC, 1976
49. Blanchard M, Main M: Avoidance of the attachment figure and social-emotional adjustment in day care infants. Dev Psychol 15:445–446, 1979
50. Vaughn B, Gove G, Egeland B: The relationship between out-of-home care and the quality of infant-mother attachment in an economically deprived population. Child Dev 51:1203–1214, 1980